MCQs in Critical Care

MCQs in Critical Care

Editor-in-Chief

Yatin Mehta
MD MNAMS FRCA FAMS FIACTA FICCM FTEE
Chairman
Medanta Institute of Critical Care and Anesthesiology
Medanta—The Medicity
Gurugram, Haryana, India

Editor

Prashant Kumar
MD IDCCM FNB (Critical Care) EDIC ADHCA DOA
Editor 'Critical Care WAarticles'
Organising Secretary 'CCW Online Quiz International®'
Senior Consultant Critical Care
Medanta—The Medicity
Gurugram, Haryana, India

Forewords

Naresh Trehan
Kapil Zirpe

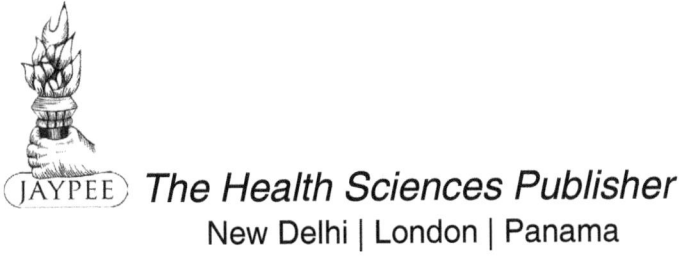

JAYPEE *The Health Sciences Publisher*
New Delhi | London | Panama

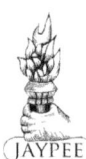 **Jaypee Brothers Medical Publishers (P) Ltd**

Headquarters
Jaypee Brothers Medical Publishers (P) Ltd.
4838/24, Ansari Road, Daryaganj
New Delhi 110 002, India
Phone: +91-11-43574357
Fax: +91-11-43574314
E-mail: jaypee@jaypeebrothers.com

Overseas Offices

JP Medical Ltd.
83 Victoria Street, London
SW1H 0HW (UK)
Phone: +44-20 3170 8910
Fax: +44(0)20 3008 6180
E-mail: info@jpmedpub.com

Jaypee-Highlights Medical Publishers Inc.
City of Knowledge, Bld. 235, 2nd Floor, Clayton
Panama City, Panama
Phone: +1 507-301-0496
Fax: +1 507-301-0499
E-mail: cservice@jphmedical.com

Jaypee Brothers Medical Publishers (P) Ltd.
17/1-B, Babar Road, Block-B, Shyamoli
Mohammadpur, Dhaka-1207
Bangladesh
Mobile: +08801912003485
E-mail: jaypeedhaka@gmail.com

Jaypee Brothers Medical Publishers (P) Ltd.
Bhotahity, Kathmandu, Nepal
Phone: +977-9741283608
E-mail: kathmandu@jaypeebrothers.com

Website: www.jaypeebrothers.com
Website: www.jaypeedigital.com

© 2018, Jaypee Brothers Medical Publishers

The views and opinions expressed in this book are solely those of the original contributor(s)/author(s) and do not necessarily represent those of editor(s) of the book.

All rights reserved. No part of this publication may be reproduced, stored or transmitted in any form or by any means, electronic, mechanical, photocopying, recording or otherwise, without the prior permission in writing of the publishers.

All brand names and product names used in this book are trade names, service marks, trademarks or registered trademarks of their respective owners. The publisher is not associated with any product or vendor mentioned in this book.

Medical knowledge and practice change constantly. This book is designed to provide accurate, authoritative information about the subject matter in question. However, readers are advised to check the most current information available on procedures included and check information from the manufacturer of each product to be administered, to verify the recommended dose, formula, method and duration of administration, adverse effects and contraindications. It is the responsibility of the practitioner to take all appropriate safety precautions. Neither the publisher nor the author(s)/editor(s) assume any liability for any injury and/or damage to persons or property arising from or related to use of material in this book.

This book is sold on the understanding that the publisher is not engaged in providing professional medical services. If such advice or services are required, the services of a competent medical professional should be sought.

Every effort has been made where necessary to contact holders of copyright to obtain permission to reproduce copyright material. If any have been inadvertently overlooked, the publisher will be pleased to make the necessary arrangements at the first opportunity. The **CD/DVD-ROM** (if any) provided in the sealed envelope with this book is complimentary and free of cost. **Not meant for sale.**

Inquiries for bulk sales may be solicited at: jaypee@jaypeebrothers.com

MCQs in Critical Care

First Edition: **2018**

ISBN: 978-93-5270-465-1

Contributors

Babu K Abraham
MD MRCP (UK)
Senior Consultant, Critical Care
Apollo Hospital
Chennai, Tamil Nadu, India

Abdul Ansari
MD IDCCM FNB (Critical Care)
Director, Critical Care
Nanavati Super Specialty Hospital
Mumbai, Maharashtra, India

Ashutosh Bhardwaj
MD IDCCM EDIC
Clinical Lead and Senior Consultant
Critical Care Medicine
Dharmshila Narayana Superspeciality Hospital
New Delhi, India

Poulomi Chatterjee
MD (Pulmonology) DNB FISDA EDARM MNCCP
Associate Consultant
Medanta—The Medicity
Gurugram, Haryana, India

Jacob George
MBBS MD (Pulmonology)
Senior Resident
DM (Critical Care)
Tata Memorial Hospital
Mumbai, Maharashtra, India

Nita George
MD (Anesthesia) FRCA EDIC CCT
Senior Consultant Intensivist and Anesthesiologist
Lakeshore Hospital
Kochi, Kerala, India

Deepak Govil
MD EDIC FCCM
Director, Institute of Critical Care
Medanta—The Medicity
Gurugram, Haryana, India

Anish Gupta
MD EDIC
Fellow
Institute of Critical Care Medicine
Max Super Speciality Hospital
Saket, New Delhi, India

Jaya Susan Jacob
MD DNB (Anesthesia)
Senior Consultant Anesthesiologist
Lakeshore Hospital
Kochi, Kerala, India

Manish Jain
MD (Med) DM (Nephrology)
Clinical Fellowship (UBC, Vancouver, Canada)
Associate Director
Division of Nephrology and Renal Transplant Medicine
Medanta—The Medicity
Gurugram, Haryana, India

Yash Javeri
DA IDCCM FICCM
Director
Apex Healthcare Consortium
New Delhi
Secretary SCCM Delhi NCR
Chairman Elect—SCCM Delhi NCR
Convener—Indian Sepsis Forum

Deven Juneja
DNB FNB EDIC FICCM FCCP FCCM
Associate Director
Institute of Critical Care Medicine
Max Super Speciality Hospital
Saket, New Delhi, India

Gaurav Kakkar
MBBS FCARCSI CCT (UK)
Senior Consultant Neuroanesthesia
Medanta Institute of Critical Care and Anesthesiology
Medanta—The Medicity
Gurugram, Haryana, India

Poonam Malhotra Kapoor
MD DNB MNAMS FIACTA FTEE
Professor
Department of Cardiac Anesthesia
Cardiothoracic Center
All India Institute of Medical Sciences
New Delhi, India

Gaurav Kochar
DA IDCCM IFCCM
Consultant Critical Care
Medanta—The Medicity
Gurugram, Haryana, India

Amol Kothekar
MD (Anesthesia), IDCCM
Associate Professor
Department of Anesthesia
Critical Care and Pain
Tata Memorial Hospital
Mumbai, Maharashtra, India

Prashant Kumar
MD IDCCM FNB (Critical Care) EDIC ADHCA DOA
Editor 'Critical Care WAarticles'
Organising Secretary 'CCW
Online Quiz International"
Senior Consultant Critical Care
Medanta—The Medicity
Gurugram, Haryana, India

Kamal Lashkari
MBBS MD (anesthesiology) IDCCM EDIC
Critical Care Specialist and Incharge ICU
Thumbay Hospital
Ajman, UAE

Qurat Ul Ain Makhdoomi
MD (Medicine)
Intensivist
Medanta—The Medicity
Gurugram, Haryana, India

RK Mani
MD MRCP (UK) FCCP FICCM
CEO-Medical Services and Chairman
Pulmonology, Critical Care and Sleep Medicine
Nayati Healthcare and Research Pvt. Ltd
Gurugram, Haryana, India
Honorary Visiting Consultant
Saket City Hospital
New Delhi, India

Mohit Mathur
MBBS MD (Anesthesiology) IDCCM EDIC
Senior Consultant
Critical Care Medicine
Max Hospital
Gurugram, Haryana, India

Chitra Mehta
DNB (Respiratory Medicine) FNB (Critical Care)
Associate Director
Department of Critical Care Medicine
Medanta—The Medicity
Gurugram, Haryana, India

Ashish Nandwani
MD (Medicine) DNB (Nephrology) FAFN
Senior Consultant (Nephrology)
Medanta—The Medicity
Gurugram, Haryana, India

Vijaya Patil
MBBS MD (Anesthesia)
Professor
Department of Anesthesiology,
Critical Care and Pain
Tata Memorial Hospital
Mumbai, Maharashtra, India

Bala Prakash
MD
Consultant, Critical Care
Apollo Hospital
Chennai, Tamil Nadu, India

Monika Rajani
MD (Microbiology)
Assistant Professor
Department of Microbiology
Career Institute of Medical
Sciences and Hospital
Lucknow, Uttar Pradesh, India

BK Rao
MD (Anesthesia)
Chairman
Department of Critical Care and
Emergency Medicine
Sir Ganga Ram Hospital
New Delhi, India

Indraneel Raut
DNB (Medicine) IFCCM EDIC
Additional Director
Jaslok Hospital
Mumbai, Maharashtra, India

Srinivas Samavedam
MD DNB FRCP FNB EDIC FICCM
Diploma in Health Care Quality Management
Diploma in Medical Law and Ethics
Head, Critical Care Unit
Virinchi Hospitals
Hyderabad, Telangana, India

Contributors

Harsh Sapra
MBBS DA
Fellowship in Neuroanesthesia and
Critical Care (RVH, Belfast, UK)
Director
Neuroanesthesia
Medanta Institute of Critical Care and Anesthesiology
Medanta—The Medicity
Gurugram, Haryana, India

Pratik Savaj
DNB (Medicine)
FNB Infectious Disease Fellow
PD Hinduja Hospital
Mumbai, Maharashtra, India

Rachit Saxena
MBBS MS MCh (CTVS)
Consultant, Cardiac Surgery
Medanta—The Medicity
Gurugram, Haryana, India

Mukta Seth
MBBS MS (OBG)
Consultant Obstetrics and Gynecology
Jeevan Anmol Hospital
New Delhi, India

Rajiv Jitendra Shah
DNB IDCCM FNB (Critical Care)
Consultant, Critical Care
Nanavati Super Specialty Hospital
Mumbai, Maharashtra, India

Ankit Sharma
MD (Anesthesia)
Assistant Professor
Anesthesia and Intensive Care
GB Pant Institute of Postgraduate Medical Education and Research
New Delhi, India

Om Shrivastav
MD (Medicine)
Consultant
Infectious Diseases and Immunology
Reliance Foundation
Sir HN Hospital, Jaslok Hospital,
Saifee Hospital, Wockhardt Hospital
Mumbai, Maharashtra, India

Amit Singh
MD IFCCM EDIC
Consultant (Critical Care)
Max Hospital
Gurugram, Haryana, India

Manish Kumar Singh
MSc (Health Statistics)
Bio-Statistician
Medanta—The Medicity
Gurugram, Haryana, India

Manoj Singh
MD DNB (Chest) FNB (Critical Care)
Consultant Chest and Critical Care
Apollo Hospital International Ltd
Gandhinagar, Gujarat, India

Mehul Solanki
MD (Internal Medicine) IDCCM FNB (Critical Care)
Consultant Critical Care
BAPS Hospital
Ahmedabad, Gujarat, India

Rajeev Soman
MD (Medicine) FIDSA
Consultant Physician
PD Hinduja Hospital, Mumbai
Jupiter Hospital
Pune, Maharashtra, India

Shrikanth Srinivasan
MD DNB FNB EDIC FICCM
Consultant and Head of Department
Critical Care Medicine
Manipal Hospitals
New Delhi, India

Saurabh Taneja
MD (Anesthesia) FNB (Critical Care Medicine) Exec MBA HCA
Consultant, Department of Critical Care and Emergency Medicine
Sir Ganga Ram Hospital
New Delhi, India

Aseem Kumar Tiwari
MD (Pathology)
Director, Blood Bank
Medanta—The Medicity
Gurugram, Haryana, India

Foreword

Knowledge and competence are tested commonly by Multiple Choice Questions (MCQs). In critical care medicine, there is a scarcity of good books on MCQs. The present book *MCQs in Critical Care* is an excellent collection. The emphasis on core concepts-based questions divided into chapters will be a very useful source of preparation for several entrance examinations and for the final examinations such as FNB (Critical Care), IDCCM, IFFCCM, EDIC etc.

I congratulate Dr Yatin Mehta, Editor-in-Chief and Dr Prashant Kumar, Editor from Medanta family for their brilliant efforts to compile the contributions from the authors. I also find commendable work of the authors from various leading centers across the country. Besides providing clinical care the additional efforts in academics goes a long way to help the young in the field to quickly grasp the concept and learn the subject.

Finally, I congratulate everyone involved directly or indirectly in the project.

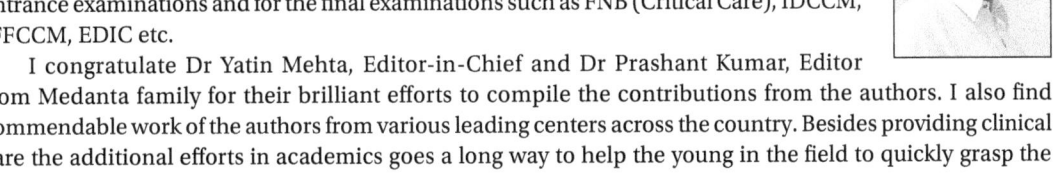

Naresh Trehan
Diplomate American Board of Cardiothoracic Surgery
Chairman and Managing Director
Medanta—The Medicity
Chairman, Medanta Heart Institute
Gurugram, Haryana, India

Foreword

It gives me a great pleasure to write the foreword for much deserved MCQ book on Critical Care.

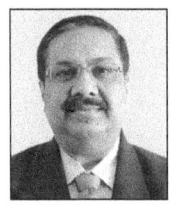

Critical care medicine has been practiced for decades in India and various certifications examinations have been conducted in this speciality since late 1900s. In India, since then very few books based on MCQs have been available for the preparations of critical care examinations. There are 21 chapters with approximately 1500 MCQs along with 2 model question papers for practicing MCQ-based exams. This book is the perfect companion as a training resource. It may be relevant to the intensive care trainees who are sitting for various critical examinations or for those who wish to improve their knowledge in constantly developing intensive care medicine practice.

I am sure, this book will be useful tool to assist in the preparations for qualifying MCQ-based examinations in critical care speciality.

Kapil Zirpe
MD FCCM FICCM
President
Indian Society of Critical Care Medicine (ISCCM)
Director and Head of the Department
Neuro-Trauma Unit
Grant Medical Foundation
Ruby Hall Clinic
Pune, Maharashtra, India

Preface

This book is the culmination of a lot of effort (academic and otherwise) by many people over a span of one year. A lot of planning and execution went into the final product. There are many books on MCQs but this book consists of each MCQs followed by a detailed evidence-based explanation (the literature) of the same. The book has been divided into different systems with relevant critical care related issues.

The chapters were allotted to experts in those fields with input from intensivists specializing in that field, so the whole science is covered adequately.

It consists of 21 chapters and 1467 MCQs. Even if one goes through the book once, it would be a full revision of the vast curriculum of Critical Care and will help the candidates appearing in FNB, IDCCM, Post MBBS certificate course, IFCCM or EDIC. Questions have been formatted into 'A' type and 'K' type. Weightage has been given to systems-based on their significance in these exams. Besides the students/fellows, it is going to be a good, read for established clinicians of all specialist including teachers of critical care medicine covering the full spectrum of the subject.

I would like to thank first of all Dr Prashant Kumar who has put in a Herculean effort for the book. I would also like to thank all the contributors who have done a tremendous job in bringing out this book, I would also like to thank my family because the time spent on the book was theirs!

This book could not have been done without the assistance of Ms Poonam Anand, my secretary and Mr Jitendar Pal Vij (Group Chairman), Mr Ankit Vij (Group President), Ms Chetna Malhotra Vohra (Associate Director-Content Strategy) and Ms Kritika Dua (Development Editor) of Jaypee Brothers Medical Publishers, New Delhi, India whose persistence finally paid off. A big thank you to Dr Naresh Trehan, CMD, Medanta—The Medicity, for his encouragement and foreword. I am thankful to Dr Qurat Ul Ain Makhdoomi for her contribution to the book.

Happy Reading!

Yatin Mehta
Editor-in-Chief

Contents

1. **Cardiology (Part I)**   1
   Poonam Malhotra Kapoor
   Cardiology (Part II)   25
   Prashant Kumar, Qurat Ul Ain Makhdoomi

2. **Respiratory**   41
   Chitra Mehta, Poulomi Chatterjee

3. **Neurointensive Care**   79
   Harsh Sapra, Gaurav Kakkar

4. **Gastrointestinal**   117
   Manoj Singh, Ashutosh Bhardwaj, Mehul Solanki

5. **Nutrition in Critical Care**   149
   Abdul Ansari, Rajiv Jitendra Shah

6. **Renal**   165
   Manish Jain, Ashish Nandwani, Gaurav Kochar

7. **Urology, Obstetrics and Gynecology**   181
   Mukta Seth

8. **Endocrinology and Metabolism**   199
   Mohit Mathur, Amit Singh, Yash Javeri

9. **Oncology**   214
   Vijaya Patil, Amol Kothekar, Jacob George

10. **Environmental Hazard, Poisoning and Acute Pharmacology**   244
    Nita George, Jaya Susan Jacob

11. **Severe Infection and Sepsis (Part I)**   270
    Rajeev Soman, Pratik Savaj
    Severe Infection and Sepsis (Part II)   287
    Bala Prakash, Babu K Abraham

12.	**Surgery and Trauma** BK Rao, Saurabh Taneja	317
13.	**Ethics, Quality Assurance and End of Life Care** RK Mani	339
14.	**General Critical Care** Deven Juneja, Anish Gupta	346
15.	**Transplantation: Heart and Liver** Rachit Saxena, Ankit Sharma, Shrikanth Srinivasan, Deepak Govil	360
16.	**Infectious Diseases** Om Srivastava, Indraneel Raut	378
17.	**Biostatistics and Research Methodology** Manish Kumar Singh	392
18.	**Transfusions in Critical Care** Aseem Kumar Tiwari, Qurat Ul Ain Makhdoomi	399
19.	**Medical Law and Ethics** Srinivas Samavedam, Kamal Lashkari	418
20.	**Infection Control in Critical Care** Monika Rajani, Yash Javeri	440
21.	**Model Question Papers**	454
	Model Question Paper I Jaya Susan Jacob, Nita George	454
	Model Question Paper II Nita George, Kamal Lashkari	487

Index *517*

CHAPTER 1

Cardiology (Part I)

Poonam Malhotra Kapoor

A Type Questions
(One best answer)

1. What does 'a' wave in CVP mean and which wave of the ECG does it follow?
   a. Passive filling of the ventricle found on the T wave
   b. The atrial kick, found just after the P wave
   c. The atrial kick, found just after the T wave
   d. The atrial kick, found after the QRS complex
   e. Contraction of the ventricle, located at the ST segment

2. Which portion of the ventricular waveform represents the preload state?
   a. Systolic peak
   b. Beginning diastole
   c. End diastolic pressure (EDP)
   d. End systolic pressure (ESP)
   e. The ventricular upstroke

3. What is the normal pressure for the pulmonary artery?
   a. 45/10/40
   b. 30/30/24
   c. 25/10/15
   d. 50/15/33
   e. 45/10/15

4. The normal pulmonary capillary wedge pressure (PCWP) is:
   a. 12–16 mm Hg mean
   b. 2–6 mm Hg mean
   c. 10–15 mm Hg mean
   d. 10–30 mm Hg mean
   e. 14–45 mm Hg

5. What is the Fick formula for cardiac output?
   a. Wt. (kg) × 3/(Ao Sat − Pa Sat) × 1.36 × hemoglobin × 10
   b. Wt. (lbs.) × 3/Ao Sat × Pa Sat) × 1.36 × 10
   c. Height × weight/stroke volume × heart rate + hemoglobin
   d. Wt. (kg) × body surface area/(Ao Sat + Pa Sat) × 80
   e. Wt. (kg.) × 3/Ao Sat × Pa Sat) × 1.36 x 20

6. What is the metric unit for vascular resistance?
   a. Dynes-5/cm
   b. Dynes·sec·cm^{-5}
   c. mm Hg
   d. Cm^2 × dynes × 5
   e. dyn·s/cm^5

7. Where, on the respiratory cycle, is the optimal measurement point for measuring atrial and wedge pressures?
   a. End inspiration
   b. You need inspiration and expiration, and average them
   c. End expiration
   d. Either one is OK, as long as you adjust the measurement scale
   e. None of the above

8. In which case might a thermodilution cardiac output be superior to a Fick?
   a. Low cardiac output state
   b. Tricuspid valve regurgitation
   c. Mitral valve stenosis

d. High cardiac output state
e. Pulmonary valve regurgitation

9. **The normal value of stroke index, postcardiac surgery is:**
   a. 60–80 mL/m²
   b. 40–60 mL/m²
   c. 30–65 mL/m²
   d. 20–30 mL/m²
   e. 10–20 mL/m²

10. **The figure shows ultrasound guided IVC imaging showing collapsibility in the:**

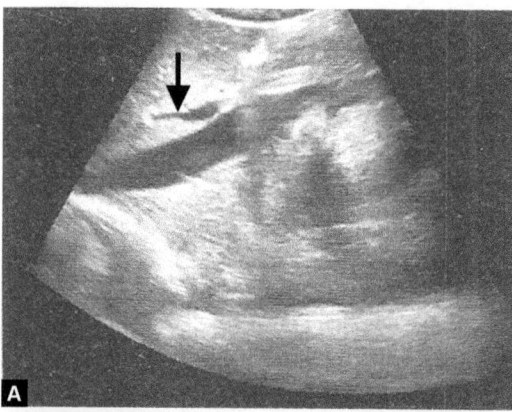

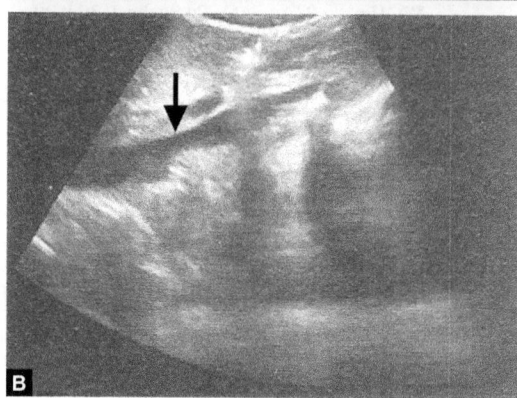

   a. Figure A only
   b. Figure B only
   c. Both Figures A and B
   d. Both are normal
   e. Both are abnormal

11. **The invasive method of diagnosing possible cause of pulmonary edema is:**
   a. Cardiac biomarkers
   b. Right heart catheterization
   c. Hemoconcentration
   d. Transthoracic echocardiography
   e. Left heart catheterization

12. **The best therapeutic options for weaning associated pulmonary edema:**
   a. Diuretics
   b. Vasodilators
   c. PEEP
   d. CPCP/BiPAP
   e. Nitroglycerin

13. **Which of the following is true regarding ECMO in adult patients with ARDS?**
   a. VA-ECMO is associated with decreased mortality compared to VV-ECMO
   b. VA-ECMO is associated with increased mortality compared to VV-ECMO
   c. Anticoagulation is required but is not associated with increased complications
   d. Transfer to a specialized center with ECMO capability is associated with decreased mortality
   e. ECMO is contraindicated after ≥ 5 days of mechanical ventilation

14. **Noninvasive ventilation indicated in:**
   a. Asthma
   b. Do-not-intubate (DNI) patients
   c. Hypoxemia
   d. All of the above
   e. None of the above

15. **Angiotensin converting enzyme inhibitors (ACEI) are indicated in:**
   a. In a 40-year-old patient with idiopathic dilated cardiomyo-pathy
   b. In a patient after a myocardial infarction
   c. A hypertensive patient with proteinuria
   d. All of the above
   e. None of the above

16. **Cautions about the use of digitalis include:**
   a. Hypokalemia
   b. Diabetes mellitus
   c. Low platelets
   d. High platelets
   e. Presence of atrial fibrillation

17. **Which of the following statements is true?**
   a. Vitamin E is of proven value in the treatment of hypertension
   b. Prazosin has survival benefit in hypertension
   c. Folic acid supplementation may be beneficial in preventing ischemic heart disease
   d. Beta carotene has beneficial effects in ischemic heart disease through its antioxidant effects
   e. All statements are true

18. Regarding Calcium channel blockers:
    a. Reduce proteinuria
    b. Short acting nifedipine increases mortality in hypertension
    c. Can be used to delay surgery in patients with aortic regurgitation
    d. All of the above
    e. None of the above

19. Side effects of thiazide diuretics include:
    a. Hypercalcemia
    b. Acute pancreatitis
    c. Hyperkalemia
    d. Hypocalcemia
    e. Hypoglycemia

20. Streptokinase treatment in acute myocardial infarction (AMI):
    a. May be associated with an anaphylactic reaction
    b. Is as effective in improving prognosis in patients with inferior as well as anterior infarctions
    c. Should be started within 1 hour of AMI
    d. Both A and B
    e. Neither A nor B

21. In the management of Central Diabetes insipidus in the cardiac patient in ICU, the dose of Desmopressin is:
    a. 2 µg/day
    b. 4 µg/day
    c. 6 µg/day
    d. 1 µg/day
    e. 5 µg/day

22. One of the following antiplatelet drugs for myocardial infarction management should be avoided in case of history of transient ischemic attach (TIA) or stroke:
    a. Aspirin
    b. Clopidogrel
    c. Prasugrel
    d. Tocagrelor

23. The most common presenting clinical symptom of acute heart failure is:
    a. Dyspnea
    b. Peripheral edema
    c. Palpitations
    d. Altered mentation

24. Oxygen, noninvasive ventilation or invasive mechanical ventilation should be considered for the management of acute heart failure, when:
    a. SBP is less than 85 mm Hg
    b. Oxygen saturation is less than < 90%
    c. Dyspnea is severe
    d. Diastolic blood pressure is less than 60 mm Hg
    e. All of the above

25. The Levine sign is typically seen in:
    a. Hypertensive crises
    b. Myocardial infarction
    c. Pulmonary hypertension
    d. Heart failure

26. Cardiogenic shock is seen typically in Killip Classification:
    a. Class I
    b. Class II
    c. Class III
    d. Class IV
    e. Class V

27. On low flow during weaning of ECMO:
    a. Heparin requirement increases
    b. High risk of clotting
    c. None of the above is correct
    d. Both (a) and (b) are correct

28. During weaning of VV-ECMO FiO2 is reduced every hourly by:
    a. 10%
    b. 20%
    c. 5%
    d. 15%
    e. 25%

29. Echocardiography in ECMO is useful in all of the following *except*:
    a. Excluding new reversible pathology
    b. LV dysfunction
    c. Undiagnosed cardiac valve pathology
    d. Limb ischemia

30. Echocardiography can help to differentiate the need for VV or VA-ECMO in conditions such as:
    a. Pneumonia
    b. Pulmonary hypertension
    c. Medication overdose
    d. Bridge to lung transplant
    e. Severe septic cardiomyopathy

31. By echocardiography, an aortic intramural hematoma may be difficult to distinguish from which of the following?
    a. A descending thoracic aortic aneurysm with mural thrombus
    b. An ascending thoracic aortic dissection

c. A descending thoracic aortic saccular aneurysm
d. Protruding mobile atheroma in the aortic arch
e. All of the above

32. **Signs of membrane failure in ECMO include:**
    a. Decreasing PO_2
    b. Increasing CO_2
    c. Signs of consumptive coagulopathy
    d. All of the above

33. **Which of the following drugs is found to be useful in idiopathic ventricular fibrillation (IVF)?**
    a. Quinidine
    b. Bisoprolol
    c. Verapamil
    d. Sotalol

34. **An 18-year-old patient develops sudden ventricular tachycardia characterized by QRS complexes of changing amplitude that appear to twist around the isoelectric line at a rate of 250/min and QT is 524 ms.**

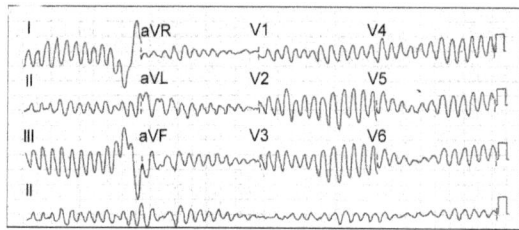

    What is the diagnosis?
    a. Torsades de pointes
    b. Ventricular fibrillation
    c. Polymorphic VT
    d. Atrial fibrillation

35. **Mr Ahmed, 56 year/M, BW-60 kg, postoperative presented in atrial fibrillation. While shifting from parenteral anticoagulation to new oral anticoagulation, it is wise to monitor his:**
    a. Creatinine clearance as Dabigatran is eliminated renally
    b. Liver function test as Dabigatran is eliminated hepatically
    c. Creatinine clearance 24 hours after last dose of Rivaroxaban
    d. Creatinine clearance as Rivaroxaban is eliminated only renally
    e. PT and INR as clinical monitoring is insufficient

36. **All the following are potential hypercoagulable states in the ICU, *except*:**
    a. Protein C deficiency
    b. Protein S deficiency
    c. Factor VII excess
    d. Factor VIII excess
    e. Splenomegaly

37. **The figure below shows dilated left atrium on a:**

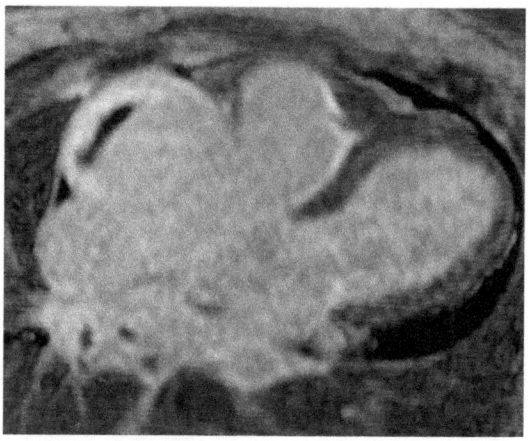

    a. 3D ECHO
    b. PET Scan
    c. CT Angio
    d. Cardiac MRI
    e. None of the above

38. **In trauma cases, transesophageal echocardiography (TEE) is a highly accurate tool for the evaluation of aortic injury and rupture. Which of the following findings is most consistent with a traumatic aortic injury of the thoracic aorta?**
    a. A sessile irregularly bordered echo density in the mid descending thoracic aorta
    b. A markedly dilated ascending aorta and aortic arch
    c. A mobile linear flap located just distal to the aortic isthmus
    d. A mural echo density in a large descending thoracic aortic aneurysm
    e. All of the above

39. **In a patient with severe dyspnea, an apical four chamber view on transthoracic echocardiography (TTE) reveals significant ECHO free space over the RA. The possible diagnosis is:**
    a. Right pleural effusion

b. Ascites
c. RA infarction
d. Tamponade
e. All of the above

40. To rule out a cardiac tamponade on a subcostal view on TTE:
    a. IVC is enlarged and collapses well
    b. IVC is not enlarged and collapsing well
    c. IVC is not enlarged and non-collapsing
    d. IVC is enlarged and non-collapsing
    e. All of the above

41. The echocardiographic view in the intensive care frequently requested for discerning the LV systolic function is:
    a. Parasternal long axis
    b. Parasternal short axis
    c. 4 Chamber view
    d. All of the above
    e. None of the above

42. In the setting of STEMI the ideally invasive arterial line, should be inserted in which artery:
    a. Radial
    b. Femoral
    c. Carotid
    d. Brachial
    e. Dorsalis pedis

43. One of the modulators for structural alteration in AF is:
    a. Coronary blood flow reserve impairment
    b. Atrial fibroses
    c. Atrial dilatation
    d. Ectopic focal discharge from pulmonary vein
    e. All of the above

44. The European guidelines for first line of antiarrhythmic drug selection in case of AF with symptomatic heart Failure is:
    a. Amiodarone
    b. Dofetilide
    c. Sotalol
    d. Flecainide
    e. All of the above

45. The chemical cardioversion with drugs in hemodynamically unstable AF patients is less successful than direct cardioversion because there is a concern with drugs of:
    a. Tolerance
    b. Proarrhythmia
    c. Longer duration
    d. Electrolyte imbalance
    e. All of the above

K Type Questions
[Marked True (T)/False (F)]

1. The lung ultrasound deciphers:
   a. Quantification of pleural effusion
   b. Quantification of pericardial effusion
   c. Sensitive in finding pneumothorax in obese patients
   d. Identification of pulmonary edema
   e. Identification of pulmonary over inflation

2. Regarding transesophageal echocardiography (TEE) in patients with atrial fibrillation:
   a. Cardioversion can be safely performed off anticoagulation if TEE is negative for thrombus
   b. Spontaneous echo contrast is common and does not offer independent prognostic value
   c. Spontaneous echo contrast is highly associated with previous stroke or peripheral embolism in patients with atrial fibrillation
   d. Surgical ligation does not exclude flow into the left atrial appendage in majority of the cases
   e. Anticoagulation before proceeding with cardioversion should be started in few selected cases only

3. Following is commonly used to measure cardiac output in the ICU:
   a. Pulse contour analysis
   b. Thermodilution
   c. Esophageal Doppler
   d. Bioimpedance
   e. Transcutaneous Doppler

4. Capnography may be used in the ICU for:
   a. Indirect CO measurement
   b. Esophageal intubation alarm
   c. Return of spontaneous circulation (ROSC) after cardiac arrest
   d. Oxygen saturation monitoring
   e. Stroke volume monitoring

5. Dynamic variables like stroke volume variation (SVV) can vary with:
   a. Lung dynamics
   b. Arrhythmias

c. Tidal volume
   d. Spontaneous breathing patient
   e. Mechanical ventilation
6. Consider the following statements about digoxin:
   a. Is indicated in patients with mitral stenosis in sinus rhythm
   b. Currently the most accepted indication is heart failure
   c. Can cause tachyarrhythmias
   d. Can cause heart block
   e. Can cause hyperkalemia
7. The side effects of ACE inhibitors are:
   a. Cough
   b. Headache
   c. Hypokalemia
   d. Worsening of renal function in patients with chronic renal failure
   e. Cause decrease in systemic vascular resistance (SVR)
8. **Amiodarone:**
   a. Can cause hypothyroidism
   b. Has a half-life of 3 days
   c. Causes prolongation of the QT interval
   d. Is useful in the treatment of atrial fibrillation
   e. Safe in pregnancy
9. **Drugs which may be used in hypertensive crisis management in a post CABG patient:**
   a. Nitroglycerin
   b. Sodium nitroprusside
   c. Sotalol
   d. Hydralazine
   e. Labetalol
10. Side effect of Amiodarone is/are:
    a. Bradycardia
    b. Shortened QT interval
    c. Thrombophlebitis
    d. Corneal deposits
    e. Diarrhea
11. The following may be used as alternatives to heparin:
    a. Low molecular weight heparin
    b. Dermatan sulfate
    c. Warfarin
    d. Hirudin
    e. Recombinant factor VIIa
12. The pathophysiology of acute heart failure includes:
    a. Renal
    b. Cardio
    c. Vascular
    d. Endocrine
    e. Cerebral
13. **Laboratory changes associated with MI are:**
    a. The CK-MB level is a fairly accurate method of diagnosing acute MI
    b. SGOT and LDH are not specific enzymes
    c. Skeletal muscle injury cannot increase the concentration of CK-MB
    d. The increase in CK-MB persists for 72 hours
    e. Plasma troponin concentration increases after 24 hours
14. **Signs of weaning failure during respiratory ECMO:**
    a. Hypoxia
    b. Hypercapnia
    c. Fluid overload
    d. Limb ischemia
    e. Infection
15. **Common complications of ECMO include:**
    a. Bleeding
    b. Thromboembolic events
    c. Sepsis
    d. Pulmonary embolism
    e. Cannula migration
16. **Following are potential hypercoagulable states in the ICU:**
    a. Protein C deficiency
    b. Protein S excess
    c. Factor VII excess
    d. Factor VIII excess
    e. Low fibrinogen levels
17. **The CHA2 – DA2 – VASC score in atrial fibrillation is labeled '1' in following cases of atrial fibrillation:**
    a. Female sex
    b. Age > 75 years
    c. Hypertension
    d. Coronary heart failure with decreased ejection fraction
    e. Male sex
18. **Following statements about arrhythmias caused by accessory pathways (AP) are correct:**
    a. Majority of APs conduct both antegradely and retrogradely

b. Around 50% of patients with pre-excitation have bypass tracts that conduct only antegradely
c. Retrograde only conduction is more common than antegrade only conduction via APs
d. In around 10% of patients spontaneous disappearance of pre-excitation may be seen
e. Pre-excitation is seen in myelinated fibers

19. **Following statements about ventricular fibrillation (VF) are true:**
    a. Ninety to ninety-five percent of individuals with VF reveal underlying structural heart disease
    b. No structural heart disease can be identified in 55% to 60% of patients
    c. According to the results of the Cardiac Arrest Survivors with Preserved Ejection Fraction Registry (CASPER) among patients with normal left ventricular function, idiopathic ventricular fibrillation (IVF) was diagnosed in 44% of patients with ventricular fibrillation without structural heart disease
    d. The diagnosis of idiopathic ventricular fibrillation (IVF) is based on the exclusion of currently known structural and primary electrical heart diseases following a complete noninvasive, invasive, and genetic workup
    e. All have atrial fibrillation first

20. **Consider the following statements related to vasodilators:**
    a. The vasodilators that are feely available and commonly used in India are sodium nitroprusside and nitroglycerin
    b. Venodilators increase the preload
    c. They can lead to loss of hypoxic pulmonary vasoconstriction
    d. They may lead to metabolic acidosis
    e. The arterial vasodilators decrease SVR and increase cardiac output

21. **The following statements are correct about the Fast-Flush Test:**
    a. It determines the dynamic response of the monitoring system to assess the distortion in the system
    b. It corresponds to a resonant frequency of 10-20 Hz
    c. Has dampening coefficient of 0.5-0.7 for arterial pressure monitoring
    d. Is excellent for filling pressure as well
    e. Corrects both under damping and over damping

22. **Regarding internal jugular vein central vein cannulation:**
    a. Internal Jugular vein is directly anterior to the carotid artery
    b. Complications are less with internal jugular vein (IJV) puncture as compared to subclavian puncture
    c. Doppler ultrasound guided puncture could reduce the time and number of attempts
    d. Success rate is higher in infants than adults
    e. It is a rapid alternative to surgical cut down

23. **Methods to evaluate regional cerebral saturation, the correct statements are:**
    a. Mixed venous saturation is most ideal
    b. BIS and NIRS correlate well in infants
    c. Lactate levels in superior vena cava are higher than inferior vena cava
    d. NIRS is 90% sensitive and specific for regional cerebral saturation monitoring
    e. BIS gives only depth of anesthesia/sedation

24. **For hypertensive emergencies in the ICU:**
    a. Sodium nitroprusside is first choice for most cases of hypertensive crisis
    b. Labetalol can be used as it maintains the cardiac output
    c. Thiocyanate toxicity is seen with labetalol
    d. Nicardipine is useful in CAD as well
    e. Clevidipine cannot be used as it is a long-acting intravenous calcium channel blocker

ANSWERS

A Type Answers

Q1. Answer b

The mechanical activity of the heart always follows the electrical activity of the heart. Since the P wave reflects atrial depolarization or contraction, look for the A wave to come directly after the P wave. In the case of a wedge pressure, there will be a delay, and the A wave may show up just after the QRS complex. The A wave is important, because it reflects the atrial kick, which drives 20–25% of the atrial blood into the left ventricle and helps establish the preload state (end diastolic pressure, EDP) of the ventricle. Line a piece of paper up to the P wave of the ECG and move the paper to the right. When you see an elevated portion of the waveform, you have found the A wave. In a case like atrial fibrillation where there is no P-wave on the ECG, there is no atrial kick, and therefore, no A wave on the atrial waveform. Sometimes in nodal rhythms A wave may be large due to atrium contracting against a closed tricuspid valve.

Q2. Answer c

EDP is an important measurement for the ventricle. The physicians routinely ask for pressures to be performed on a 40–50 mm Hg scale, and increase the paper speed to at least 50 mm/sec to assess the EDP. It reflects the preload state, and is a highly valuable measurement. It can be used to determine if patients are fluid overloaded, in heart failure, and if they can be aggressively hydrated for conditions like kidney disease. Along with isovolumetric contraction and after load, preload is a primary determinant of cardiac output.

> Mielniczuk LM, Lamas GA, Flaker GC, et al. Left ventricular end-diastolic pressure and risk of subsequent heart failure in patients following an acute myocardial infarction. Congest Heart Fail. 2007;13(4):209-14.

Q3. Answer c

The normal pressure for the pulmonary artery is approximately 25 systolic, 10 diastolic, and a mean pressure of 15. If the pulmonary artery pressures are extremely elevated, it suggests either pulmonary artery hypertension or left heart failure that is elevating right-sided pressures. It is important to obtain a wedge pressure at this point, to see if the patient has pulmonary hypertension (PHTN) or a left-sided source that is causing the pressure elevation. By calculating effective mean pulmonary artery pressures and mean wedge pressures, a pulmonary vascular resistance can be calculated to determine if there is pulmonary artery hypertension, and the severity of PHTN, should it exist. Because this pressure is elevated, the catheter should be advanced into the pulmonary capillary beds for left heart analysis.

> Rose-Jones LJ, Mclaughlin VV. Pulmonary hypertension: types and treatments. Curr Cardiol Rev. 2015;11(1):73-9.

Q4. Answer a

The normal PCWP pressure is around 12–16 mm Hg mean pressure. The PCWP is a left-sided pressure, and pathology associated with elevated wedge pressure is usually associated with left heart failure, or mitral valve stenosis. Because the wedge pressure is measured during the 'right heart catheterization,' it is more accurate to think of a 'right heart cath' as a hemodynamic study that looks at both left and right-sided pressures. Elevated wedge pressures are a classic finding for left heart failure. They may also indicate mitral valve stenosis. If the wedge pressure is associated with an elevated V wave, this is often associated with mitral valve regurgitation. When measuring the wedge pressure, there are a couple of points to remember for practice. The wedge pressure is delayed, in relationship to the right atrial pressure because it is an indirect measurement. Therefore, the A wave will usually arise shortly after the QRS complex, and the V wave will seem to be slightly before the A wave. This is important in making a diagnosis of mitral regurgitation, characterized by a classic, elevated V wave in the wedge pressure measurement. The first positive waveform after the P wave is the A wave, and the second positive waveform is the V wave.

> Muralidhar K. Central venous pressure and pulmonary capillary wedge pressure monitoring. Indian J Anaesth. 2002;46(4):298-303.

Q5. Answer a

The Fick formula has 2 variants, but both assess the same factors. They take the presumed oxygen content, i.e. the difference between arterial and venous O_2 saturation. Either (BSA × 125) or (weight in kilograms × 3)/(Ao Sat-Pa Sat) × Hemoglobin × 1.36 × 10 can be used. These are presumed values and may not be completely accurate. Many variables can influence the output, including supplemental oxygen, sedation, and septal defects. Clinical assessment may facilitate the need to calculate a thermodilution (TD) or angiographic output.

Kern M. Measurement of cardiac output in the cath lab:How accurate is it? Cath Lab Digest. 2014;22(7).

Q6. Answer b

Most computers record vascular resistance in metric units of dynes·sec·cm^{-5}. To convert Wood units to metric units, simply multiply the Wood units by 80. To convert the metric numbers to Wood units, divide the metric units by 80. If the physician is performing tests on the patient to determine response to pulmonary hypertension, they might want to use Wood units, rather than metric units, to record real-time calculations.

Kern M. measurement of cardiac output in the cath lab: How accurate is it? Cath Lab Digest 2014;22(7).

Q7. Answer c

The best area to assess hemodynamic pressures is at end expiration. This is described as the area where the measurement 'falls off the cliff.' The extremely low pressures are generated by the negative pressure created by the inspiratory effort. They can grossly distort accurate hemodynamics in patients who have significant respiratory variance. This includes patients who have sleep apnea, chronic obstructive pulmonary disease (COPD), and other lung diseases. In this patient, there is a sharp respiratory variance on the wedge pressure waveforms. It is important to make sure that the computer aligns with the expiratory measurements, and that the mean pressure is accurate, because it determines pulmonary vascular resistance. A tip to improve practice is to color in the 'valleys' that occur during the inspiratory effort and then discard them.

Kern M. measurement of cardiac output in the cath lab: How accurate is it? Cath Lab Digest 2014;22(7).

Q8. Answer d

Cardiac output (CO) can also be measured by thermodilution technique. Thermodilution CO involves the use of a catheter with a proximal and distal port, as well as a thermistor, to measure temperature changes. Saline, which may be chilled, is injected into the proximal portion of the catheter, which lies in the right atrium. The injectate mixes with blood and warms up as it passes through the pulmonary arteries. This temperature change is captured by the thermistor and an output is generated. Typically, around 4–5 injections are performed, the outliers are discarded, and an average is taken. Thermodilution cardiac output is highly useful in patients with very high cardiac outputs, because very slight changes in Ao or Pa saturation can cause large changes in cardiac output via the Fick method. The TD technique is usually contraindicated in patients with tricuspid regurgitation, because the injectate is not able to cross the right atrium and reach the pulmonary artery before it becomes too diluted.

Berthelsen PG, Eldrup N, Nilsson LB, Rasmussen JP. Thermodilution cardiac output. Cold vs room temperature injectate and the importance of measuring the injectate temperature in the right atrium. Acta Anaesthesiol Scand. 2002;46(9):1103-10.

Q9. Answer c

Variable	Formula	Normal range
Cardiac Index (CI)	Q/BSA	2.5–4.0 litre min^{-1} m^{-2}
Stroke Volume	Q/HR	60–80 mL
Stroke Index	SV/BSA	30–65 m^{-2}
Left ventricular stroke work index (LVSWI)	CI × (MAP – PAOP) × 0.0136	40–60 g m^{-1} m^{-2}

Q=Cardiac output, BSA=Body Surface Area, HR=Heart Rate, SV=Stroke Volume, MAP=Mean Arterial Pressure, PAOP=Pulmonary Artery Occlusion Pressure

Kumar P. ICU Manual. New Delhi: Jaypee Brothers Medical Publishers; 2017.

Q10. Answer b

1. Spontaneous breathing patients—fluid responsive, if (1) IVC measuring < 2 cm in diameter coupled with IVC collapse > 50% with each breath or (2) IVC collapsibility >12%

2. Mechanically ventilated patients—fluid responsive, if IVC distensibility >18%.
3. IVC collapsibility = (Max diameter - min diameter)/(mean diameter) × 100
4. IVC distensibility = (Max diameter - min diameter/min diameter) × 100
5. Caval index (the fractional change in the IVC diameter during respiration).
6. A greater than 50% decrease in IVC diameter is associated with a CVP <8 mm Hg in management of sepsis.

Doppler ultrasound can be used to measure blood velocity in descending aorta and can be used for estimating cardiac output (Figs. A and B).

_{Kumar P. ICU Manual. New Delhi: Jaypee Brothers Medical Publishers; 2017.}

Q11. Answer b

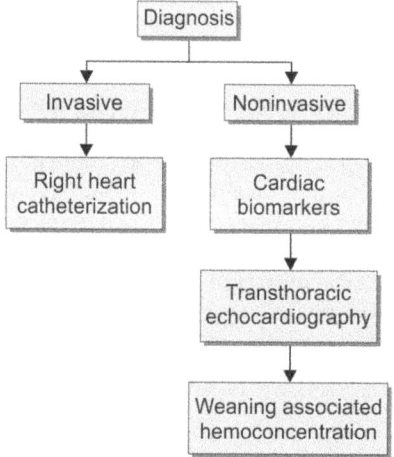

Q12. Answer a

Therapeutic options available to treat pulmonary edema: Rule out extra cardiac causes of weaning failure, Excessive preload: diuretics, Excessive afterload of myocardial ischemia: vasodilators. Use CPAP/BiPAP to prevent significant alteration in intrathoracic pressures.

_{Jean-Louis T, Monnet X, Richard C. Weaning failure of cardiac origin: recent advances. Crit Care. 2010;14(2):211-5.}

Q13. Answer d

Interest in ECMO support of severe ARDS has increased following reports of successful salvage of H1N1 patients and with advances in pump and oxygenator technology. The CESAR trial randomized 180 ARDS patients to best conventional expert treatment versus transfer to a specialized center with ECMO capabilities; significant reduction of six month mortality was seen in the specialized center. A European multicenter trial is underway to assess these findings in early severe ARDS. VV-ECMO is the preferred mode for support of acute respiratory failure. Bleeding events are responsible for the most serious complications on ECMO. ECMO support is most commonly considered within seven days of initiating mechanical ventilation, however, successful support is feasible after the initial time window.

_{Brodie D, Bacchetta M. Extracorporeal membrane oxygenation for ARDS in adults. N Engl J Med. 2011;365:1905-14.}

Q14. Answer d

There is strong evidence that non-invasive ventilation should be used for the initial management of acute respiratory failure in patients with exacerbated COPD, acute pulmonary edema, disorders with concomitant immunosuppression as well as to facilitate extubation in patients with COPD who have failed weaning attempts. In postoperative patients, noninvasive ventilation should be considered both as a prophylactic and as a therapeutic tool for improving gas exchange. Administration of noninvasive ventilation is also recommended in palliative care for hypercapnic and pulmonary edema patients.

Ambrosino N, Vagheggini G. Non-invasive ventilation in exacerbations of COPD. Int J Chron Obstruct Pulmon Dis. 2007;2(4):471-6.

Q15. Answer d

ACEI have a variety of beneficial effects. They reduce symptoms and mortality in patients with heart failure due to any cause. ACEI also have effects on ventricular remodelling after a myocardial infarction, and can reduce the risk of development of myocardial dysfunction. ACEI reduce proteinuria in normotensive diabetics with proteinuria, and hypertensives with proteinuria. There is no indication for its use in a normotensive diabetic patient without proteinuria. ACEI cause systemic vasodilatation, and are contraindicated in patients with aortic stenosis, as they can result in hypotension.

Izzo JL, Weir MR. Angiotensin-converting enzyme inhibitors. J Clin Hypertens (Greenwich). 2011;13(9):667-75.

Q16. Answer a

Hypokalemia worsens digitalis toxicity. However, in overdose, digoxin causes hyperkalemia. Elderly patients are at greater risk of digoxin toxicity because of reduced renal function. Digoxin has no effect on platelets. The presence of atrial fibrillation is an indication rather than a caution for the use of digoxin. Digoxin is used to control the ventricular rate in atrial fibrillation.

Wofford JL, Ettinger WH. Risk factors and manifestations of digoxin toxicity in the elderly. Am J Emerg Med. 1991; 9(2 Suppl 1):11-5;33-4.

Q17. Answer c

Although antioxidants such as vitamin E and beta carotene have long been thought to be beneficial in the treatment of cardiovascular disease, there is no convincing trial evidence of such benefit. Elevated homocysteine levels increase cardiovascular risk by its procoagulant effects. Folate deficiency may result in elevated homocysteine levels, and it is thought that in patients who are folate deficient, folic acid supplementation may be of use. Again, there is no definite evidence. Nicotinic acid is an effective, but poorly tolerated, cholesterol lowering agent.

Ganguly P, Alam SF. Role of homocysteine in the development of cardiovascular disease. Ganguly and Alam Nutrition Journal. 2015;14(6):2-10.

Q18. Answer d

Though calcium channel antagonists are effective anti-anginal agents, there is little evidence that they affect survival in patients with ischemic heart disease. There is some evidence that Diltiazem prevents reinfarction in patients with non Q MI. Calcium channel blockers reduce proteinuria in patients with diabetes. Short acting Nifedipine, although an effective antihypertensive agent, increases mortality in patient with hypertension and should not be used. Nifedipine is used in patients with aortic regurgitation to reduce symptoms and delay surgery.

Sleight P. Calcium antagonists during and after myocardial infarction. Drugs. 1996;51(2):216-25.

Q19. Answer b

The most important side effects of thiazides are orthostatic hypotension, photosensitivity, hypokalemia, and anorexia and epigastric distress. Hepatic dysfunction, acute pancreatitis, and erythema multiform are known to occur. There are concerns that thiazides can cause hyperglycemia and worsen diabetes, but this effect is clinically not of importance.

Dutta SK, Mobrahan S, Iber FL. Associated liver disease in alcoholic pancreatitis. Am J Dig Dis. 1978;23(7):618-22.

Q20. Answer d

Apart from the fact that streptokinase is effective only if given intravenously, it causes bleeding, and if given by the intramuscular route will result in the formation of a muscle hematoma. It is well known to cause anaphylactic reactions. Treatment with streptokinase is associated with a 25% reduction in mortality. There are long-term survival benefits. There is no benefit seen with streptokinase treatment in non ST elevation MI. Streptokinase is equally effective in all types of ST elevation MI. Percutaneous coronary intervention (PCI), also known as coronary angioplasty, is a nonsurgical technique for treating obstructive coronary artery disease, including unstable angina, acute myocardial infarction (MI), and should be performed within 90 minutes of first medical contact.

Rubboli A, Capecchi A, Pasquale GD. Utilizing enoxaparin in the management of STEMI. Vasc Health Risk Manag. 2007;3(5): 691-700.

Q21. Answer b

Management of Diabetes Insipidus

Central Diabetes Insipidus (DI)
- Desmopressin – intranasal or 4 µg/day IV or SC in divided doses
- Low salt diet + low dose thiazides diuretics

Partial Central DI
- Chlorpropamide, clofibrate, carbamazepine
  These drugs stimulate Arginine Vasopressin (AVP) secretion or its action on Kidney
  NSAIDs – They impair prostaglandin synthesis and potentiate AVP action.

Mishra G, Chandrashekhar SR. Management of diabetes insipidus in children. Indian J Endocrinol Metab. 2011;15(Suppl3): S180-S187.

Q22. Answer c

Prasugrel: The loading dose of Prasugrel is 60 mg followed by 10 mg daily. Prasugrel should not be given in patients with history of TIA or stroke

Ticagrelor: The loading dose of Tricagrelor is 180 mg followed by 90 mg twice. When using Ticagrelor, the recommended maintenance dose of Aspirin is 81 mg daily.

Alexander W. FDA Advisory Committee Meeting on Prasugrel For Acute Coronary Syndromes. P T. 2009;34(3):155-6.

Q23. Answer a

Dyspnea is the most common symptom and is present in 90% cases. Dyspnea typically is present at rest or with minimal exertion. Patients also may present with signs and symptoms related to systemic venous congestion such as peripheral edema. In elderly patients, atypical manifestations such as fatigue, depression, altered mental status or sleep disruptions can occur.

Kamal AH, Maguire JM, Wheeler JL. Currow DC, Abernethy AP. Dyspnea Review for the Palliative Care Professional: Treatment Goals and Therapeutic Options. J Palliat Med. 2012;15(1):106-14.

Q24. Answer e

Oxygen therapy should be individualised based on clinical condition.

O₂/NIV/Invasive mechanical ventilation	Oxygen saturation (Sao$_2$) < 90%
Consider vasopressors/ nonvasodilating inotrope/right heart catheterization/ mechanical circulatory support (e.g. IABP, ventricular assist device)	SBP < 85 mm Hg
Diuretics right heart catheterization	Urine output < 20 mL/hr

Increasing dissolved oxygen in plasma by oxygen therapy may also be used to offset the effects of hypoperfusion to some extent (stagnant hypoxia) and may well be important in certain situations (cardiogenic shock), although the effect is only marginal. Increased inspired oxygen will only marginally mitigate the effects of anemic hypoxia but, because the CaO_2 in patients with anemia is less than that in patients with normal haemoglobin, the effect of additional oxygen carried in solution may become more important in these situations.

> Kumar P. ICU Manual. New Delhi: Jaypee Brothers Medical Publishers; 2017.
>
> BTS guideline for oxygen use in adults in healthcare and emergency settings. June 2017 Volume 72 Supplement 1. Available from: https://www.brit-thoracic.org.uk/document-library/clinical-information/oxygen/2017-emergency-oxygen-guideline/bts-guideline-for-oxygen-use-in-adults-in-healthcare-and-emergency-settings/(Accessed 28 December 2017).

Q25. Answer b

Levine's sign is a clenched fist held over the chest to describe ischemic chest pain. Patients are anxious and restless and describe their pain with a clenched fist held against the sternum. Those presenting with failure may have cold and clammy extremities. As the referred pain associated with ischemia radiates to the area of the left proximal forelimb, the right, unaffected arm is used to produce the gesture. This clenched fist signal may be seen in patients with acute coronary syndrome (myocardial infarction and angina pectoris). A variant of this sign which uses the entire palm instead of the clinched fist over the chest is commonly known as the 'Palm Sign'.

> Murday A. Optimal management of acute ventricular septal rupture. Heart. 2003;89(12):1462-6.

Q26. Answer d

The classification or index of heart failure severity in patients with acute myocardial infarction (AMI) was proposed by Killip and Kimball aiming at assessing the risk of in-hospital death and the potential benefit of specific management of care provided in Coronary Care Units (CCU).

Killip's class
I. No congestive heart failure
II. Mild congestive heart failure, rales, S3. congestion on Chest X-ray
III. Pulmonary edema
IV. Cardiogenic shock

The Killip and Kimball classification performs relevant prognostic role in mortality at mean follow-up of 05 years post-AMI, with a similar pattern between NSTEMI and STEMI patients.

> de Mello BHG, Oliveira GBF, Ramos RF. Validation of the Killip-Kimball Classification and Late Mortality after Acute Myocardial Infarction. Arq Bras Cardiol. 2014;103(2):107-17.

Q27. Answer d

Weaning of VV-ECMO by reducing the pump flow was preferred technique in the past and is seldom practiced now. The reason for not using this technique is when one come on low flow there is high risk of clotting and usually heparin requirement increases. The weaning procedure is similar to VA-ECMO except the weaning can be done quickly. Flow can be reduced even by 20 mL/kg/min (as compared to 10 mL/kg/min of VA-ECMO) and even the time between the changes can be reduced. For VV-ECMO, idling may be reached at 40 to 50 mL/kg/min.

> Kapoor PM. Manual of extracorporeal membrane oxygenation in the ICU. New Delhi: Jaypee Brothers Medical Publishers; 2013.

Q28. Answer c

Usually the ECMO FiO_2 is reduced by 5% per hour or even 30 minutes. Ventilator setting is upgraded to moderate level. Once the FiO_2 requirement is 21% then the sweep gas flow is being reduced by 10% per hour or half hourly. Adjusting heparin dose is not required as there is no change in pump flow. Alternatively, few centers only decreases sweep gas flow by 10% per hour without changing FiO_2 of ECMO. ECMO FiO_2 is always kept 100%.

> Kapoor PM. Manual of extracorporeal membrane oxygenation in the ICU. New Delhi: Jaypee Brothers Medical Publishers; 2013.

Q29. Answer d

Echocardiography helps exclude new reversible pathology, which may account for a patient's hemodynamic instability (such as cardiac tamponade, undiagnosed cardiac valve pathology, and LV dysfunction), avoiding the need for ECMO support.

Kapoor PM. Manual of extracorporeal membrane oxygenation in the ICU. New Delhi: Jaypee Brothers Medical Publishers; 2013.

Q30. Answer d

Echocardiography plays a crucial role at every step of ECMO support. At the time of consideration, it can confirm the diagnosis and help in defining the choice between VV and VA-ECMO. By assessing cardiac function, echocardiography can help determine whether VV-ECMO is sufficient or whether VA-ECMO should be considered in conditions such as pneumonia with severe septic cardiomyopathy. Although, it is unlikely that utilization of echocardiography by itself will directly improve the outcome of patients supported on ECMO, echocardiography may help to reduce complications and guide clinicians in the daily management of these complex patients. It provides guidance at the time of cannulation. Once the patient is on ECMO support, it procures valuable information pertaining to recovery and possible complications. It is essential during the weaning phase for VA-ECMO.

Douflé G, Roscoe A, Billia F, Fan E. Echocardiography for adult patients supported with extracorporeal membrane oxygenation. Crit Care. 2015;19:326.

Q31. Answer a

Aortic intramural hematoma is characterized by echocardiography as a circumferential or crescent-shaped smooth-margined thickening of the aortic wall without an intimal flap. The degree of aortic wall thickening should be >5–7 mm. Intimal calcium may be displaced by the accumulation of hematoma. Echolucent areas in the aortic wall may be seen suggestive of noncommunicating blood in the medial hematoma. An intramural hematoma is generally continuous over a relatively localized or extensive portion of the aorta. Aortic atheromatous disease and aortic aneurysms with mural thrombus can be commonly encountered diagnostic challenges. Important distinguishing features of intramural hematoma are its smooth aortic wall contour, continuous nature, and its echogenic border due to displaced intimal calcium. In contrast, aneurysms with mural thrombus have irregular borders, and the thrombus is located above the calcified intima. Aortic atheromatous disease often has irregular borders with protruding and/or mobile components, scattered areas of calcification, and is not continuous.

Nishigami K. Echocardiographic characteristics of aortic intramural hematoma for the differentiation from atheromatous plaques and mural thrombi in the aorta. Journal of Echocardiography. 2011;9(4):167-8.

Q32. Answer d

Earliest sign of oxygenator failure will be rising delta pressure, i.e. the pressure difference between the inlet and outlet of the oxygenator. The preoxygenator increases as the resistance of the oxygenator increases while the postoxygenator pressure decreases leading to increased delta pressure. The other signs of membrane failure include deterioration in gas exchange (rising carbon dioxide and decreasing pO_2 in postoxygenator blood gas), plasma leak, increased platelet consumption and picture of consumptive coagulopathy.

Tamari Y, Tortolani AJ, Maquine M, et al. The effect of high pressure on microporous membrane oxygenator failure. Artif Organs. 1991 Feb;15(1):15-22.

Q33. Answer a

IVF has a high recurrence rate.

The recommended therapy is implantation of implantable cardioverter defibrillator (ICD). Currently, recommendations for a specific drug therapy are not available. Antiarrhythmic agents had no effect on the recurrence rate. In a study by Belhassen et al. patients with IVF have received oral quinidine guided by serial electrophysiological studies. In patients receiving continuous quinidine treatment, no recurrences of VF were reported during a mean follow-up period of 9.1 ± 5.6 years. In a subset of patients, these promising results were confirmed during long-term follow-up. Currently, pharmacologic therapy serves as an adjunct to ICD therapy in patients with multiple ICD discharges.

Belhassen B, Viskin S, Fish R, et al. Effects of electrophysiologic guided therapy with Class IA antiarrhythmic drugs on the long-term outcome of patients with idiopathic ventricular fibrillation with or without the Brugada syndrome. J Cardiovasc Electrophysiol. 1999; 10(10):1301-12.

Q34. Answer a

Torsades de pointes: VT characterized by QRS complexes of changing amplitude that appear to twist around the isoelectric line and occur at rates of 200 to 250/minute and QT intervals generally >500 ms. Polymorphic VT in the absence of QT prolongation is not considered as Torsades de pointes.

Kumar P. ICU Manual. New Delhi: Jaypee Brothers Medical Publishers; 2017.

Q35. Answer a

Dabigatran is oral direct thrombin inhibitor anticoagulant. Absorption is rapid with peak plasma concentrations reached at 4-6 hours. Its oral bioavailability is low, but shows minimal interindividual variability. Dabigatran specifically and reversibly inhibits thrombin, the key enzyme in the coagulation cascade. The anticoagulant effect correlates adequately with the plasma concentrations of the drug, demonstrating effective anticoagulation combined with a low risk of bleeding. Dabigatran is mainly eliminated by renal excretion (a fact which affects the dosage in elderly and in moderate-severe renal failure patients), and no hepatic metabolism by cytochrome *P450* isoenzymes has been observed, showing a good interaction profile. Rivaroxaban is also factor Xa (FXa) direct inhibitor anticoagulant drug. It produces a reversible and predictable inhibition of FXa activity with potential to inhibit clot-bound FXa. Its pharmacokinetic characteristics include rapid absorption, high oral availability, high plasma protein binding and a half-life of approximately 8 hours. Rivaroxaban elimination is mainly renal, but also through faecal matter and by hepatic metabolism.

Baines OJP, Grana CE, Botella JA, García VI. Pharmacokinetics and pharmacodynamics of the new oral anticoagulants dabigatran and rivaroxaban. Farm Hosp. 2009;33(3):125-33.

Q36. Answer e

Hypercoagulable states in anesthesia and critical care

Acquired: Age, previous thrombosis, immobilization, major surgery, orthopaedic surgery, malignancy, oral contraceptives, pregnancy, hormonal replacement therapy, antiphospholipid syndrome, essential thrombocythemia, polycythemia vera, paroxysmal nocturnal hemoglobinuria, splenectomy

Inherited: FVL G1691A, protein C deficiency, protein S deficiency, antithrombin deficiency, dysfibrinogenemia, prothrombin mutation G20210A.

Mixed or unknown: Hyperhomocysteinemia, high levels of factor VIII, APC-resistance in the absence of FVL, High levels of factor IX, factor XI and TAFI.

Bande BD, Bande SB, Mohite S. The hypercoagulable states in anesthesia and critical care. Indian J Anaesth. 2014;58(5):665-71.

Q37. Answer d

Cardiac magnetic resonance imaging (MRI) uses a powerful magnetic field, radiowaves and a computer to produce detailed pictures of the structures within the heart. It is used to detect or monitor cardiac disease and to evaluate the heart's anatomy and function in patients with congenital heart disease. Cardiac MRI (CMRI) does not use ionizing radiation, and it may provide images of the heart that are better than other imaging methods for certain conditions. Atrial dilatation can be both the cause and effect of atrial fibrillation (AF). Atrial enlargement is an important marker of left atrium (LA) structural remodeling and predictor of AF (re) occurrence and mortality. Hence, accurate assessment of LA dimensions is critical for AF assessment. CMRI with its high spatial and temporal resolution allows accurate delineation of the LA, LAA and pulmonary veins (PV) morphology. CMRI is today the gold standard for cardiac volumes and has shown excellent correlation with cadaveric casts. Despite the irregular rhythm, CMRI is able to measure accurate atrial and ventricular volumes.

Prabh S, Voskoboinik A, Kaye DM. Atrial Fibrillation and Heart Failure Cause or Effect? Heart, Lung and Circulation. 2017;26(9):967-74.

Q38. Answer c

TEE imaging of the aorta is a highly accurate method of aortic evaluation in patients with deceleration and blunt chest trauma. Characteristic echocardiographic findings suggestive of aortic injury include the presence of an intraluminal flap located near or just distal to the aortic isthmus, or near the gastroesophageal junction. The intraluminal flap is usually mobile, may be extensive or localized to a short segment of the aorta, and usually occurs at points of attachment such as the sinuses of Valsalva, the isthmus, and the diaphragm. Alternatively, intraluminal masses suggestive of discrete thrombus formation can be seen and typically occur at the arch, isthmus, or near the diaphragm; in these cases, development of aortic thrombus occurs in areas overlying intimal tears or injury. A sessile irregularly bordered echodensity located in the mid descending thoracic aorta is descriptive of aortic atheromatous disease. The presence of a dilated ascending aorta alone is not consistent with aortic injury. A mural echodensity in a large descending thoracic aortic aneurysm is most suggestive of mural thrombus.

Patil TA, Nierich A. Transesophageal echocardiography evaluation of the thoracic aorta. Ann Card Anaesth. 2016; 19(Suppl 1):S44-S55.

Q39. Answer a

The right lung is very close to the RA. An echo-free space seen over the RA in an apical four-chamber view is consistent with right pleural effusion. Right pleural effusion may also present as an echo-free space next to the RA. Of course, pericardial effusion (PE) will present similar findings of echo-free spaces next to RA or RV and therefore, examination from the back with the patient sitting up becomes important for differentiation, as mentioned previously.

Price S, Platz E, Cullen L, et al. Expert consensus document: Echocardiography and lung ultrasonography for the assessment and management of acute heart failure. Nature Reviews Cardiology. 2017;14:427-40.

Q40. Answer b

To make a rapid diagnosis of tamponade in a patient with pericardial effusion, it is important to perform a subcostal examination to image the inferior vena cava (IVC). If the IVC is not enlarged (< 20 mm) and collapses well (around 50% or more) during respiration, tamponade can be immediately excluded because these findings indicate there is no elevation of RA pressure which occurs in tamponade. An exception is a patient with hypovolemia due, e.g. to diuresis induced by a diuretic, hemorrhage, or inadequate fluid intake. In this situation, because of low blood volume status, the IVC is not enlarged and may also show some collapse, even though tamponade may have developed.

Pérez-Casares A, Cesar S, Brunet-Garcia L, et al. Echocardiographic Evaluation of Pericardial Effusion and Cardiac Tamponade. Front Pediatr. 2017;5:79.

Q41. Answer d

Information	Echocardiographic view
LV systolic function	Parasternal long axis and short axis view, 2, 3 and 4-chamber view
Cardiac output	4-chamber view
Right heart assessment	Parasternal long axis and short axis view, 4-chamber view
Pericardial disease	Parasternal long axis and short axis view, 4-chamber view, subcostal view
Valvular disease	Parasternal long axis and short axis view, 4-chamber view
Volume status and responsiveness	4-chamber view, inferior vena cava

Walley PE, Goodgame B, Punjabi V, et al. A practical approach to goal directed echocardiography in the critical care setting. Crit Care. 2014;18(6):681.

Q42. Answer a

In the setting of STEMI, radial access for primary PCI is the best option to avoid procedural bleeding depending on operator expertise and preference. In patients with STEMI and AF at low risk of bleeding (HAS-BLED 0-2), the initial use of triple therapy [oral anticoagulants (OAC), aspirin, and clopidogrel] should be considered for 6 months following PCI irrespective of stent type; this should be followed by long-term therapy (up to 12 months) with OAC and clopidogrel 75 mg/day (or alternatively, aspirin 75–100 mg/day).

Alizadehasl A, Ziyaeifard M, Peighambari M, et al. Avoiding heparinization of arterial line and maintaining acceptable arterial waveform after cardiac surgery: A randomized clinical trial. Res Cardiovasc Med. 2015;4(3):e28086.

Q43. Answer a

Triggers, modulators and structural/functional alteration in Atrial Fibrillation

Triggers: Acute/chronic atrial stretch, Ectopic focal discharge from pulmonary vein.

Modulators: Autonomic nervous system

Structural/functional alterations: Atrial dilatation (macro-manifestation), atrial fibrosis (macro-manifestation), myocardial perfusion abnormalities (microvascular manifestation), coronary blood flow reverse impairment (Microvascular manifestation).

Csepe TA, Kalyanasundaram A, Hansen BJ, et al. Fibrosis: a structural modulator of sinoatrial node physiology and dysfunction. Front Physiol. 2015;6:37.

Q44. Answer a

The European guidelines suggest that disopyramide be considered for patients with a vagal trigger associated with AF, whereas disopyramide and quinidine, procainamide, are completely omitted from the US guidelines. Dofetilide is not approved for use in Europe but is indicated in all clinical categories in the US guidelines. Both guidelines agree on the use of sotalol, amiodarone, and dronedarone for patients with coronary artery disease and amiodarone for patients with symptomatic congestive heart failure.

Amin A, Houmsse A, Ishola A, et al. The current approach of atrial fibrillation management. Avicenna J Med. 2016;6(1):8-16.

Q45. Answer b

Chemical cardioversion: It can be accomplished with intravenous or oral antiarrhythmic drugs. In general, the conversion success of antiarrhythmic drug therapy is significantly higher for acute (< 7 days) compared with longer-duration AF. Drugs used for chemical cardioversion are: ibutilide, amiodarone, flecainide, propafenone and vernakalant. Chemical cardioversion is simple but less efficacious (50% success) as compared to electrical cardioversion (80–89% success). With drugs, pro-arrhythmic effect is a concern.

Raghavan AV, Decker WW, Meloy TD. Management of Atrial Fibrillation in the Emergency Department. Emergency Medicine Clinics of North America. 2005;23(4):1127-39.

K Type Answers

Q1. Answer TTFTF

Utilities of thoracic ultrasound: Diagnosis of pleural effusion, Quantification of pleural effusion, Characterization of pleural effusion, Identification of pleural masses, Identification of parenchymal disease (infection or masses), Identification of pulmonary edema.

Limitations of lung ultrasound: The learning curve for acquiring skills for diagnosing pleural effusion, lung consolidation and alveolar-interstitial syndrome is short. But learning time for acquiring skills required for diagnosing pneumothorax is probably longer. Obese patients are frequently difficult to examine using lung ultrasound because of the thickness of their rib cage. The presence of subcutaneous emphysema or large thoracic dressings alters or precludes the propagation of ultrasound beams to the lung periphery. Lung ultrasound cannot detect lung over-inflation resulting from an increase in intrathoracic pressures.

Saraogi A. Lung ultrasound: Present and future. Lung India. 2015;32(3):250-7.

Q2. Answer FFTTF

Patients undergoing cardioversion are treated conventionally with therapeutic anticoagulation for three weeks before and four weeks after cardioversion to decrease the risk of thromboembolism. TEE guided strategy has been proposed as an alternative that may lower stroke and bleeding events. Patients without atrial cavity thrombus or atrial appendage thrombus by TEE are cardioverted on achievement of therapeutic anticoagulation, whereas cardioversion is delayed in higher risk patients with thrombus. In patients with permanent atrial fibrillation, the presence of severe spontaneous contrast or smoke is a marker of increased risk of thromboembolic events. Electrical cardioversion causes left atrial appendage (LAA) stunning with increased severity of echo contrast immediately after the procedure. There have been published series of cases of embolic stroke after cardioversion in patients with negative TEE for LA thrombus who are not anticoagulated. For this reason, patients should have therapeutic levels of anticoagulation before proceeding with cardioversion. Patients with surgical LAA ligation show a high incidence of residual flow between the LA and LAA.

Mathuria N. Role of TEE before atrial fibrillation ablation: Is less really more? Heart Rhythm. 2016;13(1):20.

Q3. Answer TTFFT

Pulse contour analysis monitors increase in SV reasonably accurately in addition to SVV which is a good preload indicator. Cardiac output noninvasive measurement is well known today. One such method is in which electrodes are placed in the neck and thorax region and the fluctuations in electrical impedance are measured. The change in aortic flow is measured by the change in the thoracic bioimpedance through the cardiac cycle. Esophageal Doppler measures blood flow velocity in the descending aorta by a Doppler probe kept in the esophagus 40 cm from the mouth. It is a useful monitor for measuring cardiac output. It has been used for high-risk surgical patients but its use in critical care is less common. Transcutaneous Doppler monitoring by an external probe can measure transpulmonary and transaortic cardiac output. Unfortunately, the bioimpedance (BoMed®) had problems with its reliability and was never accepted into clinical practice. Nexfin measure arterial blood pressure using a finger cuff. It is able to track blood pressure from the digital artery in real time.

Critchley LAH. Minimally Invasive Cardiac Output Monitoring in the Year 2012. Available from: https://www.intechopen.com/books/artery-bypass/minimally-invasive-cardiac-output-monitoring-in-the-year-2012 (Accessed 28 December 2017).

Q4. Answer TTTFF

Uses of capnography in the ICU: Detection of ROSC after cardiac arrest, detection of esophageal intubation and accidental extubation, diagnosing air and pulmonary embolism, indirect indicator of cardiac output.

Noninvasive monitoring of cardiac output based on principle for capnography: Based on the well-known accepted Fick's Principle, Novametrix introduced NICO (Novametrix NICO®) cardiac output measurement device that uses partial CO_2 breathing to determine cardiac output noninvasively. The NICO® Cardiopulmonary Management System provides continual cardiac output monitoring. These measurements are accomplished and measured by the proprietary NICO Sensor, which periodically adds a rebreathing volume into the breathing circuit. In addition, NICO provides non-invasive measurement of airway dead space. If arterial carbon dioxide tensions are known, physiological dead space can be calculated easily. Traditional capnography cannot be used to measure stroke volume or cardiac output.

Kerslake I, Kelly F. Uses of capnography in the critical care unit. BJA Education. 2017;17(5):178-83.

Q5. Answer TTTTF

Limitations of SVV: (1) They can vary with tidal volume, peak inspiratory pressure and lung dynamics. (2) Can vary with cardiac arrhythmias. (3) Only validated in mechanically ventilated patients can be monitored. Spontaneously breathing patients may have irregular rate and tidal volumes interfering with the interpretation. The minimum tidal volume should be 8 mL/kg.

Song Y, Kwak YL, Song JW, Kim YJ, Shim JK. Respirophasic carotid artery peak velocity variation as a predictor of fluid responsiveness in mechanically ventilated patients with coronary artery disease. BJA: British Journal of Anaesthesia. 2014;113(1):61-66.

Q6. Answer FFTTF

Digoxin has complex pharmacodynamics and pharmacokinetics. It has cardiac inotropic effects, can cause heart block, and in overdose can result in various types of tachyarrhythmias. There has been much controversy about the use of digoxin in heart failure. When digoxin was first discovered it was found to be effective in congestive heart failure. Subsequently there were concerns that although it improves symptoms it may increase mortality. The Digitalis Investigation Group or DIG trial showed that digoxin improved symptoms and reduced hospital admissions, but neither increased nor decreased mortality. It is used in resistant heart failure as an add-on drug to more beneficial drugs like angiotensin-converting-enzyme (ACE) inhibitors and spironolactone, and is no longer a first line drug in heart failure. However, in mitral stenosis with atrial fibrillation, it is useful in reducing the ventricular rate. There is no indication for its use in patients with mitral stenosis who are in sinus rhythm. The only still generally valid indication for a long-term digoxin treatment is chronic tachycardia atrial fibrillation (but not hyperthyroidism or Wolff-Parkinson-White syndrome). Digoxin therapy of left ventricular insufficiency in persons with normal sinus rhythm is controversial. Apparently, only a minority of the patients has drawn clinically relevant advantages from it.

Currie GM, Wheat JM, Kiat H. Pharmacokinetic considerations for digoxin in older people. Open Cardiovasc Med J. 2011;5:130-5.

Q7. Answer TFFTT

Headache is not a recognized side effect of ACE inhibitors. Cough is common, and is an indication to switch over to an angiotensin receptor blocker. Hyperkalemia is a known side effect, especially in patients on spironolactone and those in renal failure. ACE inhibitors are useful even in late stages of renal failure; however worsening of renal function can occur, due to changes in intrarenal autoregulation. If renal function deteriorates, the ACE inhibitor may need to be discontinued. First dose hypotension is a well-known side effect, and patients are therefore advised to take the first dose while lying in bed.

Francisco AM, García-Luque A, Fernández M, Puerro M. Side Effects of angiotensin converting enzyme inhibitors and angiotensin II receptor antagonists: are we facing a new syndrome. Am J Card 2012;110(10):1552-3.

Q8. Answer TFTTF

Amiodarone can cause both hypo-and hyperthyroidism. It has a very long half-life of nearly 100 days. It causes prolongation of the QT interval, and can be arrhythmogenic. It is used to convert atrial fibrillation to sinus rhythm, and therefore has a place in medical cardioversion of acute atrial fibrillation. Fetal thyroid abnormalities are known to occur, and the drug is contraindicated in pregnancy.

Loh K. Amiodarone-induced thyroid disorders: a clinical review. Postgraduate Medical Journal. 2000;76:133-40.

Q9. Answer TTFFT

Drugs used in the management of hypertensive crisis: Sodium Nitroprusside, Labetalol, Nitroglycerin, Urapidil, Fenoldopam, Nicardipine, Clevidipine, Enalapril, Intravenous Hydralazine etc. Hydralazine reduces peripheral vascular resistance leading to a reflex tachycardia that can increase cardiac output. Therefore, hydralazine would not be a good choice in a patient with ischemic heart disease who may not tolerate the increased myocardial oxygen consumption. Because of the proarrhythmic effects of sotalol, ordinary beta-blockers are a safer alternative to sotalol after surgery.

Powers DR, Papadakos PJ, Wallin JD. Parenteral hydralazine revisited. J Emerg Med. 1998;16:191-6.

Varon J, Marik PE. Clinical review: The management of hypertensive crises. Crit Care. 2003;7(5):374-84.

Q10. Answer TFTTF

Amiodarone lowers the incidence of postoperative AF by about 40 to 50%. Adverse effects of amiodarone are hypotension, circulatory collapse, bradycardia, nausea, flushing, Torsades De Pointes, thyroid disease, pulmonary fibrosis, corneal deposits etc.

Giardina EG, Zimetbaum PJ, Monitoring and management of amiodarone side effects. Available from: https://www.uptodate.com/contents/monitoring-and-management-of-amiodarone-side-effects (Accessed 29 November 2017).

Mäntyjärvi M, Tuppurainen K, Ikäheimo K. Ocular side effects of amiodarone. Surv Ophthalmol. 1998;42(4):360-6.

Q11. Answer TTFTF

The ideal anticoagulation strategy for cardiac surgery with CPB does not exist. Heparin and protamine remain the gold standard for anticoagulation therapy. Bivalirudin is the most promising molecule despite its high cost and lack of a readily available antagonist.

Bouraghda A, Gillois P, Albaladejo P. Alternatives to heparin and protamine anticoagulation for cardiopulmonary bypass in cardiac surgery. Can J Anaesth. 2015;62(5):518-28.

Q12. Answer TTTFF

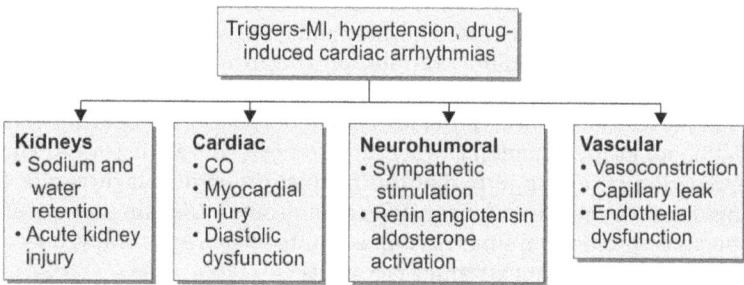

Arrigo M, Parissis JT, Akiyama E, Mebazaa A. Understanding acute heart failure: pathophysiology and diagnosis. European Heart Journal Supplements 2016;18(1):G11-G18.

Q13. Answer TTFTF

CK and CK-MB were the most commonly used serologic tests for the diagnosis of myocardial infarction prior to the widespread adoption of troponin. Their use has markedly diminished over time. They are discussed here predominantly for those areas of the world where cardiac troponin assays are not yet in use. Some clinicians prefer the use of CK-MB for the detection of early reinfarction. LDH was commonly used in the past in combination with aspartate aminotransferase (AST or SGOT) and CK-MB to diagnose MI. LD consists of M (muscle) and H (heart) subunits that give rise to five isoenzymes. The heart primarily contains LD1 and some LD2. Red cells, kidney, stomach, and pancreas are other important sources of LD1. In contrast, LD5 predominates in skeletal muscle and liver. LD activity rises to abnormal levels approximately 10 hours after the onset of MI, peaks at 24 to 48 hours, and remains elevated for six to eight days. However, since troponins are more specific than LD and remain elevated for 5 to 10 days, current recommendations suggest that LD no longer has a role in the diagnosis of MI. Skeletal muscle injury elevates CK-MB. The proportion of CK that is CK-MB can be as high as 50 percent with chronic skeletal muscle injury, such as dermatomyositis/polymyositis, due to increased production of B chain CK protein. So the proportion factor may mislead in such cases.

Chan D. Leong LN. Biomarkers in acute myocardial infarction. BMC Med. 2010;8:34.

Q14. Answer TTTFF

Sometime weaning and trial off may not be successful and we need to go back on ECMO support. Signs of weaning failure during cardiac ECMO (VA-ECMO) are inappropriate tachycardia, hypotension drop in mixed venous saturation below 60% with or without worsening echocardiography. Signs of weaning failure during respiratory ECMO (VV-ECMO) are hypoxia or hypercapnia. The reason for weaning failure should be established and corrected if possible. The reason for weaning failure are that heart or lung have still not recovered completely to tolerate weaning, inadequate ventilator setting, presence of fluid overload and mucus plug. Persistent pulmonary hypertension, underlying other congenital heart disease can also be the cause for weaning failure. If the cause of weaning failure is identified then retry for weaning should be given after correction of the cause. If no factors are discovered then one should retry weaning after 24 to 36 hours.

Aokage T, Palmér K, Ichiba S, Takeda S. Extracorporeal membrane oxygenation for acute respiratory distress syndrome. Journal of Intensive Care. 2015;3:17.

Q15. Answer TTFFF

ECMO is associated with significant complications related to the critically ill patient subset in which it is used and the therapy itself. Common complications include bleeding, thromboembolic events, and sepsis. Less common complications include limb ischemia, hemolysis, and mechanical failure (such as oxygenator or cannula or device thrombosis). Rarer but potentially catastrophic complications include intracerebral bleeding, circuit rupture, accidental decannulation, and air embolism.

>Cheng R, Hachamovitch R, Kittleson M, et al. Complications of extracorporeal membrane oxygenation for treatment of cardiogenic shock and cardiac arrest: a meta-analysis. Ann Thorac Surg. 2014;97:610-6.

Q16. Answer TFTTF

Established or potential hypercoagulable states are activated protein C resistance, Alpha-macroglobulin deficiency, Anticardiolipin antibodies, antithrombin deficiency, dysfibrinogenemia, factor V Leiden, Factor V deficiency, excess, Factor VII excess, Factor VIII excess, Factor IX excess, Heparin cofactor II deficiency, Hyperhomocysteinemia, Hyperfibrinogenemia, Lupus Anticoagulants, PAI - 1 excess, Plasminogen deficiency, Protein C deficiency, Protein S deficiency, Prothrombin G 20210A, tPA deficiency, TFPI deficiency, Thrombomodulin deficiency etc.

>Bande BD, Bande SB, Mohite S. The hypercoagulable states in anaesthesia and critical care. Indian J Anaesth. 2014;58(5): 665-71.

Q17. Answer TFTTF

Predictor	Score
CHF, decreased ejection fraction	1
Hypertension	1
Age > 75 years	2
Diabetes mellitus	1
Vascular disease	1
Stroke/TIA	2
Age 65–74 years	1
Sex, Female	1
Maximum potential score	9

>Wasmer K, Köbe J, Dechering D, et al. CHADS(2) and CHA(2)DS (2)-VASc score of patients with atrial fibrillation or flutter and newly detected left atrial thrombus. Clin Res Cardiol. 2013;102(2):139-44.

Q18. Answer TFTTT

The vast majority of A-V bypass tracts conduct both antegradely and retrogradely. Less than 5% of patients with preexcitation have bypass tracts that conduct only antegradely. This is much less common than the converse situation of retrogradely conducting bypass tracts in the absence of antegrade preexcitation (i.e. so-called concealed bypass tracts).

In patients who manifest only antegrade conduction over their bypass tract, spontaneous circus movement tachycardia, either antidromic or orthodromic, is not usually observed, but when it is, it is antidromic. The primary rhythm disturbance they manifest is atrial fibrillation. Over time antegrade conduction over an A-V bypass tract may disappear. Chen et al. noted a loss of pre-excitation in one fifth of symptomatic patients with WPW. Only 7.8% lost retrograde conduction. Spontaneous loss of pre-excitation has been observed in one fifth to one half of children with WPW.

>Skinner JR, Sharland G. Detection and management of life threatening arrhythmias in the perinatal period. Early Hum Dev. 2008;84(3):161-72.

Q19. Answer TFTTF

VF in patients without structural heart disease is rare. 90–95% of individuals with ventricular fibrillation reveal underlying structural heart disease.
- No structural heart disease can be identified in only 5% to 10% of patients
- According to the results of CASPER among patients with normal left ventricular function, a causal diagnosis for VF can be found in 56%. Most diagnoses were primary electrical diseases (catecholaminergic polymorphic VT [CPVT], long QT syndrome, early repolarization syndrome,

and Brugada syndrome [69%]). In 31% of patients, a subtle structural heart disease (i.e. coronary spasm, subclinical arrhythmogenic right ventricular cardiomyopathy and myocarditis) was identified. In addition, IVF was diagnosed in 44% of patients with VF without structural heart disease.
- The diagnosis of IVF is based on the exclusion of currently known structural and primary electrical heart diseases following a complete noninvasive, invasive, and genetic workup.

    Axel Sarrias, Roger Villuendas, Felipe Bisbal, et al. From Atrial Fibrillation to Ventricular Fibrillation and Back. Circulation. 2015;132:2035-36.

Q20. Answer TFTFT

Severe acute pulmonary hypertension may contribute to the development or worsening of right ventricular (RV) failure. Pulmonary hypertension and RV failure may reduce left ventricular (LV) filling, LV systolic and diastolic pressures, and cardiac output and lead to systemic hypotension. Decreased arterial blood pressure may compromise LV and RV coronary perfusion at a time when RV end-diastolic pressures and RV myocardial oxygen consumption are increased due to increased RV wall tension, thereby leading to RV ischemia. RV ischemia exacerbates RV failure, causing a further reduction in cardiac output and blood pressure. Concomitant LV dysfunction further impairs RV performance due to the loss of the interventricular septal contributions to RV function, which are largely determined by LV function. One of the key interventions to break this vicious cycle is to reduce the RV afterload, for example, by decreasing pulmonary vascular resistance (PVR), thereby enabling the RV to pump more blood forward. Although systemic vasodilators may reduce PVR, concomitant reduction of systemic blood pressure not only decreases the RV coronary perfusion pressure but also decreases LV contraction, which adversely affects RV function. Inhalation of nitric oxide (NO) produces selective pulmonary vasodilation without reducing the systemic arterial pressure in patients with pulmonary hypertension. Although the only current Food and Drug Administration-approved indication of inhaled NO is persistent pulmonary hypertension of newborns, off-label use of inhaled NO is widespread. However, inhaled NO is very expensive; despite the need to treat RV dysfunction in patients undergoing cardiac surgery, as well as patients undergoing heart and lung transplantation or requiring the placement of a ventricular assist device, there is no established consensus concerning the use of pulmonary vasodilators for these indications.

    Fumito I, Warren ZM. Inhaled Pulmonary Vasodilators in Cardiac Surgery Patients: Correct Answer Is 'NO'. Anesthesia and Analgesia 2017;125(2):375-7.

Q21. Answer TTTFF

Fast-flush test is a method of determining the dynamic response of the monitoring system to assess the amount of distortion existing in the system. The fast-flush valve is opened for a short time and the resulting flush artifacts are examined (see Figure on page 23). An optimal fast-flush test results on one undershoot followed by small overshoot, and then followed by the waveform. An adequate fast-flush test usually corresponds to a resonant frequency of 10-20 Hz with a damping coefficient of 0.50.7 for peripheral arterial pressure monitoring. The arterial trace should normalize within three oscillations in an optimally dampened system.

Table: Causes of dampening

Overdamping	Underdamping
Air bubbles	Excessive tubing length
Clot	Patient on inotropes
Kink	
Deflated pressure bag	
Over complaint tubing	
Poor connections of stopcock	

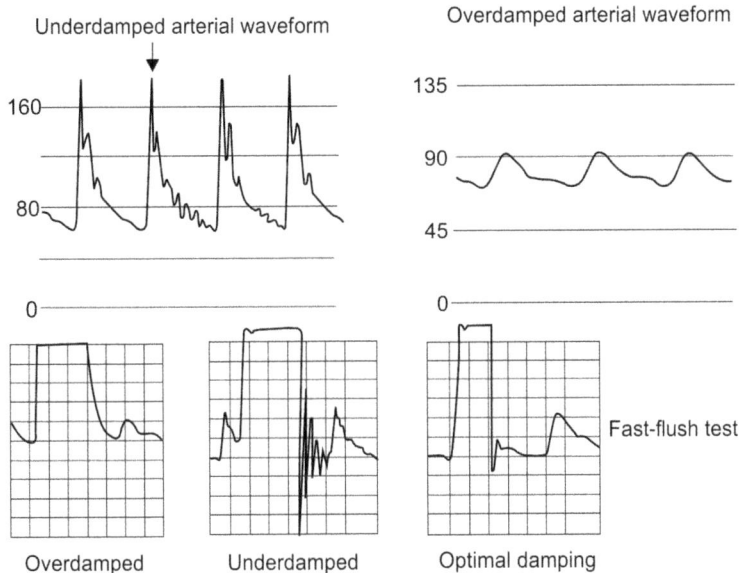

Fast-Flush test should be done in the following circumstances: every 8 hourly, when significant change appears in patient hemodynamic status, after zeroing and sampling, change in tubing, damped waveform seen on the monitor.

_{Kumar P. Peripheral arterial catheterization. In: Kumar P (Ed.). ICU Manual. 1st Edition. India: Jaypee Brothers Medical Publishers (P) Ltd, 2017; p 18-23.}

Q22. Answer TTTFF

The IJV provides a useful and reliable site with a low failure rate and its cannulation is traditionally performed with the aid of both palpation and anatomical landmarks. Various approaches may be used to reach the IJV. Variations between the carotid artery and the IJV, and the depth and size of the IJV may account for failure to locate the vein, and these factors were found to be independent of age and size. The IJV was found directly anterior to the carotid artery, at the level between the two heads of the sternocleidomastoid muscle, in about 50% of cases, and anterior or anterolateral at the level of the cricoid cartilage in about 30% of the cases. Doppler ultrasound guided puncture could reduce the time and the number of attempts for successful cannulation. Direct two-dimensional ultrasound identification proved to be more precise and efficient, especially in small children, and it is now recommended when difficulties are anticipated, complications have been encountered, or when repeated IJV cannulation is required.

Using ultrasound guided IJV cannulation in infants can be 100% successful with ultrasound, as compared with a 75% success rate using a traditional palpation method. Incidence of carotid artery punctures may be 0% versus 25% respectively. In 2002, these findings were repeated by Asheim and coworkers, who found a 100% success rate in 45 consecutive children and a median time to aspirate blood from the IJV of 12 s. Complications include arterial puncture, haematoma formation and catheter malposition, but thrombosis and pneumothorax are rarely reported.

_{Haas NA. Clinical review: Vascular access for fluid infusion in children. Crit Care. 2004;8(6):478-84.}

Q23. Answer FTTFT

In a study of 20 neonates and small infants, venous oxygen saturation was lower and lactate level higher from the superior vena cava compared with the inferior vena cava. Cerebral tissue oxygenation was analyzed by near-infrared spectroscopy. Based on these measurements, the authors concluded that mixed venous saturation alone is inadequate to evaluate regional cerebral saturation.

Redlin M, Koster A, Huebler M, et al. Regional differences in tissue oxygenation during cardiopulmonary bypass for correction of congenital heart disease in neonates and small infants: Relevance of near-infrared spectroscopy. J Thorac Cardiovasc Surg. 2008;136:962-7.

Q24. Answer TTFTF

A great number of medications are available for the treatment of hypertensive emergencies. Sodium nitroprusside is a first-choice for the majority of hypertensive emergencies, and it acts within seconds as a potent arterial and venous dilator. The most important disadvantage is thiocyanate toxicity. The toxicity is more likely to occur if patients have hepatic or renal failure and when the agent is administered for more than 48–72 h. Labetalol can be used to treat hypertensive emergencies through IV administration with a non-selective β-blocker and a1 adrenergic receptor blocker with 6.9:1 ratio of antagonism reducing the systemic vascular resistance but maintaining the cerebral, renal, and coronary blood flow. It is interesting that despite the β-blocking effect it maintains also the cardiac output. Nitroglycerine is a venodilator that mainly reduces the preload and decreases the cardiac oxygen demands, and it is often used in hypertensive crises. This agent is used primarily in acute myocardial infarction and acute pulmonary edema along with other antihypertensive regimens. Other agents that can be used in hypertensive emergencies include nicardipine (dihydropyridine calcium channel blocker), which is a useful agent for patients with coronary artery disease due to its beneficial effect on coronary blood flow or clevidipine, which is a new short-acting intravenous dihydropyridine calcium channel blocker. Enalapril is an angiotensin-converting enzyme inhibitor, but it is not recommended since it can aggravate renal blood flow, and the potential of renal failure in patients with hypertensive emergency is high. Fenoldopam is an important medication, and it acts through peripheral dopamine-1 receptors as a vasodilator and as a diuretic.

Goswami S, Gupta MK, Mehta Y. Hypertensive urgencies and emergencies. In: Chawla R, Todi S (Eds). ICU protocol book 2nd Edition. Springer India (pub); 2018 (in press).

Cardiology (Part II)

Prashant Kumar, Qurat Ul Ain Makhdoomi

A Type Questions
(One best answer)

1. Common causes of pulmonary artery hypertension in the intensive care unit are the following *except*:
   a. Acute respiratory distress syndrome
   b. Pulmonary embolism
   c. Interstitial lung disease
   d. Lobar pneumonia
   e. Chronic obstructive pulmonary disease

2. The most appropriate ventilation strategy in pulmonary artery hypertension (PAH) is:
   a. Low tidal volume, low PEEP, permissive hypercapnia
   b. High tidal volume, low PEEP, permissive hypercapnia
   c. Low tidal volume, low PEEP, without permissive hypercapnia
   d. Low tidal volume, high PEEP, permissive hypercapnia
   e. High tidal volume, high PEEP, permissive hypercapnia

3. Pulmonary Embolism with shock can initially be best treated by:
   a. Large fluid bolus, norepinephrine, dobutamine, fibrinolytics
   b. Small fluid bolus, norepinephrine, dobutamine, fibrinolytics
   c. Small fluid bolus, norepinephrine, dobutamine, anticoagulation
   d. Large fluid bolus, norepinephrine, dobutamine, anticoagulation
   e. Large fluid bolus, norepinephrine, dobutamine, no fibrinolytics

4. Right ventricular infarction is most commonly associated with myocardial infarction involving:
   a. Anterior wall
   b. Posterior wall
   c. Lateral wall
   d. Anteroseptal wall
   e. Inferior wall

5. A 45-year-old man is found collapsed at home. There is no history available. His ECG is shown below:

   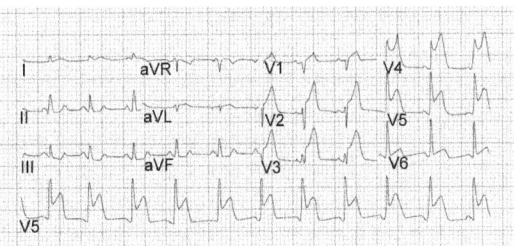

   What is the diagnosis?
   a. Anterolateral ST elevation
   b. Atrial fibrillation with fast ventricular rate
   c. Polymorphic VT or torsades de pointes
   d. Wolff Parkinson-White syndrome
   e. S1Q3T3

6. Temporary transvenous pacing lead was placed in a case of acute coronary syndrome with high grade AV block. Chest X-ray shows the right ventricular position as shown in the picture below:

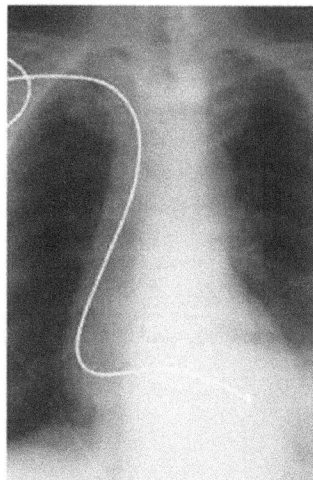

The pattern on 12 lead ECG in this lead position is:
a. Normal ECG
b. ST elevation pattern in lateral leads
c. Left bundle branch block (LBBB)
d. Right bundle branch block (RBBB)
e. Short PR interval with prominent R in V1

7. A 79-year-old undergoes primary percutaneous coronary intervention (PCI) for anterior wall myocardial Infarction. He required Intubation and mechanical ventilation due to cardiogenic shock. Percutaneous tracheostomy is planned due to difficult weaning. The following is an appropriate strategy for dual antiplatelet in case of drug eluting stents (DES):
a. Dual antiplatelet therapy (DAPT) are not required for DES placed in stable ischemic heart disease (SIHD)
b. Aspirin may reasonably be continued while Clopidogrel is stopped for 3-5 days before planned procedure; there is no need to restart Clopidogrel if no stent thrombosis is detected in the interval
c. Aspirin may reasonably be continued while Clopidogrel is stopped for 3-5 days before planned procedure; Clopidogrel to be restarted post procedure as before and completed for at least 6 months as scheduled
d. In case of bare metal stent the minimum duration of DAPT is at least 12 months
e. In case of bleeding in patients on DAPT, platelet transfusions have no role due to long half-life of antiplatelet drugs

8. The maximum incidence of peripartum Cardiomyopathy occurs at the following stage of pregnancy:
a. 32 weeks
b. 37 to 40 weeks (term)
c. During delivery
d. Postpartum (up to 4 weeks of delivery)
e. Late (4 weeks to 20 weeks of delivery)

9. A 45-year-old patient who was hospitalized following the ingestion of 100 tablets of 0.25 mg digoxin. Serum digoxin level was found to be 12.6 ng/mL. The ECG recorded AF with PVC.

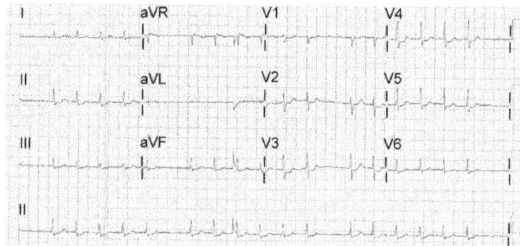

What is the therapeutic window of digoxin?
a. 0.10-0.5 ng/mL
b. 0.5-2 ng/mL
c. 2-6 ng/mL
d. 6-12 ng/mL
e. >12.0 ng/mL

10. Typical heparin induced thrombocytopenia (HIT) occurs after the following days of starting heparin:
a. 1-2
b. 2-5
c. 4-10
d. 21-28
e. ≥ 28

11. A 74-year-old hypertensive woman was admitted through the emergency department for epigastric pain and dyspnea that had started two days ago. The blood pressure was 90/60 mm Hg and echocardiography shows as below:

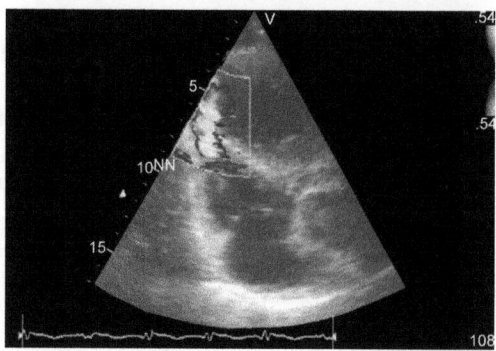

One of the following is most appropriate initial strategy to manage shock in this condition:
   a. Inotropic support without intra-aortic balloon pump (IABP)
   b. Extracorporeal membrane oxygenation (ECMO)
   c. Early surgery
   d. Trans catheter closure using Amplatzer®
   e. Inotropic support with Intra-aortic balloon pump (IABP)

12. A 65-year-old male is ventilated in the ICU following an emergency laparotomy for perforated sigmoid diverticulum. He has critical aortic stenosis (AS) and is being considered for an aortic valve replacement. Management strategy which is not appropriate:
   a. To reduce BP, calcium channel blockers (CCB) are preferred over ACE inhibitors
   b. Aggressive use of anti arrhythmics to maintain normal sinus rhythm
   c. Maintenance of a high left ventricular preload
   d. Avoidance of diuretics
   e. Beta-blockers should be avoided or used in low doses

13. Regarding the arterial pressure waveform in the hypovolemic mechanically ventilated patients which is correct?
   a. Changes in systolic pressure better reflect hypovolemia as compared to changes in pulse pressure across the respiratory cycle
   b. PPV is an indicator of volume status
   c. Pulse pressure is directly proportional to stroke volume
   d. The maximum fall in systolic pressure coincides temporally with the peak inspiratory pressure

14. A 45-year-old man is admitted into ICU following abdominal surgery. He has oliguria, hypotension and tachycardia 135 bpm, BP systolic 80/40 mm Hg. An esophageal Doppler probe is used showing corrected flow time (FTc) 256 ms (normal value 330 to 360 ms), Peak Velocity (PV) 55cm/s (normal value 90–120 cm/s). Stroke volume 39 mL (Normal value 60 to 100 mL). Which one of the following is most appropriate diagnosis?
   a. Intraoperative myocardial infarction
   b. Massive pulmonary embolism
   c. Hypovolemia
   d. Septic shock
   e. Abdominal compartment syndrome

15. Which of the following best distinguishes a condition of non- ST segment elevation MI from unstable angina?
   a. Severe chest pain
   b. ST segment depression in two or more contiguous leads of ECG
   c. Raised troponin level
   d. Chest pain lasting more than 15 minutes
   e. NT pro BNP level

16. A 28-year-old previously well woman is seen in the emergency room with sudden onset palpitation. The ECG shows atrial fibrillation (AF) with a ventricular rate of 140 bpm. On examination, she complains of a feeling of breathlessness but is able to talk in sentences. She also feels very mild pain in the chest. The most appropriate first line treatment of her arrhythmia would be:
   a. Oral digoxin 250–500 over 30 minutes
   b. Intravenous metoprolol 2.5–5 mg over 1 minute
   c. Intravenous flecainide 100–150 mg over 30 minutes
   d. Synchronized cardioversion under sedation
   e. Intravenous verapamil 5 m intravenous bolus

17. The following assumptions regarding cardiac output is correct when determining from esophageal Doppler probe *except*:
   a. Changes in Stroke Distance (SD) is directly related to Stroke volume (SV)
   b. Estimate of cross sectional area may be an important source of error
   c. The device has errors in high and low cardiac output
   d. Corrected flow time (FTc) < 330 ms indicates good ventricular fillings
   e. Peak velocity is generally less in the old than in young individuals

18. A 36-year-old previously healthy male who takes care of a horse presented to the medical casualty ward with a one-day history of fever, arthralgia and severe myalgia. He developed hypotension on the second day of illness. ECG showed sinus tachycardia with ST segment depression in lateral leads which evolved into rapid AF in the subsequent days. 2D echocardiogram showed dilated cardiac chambers with severe global hypokinesia and an ejection fraction of 20%. Leptospirosis was confirmed by positive leptospira IgM

and negative IgG. He develops shock and multiorgan failure.

One of the following is False in this condition:
a. Milrinone is less proarrhythmic than Dobutamine
b. Aldosterone antagonist spironolactone has have symptomatic and survival benefit
c. Immunosuppressive therapy may be started in secreted patients who have connective tissue diseases also
d. Beta-blockers are contraindicated
e. Intra-aortic balloon counter pulsation (IABP) is an option for patient unresponsive to pharmacologic therapy

19. A 44-year-old man with dilated cardiomyopathy is on the waiting list for heart transplantation. His condition is refractory to maximal medical therapy, and placement of a left ventricular assist device (LVAD) is considered. One of the following is false about LVAD:
a. Third generation LVAD produce pulsatile flow to mimic normal physiology
b. Echocardiography is an important imaging modality used to determine the indication of left ventricular assist device (LVAD)
c. The LVAD takes blood from the left ventricle and delivers into the aorta
d. Approximately one-fourth of VAD patients suffer from gastrointestinal bleeding
e. LVADs may be used as a bridge to transplant for candidates awaiting heart transplantation

20. Regarding the physics of direct arterial blood pressure measurement, which is correct?
a. The natural frequency of system should be at least 4 times the fundamental frequency of arterial wave
b. The catheter connect the arterial cannula to the transducer should be short, stiff and wide to increase natural frequency
c. The fluid used within the tubing should be of high density
d. Clot causes under damping

K Type Questions
[Marked True (T)/False (F)]

1. Hemodynamic effects of the intra-aortic balloon pump (IABP) are the following:
a. Increase of afterload
b. Reduction of preload
c. Improvement in cardiac output
d. Increase in systolic blood pressure
e. Improvement of coronary blood flow

2. Fibrinolytic agent given as single bolus dose:
a. Streptokinase
b. Tenecteplase
c. Reteplase
d. Alteplase
e. Fondaparinux

3. Consider the following statements about natriuretic peptides:
a. Natriuretic peptides are released in response to Atrial and ventricular wall stretch
b. Marked elevation in natriuretic peptides are also a prognosticator
c. NT-pro brain natriuretic peptide (BNP) level up to 350 normal for all age groups
d. BNP and NT-proBNP can be collectively used to differentiate systolic heart failure from preserved ejection failure heart failure
e. BNP level of less than 100 is reasonably able to rule out heart failure

4. Hemodynamic profiles used to describe acutely decompensated heart failure (ADHF):
a. Warm and wet
b. Warm and red
c. Cold and wet
d. Cold and dry
e. Warm and friable

5. Regarding atrial fibrillation (AF) in sepsis:
a. Vernakalant is a new oral antiarrhythmic which has been found effective in AF of more than 7 days of duration
b. Amiodarone has less negative inotropic effects compared to B-blockers and calcium channel blockers
c. The incidence of AF is higher in sepsis when compared to patients without sepsis
d. Synchronized cardioversion is the treatment of choice for hemodynamically unstable patients
e. Short-term anticoagulation therapy is considered for persistent AF to avoid risk of bleeding

6. Mark the following statements as True or False:
a. A normal electrocardiogram (ECG) can exclude acute myocardial Infarction
b. ST elevation myocardial infarction (STEMI) in whom the time in whom expected time to primary PCI is greater than 120 minutes

should be considered for fibrinolytic therapy within 30 minutes
   c. Cardiogenic shock is most often associated with anterior wall myocardial infarction (AWMI)
   d. Advanced atrioventricular block is not a contraindication to B-blockers in the first 24 hours.
   e. Nitrates are useful in RV infarction because of its propensity to increase RV preload and hence cardiac output

7. Typical characteristics of pulmonary hypertension (PH) due to lung disease are:
   a. Echocardiography is gold standard for diagnosis of PH
   b. PAP of more than 35 mm Hg must be specifically addressed for its long-term adverse effects
   c. PH is poor prognostic factor in both chronic obstructive pulmonary disease (COPD) and interstitial lung disease (ILD)
   d. Bosentan is the therapy of choice with excellent long-term results for COPD with documented chronic hypoxemia
   e. PH is more prevalent in advanced COPD than ILD

8. Features typical of Takotsubo cardiomyopathy:
   a. Involvement of left ventricular apex
   b. ECG changes undifferentiated from myocardial infarction
   c. Gradual onset
   d. Chest pain or discomfort similar to myocardial infarction
   e. Coronary insufficiency on angiography

9. An 82-year-old lady, a known case of diabetes mellitus, CAD, and post CABG (15 years ago) brought to emergency with complaints of breathlessness, decreased urine output and weakness. She was diagnosed as carcinoma breast which was treated by surgery, chemotherapy and radiotherapy 10 years ago. She has a baseline ejection fraction of 20%. USG chest revealed large pleural effusion of the right side. Diagnostic/therapeutic thoracentesis reveled total protein 3.5 gm/dL (serum protein 5.0 gm/dL), LDH 300 U/L (Serum LDH 350U/L), NT pro BNP 1500 few pus cells, no micro-organism, no AFB, no fungal elements, no malignant cells. In the past 2 days 750 mL of pleural fluid was drained in the chest drain bag. Serum NT pro BNP was 18000 pg/mL. She has received aggressive diuretic therapy in the last few days. The following characteristics of pleural effusion support cardiac etiology despite of exudative characteristics in these settings:
   a. Post CABG status
   b. Carcinoma breast in the past
   c. NT pro BNP in pleural fluid 1500 pg/mL
   d. Total protein in pleural fluid 2.5 gm/dL
   e. Serum NT pro BNP was 18000 pg/mL

10. An 64-year-old male, CAD, TVD HTN, DM, post CABG patient presented with shortness of breath, bilateral leg swelling and severe weakness. He complains of passage of blood in stool. LV EF is 55%. He is taking Aspirin 150 mg once a day in the last 2 years. On arrival his Hb was 4.5 gm/dL and was transfused 2 units of Packed Red Blood Cells. Iron studies reveal- Serum Iron- 46 microgram/dL (49-181), Ferritin 20.70 (17-464), Vitamin B12 839 (261-462).
    There is splenomegaly. Upper GI endoscopy reveal grade I varices with no stigmata of recent bleeding. USG abdomen reveals liver parenchymal disease mild splenomegaly with ascites. Approach to manage upper gastrointestinal bleeding due to antiplatelet therapy includes:
    a. Packed red blood transfusion to correct blood loss
    b. Reversal of the effect of co-prescribed anticoagulants should also be considered
    c. Upper GI endoscopy is avoided in active bleeding
    d. Platelet transfusion is contraindicated due to risk of thrombosis in such cases
    e. Decisions to withhold anti-platelet drugs with due consideration

11. Cardiologists may use one of the following strategies to reduce the chances of contrast induced nephropathy (CIN) following percutaneous coronary intervention:
    a. Judicious hydration possibly guided by patient's hemodynamic status
    b. No role of minimizing the volume of contrast agent
    c. Stopping nephrotoxic agents
    d. Allow intervals between two contrast exposures

e. N-Acetylcysteine 600 mg for two days including the day of the procedure

12. **Correct indication(s) for temporary transvenous pacing:**
    a. Symptomatic bradycardia unresponsive to temporary transcutaneous pacing
    b. Symptomatic bradycardia not responding to drugs
    c. Atrial fibrillation waiting for cardioversion
    d. Hemodynamically unstable patient with hypokalemia where defibrillation is contraindicated
    e. Bradycardia with severe coagulopathy

13. **Regarding arterial pressure waveform:**
    a. In severe sepsis there is a delayed dicrotic notch
    b. Hypovolemia is characterized by an increase in pulse pressure
    c. Stroke volume can be obtained from the area under the entire waveform
    d. Dicrotic notch is delayed in hypovolemia

14. **Regarding postoperative atrial fibrillation (AF):**
    a. Overall incidence in the noncardiac surgery is low compared to cardiac surgery
    b. It most commonly occurs on the 7th postoperative day
    c. Generally it resolves spontaneously
    d. It increase the risk of stroke three fold
    e. Incidence has no relation with age

15. **The following can be assessed from transpulmonary thermodilution method (TPTD):**
    a. Preload
    b. Cardiac Index
    c. Estimate of pulmonary edema
    d. An estimate of total circulating blood volume

16. **Mark True or False on drug class and the respective examples in the following pairs:**
    a. Direct Thrombin Inhibitor—Ximelagatran
    b. Factor Xa Inhibitor—Tenecteplase
    c. P2Y12 Inhibitor—Prasugrel
    d. Glycoprotein IIb/III inhibitors—Tirofiban
    e. Recombinant tPA—Fondaparinux

17. **According to the American Heart Association (AHA) guidelines which of the followings are correct?**
    a. Heart failure with reduced ejection failure (HFrEF) is when left ventricular ejection fraction is less than 40%
    b. Heart failure with preserved ejection fraction (HFpEF) is when left ventricular ejection fraction is more than 50%
    c. Heart failure with reduced ejection fraction (HFrEF) borderline is defined as ejection fraction 41% to 49%
    d. Heart failure with reduced ejection failure (HFrEF) was earlier called as systolic heart failure
    e. Heart failure with preserved ejection fraction (HFpEF) was earlier called as diastolic heart failure

18. **About Milrinone:**
    a. Increases blood pressure by vasoconstriction
    b. Increases cardiac output by inotropy
    c. less tachycardia than b-agonists
    d. Thrombocytopenia and hepatic dysfunction are known adverse effects
    e. Commonly prescribed dose is 50 mg/kg loading followed by 0.375–0.75 mcg/kg/min IV

19. **About pulmonary artery occlusion pressure (PAOP):**
    a. PAOP is a static parameter
    b. PAOP is generally considered not good predictor of volume responsiveness
    c. Pulmonary artery wedge pressure (PAWP), and pulmonary artery occlusion pressure (PAOP) are one and the same thing
    d. In normal hearts pulmonary artery wedge pressure (PAWP) is more than left ventricular end diastolic pressure (LVEDP)
    e. In mitral stenosis PAWP is more than LVEDP

20. **Mark True or False about thrombolytic therapy for pulmonary embolism (PE):**
    a. There is a 10% risk of clinically significant bleeding
    b. Tenecteplase is US FDA approved drug for acute PE
    c. Significant RV dysfunction and myocardial necrosis is an indication of thrombolysis
    d. Systemic hypotension is an absolute contraindication to thrombolysis

ANSWERS

A Type Answers

Q1. Answer d

Causes of pulmonary artery hypertension in the ICU:
1. Pulmonary hypertension due to left heart disease: Systolic dysfunction, diastolic dysfunction, valvular disease: Mitral stenosis, mitral regurgitation
2. Pulmonary hypertension due to lung diseases and/or hypoxia: Chronic obstructive pulmonary disease, interstitial lung disease, sleep-disordered breathing, alveolar hypoventilation disorders
3. Unclear and/or multifactorial mechanisms: Hematological disorders: myeloproliferative disorders, systemic disorders: sarcoidosis, vasculitis, metabolic disorders: glycogen storage disease
4. Others: Tumor obstruction, fibrosing mediastinitis, chronic renal failure on dialysis

Triggers of right ventricle failure in the ICU: Sepsis, arrhythmias, pericardial effusion, anemia, hypoxemia, acidosis, metabolic abnormalities, withdrawal of pulmonary vasodilators, pulmonary embolism, and myocardial infarction. A French series of 46 patients with PAH admitted to the ICU for right ventricle failure found a causative factor in 41% of patients.

Sztrymf B, Souza R, Bertoletti L, et al. Prognostic factors of acute heart failure in patients with pulmonary arterial hypertension. Eur Respir J. 2010;35(6):1286-93.

Q2. Answer c

Mechanical ventilation may have untoward hemodynamic effects in patients with PAH. Increases in lung volume and decreases in functional residual capacity can increase pulmonary vascular resistance (PVR) and right ventricular afterload. In patients with normal right ventricular function, transient increases in PVR are inconsequential. However, in patients with pre-existing or impending right ventricular failure, lung hyperinflation and either inadequate or excessive PEEP can fatally reduce cardiac output. The elevated pulmonary artery pressure (PAP) correlated directly with increased right atrial pressure and PVR. Right ventricular outflow impedance in mechanically ventilated patients increases as tidal volume is progressively increased and this is ameliorated with the application of low levels of PEEP between 3 cm H_2O and 8 cm H_2O. Optimal ventilator management of patients with PAH may be with low tidal volumes and relatively low PEEP. This strategy of low tidal volume ventilation is similar to the strategy used to ventilate patients with ARDS, but care should be taken to avoid permissive hypercapnia, which may have untoward hemodynamic effects, including increased PAP, arrhythmia and vasodilatation.

Zamanian RT, Haddad F, Doyle RL, et al. Management strategies for patients with pulmonary hypertension in the intensive care unit. Crit Care Med. 2007;35(9):2037-50.

Q3. Answer b

Traditionally, volume expansion with 1 to 2 L of crystalloid is the initial treatment for hypotension in patients with undifferentiated shock. However, in hypotensive patients with moderate-to-severe RV dysfunction; the aggressive fluid administration may lead to further increased RVEDP as well as decreased RV coronary perfusion pressure, ultimately resulting in RV ischemia and further deterioration in RV function. Fluids should be used with caution, and early consideration should be given to vasopressor therapy. Norepinephrine, epinephrine, and high-dose dopamine have demonstrated favorable hemodynamic effects in the setting of acute PE and circulatory failure. Anticoagulation with heparin should be begun while pursuing the diagnostic workup. Thrombolytic therapy causes rapid lysis of clot and more rapid improvement in RV hemodynamics. Thrombolytic therapy is recommended as standard, first-line treatment in patients with massive PE, unless contraindicated. The role of thrombolytic therapy for submassive PE is controversial.

Sekhri V, Mehta N, Rawat N, et al. Management of massive and nonmassive pulmonary embolism. Arch Med Sci. 2012;8(6):957-69.

Q4. Answer e

Right ventricle myocardial infarctions (RVMIs) accompany inferior wall ischemia in up to one-half of cases. Nearly 70% of all AMIs involve some or part of the left ventricle. Left ventricle can be involved in different proportions in all other MI due to its large share of heart muscle as a whole.

Ondrus T, Kanovsky J, Novotny T, et al. Right ventricular myocardial infarction: from pathophysiology to prognosis. Exp Clin Cardiol. 2013;18(1):27-30.

Q5. Answer a

12 lead ECG showing an anterolateral ST elevation myocardial infarction. ST segment is showing elevation in precordial leads V1 to V5.

Septal leads = V1-2

Anterior leads = V3-4

Lateral leads = V5-6

Anterior Myocardial Infarction. Available from: https://lifeinthefastlane.com/ecg-library/anterior-stemi/ (Accessed 28 December 2017).

Q6. Answer c

The universally accepted rule that RV pacing will produce LBBB and left ventricle (LV) pacing of an RBBB pattern on a surface ECG. Paced RBBB morphology in patients with RV apical pacing is usually indicative of inadvertent LV pacing through intracardiac defects such as patent foramen ovale, a ventricular septal defect. Sometimes it may represent coronary sinus pacing.

Jain R, Mohanan S, Haridasan V, et al. Change in QRS morphology in right ventricular apical pacing: is it a red flag sign? Heart Asia. 2014;6(1):152-4.

Q7. Answer c

Noncardiac surgery is often required in patients taking DAPT after PCI with stenting. Cessation of DAPT prior to the recommended duration of its use, as well as the prothrombotic and proinflammatory state associated with surgery; contribute to an increased risk of adverse cardiovascular events such as stent thrombosis, myocardial infarction, or even death. On the other hand, for some patients such as those undergoing neurosurgical procedures, the risk of bleeding attributable to DAPT may be greater than the risk of adverse cardiovascular events without such therapy. Best is to defer elective noncardiac surgery for at least 12 months, as opposed to operating sooner, irrespective of stent type. In patients who cannot wait at least 12 months for noncardiac surgery an attempt to defer surgery for at least 30 days after bare metal stent placement and at least six months after DES placement is preferred. For most patients undergoing noncardiac surgery who are taking DAPT after PCI with stenting because they have not reached the recommended duration of such therapy, continuing DAPT, as opposed to stopping it prior to surgery is recommended. In patients for whom the risk of bleeding is likely to exceed the risk of a perioperative event due to the premature cessation of DAPT; aspirin alone is continued. In patients for whom a bleeding complication could be catastrophic, such as patients undergoing neurosurgical, prostate or posterior chamber eye procedures, stopping both antiplatelet agents might be reasonable.

Mahmoud KD, Sanon S, Habermann EB, et al. Perioperative cardiovascular risk of prior coronary stent implantation among patients undergoing noncardiac surgery. J Am Coll Cardiol. 2016;67:1038.

Q8. Answer d

Peripartum cardiomyopathy occurs in the first 4 months postpartum; fewer than 10% of cases occur prepartum. Common symptoms include dyspnea, cough, orthopnea, hemoptysis, and paroxysmal nocturnal dyspnea. Most affected patients have New York Heart Association (NYHA) class III or IV function. Additional symptoms include nonspecific fatigue, malaise, palpitations, chest and abdominal discomfort, and postural hypotension. Diagnosis requires a high degree of suspicion, because symptoms of peripartum cardiomyopathy can be confused with physiologic changes associated with advanced pregnancy. Common signs of peripartum cardiomyopathy include displacement of the apical impulse, presence of S3, and evidence of mitral or tricuspid regurgitation. Engorgement of the neck veins, pulmonary crepitations, hepatomegaly, and pedal edema may also be present.

Sliwa K, Hilfiker-Kleiner D, Petrie MC, et al. Current state of knowledge on aetiology, diagnosis, management, and therapy of peripartum cardiomyopathy: a position statement from the Heart Failure Association of the European Society of Cardiology Working Group on peripartum cardiomyopathy. Eur J Heart Fail. 2010;12(8):767-78.

Q9. Answer b

Serum digoxin level: Therapeutic levels are 0.6–1.3 to 2.6 ng/mL. Levels associated with toxicity overlap between therapeutic and toxic ranges. False-negative assay results may occur with acute ingestion of non-digoxin cardiac glycosides (e.g. herbal compounds, such as foxglove or oleander). Levels determined less than 6–8 hours after an acute ingestion do not necessarily predict toxicity. The best way to guide therapy is to follow the digoxin level and correlate it with serum potassium concentrations and the patient's clinical and ECG findings. Assuming that the digoxin level was drawn at the correct time, at steady state, and under conditions of stable renal function, there is a linear relationship between digoxin dose and serum concentration.

Goldberger ZD, Goldberger AL. Therapeutic ranges of serum digoxin concentrations in patients with heart failure. Am J Cardiol. 2012;109(12):1818-21.

Q10. Answer c

Heparin induced thrombocytopenia is a complication of heparin therapy. There are two types of HIT. Type 1 HIT presents within the first 2 days after exposure to heparin and the platelet count normalizes despite continued heparin therapy. Type 1 HIT is a nonimmune disorder that results from the direct effect of heparin on platelet activation.

Type 2 HIT is an immune-mediated disorder that typically occurs 4–10 days after exposure to heparin and has life- and limb-threatening thrombotic complications. In general medical practice, the term HIT refers to type 2 HIT.

HIT must be suspected when a patient who is receiving heparin has a decrease in the platelet count, particularly if the fall is over 50% of the baseline count, even if the platelet count nadir remains above 150 × 10^9/L. Clinically, HIT may manifest as skin lesions at heparin injection sites or by acute systemic reactions (e.g. chills, fever, dyspnea, chest pain) after administration of an intravenous bolus of heparin.

Warkentin TE, Greinacher A. Heparin-induced thrombocytopenia: recognition, treatment, and prevention: the Seventh ACCP Conference on Antithrombotic and Thrombolytic Therapy. Chest. 2004;126(3 Suppl):311S-337S.

Q11. Answer e

The treatment of patients with ventricular septal defect (VSD) depends on the type of defect, its size, shunt severity, PAP, vascular resistance and associated acquired complications including double chambered right ventricle, aortic regurgitation, and pulmonary hypertension (PH). Observational data suggest that surgical closure decreases the risk of endocarditis by at least half. Observational series also suggest that surgical closure in patients with significant shunts reduces PAP and improves long-term survival. Therefore, repair of VSD should be considered in all adult patients who are symptomatic or have signs of left ventricular volume overload without irreversible pulmonary vascular disease and for those with complications related to the VSD, such as progressive aortic valve regurgitation. Observation is reserved for (1) asymptomatic patients with no evidence of left ventricular volume overload and (2) medical management is suggested for patients with symptoms and/or left ventricular volume overload who are not candidates for repair such as those with large defects and severe irreversible PH (Eisenmenger complex). Application of IABP results in better clinical improvements.

Ammash NM, Warnes CA. Ventricular septal defects in adults. Ann Intern Med. 2001;135:812.

Q12. Answer a

The patient with severe aortic stenosis is relatively 'afterload fixed and preload dependent'. Thus all afterload reducing agents (ACE inhibitors, CCB) are contraindicated. Only in mild AS, CCB have been used but not suggested. However, in patients with mild-to-moderate AS vasodilators such as hydralazine can increase cardiac output. Nitrates and diuretics can be used to treat angina and congestion, but with great care, as they may provoke a decrease in cardiac output. To treat hypertension low dose ACE inhibitors are considered better than CCB.

Carabello BA, Paulus WJ. Aortic stenosis. Lancet. 2009;373(9667):956.

Q13. Answer c

Pulse pressure is the difference between the systolic and diastolic pressure. It is measured in millimeters of mercury (mm Hg). For example, if resting blood pressure is 120/80 mm Hg, pulse pressure is 40 mm Hg. Pulse pressure is proportional to stroke volume, or the amount of blood ejected from the left ventricle during systole and inversely proportional to the compliance of the aorta. A pulse pressure is considered abnormally low if it is less than 25% of the systolic value. The most common cause of a low (narrow) pulse pressure is a decrease in left ventricular stroke volume. If the pulse pressure is extremely low, i.e. 25 mm Hg or less, the cause may be low stroke volume, as in congestive heart failure and/or cardiogenic shock. A chronically increased stroke volume is also a technical possibility, but very rare in practice.

Franklin SS, Gustin W, Wong ND, et al. Hemodynamic patterns of age-related changes in blood pressure. The Framingham Heart Study. Circulation. 1997;96(1):308.

Q14. Answer c

Esophageal Doppler hemodynamic parameters interpretation:
- Stroke volume (SV) measured by stroke distance × aortic root diameter—indicates blood ejected per beat of heart
- Peak velocity (PV)—indicates contractility
- Corrected (systolic) flow time (FTc)—indicates preload
- This patient is having low SV/SD and FTc was short indicating an increased afterload. The most common cause of this is hypovolemia.

Morris C. Oesophageal Doppler monitoring, doubt and equipoise: evidence based medicine means change. Anaesthesia. 2013;68(7):684-8.

Q15. Answer c

Cardiac troponins are sensitive markers for minor degrees of myocardial damage and elevated values can diagnose MI with high degrees of sensitivity and specificity.

Shyu KG, Kuan PL, Cheng JJ, et al. Cardiac troponin T, creatine kinase, and its isoform release after successful percutaneous transluminal coronary angioplasty with or without stenting. Am Heart J. 1998;135(5 Pt 1):862.

Q16. Answer d

Atrial fibrillation (AF) is the most frequent arrhythmia treated with electrical cardioversion. When monophasic waveforms are used, 100 to 200 joules (watt-seconds) is often adequate to restore sinus rhythm, although >200 joules may be required, particularly for AF of long duration. The overall success rate (at any level of energy) of electrical cardioversion for AF is 75 to 95% and is related inversely both to the duration of AF and to left atrial size.

Gurevitz OT, Ammash NM, Malouf JF, et al. Comparative efficacy of monophasic and biphasic waveforms for transthoracic cardioversion of atrial fibrillation and atrial flutter. Am Heart J. 2005;149(2):316.

Q17. Answer d

Corrected flow time (FTc) indicates preload (normal = 0.33–0.36 s). Corrected flow time (FTc) by esophageal Doppler is considered to be a 'static' preload index. FTc predicts fluid responsiveness. However, FTc should be used in conjunction with other clinical information.

Lee JH, Kim JT, Yoon SZ et al. Evaluation of corrected flow time in esophageal doppler as a predictor of fluid responsiveness. British Journal of Anaesthesia. 2007;99(3):343-8.

Q18. Answer d

There is definite cardiac involvement in leptospirosis, which even though not symptomatically evident, may add to the morbidity or be contributory to the mortality associated with the disease. There is a possibility of dilated cardiomyopathy as a delayed consequence of severe myocarditis. Medical therapy is recommended such as beta-blocker or ACE inhibitor administration. ICD may be needed for arrhythmias.

Shah K, Amonkar GP, Kamat RN, et al. Cardiac findings in leptospirosis. J Clin Pathol. 2010;63(2):119-23.

Q19. Answer a

Short-term circulatory assist devices improve cardiovascular hemodynamics. The LVAD can be used two ways: (1) Bridge-to-transplant, which means it can help a patient survive until a donor heart becomes available. This option may be appropriate for people whose medical therapy has failed and who are hospitalized with end-stage systolic heart failure. (2) Destination therapy, which is an alternative to heart transplant. Destination therapy provides long-term support in patients who are not candidates for transplant. Both continuous and non-pulsatile devices are available, each with different effects on a patient's physiology. In general, these effects are not clinically significant with the exception of bleeding events which are more common with continuous-flow devices in some series. Both devices increase survival beyond medical management. Continuous-flow devices are smaller and are associated with less overall morbidity than pulsatile devices. Reduced pulsatility in patients supported with the continuous-flow LVAD HeartMate II is associated with an increased risk of nonsurgical bleeding.

Simon D, Fischer S, Grossman A, et al. Left ventricular assist device-related infection: treatment and outcome. Clin Infect Dis. 2005;40(8):1108.

Q20. Answer b

Every material has a frequency at which it oscillates freely. This is called its natural frequency. If a force with a similar frequency to the natural frequency is applied to a system, it will begin to oscillate at its maximum amplitude. This phenomenon is known as resonance. Resonance may occur when the frequency of the pressure waves in the incoming impulse matches the natural frequency of the transducer thereby causing superimposition of pressure waves. The natural frequency of the system may be increased by using a stiff diaphragm and short wide-bore tubing. If the natural frequency of measuring system lies close to the frequency of any of the sine wave components of the arterial waveform, then the system will resonate, causing excessive amplification, and distortion of the signal. In that case, an erroneously wide pulse pressure and elevated systolic blood pressure would result. Tubing system should have very high natural frequency—at least eight times the fundamental frequency of the arterial waveform (the pulse rate). Therefore, for a system to remain accurate at heart rates of up to 180 bpm, its natural frequency must be at least: (180 bpm × 8)/ 60 secs = 24 Hz. Damping reduces the high-frequency noise to allow a more accurate reproduction of the wave form. Too little damping allows oscillations which distort the results while too much damping delays the signal.

Wilkinson MB, Outram M. Principles of pressure transducers, resonance, damping and frequency response. Anaesthesia & Intensive Care Medicine. 2009;10(2):102-5.

K Type Answers

Q1. Answer FTTFT

Hemodynamic effects of the intra-aortic balloon pump include: (1) Reduction in systolic blood pressure. (2) Fall in end-diastolic aortic pressure. (3) Shortening of the isometric phase of left ventricular contraction (4) Reduction in left ventricular wall stress. (5) Increase in left ventricular ejection fraction. (6) Reduction of preload/afterload.(7) Increase in DPTI/TTI ratio. (8) Improvement of coronary flow. (9) During hemorrhagic shock, an improvement in vasoregulatory control of splanchnic blood flow

Prondzinsky R, Unverzagt S, Russ M, et al. Hemodynamic effects of intra-aortic balloon counter pulsation in patients with acute myocardial infarction complicated by cardiogenic shock: the prospective, randomized IABP shock trial. Shock. 2012;37(4):378-84.

Q2. Answer FTFFF

Streptokinase—20,000 IU by bolus followed by 2,000 IU/min for 60 minutes.

Tenecteplase—70 to less than 80 kg: 40 mg IV bolus administered over 5 seconds.

Reteplase—10 units IV bolus (over 2 minutes), then Second dose given 30 minutes after first (for total cumulative dose of 20 units).

Alteplase—0.9 mg/kg (not to exceed 90 mg total dose), with 10% of the total dose administered as an initial intravenous bolus over 1 minute and the remainder infused over 60 minutes.

Fondaparinux—It is a synthetic and specific inhibitor of activated Factor X (Xa) not a fibrinolytic drug.

Ali MR, Hossain MS, Islam MA, et al. Aspect of Thrombolytic Therapy: A Review. Scientific World Journal. 2014:8.

Q3. Answer TTFFT

The natriuretic peptide system impacts salt and water handling and pressure regulation and may influence myocardial structure and function. Both atrial natriuretic peptide (ANP) and BNP are increased in heart failure (HF), as ventricular cells are recruited to secrete both ANP and BNP in response to the high ventricular filling pressures. The plasma concentrations of both hormones are increased in patients with asymptomatic and symptomatic left ventricular dysfunction, permitting their use in diagnosis. In an analysis of more than 4,000 patients from the Val-HeFT trial, those with a baseline plasma BNP concentration in the highest quartile (≥238 pg/mL) had a significantly greater mortality at two years than those with a plasma BNP in the lowest quartile (<41 pg/mL) (32.4 versus 9.7%). Normal plasma BNP values increase with age and are higher in women than men. It cannot be collectively used to differentiate systolic heart failure from heart failure with preserved ejection. A normal value of BNP is used to exclude heart failure.

> Kinnunen P, Vuolteenaho O, Ruskoaho H. Mechanisms of atrial and brain natriuretic peptide release from rat ventricular myocardium: effect of stretching. Endocrinology. 1993;132(5):1961.

Q4. Answer TFTTF

Clinical assessment of hemodynamic profiles (ADHF): The assessment of patients with HF is based on whether clinical symptoms indicate that filling pressure is or is not elevated (wet or dry) and perfusion is or is not adequate (warm or cold), with combinations of these parameters yielding four possible hemodynamic profiles.
- Dry-warm—PCWP normal, CI normal
- Wet-warm—PCWP elevated CI normal
- Dry-cold—PCWP low/normal, CI decreased
- Wet-cold—PCWP elevated, CI decreased

> Fonarow GC, Weber JE. Rapid clinical assessment of hemodynamic profiles and targeted treatment of patients with acutely decompensated heart failure. Clin Cardiol. 2004;27(Suppl V):V1-V9.

Q5. Answer FTTTF

Vernakalant is indicated for the rapid conversion of recent onset of AF to sinus rhythm in adults for non-surgery patients that lasts for less than 7 days of duration and post-cardiac surgery patients with AF lasting less than 3 days of duration. Intravenous amiodarone may be an effective short-term agent for ventricular rate control in acutely ill or postoperative patients. Intravenous amiodarone is generally well tolerated in critically ill patients who develop rapid atrial tachyarrhythmias refractory to conventional treatment and may be less likely to cause systemic hypotension than intravenous calcium channel blockers or beta-blockers. Sepsis patients have higher incidence of AF which exhibited higher rates of mortality and stroke, and heart failure risk. Synchronized cardioversion is the treatment of choice for hemodynamically unstable patients which also acts faster than chemical cardioversion.

> Katritsis DG, Gersh BJ, Camm AJ. Anticoagulation in atrial fibrillation—current concepts. Arrhythm Electrophysiol Rev. 2015;4(2):100-7.

Q6. Answer FTTFF

Patients presenting to emergency departments with a complaint of chest pain and who ultimately have a myocardial infarction (MI) may have a normal initial ECG in the following circumstances: (1) If the MI is very small, the magnitude of ECG changes may be undetected. It has been suggested that, in some infarcts, at least 3% of the left ventricle must be involved for ECG changes to develop. (2) The traditional 12-lead ECG generously interrogates the anterior wall, apex, and inferior wall. Infarctions in the lateral and posterior segments of the left ventricle, however, are not directly interrogated by conventional ECGs. It has been estimated that up to 50% of infarctions in the left circumflex distribution may be electrocardiographically normal. (3) Patients may present so early in the course of their MI that ECG disturbances are not yet apparent. Such patients are destined, often within a short time, to develop recognizable ECG abnormalities. Reperfusion strategy, for ST elevation or LBBB on ECG presenting within 12 hours pain onset (Benchmark)- call-to-needle time of under 60 minutes, with door-to-needle time within 30 minutes of patient arrival (thrombolysis), or door- to-skin time within 90 min [percutaneous coronary intervention (PCI)]. Left ventricular dysfunction (LVD) is the most frequent cause of cardiogenic shock occurring in 74.5% of patients. This was followed by acute mitral regurgitation (8.3%), ventricular septal rupture (4.6%), isolated right ventricular shock (3.4%), tamponade or cardiac rupture (1.7%), and other causes (8%). Infarctions were located anteriorly in most of the patients (55%) in the SHOCK trial registry.

> Cweres L, Cooke D, Zalenski R, et al. Myocardial infarction with an initially normal electrocardiogram—angiographic findings. Clin Cardiol. 1995;18:563-8.
>
> Hochman JS, Boland J, Sleeper LA, et al. Current spectrum of cardiogenic shock and effect of early revascularisation on mortality. Results of an international registry. SHOCK registry investigators. Circulation. 1995;91:873-81.

Q7. Answer FTTFT

Patients with PH due to diffuse lung disease (e.g. COPD, ILD, or overlap syndromes) or conditions that cause hypoxemia (e.g. obstructive sleep apnea, alveolar hypoventilation disorders) are classified as having group 3 PH.

Clinical classification of pulmonary hypertension (NICE, 2013):
- Group 1: Pulmonary arterial hypertension (PAH)-idiopathic
- Group 2: Pulmonary hypertension owing to left heart disease
- Group 3: Pulmonary hypertension owing to lung diseases and/or hypoxia
- Group 4: Chronic thromboembolic pulmonary hypertension (CTEPH)
- Group 5: Pulmonary hypertension with unclear multifactorial mechanisms.

In group 3 PH have mild-to-moderate elevations in mPAP (25 to 35 mm Hg) compared to group 1 where mean mPAP is 50 mm Hg. If echocardiogram is suggestive of mild pulmonary hypertension (e.g. PASP 20 to 39 mm Hg) in the absence of any other etiology for PH, then most clinicians do not proceed with right heart catheterization (RHC), but rather observe patients for progressive symptoms over time. RHC is the gold standard for evaluation. The dual endothelin receptor antagonist, bosentan, is an orally active therapy, which is effective in the treatment of PH in idiopathic and familial PH, in PH associated with connective tissue disease and in PH which may develop in association with other conditions. COPD with hypoxemia may better be treated by supplementary oxygen therapy first.

> Klings ES. Pulmonary hypertension due to lung disease and/or hypoxemia (group 3 pulmonary hypertension): Epidemiology, pathogenesis, and diagnostic evaluation in adults. Available from: https://www.uptodate.com/contents/pulmonary-hypertension-due-to-lung-disease-and-or-hypoxemia-group-3-pulmonary-hypertension-epidemiology-pathogenesis-and-diagnostic-evaluation-in-adults (Accessed 28 December 2017).

Q8. Answer TTFTF

Stress cardiomyopathy (also called apical ballooning syndrome, Takotsubo cardiomyopathy, broken heart syndrome, and stress-induced cardiomyopathy) is a syndrome characterized by transient regional systolic dysfunction of the left ventricle (LV), mimicking myocardial infarction, but in the absence of angiographic evidence of obstructive coronary artery disease or acute plaque rupture. In most cases of stress cardiomyopathy, the regional wall motion abnormality extends beyond the territory perfused by a single epicardial coronary artery. The term 'takotsubo' is taken from the Japanese name for an octopus trap, which has a shape that is similar to the systolic apical ballooning appearance of the LV in the most common and typical form of this disorder; mid and apical segments of the LV are depressed, and there is hyperkinesis of the basal walls. A midventricular type and other variants have also been described.

> Kurowski V, Kaiser A, von Hof K, et al. Apical and midventricular transient left ventricular dysfunction syndrome (takotsubo cardiomyopathy): frequency, mechanisms, and prognosis. Chest. 2007;132(3):809.

Q9. Answer FFTFT

The pleural NT-proBNP levels are elevated in all patients who have transudate. Therefore if the NT-proBNP levels of pleural effusion are within the normal range, transudate resulting from congestive heart failure can be ruled out. Inclusion of pleural fluid NT-proBNP measurement in the routine diagnostic panel would enhance discrimination among the different causes of pleural effusions.

> Tomcsanyi J, Nagya E, Somloia M, et al. NT-brain natriuretic peptide levels in pleural fluid distinguish between pleural transudates and exudates. Eur J Heart Fail. 2004;6:753-6.

Q10. Answer TTFFT

Gastrointestinal bleeding is a relatively common complication in patients receiving antiplatelet therapy and is associated with an increased risk of recurrent ischemic events and mortality. Prophylaxis with antisecretory drugs such as PPIs reduces the risk of GIB. Early endoscopy is useful for both the diagnosis and the therapeutic management of GIB. Antiplatelet therapy should be resumed immediately after endoscopic hemostasis of GIB, unless the bleeding is life threatening. Aspirin inhibits platelet activation by inactivating platelet cyclooxygenase. Aspirin has a rapid onset of action after oral administration (<1 hour but 3–4 hours with enteric-coated preparations) and has a plasma half-life of 20 minutes. However, laboratory evidence of platelet inhibition may persist for 4 days because the effect of aspirin on individual platelets is irreversible.

Yasuda H, Matsuo Y, Sato Y, et al. Treatment and prevention of gastrointestinal bleeding in patients receiving antiplatelet therapy. World J Crit Care Med. 2015;4(1):40-6.

Q11. Answer TFTTF

Prevention of CIN: (1) Identifying patients at risk: All patients with eGFR <60 mL/min/1.73 m^2 and comorbidities including diabetes, heart failure, liver failure, or multiple myeloma. (2) Preventive measures: Avoid volume depletion and NSAIDs, low dose iso-osmolal agent. Fluid administration 3 mL/kg crystalloid over one hour preprocedure and 1 to 1.5 mL/kg/hour during and for four to six hours postprocedure, with administration of at least 6 mL/kg postprocedure. (3) Sodium bicarbonate, acetylcysteine, statins, diuretics and ascorbic acid are not recommended.

KDIGO Clinical Practice Guideline for Acute Kidney Injury. Kidney Int Suppl. 2012;2(Suppl 1):8.

Q12. Answer TTFTF

Transvenous cardiac pacing: (1) Indications: Bradycardias, symptomatic sinus node dysfunction, second- and third-degree heart block, atrial fibrillation with a slow ventricular response, new left bundle branch block, bifascicular block, alternating bundle branch block, malfunction of an implanted pacemaker, tachycardias, supraventricular dysrhythmias, ventricular dysrhythmias. (2) Contraindications: Prosthetic tricuspid valve, severe hypothermia. (3) Complications: Inadvertent arterial puncture, venous thrombosis/thrombophlebitis, pneumothorax/other anatomic injury, ventricular arrhythmia, misplacement of the pacing catheter, myocardial/pericardial, perforation, entanglement of the pacing catheter. Coagulopathy is relative contraindication.

Aguilera PA, Durham BA, Riley DA. Emergency transvenous cardiac pacing placement using ultrasound guidance. Ann Emerg Med. 2000;36:224-7.

Q13. Answer TFFT

Arterial waveforms may provide a deeper insight into overall hemodynamic status. Vasodilatation usually causes lower systolic/diastolic pressures associated with a wide pulse pressure (PP) and delayed dicrotic notch. Vasoconstriction is usually associated with a narrow PP. Regular calibration is essential when pulse contour analysis is used to measure cardiac output.

Midway through the downstroke, a notch, called the *dicrotic notch*, may be visible, indicating closure of the aortic valve. The dicrotic notch also represents the beginning of diastole. The remainder of the waveform's downstroke represents blood flow into the arterial tree, with the lowest point representing diastole. Arterial catheterization can also help to guide volume replacement and monitor patients with hypovolemic or septic shock during the administration of pressor or inotropic agents.

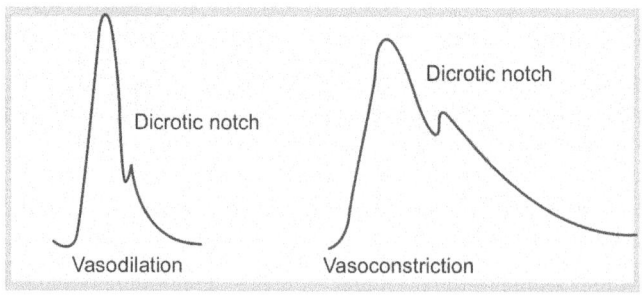

Stroke volume can be obtained by area under the systolic portion of the waveform:

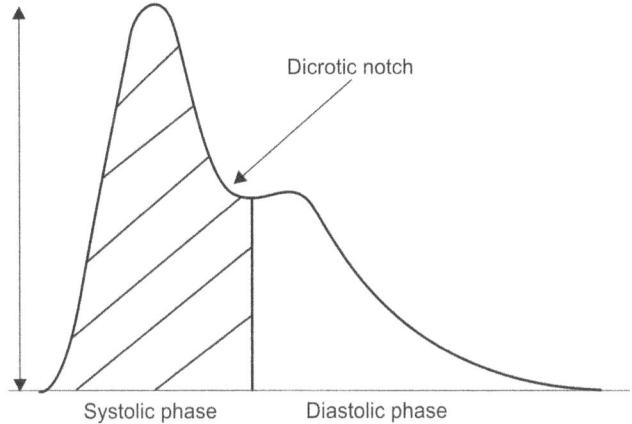

Nirmalan M, Dark PM. Broader applications of arterial pressure wave form analysis. Anesthesia Critical Care & Pain. 2014;14(6):285-90.

Q14. Answer TFTTF

Atrial fibrillation (AF) and atrial flutter (AFl) occur frequently after cardiac surgery. Its reported incidence ranges from 0.4% to 26% in patients undergoing non-cardiac non-thoracic surgery. AF occurs in 15–40% of patients in the early postoperative period following coronary artery bypass graft surgery (CABG in 37–50% after valve surgery, and in as many as 60% undergoing valve replacement plus CABG. The incidence is less in beating heart surgery than CABG on cardiopulmonary bypass (CPB). The incidence increases with increasing age. Atrial arrhythmias occur most often within the first few days after surgery. In a prospective, multicenter study of 4,657 patients undergoing surgery, the majority of first episodes of AF occurred by day two, while the majority of recurrent episodes occurred by day three. Forty-three percent of patients with AF had more than one episode.

Maisel WH, Rawn JD, Stevenson WG. Atrial fibrillation after cardiac surgery. Ann Intern Med. 2001;135(12):1061.

Q15. Answer TTTF

Transpulmonary thermodilution method (TPTD) is a safe, multiparametric advanced cardiopulmonary monitoring technique that provides important parameters required for making decisions in critically ill patients. The TPTD provides more reliable indicators of preload than filling pressures, the unique measurement of extravascular lung water (EVLW) and comparable accuracy in measuring cardiac output (CO). TPTD-guided algorithms have been shown to improve the management of high-risk surgical and critically ill patients.

Intermittent measurement of the CO by TPTD when coupled with pulse contour analysis, offer automatic calibration of continuous CO, as well as accurate assessment of volumetric preload, fluid responsiveness and EVLW.

Sakka SG, Reuter DA, Perel A. The transpulmonary thermodilution technique. J Clin Monit Comput. 2012;26(5):347-53.

Q16. Answer TFTTF
- Direct Thrombin Inhibitor—Ximelagatran
- Factor Xa Inhibitor—Fondaparinux
- P2Y12 Inhibitor—Prasugrel
- Glycoprotein IIb/III inhibitors—Tirofiban
- Recombinant tPA—Tenecteplase

Q17. Answer TTTTF
Definitions of HFrEF and HFpEF

Classification	EF (%)	Description
Heart failure with reduced ejection fraction (HFrEF)	≤40	Also referred to as systolic HF. Randomized controlled trials have mainly enrolled patients with HFrEF, and it is only in these patients that efficacious therapies have been demonstrated to date.
Heart failure with preserved ejection fraction (HFpEF)	≥50	Also referred to as diastolic HF. Several different criteria have been used to further define HFpEF. The diagnosis of HFpEF is challenging because it is largely one of excluding other potential noncardiac causes of symptoms suggestive of HF. To date, efficacious therapies have not been identified.
a. HFpEF, borderline	41 to 49	These patients fall into a borderline or intermediate group. Their characteristics, treatment patterns, and outcomes appear similar to those of patients with HFpEF.
b. HFpEF, improved	>40	It has been recognized that a subset of patients with HFpEF previously had HFrEF. These patients with improvement or recovery in EF may be clinically distinct from those with persistently preserved or reduced EF. Further research is needed to better characterize these patients.

2013 ACCF/AHA Guideline for the Management of Heart Failure: Executive Summary. Journal of the American College of Cardiology. 2013;62(16):0735-1097.

Q18. Answer FTTTF

Milrinone is a phosphodiesterase 3 inhibitor which increases the heart's contractility and decrease pulmonary vascular resistance. Milrinone also causes vasodilatation which helps alleviate increased pressures (afterload) of the heart, thus improving its pumping action. Amrinone and milrinone can cause thrombocytopenia. Loading dose 50 mcg/kg administered over 10 minutes followed by a maintenance dose titrated according to hemodynamic and clinical response; Maintenance dose: IV infusion: 0.375 to 0.75 mcg/kg/minute; lower initial doses of 0.1 mcg/kg/minute (with final maintenance doses of 0.2 to 0.3 mcg/kg/minute) have also been recommended. It can lead to hypotension which can be alleviated by coadmistering norepinephrine.

Abraham WT, Adams KF, Fonarow GC, et al. ADHERE Scientific Advisory Committee and Investigators, ADHERE Study Group. In-hospital mortality in patients with acute decompensated heart failure requiring intravenous vasoactive medications: an analysis from the Acute Decompensated Heart Failure National Registry (ADHERE). J Am Coll Cardiol. 2005;46(1):57.

Q19. Answer TTTFT

The pulmonary wedge pressure or PWP, or cross-sectional pressure (also called the pulmonary arterial wedge pressure or PAWP, pulmonary capillary wedge pressure or PCWP, or pulmonary artery occlusion pressure or PAOP), is the pressure measured by wedging a pulmonary catheter with an inflated balloon into a small pulmonary arterial branch. It estimates the left atrial pressure. PAOP is a static parameter generally considered not good predictor of volume responsiveness. PAWP and PAOP is one and the same thing. In normal hearts pulmonary artery wedge pressure (PAWP) is less than left ventricular end diastolic pressure (LVEDP) by 2–3 mm Hg. In mitral stenosis PAWP is more than LVEDP.

Chaliki HP, Hurrell DG, Nishimura RA, et al. Pulmonary venous pressure: relationship to pulmonary artery, pulmonary wedge, and left atrial pressure in normal, lightly sedated dogs. Catheter Cardiovasc Interv. 2002;56(3):432-8.

Q20. Answer FTTF

Thrombolysis in PE: (1) used in massive or high risk PEs, (2) can be used up to 14 days after symptoms begin, (3) PE resolve more quickly than with heparin alone, (4) as successful as embolectomy in massive PE (earlier the better), (5) indicated in patients with RV compromise + hemodynamically unstable, (6) rTPA 1.5 mg/kg is maximum dose (as good through peripheral IV or CVL), (7) alteplase 100 mg (0.6 mg/kg) as a continuous infusion over 2 hours.

Contraindications: Absolute (1) bleeding, (2) recent stroke, (3) HI, (4) current GI bleeding. Relative (1) PUD, (2) surgery within 7 day, (3) prolonged CPR.

Major hemorrhage following thrombolytic therapy for acute PE is a common complication that warrants specific evaluation of patient risk factors prior to determining appropriate candidacy for thrombolytic therapy.

The increased fibrin specificity and single bolus administration of TNK-tPA do not increase the risk of intracranial hemorrhage but are associated with less non-cerebral bleeding, especially amongst high-risk patients. A total of 4.66% of patients in the TNK-tPA group experienced major non-cerebral bleeding, in comparison with 5.94% in the rt-PA group.

Wang TF, Squizzato A, Dentali F, et al. The role of thrombolytic therapy in pulmonary embolism. Blood. 2015;125(14):2191-9.

CHAPTER 2

Respiratory

Chitra Mehta, Poulomi Chatterjee

A Type Questions
(One best answer)

1. Which of the following statements is correct?
   a. The alveolar PO_2 and PCO_2 are determined by the relationship between alveolar ventilation and perfusion
   b. A V/Q mismatch always results in low PaO_2 coupled with elevated $PaCO_2$
   c. Alveoli with high V/Q ratios can compensate for alveoli with low V/Q ratios
   d. A doubling of alveolar PO_2 has an impact on oxygen content of the blood

2. Which of the following statements is true?
   a. Normal PaO_2 varies with age and supine position
   b. Normal $PaCO_2$ varies with age but not body position
   c. The Normal pH is close to 7.4 and is likely to vary with age
   d. Normal PaO_2 is about 90 mm Hg and normal $PaCO_2$ is 40 mm Hg

3. Which of the following pathophysiological mechanisms does not result in hypercapnia?
   a. Low V/Q mismatch
   b. Hypoventilation
   c. Right to left shunt
   d. Diffusion impairment
   e. High partial pressure of inspired CO_2

4. A 62-year-old gentleman, reformed smoker, known case of Chronic Obstructive Pulmonary Disease (COPD) presented to Emergency Room (ER) with history of increased cough, dyspnea and high fever (39°C). His presenting arterial blood gas (ABG) showed PaO_2:182 mm Hg, $PaCO_2$: 88 mm Hg, pH: 7.27, HCO 32. X-ray chest showed hyperinflated lungs. Which of the following interventions would you not do to bring down the CO_2?
   a. Nebulized bronchodilators and steroids
   b. Apply bi-level positive airway pressure
   c. Give paracetamol to control the temperature
   d. Give high caloric diet to build up his respiratory muscles

5. A 45-year-old gentleman is brought to ER in a stuporous state. ABG on room air shows PaO_2 of 58, $PaCO_2$ of 68 and pH of 7.21. An X-ray chest does not show any abnormality. On auscultation patient has noisy breathing. Following steps are important in the management:
   a. Patient has acute asthma, should be started on bronchodilators and steroids
   b. Patient should be given noninvasive ventilation (NIV)
   c. Patient should undergo Computerized Tomographic Pulmonary Angiography (CTPA) to rule out pulmonary embolism (PE)
   d. A drug overdose should be suspected

6. What is not true about PE in a pregnant patient?
   a. It has been attributed to hypercoagulable state associated with pregnancy
   b. Incidence increases with caesarian section, increased maternal age, multiparity, obesity, suppression of lactation with estrogen

c. D-dimer is very useful in this setting
   d. CT angiography is now recommended as the first screening examination

7. A 51-year-old morbidly obese lady, known asthmatic, was received in ICU after laparoscopic cholecystectomy. She was successfully extubated the next day. But within few hours she looked lethargic, and ABG done at that time showed pH of 7.24, PO$_2$ of 56, PCO$_2$ of 98 mm Hg (patients baseline PaCO$_2$ was 50 mm Hg). Patient was immediately put on NIV with 16/6 settings, and nebulization was ordered. ABG done after an hour showed pH of 7.25, PaO$_2$ of 70, PCO$_2$ of 86 mm Hg. Patient still looked fatigued. What is the next best step?
   a. Intubate the patient
   b. Increase the IPAP to 20 and repeat ABG after an hour
   c. Continue the same setting and observe
   d. Change to full face mask

8. Acute obstruction of the trachea is a life-threatening emergency. The critical narrowing of trachea occurs at:
   a. Less than 30 mm
   b. Less than 40 mm
   c. Less than 10 mm
   d. Cannot be quantified

9. What is not true for extracorporeal membrane oxygenation (ECMO) used for pulmonary reasons?
   a. In pure pulmonary pathology VV ECMO is the procedure of choice
   b. Incidence of neurological complication is about 50% if V-A ECMO is used
   c. Incidence of neurological complication is 10% if ECMO is instituted for pulmonary reasons
   d. V-A ECMO is initiated during cardiopulmonary resuscitation (CPR)

10. Sudden fall in respiratory compliance on ventilator can be due to all *except*:
    a. Pneumothorax
    b. Pleural effusion
    c. Pulmonary embolism
    d. Lung collapse
    e. Bronchospasm

11. A 68-year-old patient with massive hemoptysis presents to ER. He is immediately intubated and shifted to ICU. He has high FiO$_2$ requirement, the next step should be:
    a. Auscultation
    b. X-ray chest
    c. Change the single lumen tube to the double lumen tube.
    d. Bronchoscopy
    e. CT Chest

12. Under which condition is prone ventilation not advisable?
    a. Post cardiac surgery patients
    b. Presence of contraindications
    c. No benefit observed with the therapy
    d. Early ARDS

13. A 56-year-old man, chronic smoker, presents with massive haemoptysis requiring intubation and mechanical ventilation. On CT angiography of chest, he is found to have blush around the left bronchial artery with a left lingular SOL. He is sent for arterial embolization. Next day when you examine the patient, he is found to have paraplegia. What may be the possible cause?
    a. Critical illness neuropathy
    b. Eaton-Lambert syndrome
    c. Anterior spinal cord infarction
    d. Paraneoplastic Guillain-Barré syndrome

14. Which of the following would you associate with acute PE?
    a. Warburg effect
    b. Anton's syndrome
    c. Sign of Leser-Trelat
    d. McConnell's sign

15. A lung transplant recipient may be asymptomatic while having acute rejection. Which of the following makes you suspect the presence of acute rejection?
    a. Basophilic predominant inflammatory response
    b. Monocytic predominant inflammatory response
    c. Lymphocytic predominant inflammatory response
    d. Eosinophilic predominant inflammatory response
    e. Neutrophilic predominant inflammatory response

16. Which of the following sign is more predictive of re-expansion pulmonary edema (REPE) in a patient undergoing thoracentesis?
    a. Cough
    b. Shortness of breath

c. Hemoptysis
d. Chest pain

17. A 55-year-old man presents with acute febrile illness with respiratory failure. His X-ray chest shows bilateral mid zone and lower zone infiltrates. He needed intubation, and was found to have refractory hypoxemia, despite open lung approach, recruitment maneuvers and prone ventilation. He is initiated on VV-ECMO. Few days later he suddenly desaturates (on constant blood flow and sweep gas flow parameters). Clinically his left hemithorax is found to be moving less. Which single test would help us in diagnosing pneumothorax?
    a. X-ray chest
    b. CT chest
    c. Ultrasound of chest
    d. Bronchoscopy

18. Following are true for postoperative complications except:
    a. It is pulmonary abnormality that produces clinically significant and identifiable disease in the postoperative period
    b. It does not adversely affect the clinical outcome
    c. It has a prevalence of 2 to 40%
    d. It is associated with hospital readmissions

19. Perioperative atelectasis can be made out in ICU with the help of following except:
    a. Plain radiograph
    b. HRCT chest
    c. Lung ultrasound
    d. MRI lung
    e. Pulmonary function test (PFT)

20. What is the current status on use of pulmonary clearance medications in the acutely ill patient?
    a. It is now a standard of care and universal recommendation
    b. It is harmful as it may induce bronchospasm in an acutely ill patient
    c. It is meant to be used as a part of long term care of patients with chronic lung disease
    d. It is not recommended for general use in critically ill patients

21. What all interventions are different in managing a patient with refractory asthma in ICU as compared to a patient with acute asthma?
    a. Nebulized bronchodilator therapy
    b. Parenteral steroids
    c. Mepolizumab and Reslizumab
    d. Specialist physiotherapy

22. A 45-year-old lady, known asthmatic, presented to ER with acute asthma. She was recently diagnosed to have rheumatoid arthritis and was prescribed aspirin on SOS basis. She was treated with standard treatment of bronchodilators, steroids, parenteral intravenous fluids and supplemental oxygen. What further instruction would you leave with the ICU resident for the night?
    a. To procure a HRCT chest in case dyspnea persists
    b. To record peak expiratory flow rates two hourly
    c. To add a mucolytic agent
    d. To avoid use of aspirin in this patient

23. A 30-year-old man, intravenous drug abuser presents to the ER with pleuritic chest pain and dyspnea of few days duration. He had complaints of nonproductive cough, weight loss and a growth in his groin for last few weeks. Patient was hypoxic, normotensive. He required 40% FiO$_2$ for oxygenation. CECT chest showed diffuse mediastinal lymphadenopathy with multiple pulmonary nodules, septal thickening and patchy interstitial opacities. Ultrasound of pelvis and scrotum showed a complex mass at the right edge of mons pubis extending up to the inguinal region. His total WBC counts were 6.26 k/μL. Appropriate next step would be to:
    a. Start him on high flow nasal cannula therapy (HFNC)
    b. Start him on Inj Tecpime and Vancomycin
    c. Start him on Antitubercular therapy
    d. Initiate mechanical ventilation and EBUS guided FNA of the lymph node
    e. Perform the biopsy of inguinal mass

24. A 70-year-old man, reformed smoker, hypertensive, with old CVA was shifted to ICU from the ward with acute respiratory distress and hypotension. He was being treated for community acquired pneumonia for last few days. He was not receiving deep venous thrombosis prophylaxis. On arrival, his temperature was 37°C, HR was 50/min, BP 97/56 mm Hg, respiratory rate of 36 breaths/min. He had O$_2$ saturation of 70% through nonrebreather mask. He was immediately

intubated, and started on vasopressors after fluid challenge failed. Bedside ultrasound revealed a severely dilated right ventricle with flattened septum. A portable anteroposterior chest radiograph did not show any opacity. An electrocardiogram showed ST-T changes in the inferior leads and troponin was greater than 10 ng/mL. What will be your appropriate next step?
   a. Perform a CT pulmonary angiography
   b. Immediate thrombolysis for suspected pulmonary embolism (PE) in a hemodynamically unstable patient
   c. Formal echocardiography
   d. Intra-aortic balloon pump (IABP) insertion

25. A 60-year-old man, awaiting liver transplant for hepatitis C-related cirrhosis, presented to ER with 3 weeks history of shortness of breath, nonproductive cough and pleuritic chest pain. There was no history of fever, sore throat, abdominal pain. He was a reformed smoker. He deteriorated within 2 days of admission and required to be put on mechanical ventilation. CT chest and abdomen showed multiple pulmonary nodules with ground glass opacities with interstitial predominance. There were two lesions in the liver showing arterial hyperenhancement, and were thought to be hepatocellular carcinoma. He had normal white cell count, stable thrombocytopenia, and elevated bilirubin of 4.5 mg/dL. What holds most true in this situation?
   a. He should have detailed bubble echocardiography for diagnosis of hepatopulmonary syndrome
   b. He should be started on steroids
   c. An extensive work up is essential in this case
   d. He should be given broad spectrum antibiotics and empiric anti tubercular therapy

26. Following are the extrapulmonary causes of hypercapnic respiratory failure except:
   a. Primary alveolar hypoventilation
   b. Thoracoplasty
   c. Polymyositis
   d. Vocal cord tumor
   e. Sepsis and capillary leak syndrome

27. About 10 to 20% of patients having obstructive sleep apnea (OSA) have a coexistent obesity hypoventilation syndrome (OHS). The prevalence of OHS in ICU is not exactly known. Most patients having OHS have OSA as well. Sleep related hypoventilation is present in about 10% of patients without OSA. Evaluation for OHS should start in obese individuals in all except:
   a. Unexplained awake SpO_2 on air less than 95% or an overnight Nadir saturation of 80%
   b. A raised bicarbonate on venous blood sample
   c. Right heart failure or pulmonary hypertension
   d. Unexplained dyspnea on exertion
   e. Snoring

28. Pulmonary artery hypertension (PAH) is characterized by elevated pulmonary vascular resistance. It progresses rapidly if left untreated leading to right heart failure and death. Drugs targeting the abnormalities in the prostacyclin pathway remain major therapeutic options to treat PAH. Following statements are true except:
   a. Inhaled treprostinil (tricyclic analogue of prostacyclin) is recommended for NHYA class III
   b. Selexipag is FDA approved for NHYA class III PAH
   c. Preferred treatment of choice for NHYA class II or III PAH is ambrisentan plus tadalafil
   d. Oral Calcium channel blocker (CCB) is the first drug of choice
   e. All patients with pulmonary hypertension should receive influenza and pneumococcal vaccines

29. A large spontaneous, non-recurring pneumothorax resolves spontaneously in how much time?
   a. 6 to 12 weeks
   b. 11 to 13 days
   c. 4 to 6 weeks
   d. Partial resolution only

30. A 30-year-old lady, known case of bronchial asthma gets admitted to ICU with severe asthma. Her ABG shows pH 7.36 PO_2 of 80, $PaCO_2$ of 40 mm Hg. She has diaphoresis and her heart rate is 150 per minute. A decision to intubate is taken. Within 20 minutes of intubation she goes into cardiac arrest. What may be the most likely reason for it?
   a. Pneumothorax

b. Acute coronary syndrome
c. Aspiration
d. Circulatory arrest with electromechanical dissociation
e. Esophageal intubation

31. A 32-year-old gentleman, non-smoker, is admitted to ICU with left sided chest pain. X-ray chest shows small left pneumothorax with less than 3 cm from apex to cupola. He is not in respiratory failure. How will you manage the patient?
    a. Observation with oxygen
    b. One time needle aspiration of air
    c. Chest tube insertion
    d. Chest tube drainage with negative pressure suction

32. A 45-year-old obese lady with long standing history of asthma undergoes gastric bypass surgery. She is extubated on OT table and transferred to ICU for observation. After few hours patient looks fatigued. An ABG done at this point shows a pH of 7.18 PaO_2 of 72 and $PaCO_2$ of 92. You order nebulized bronchodilators and connect her to NIV with IPAP of 16 and EPAP of 6 cm of H_2O. You check her preanesthetic check-up (PAC) chart and found her baseline PCO_2 to be around 55 mm of Hg. ABG repeated an hour later shows pH of 7.22 and PCO_2 of 84 and PO_2 of 64. Patient is still drowsy. What should be your next step?
    a. Nebulize her aggressively and use parenteral steroids
    b. Increase noninvasive setting to 20/6 and repeat ABG
    c. Intubate the patient
    d. Continue current settings and repeat ABG after 1 to 2 hours

33. A 65-year-old alcoholic man, who stopped drinking 1 week ago, complains of malaise, anorexia, weakness and epigastric pain since 7 days. Antacids relieved the pain but other symptoms persisted. He was confused when brought to the emergency. Physical examination revealed generalized muscle weakness and hyporeflexia. ABG specimen showed acute hypercapnic respiratory failure, the patient was intubated and mechanically ventilated. Which of the following treatments is likely to be most beneficial in correcting his ventilatory failure?

a. Corticosteroids
b. Folic acid supplementation
c. Activated charcoal
d. Phosphate supplementation
e. Plasmapheresis

34. A 78-year-old male is admitted to the ER complaining about shortness of breath, fever, chills and cough with purulent expectoration since 2 days. He is a non-smoker with no known comorbidities. The patient looks tired but not confused. Vital signs are blood pressure 110/70 mm Hg, pulse rate 115 beats per min, breathing rate 34 breaths per min, and temperature 38.9 ° C. Bronchial breath sounds are heard on auscultation of the right chest. Blood tests reveal a white blood cell count of 9000×10^9 per L with toxic granules, hematocrit 46%, urea 22 mmol/L, creatinine 160 μ mol/L, sodium 140 mmol/ L and oxygen saturation (room air) 93%. A chest radiograph demonstrates moderate cardiomegaly and a right lower lobe infiltrate with air bronchograms. Which one of the following is the appropriate management decision for this patient?
    a. Treat as an outpatient, take blood and sputum cultures, start empirical antibiotic therapy
    b. Treat as an outpatient, start empirical antibiotic therapy
    c. Admit to hospital, take blood and sputum cultures and Gram stains, start antibiotic therapy according to results
    d. Admit to hospital, start empirical antibiotic therapy within 4 hour of admission
    e. Admit in the intensive care unit, start empirical antibiotic

35. A 43-year-old male patient on mechanical ventilation for acute respiratory distress syndrome (ARDS) develops a left-sided pneumothorax. Which of the following measures should be taken at this time?
    a. Insertion of a small-bore chest tube
    b. Pleural puncture and aspiration of the air
    c. Double-lumen intubation and reduction of positive end-expiratory pressure
    d. Increase in inspiratory oxygen fraction by 10%
    e. Surgical closure of the leak by video-assisted thoracoscopic surgery

36. A 60-year-old former smoker with COPD is referred to the ICU because of an acute exacerbation, presenting with increased dyspnea and purulent sputum. Inhalation of salbutamol, intravenous antibiotics and corticosteroids, did not help and his condition worsens gradually over 30 min. He has not eaten or drunk for the last 5 hours. On ABG analysis, pH is 7.25, PaO_2 is 6.6 kPa (49.5 mm Hg) and $PaCO_2$ is 8.0 kPa (60 mm Hg). He is agitated but cooperates with inhalation and opens his eyes on request. His respiratory rate is 26 breaths per min. Which therapeutic option is most appropriate in this situation?
    a. Add inhaled short-acting anticholinergic and low-dose (2.5 mg) morphine IV
    b. Start BIPAP and oxygen
    c. Intubate and start mechanical ventilation
    d. Start CPAP and oxygen
    e. Add salbutamol IV and low-dose (2.5 mg) morphine IV

37. A middle aged otherwise healthy male presents to the ER with new onset of shortness of breath on mild exertion and a 5-day history of right calf swelling. His blood pressure is 80/55 mm Hg; his pulse rate is 140 beats per min but regular. ABG reveal a PaO_2 7.0 kPa (50 mm Hg), $PaCO_2$ of 3.7 kPa (28 mm Hg) and pH of 7.48. NT ProBNP and D-dimer are both elevated three-times above normal. A CT angiogram (angio-CT) confirms massive embolism of the common pulmonary artery. Which of the following is the appropriate initial therapy for this patient?
    a. Surgical embolectomy of the pulmonary artery.
    b. 10-mg bolus of recombinant tissue-type plasminogen activator (rTPA) intravenously, then 90 mg over 2 hours
    c. 15 000 IU low molecular weight heparin subcutaneously once daily
    d. 5000 IU heparin intravenously, followed by 25 000 IU over 24 hours
    e. Pulmonary artery catheter and selective intra-arterial thrombolysis.

38. A 65-year-old male, well controlled diabetic, presents to his primary care physician with cough, sputum production and fever up to 39.5°C in the past 36 hours. He has COPD (Global Initiative for Chronic Obstructive Lung Disease grade 4), and uses daily tiotropium and salbutamol as needed. He is allergic to amoxicillin. On examination, he has a respiratory rate of 30 breaths per min and pulse of 110 beats per min, with a blood pressure of 130/90 mm Hg. He is oriented. On auscultation, he has bilateral rhonchi and crepitation on the right lung base. His laboratory tests show a TLC of 16 000 cells per μL, C-reactive protein 50 mg/L, blood urea concentration 20 mmol/L and SpO_2 84%, at room air. Chest X-ray shows consolidation in the right upper and lower lung zones. Which is the most appropriate antibiotic regimen for this patient?
    a. Intravenous aztreonam and moxifloxacin
    b. Intravenous moxifloxacin and azithromycin
    c. Oral ciprofloxacin
    d. Oral azithromycin
    e. Intravenous ceftriaxone and azithromycin

39. Which one of the following correctly defines oxygen delivery (DO_2)?
    a. $1.36.Hb.SaO_2$
    b. $DO_2=(MAP- PCWP)/CO$
    c. $DO_2=CaO_2.CO$
    d. $DO_2= (MAP-RAP)/CO$
    [MAP: mean arterial pressure; RAP: right atrial pressure; CO: cardiac output; PCWP: pulmonary capillary wedge pressure; CaO_2: arterial oxygen content]

40. A 68-year-old male with COPD was admitted to the hospital 3 days ago with right lower lobe pneumonia accompanied by dyspnea. A sputum Gram stain showed Gram-positive cocci in pairs. He required oxygen (3 L/min) and was treated with intravenous ceftriaxone. He is afebrile (for the past 24 hours), has no cough or sputum, and is not dyspneic. His oxygen saturation on room air is 95%. A repeat chest radiograph shows a slight increase in the size of his right lower lobe infiltrate. What is the best clinical approach in the management of this patient?
    a. Switch to oral therapy with amoxicillin
    b. Order a CT scan of the chest
    c. Continue IV ceftriaxone
    d. Do a bronchoscopy
    e. Change therapy to IV erythromycin and imipenem

41. A 52-year-old woman with COPD and diabetes is admitted to the hospital with an exacerbation. The clinical examination and the chest radiograph show a consolidation of the left lower lobe. She is admitted to the ICU and intubated in view of worsening respiratory acidosis. She is treated with an intravenous antibiotic, steroids and inhaled bronchodilators. The lung consolidation resolves after 14 days but several attempts to resume spontaneous breathing fail because of tachypnea, unbearable dyspnea and elevation of $PaCO_2$. Which is the most appropriate test for identifying the cause of weaning failure?
    a. Electrophysiological studies of peripheral nerves and muscles
    b. Body composition analysis
    c. Hypercapnic response test
    d. Hypoxic response test
    e. Muscle biopsy

42. A 35-year-old obese female, a known asthmatic, is admitted to hospital with severe dyspnea with a cough, wheeze. The patient is treated for an asthmatic exacerbation with corticosteroids and nebulized bronchodilators. She shows progressive increase of dyspnea, cough and expectoration, and bilateral consolidation on X-ray. Gram stain is negative. She got intubated, transferred to the ICU and placed on broad-spectrum antibiotics. Despite assisted ventilation, she continues to deteriorate over the next few hours with severe hypoxemia (PaO_2 46 mm Hg) on FIO_2 60.0). Which one of the following is the next, most appropriate additional treatment?
    a. Vancomycin
    b. ECMO
    c. Prone ventilation
    d. High-dose inhaled corticosteroids

43. A 67-year-old male with LV Dysfunction is admitted with acute pulmonary edema. He has a blood pressure of 140/100 mm Hg, SpO_2 of 87%, PaO_2 56 mm Hg, $PaCO_2$ 25 mm Hg and pH of 7.33 in room air. After starting therapy with nitrates, oxygen and diuretics, the emergency department team request your advice on the use of NIV or CPAP therapy. Which of the following statements is true?
    a. NIV increases the risk of acute myocardial infarction
    b. Intubation rate is reduced by use of NIV
    c. NIV reduces breathlessness
    d. NIV reduces mortality as compared to CPAP

44. A 54-year-old man is admitted to the hospital with complaints of recurrent hematemesis and syncope. He has history of no other serious diseases. Endoscopy reveals a gastric ulcer with no active bleeding. Lab results show severe anemia with a Hb of 4.4 g/L. Coagulation studies are normal. He receives 10 units packed red blood cells and 8 units fresh frozen plasma. The total amount of fluid replaced is 6.5 L in 9 hours. After transfusion of the last unit of packed red blood cells, the patient becomes severely dyspneic, febrile (39°C) and hypoxemic (oxygen saturation on 5 L oxygen by face mask 88%). An echocardiogram shows normal left ventricular function but the pulmonary arterial pressure is elevated (PASP 50 mm Hg), and the right atrium and ventricle are dilated. A CT angiogram of the chest rules out PE but reveals diffuse infiltrates. What is the likely diagnosis?
    a. Diffuse alveolar hemorrhage secondary to coagulopathy after high-volume transfusion
    b. Volume overload
    c. Activation of granulocytes by transfused biologically active substances
    d. Transfusion-associated systemic infection

45. A 28-year-old female has suffered severe peripartum bleed. She received 25 packed red blood cell transfusions and 6 fresh frozen plasma transfusions. After delivery, she required mechanical ventilatory support for severe Type 1 respiratory failure. She is deeply sedated and paralyzed. On the fourth day of mechanical ventilation, her arterial blood gas analysis shows a PaO_2 of 92 mm Hg, $PaCO_2$ of 45 mm Hg and pH of 7.34: on an inspiratory oxygen fraction (FIO_2) 0.9; assist control with tidal volume 430 mL and respiratory rate of 16 breaths per min; inspiratory time (tI)/expiratory time (tE) ratio 1/2; and PEEP 10 cmH_2O. Plateau pressure is 32 cmH_2O. She weighs 62 kg. Her chest X-ray show bilateral diffuse infiltrates. What would be the most appropriate next step for this patient?
    a. Switch to inverse ratio ventilation (t I/t E 2/1)

b. Decrease ventilator frequency to 15 breaths per min
c. Decrease PEEP to 8 cm H_2O
d. Decrease tidal volume to 360 mL

46. A 28-year-old primigravida woman in her 26th week of pregnancy is seen in the emergency with a complaint of sudden onset of shortness of breath, dry cough and sharp pain over the left chest. On examination, there are crepitations at the base of the left lung. Her left calf is tender and warm. Her arterial blood gas results are PaO_2 80 mm Hg, $PaCO_2$ 32 mm Hg and pH 7.45. D-dimers are positive. What is the next test you should ask for in this patient?
    a. Conventional pulmonary angiography
    b. CTPA
    c. Compression ultrasound of the lower limbs
    d. Ventilation–perfusion lung scanning

47. A 38-year-old female presents to the emergency with fever high grade and dry cough since the last 48 hours. On physical examination, she presents end-inspiratory crepts at the left lung base on auscultation, with no other abnormal findings. Chest X-ray reveals a small consolidation in the left lower zone. Her SpO_2 was 95% at room air. Which of the following investigations should be done next for the management of this patient?
    a. No further tests are required
    b. Pneumococcal urine antigen test
    c. Sputum sampling for Gram stain and culture
    d. Blood cultures

48. A 50-year-old female received a platelet transfusion because of severe thrombocytopenia after chemotherapy for breast cancer. 2 hrs later, she complains of an acute onset of shortness of breath. SpO_2 is 74%, and arterial blood gas analysis reveals PaO_2 of 48 mm Hg, $PaCO_2$ of 28 mm Hg and pH 7.48. Her blood pressure is 150/90 mm Hg, heart rate is regular at 124 beats per min and temperature is 38°C. The patient is transferred to the ICU and started on NIV (inspiratory oxygen fraction 0.6, spontaneous/timed mode, EPAP 8 cmH_2O, IPAP 14 cmH_2O, frequency 16 breaths per min). The chest X-ray shows bilateral diffuse pulmonary infiltrates. Arterial blood gases after 1 hour on NIV are PaO_2 64 mm Hg, $PaCO_2$ 30 mm Hg and pH 7.46. What is the next step in the management of this patient?
    a. Increase IPAP to 16 cmH_2O
    b. Request an echocardiography
    c. Proceed with current management
    d. Intubate and place the patient on invasive mechanical ventilation

49. A 69-year-old woman with severe COPD on long-term corticosteroids is admitted to the hospital with type 2 respiratory failure. She was put on mechanical ventilation, on the 6th day of ventilation, the patient had a spike of fever with a temperature of 39°C and increased purulence of sputum. Her leukocyte count is 20000/µL. Chest X-ray shows new bilateral lower-zone patchy consolidation. She is treated with amikacin and imipenem. After 2 days, her fever is down and her sputum become slightly less purulent but her infiltrates persist and she still requires ventilatory support. A sputum culture obtained shows Escherichia coli that is sensitive to both medications. Which is the most appropriate decision in the further management of this patient?
    a. Continue amikacin and imipenem, and add fluconazole
    b. Discontinue amikacin and continue imipenem
    c. Continue amikacin and imipenem
    d. Continue amikacin and imipenem, add a macrolide

50. A 68-year-old female with very severe COPD (FEV 1 30% predicted) is admitted to the hospital with a 5-day history of progressive dyspnea that has made it nearly impossible for his daily activities. He is already on long-term oxygen treatment at 2 L/min since 3 months, his ABG on 2 L/min oxygen were pH 7.37, PaO_2 60 mm Hg and $PaCO_2$ 58 mm Hg. On admission, he has increased cough and increased purulence of sputum. His medications include inhaled salbutamol and ipratropium. On examination, the patient's respiration rate is 34 breaths per min, blood pressure is 148/80 mm Hg and pulse rate is 120 beats per min, auscultation reveals diffusely reduced breath sounds and wheezing on forced expiration. He looks cachectic, sitting in tripod position with pursed-lip breathing. The physical examination is otherwise unremarkable. ABG

on 2 L/min nasal oxygen show a PaO₂ of 6.0 kPa (45 mm Hg), PaCO₂ of 8.8 kPa (66 mm Hg) and pH of 7.31. Which of the following therapies is not likely to benefit this patient?
   a. Noninvasive bi-level ventilation
   b. Systemic corticosteroids
   c. Continue therapy with an inhaled β 2 -agonist and ipratropium
   d. Increasing nasal oxygen to 5 L /min

51. Which of the following is associated with a decreased risk of upper limb catheter associated DVT?
   a. Diameter of the central venous catheter (smaller versus larger)
   b. Infection of the catheter
   c. duration of catheter use (long versus short)
   d. Antecubital versus subclavian or internal jugular venous access for central venous catheter insertion

52. A 38-year-old otherwise healthy man is admitted in the ICU with respiratory failure associated to pneumonia. He is on mechanical ventilation, volume control mode, with a tidal volume of 6 mL/kg of predicted body weight, PEEP of 16 cm H_2O, and FIO_2 100%. His SPO_2 is hovering around 88–90%. He is hemodynamically stable; his peak pressure is around 37 cm H_2O and plateau pressure of around 29 cm H_2O. What next is to be done?
   a. Airway pressure release ventilation
   b. High frequency oscillatory ventilation
   c. Inhaled nitric oxide
   d. Prone positioning

53. A 63-year-old male with no known comorbidity underwent colectomy for colonic cancer. Preoperative assessment of lungs showed normal gas exchange and spirometry. What is the most appropriate perioperative ventilator settings?
   a. Tidal volume of 10 to 12 mL/kg and maintaining end inspiratory plateau pressure of <30 cm of water
   b. Tidal volume of 6 to 8 mL/kg and maintaining end inspiratory plateau pressure of <45 cm H_2O
   c. Tidal volume of 10 to 12 mL/kg and maintaining end inspiratory plateau pressure of <45 cm H_2O
   d. Tidal volume of 6 to 8 mL/kg and maintaining end inspiratory plateau pressure of < 30 cm H_2O

54. A patient was on mechanical ventilation, suddenly the ventilator alarms were activated. The table shows the pre-alarm and post-alarm ventilator mechanics:

Pre-alarm	Post-alarm
Ppeak 24 cm	42 cm
Pplat 18 cm	23 cm

What is the most appropriate next step?
   a. Laryngoscopic evaluation of tube placement
   b. Endotracheal tube suctioning
   c. IV Diuretics
   d. Emergency tube thoracostomy

55. A 24-year-old female diagnosed with H1N1 pneumonia complicated ARDS is not maintaining on 100% oxygen on the ventilator with plateau pressure of 36 cm H_2O. Next plan is to initiate venovenous VV ECMO, which of the following is expected?
   a. Continued requirement of 100% oxygen
   b. No need for oxygen or PEEP from the ventilator
   c. Ability to change tidal volume as per the PCO_2
   d. PCO_2 can be controlled by flow of ECMO alone

56. A new antibiotic is being tested in patients with ventilator associated pneumonia (VAP). In normal subjects, the $t_{1/2}$ is 2.5 hours, volume of distribution is 11 L. Assuming normal renal and hepatic functions. What is the dosage adjustment required in this critically ill patient?
   a. No change in dosage (2 g q8h)
   b. Decrease dosing interval (2 g q12h)
   c. Administer a loading dosage (3 g at first dose)
   d. Decrease the dose (1 g q8h)

57. A 68-year-old male patient with very severe COPD (GOLD Stage 4) on long-term home oxygen therapy and domiciliary BiPAP since 4 years persists with recurrent exacerbations. Presently is hospitalized with respiratory failure. Which of the following statements is/are false?
   a. Whether to admit in the ICU should be based on the patient's quality of life and the will to live.

b. Recurrent exacerbations in patients who have been previously treated in an ICU are commonly due to Gram-negative
c. Should not be put on invasive ventilation because the probability of their extubation is low
d. Patients with very severe COPD with history of ventilation have a lower 5-year survival rate.

58. A 46-year-old male patient with no other known comorbidities, is admitted in ICU with H1N1 pneumonia with ARDS. Presently, he was desaturating on a FiO_2 of 65%. The resident performed a recruitment maneuver, the SPO_2 improved to 95%. Which of the following is/are NOT improved following recruitment?
    a. Peak Inspiratory Flow Rate
    b. Airway plateau pressure
    c. End tidal CO_2
    d. Peak airway pressure

K Type Questions
[Mark True (T)/False (F)]

1. $β_2$ adrenergic agents relieve airway obstruction caused due to smooth muscle contraction in asthmatics. What is true of them?
    a. There are two types of $β_2$ adrenergic agents: short acting and long acting
    b. They should be administered to patients by inhalational, subcutaneous or intravenous routes
    c. The major side effect of $β_2$ adrenergic agents are tremors, hypokalemia, cardiac stimulation and lactic acidosis
    d. A small volume nebulizer is better than metered dose inhaler with spacer for delivery of $β_2$ agonists in patients with acute asthma

2. The 'crazy-paving' pattern on CT chest is:
    a. Diagnostic of Alveolar proteinosis
    b. May indicate infection, neoplastic, inhalational and other disorders of lung.
    c. Refers to ground glass attenuation with superimposed interlobular septal thickening
    d. Is a sufficient finding to treat the patient

3. All are true for re-expansion pulmonary edema (REPE) except:
    a. Mortality may occur in up to 20% of cases
    b. The incidence is about 10%
    c. Risk factors are large pneumothorax or pulmonary collapse of more than 7 days duration
    d. Drainage of pleural effusion more than 3 liters in one sitting

4. A lung transplant (LTx) recipient patient gets admitted with acute breathlessness associated with low grade fever. He had undergone lung transplant 6 months back. He was stabilized on high flow nasal O_2 therapy. He undergoes bronchoscopy and transbronchial biopsy reveals bronchiolitis obliterans syndrome. His steroids doses were jacked up, and the other two immunosuppressants (calcineurin inhibitors, cytostatic agent) were continued. What drug would you add to prevent/ treat chronic rejection (CR)?
    a. Monoclonal agents directed against interleukin-2 receptor of T cells (IL2RA)
    b. Lymphocyte depleting agents
    c. Neomacrolide antibiotics
    d. Montelukast

5. Which statement holds true if there is coexistent bronchiectasis in patients with COPD admitted to ICU with acute respiratory failure?
    a. Associated with more severe exacerbation
    b. Associated with higher mortality
    c. Associated with increased risk of MDR
    d. There is no difference

6. Mechanical ventilation has been recognized to have a potential of worsening lung function and causing ventilator induced lung injury (VILI). VILI is determined by several parameters. What is true of VILI?
    a. Stress, strain, driving pressure are main determinants
    b. Strain is ratio of end inspiratory lung volume and the end expiratory lung volume
    c. Stress is the linear deformation of the lung
    d. Static strain is more important than the dynamic strain
    e. Stress is represented by transpulmonary pressure

7. Following are the causes of respiratory alkalosis with widened A-a oxygen gradient:
    a. Chronic interstitial lung disease (ILD)
    b. Pulmonary embolism
    c. Hepatic failure with normal lungs
    d. Right to left shunt
    e. High altitude

8. Pregnancy results in following changes in the cardiopulmonary physiology:
   a. Decrease in forced expiratory volume in 1 second (FEV_1)
   b. Functional residual capacity increase by 15–25%
   c. Normal PCO_2 during pregnancy is 27 to 34 mm Hg
   d. Minute ventilation increases by 20 to 40%
   e. Normal PaO_2 in pregnant women ranges from 100 to 110 mm Hg

9. Small proportion of pregnant patient develops tocolytic induced pulmonary edema that is characterized by:
   a. Risk factors include multiple gestation, large volume of crystalloid infusion and pre-eclampsia
   b. Risk comes down by maintaining the maternal heart rate under 120 and limiting the intravenous phase β adrenergic therapy to less than 24 to 48 hours
   c. Use of concomitant steroids to enhance fetal lung development is contraindicated
   d. Clinical improvement takes about 72 hours after the drug is discontinued
   e. Tocolytic therapy is not safe in patients with underlying cardiac disease

10. Following are the absolute contraindications to thrombolytic therapy in PE:
    a. Previous hemorrhagic stroke
    b. Active internal bleeding
    c. Pregnancy
    d. Uncontrolled severe hypertension
    e. Intracranial surgery

11. Bronchopleural fistula (BPF) is a commonly encountered problem in ICU. It may be found to present as a complication of a therapeutic or diagnostic procedures like thoracic surgery or due to mechanical ventilation. It may be detected if there is incomplete expansion of lung post chest tube insertion, especially in a chest trauma patient. Following statements hold true for BPF in ICU:
    a. BPF should be aggressively and surgically managed due to associated morbidity
    b. Pleurodesis is helpful in this setting
    c. In ARDS, approximately 25% of minute ventilation leaks through the BPF
    d. Negative pressure application to chest tube in BPF is associated with inappropriate cycling of the ventilator
    e. High frequency ventilation is preferred over conventional ventilation

12. Respiratory muscle weakness is frequently responsible for failure to wean patient from mechanical ventilation. It has a multifactorial etiology like:
    a. Hypothyroidism
    b. Chronic renal failure
    c. Corticosteroids
    d. Hyponatremia
    e. Critical illness neuropathy

13. Liberation from mechanical ventilation is an important process in care of critically ill patients. What is true for carrying out weaning from mechanical ventilation?
    a. Protocol based ventilatory management team lead to better outcome
    b. Spontaneous breathing trial (SBT) is found to be superior to pressure support or SIMV weaning
    c. Early identification and correction of adrenal insufficiency is associated with favorable weaning with shorter weaning times
    d. 120 minutes trial are better than 30 minutes trials
    e. Twice daily spontaneous breathing trials does not offer any advantage over once daily trial

14. Various industrial processes are associated with generation of potentially unhealthy gases which lead to acute inhalational injury if inhaled in large amounts. Approximately 44% of such injuries are related to workplace exposure, and 60% are related to exposure to a chemical in general environment. Smoke inhalation is also responsible for large number of acute inhalational injury cases. Other peculiarities of this injury are:
    a. Asphyxiants result in dilution of oxygen in ambient atmospheric air resulting in fall in FiO_2
    b. Chemical asphyxiants lead to decrease in oxygen carrying capacity
    c. Carbon monoxide is the most frequent simple asphyxiants
    d. In carbon dioxide asphyxiation symptoms appear rapidly once FiO_2 is less than 0.21 due to increase in ambient CO_2
    e. Severity of symptoms in CO poisoning correlates with carboxyhemoglobin levels better than with duration of exposure

15. **Less than 2% of women in the perinatal period require intensive care admission. Respiratory failure is the most frequent indication for ICU care. What holds true in such patients?**
    a. Pneumonia is the third leading cause of obstetric maternal deaths
    b. The first choice of antibiotic for pneumonia is a beta lactam in pregnant patient
    c. PE is the main reason for CPR in peripartum period
    d. D-dimer is most reliable in pregnancy
    e. The oxygenation goals for all causes of respiratory failure in pregnancy should be maternal SpO_2 of 95% or a PaO_2 of equal to or greater than 70 mm of Hg

16. **Hepatopulmonary syndrome (HPS) is characterized by oxygenation defect due to intrapulmonary vascular dilatation on a background of liver disease. Following statements are true regarding HPS:**
    a. Oxygenation failure in hepatopulmonary syndrome occurs secondary to intrapulmonary shunting as well as diffusion impairments
    b. Platypnea and orthodeoxia are characteristics of intrapulmonary shunting in HPS
    c. Pulmonary function test normalizes after liver transplantation
    d. Contrast enhanced transthoracic echocardiogram (CETE) and lung perfusion scan are utilized for diagnosing HPS
    e. Survival rate of HPS without liver transplant has been found to be 23% when compared to 76% post liver transplantation

17. **National Healthcare safety network (NHSN) in 2013 had come up with the definition of ventilator associated events (VAE) supplanting the previous definition of ventilator associated pneumonia (VAP). This 3-tiered definition of pneumonia is characterized by:**
    a. It provides defined objective criteria which can capture all preventable complications in electronic medical record (EMR) of patients
    b. To qualify as a VAC patient must have had 4 to 5 days of mechanical ventilation with either stable or reducing FiO_2 requirements before the days of increased oxygenation
    c. VAC suggests a causal relationship between VAE and infectious disease
    d. Most of the patients meeting the criteria for VAE are afflicted by a noninfectious cause
    e. The current VAE lacks a radiographic component

18. **Several clinical criteria have been proposed to identify patients who can be safely weaned from the ventilator. What are the minimum required criterions that must be met before weaning is initiated:**
    a. Cause of respiratory failure has improved
    b. pH more than 7.25
    c. Hemoglobin more than 8 to 10 milligram per deciliter
    d. Core temperature less than 38°C to 38.5°C degree centigrade
    e. Ability to initiate an inspiratory effort

19. **NIV in acute respiratory failure not only decreases complication rate of mechanical ventilation but also reduces mortality and shortens ICU and hospital length of stay. NIV is contraindicated in many situations like:**
    a. Severe upper GI bleeding
    b. Poor bulbar function
    c. Hypotension
    d. Severe encephalopathy
    e. Severe arrhythmias

20. **ARDS is one of the most commonly encountered clinical diagnoses in ICU. It was first reported in a clinical case series of 12 patients in 1994. Sometimes it becomes difficult to distinguish it from other causes of respiratory failure like cardiogenic edema or massive aspiration. Which of the following points support an underlying ARDS process?**
    a. Pulmonary capillary wedge pressure of more than 18 mm Hg
    b. A low neutrophil count in BAL
    c. Protein (lavage/serum) ratio of >0.7
    d. In early ARDS chest X-ray abnormalities are more pronounced than hypoxemia

21. **It was a common belief that oxygen protected cell from injury but the accumulated evidence has proven that, oxygen in fact may be responsible for much of the cell injury especially pulmonary, in critically ill patients. Pulmonary oxygen toxicity is characterized by:**
    a. Lungs are well endowed with antioxidant activity in the form of Vitamin C and glutathione normally

b. Inhalation of 100% oxygen by healthy volunteers even for brief periods of time (6 to 12 hours) results in tracheobronchitis and absorption atelectasis
c. The toxic level of FiO_2 has been identified as 0.7
d. Antioxidant protection of lung to decrease the risk of oxygen toxicity is not possible

22. **Infrared capnography is used to measure PCO_2 in the exhaled gas. When gas exchange is presumably normal, the PCO_2 at the end of expiration ($ETCO_2$) is equivalent to PCO_2 in end capillary blood. What statements hold true regarding measurement of PCO_2 and $ETCO_2$?**
    a. Under normal circumstances $ETCO_2$ is 2 to 3 mm of Hg lower than $PaCO_2$
    b. As the V/Q mismatch increases $ETCO_2$ increases relative to $PaCO_2$
    c. $PaCO_2$-$P_{ET}CO_2$ difference exceeds 3 millimeters of mercury in presence of open ventilator circuit, obstructive lung disease and PE
    d. $PaCO_2$-$ETCO_2$ is negative in presence of high cardiac output and higher FIO_2

23. **Optical and colorimetric techniques have made noninvasive monitoring of blood gases (PO_2, PCO_2) possible in ICU. These monitoring techniques are an integral part of daily ICU care. Which statements holds true for oximetry in ICU?**
    a. It utilizes the Lambert-Beer law for detection of hemoglobin in its different forms
    b. It helps in detecting four different forms of hemoglobin- oxygenated hemoglobin (HbO_2), deoxygenated hemoglobin (Hb), carboxyhemoglobin (COHb) and methemoglobin (metHb)
    c. It utilizes red and infrared regions of light
    d. Percentage (%) saturation = Hb/ HbO_2 + Hb × 100
    e. One side of the finger probe has photo transmitter and the other side has a photodetector

24. **Which statements hold true regarding Alveolar- arterial oxygen gradient (A-a DO_2):**
    a. A-aDO_2 = [FiO_2(PB-PH_2O)-($PaCO_2$/RQ)]-PaO_2
    b. A-aDO_2 increases with age and FiO_2
    c. RQ is defined as the relative exchange of oxygen and carbon dioxide across the alveolar capillary interface
    d. A-aDO_2 is a measure of intrapulmonary shunting
    e. Increasing FiO_2 changes A-aDO_2 by resulting in regional hypoxic vasoconstriction in the lungs

25. **We often use partial pressure of oxygen in arterial blood (PaO_2) as an indicator of oxygenation. It is in fact the oxygen content which is the main indicator of oxygenation. Normal values of carbon dioxide and oxygen transport parameters as derived with the help of Pulmonary artery catheter are:**
    a. Oxygen uptake = 200 to 270 mL per minute
    b. Respiratory quotient = 0.75 to 0.85
    c. Oxygen extraction ratio = 0.3 to 0.4
    d. Oxygen delivery = 900 – 1100 mL per minute
    e. Carbon dioxide elimination =162 to 220 mL per minute

26. **DHI is a common phenomenon in patients with obstructive airway disease on mechanical ventilation. What holds true for DHI?**
    a. Auto PEEP or intrinsic PEEP is usually measured by expiratory hold maneuver
    b. DHI may be reflected by peak pressures
    c. DHI can be decreased by decreasing minute ventilation and by changing to decelerating pattern of flow
    d. Work of breathing in triggering the ventilator can be countered by adding external PEEP up to 80% of the auto peep
    e. DHI is clinically recognized by noticing visible respiratory efforts but not triggering of ventilator in a patient on ACV/PS/SIMV mode

27. **Pneumothoraces in ICU are encountered routinely. These are usually related to some intervention. These are usually characterized by:**
    a. It effects the prognosis of the patient
    b. Small Pneumothorax can be treated with needle aspiration
    c. Chest tube should be inserted into the fourth or fifth intercostal space in the anterior or midaxillary line
    d. Large bore tube should be used for drainage of Pneumothorax
    e. Removal of chest tube should be done during end inspiration only

28. **A 54-year-old man renal transplant recipient is admitted to ICU with history of fever,**

dry cough and progressively worsening shortness of breath. He has been on triple immunosuppressants ever since he had transplant 3 years back. He did not have any other complaints. He was hemodynamically stable. He required 60% FiO_2 and 60 lpm of flow on high flow nasal cannula (HFNC) for stability. His X-ray chest showed features of bilateral pneumonia. What may be the possible etiological organisms?
   a. Cytomegalovirus and other herpes virus
   b. Aspergillus
   c. Mucor
   d. Pneumocystis carinii
   e. staphylococcus aureus

29. Treatment guidelines for PE recommend:
   a. In patients with acute PE and active cancer, use of direct acting oral anticoagulants (DOAC) is recommended
   b. Unfractionated heparin should be the initial agent of choice for anticoagulation in PE
   c. Systemic thrombolysis should be limited to high-risk, hemodynamically unstable PE or select intermediate PE with a low bleeding risk
   d. Alteplase (t-PA) and tenecteplase are two FDA approved agents recommended for thrombolysis in PE
   e. Surgical thrombectomy should be reserved for patients with cardiogenic shock and end organ damage

30. PE is a challenging diagnosis. Symptoms are usually vague or non-existing, with features of many other common diagnosis. In North Americans it has been found to be the third most common cause of cardiovascular death, after myocardial infarction and stroke. Following are the characteristics of PE:
   a. Patients with low risk PE have a one year survival rate of more than 95%, and patients with high-risk PE and hemodynamic instability has a 90 day mortality of 40% approximately
   b. The two most common predictive values used for PE are the Wells score and the revised Geneva score
   c. D-dimer levels are helpful in diagnosing PE
   d. Performance of CTPA and VQ scanning for diagnosing PE is equivalent
   e. A negative venous ultrasound is not sufficient to rule out PE in majority of patients

31. A humidifier should be able to deliver inspired gas at 32°C to 36 °C with a water content of 30 – 43 gm/m³. There are various options available to achieve this effect: cold water humidifier, hot water humidifier and heat and moisture exchanger (HME). Following holds true for them:
   a. Cold water humidifier are the simplest effective and most economical to use
   b. Hot water humidifier may be a potential source of infection
   c. HMEs are considered as the gold standard for humidification of inspired air
   d. HME increase dead space and increase the risk of nosocomial pneumonia
   e. Hygroscopic HMEs are more effective than hydrophobic HMEs

32. The upper airway normally moistens, warms and then filters the inspired gas. Normal physiology of respiratory tract for this function includes:
   a. Mucociliary system includes cilia in the watery (sol) layer moving the viscous mucus layer (gel)over it towards the glottis
   b. Isothermic saturation boundary (i.e. absolute humidity of 43 gm/m³ 100% relative humidity at 37°C) exist at the level of glottis
   c. Under the resting condition the normal respiratory tract looses approximately 250 mL of water and 350 kcal (1.50 KJ) of energy in a day
   d. High FiO_2 has no effect on mucociliary function
   e. Minimum relative humidity required is 50%

33. PEEP during mechanical ventilation is characterized by:
   a. When PEEP is maintained during expiration in a spontaneously breathing patient the term 'continuous positive airway pressure (CPAP)' is used
   b. Role of PEEP is to increase FRC, maintain recruitment of alveoli and minimize intra-pulmonary shunt
   c. PEEP has a direct effect on reducing extra-vascular lung water
   d. PEEP may reduce oxygen delivery
   e. In COPD patients extrinsic PEEP (PEEPe) should be less than intrinsic PEEP (PEEPi)

34. A 45-year-old gentleman known case of childhood asthma presents to ICU with acute exacerbation. He is conscious though bit

lethargic. His ABG shows pH of 7.15 PCO$_2$ of 120 PaO$_2$ of 62 on 2 liters per minute of oxygen. His X-ray chest shows hyper inflated lungs. What is the recommended management for this patient?
   a. Administer nebulized ipratropium bromide every 8 hourly along with nebulized salbutamol 2-4 hourly
   b. Patient needs to be intubated and put on mechanical ventilation.
   c. Nebulized mucolytic agent like n-acetylcysteine should be started as early as possible
   d. Respiratory stimulants should be added
   e. Noninvasive ventilation with 20/6 of setting should be started

35. Radiation therapy forms one of the pillars for primary adjuvant therapy for various thoracic malignancies. Lungs however have been found to be very sensitive to ionizing radiation. Radiation pneumonitis is a well-known complication of patients receiving thoracic radiation for lung, breast, esophageal, hematological and thymic malignancies. Radiation induced lung injury is characterized by:
   a. Characteristics of radiation pneumonitis are different for pulmonary and nonpulmonary tumors of the thorax
   b. Radiation pneumonitis is most commonly graded as per common toxicity criteria for adverse events
   c. Radiation pneumonitis depends on the volume of normal lung receiving 20 Gy or more of radiation
   d. Radiation pneumonitis has no correlation with the concomitant chemotherapeutic agent being used for malignancy
   e. Long course (8-12 weeks) of high dose steroids is usually needed

36. Portable ultrasound is now regarded as the modern stethoscope, and most important clinical tool of current time interventions. Addition of lung ultrasound to protocols has made the use of ultrasound more holistic. Various protocols have been devised for evaluation of different conditions like:
   a. FALLS protocol for evaluation of cardiac arrest patients
   b. BLUE protocol for evaluation of respiratory failure
   c. SEMAME protocol for cardiac arrest
   d. RUSH protocol for hypotensive patients

37. Postextubation laryngeal edema is characterized by the following:
   a. It can be predicted by cuff leak test or laryngeal ultrasound in high-risk cases
   b. Risk factors are female gender, larger endotracheal tube size and prolonged intubation
   c. Nebulized corticosteroids can prevent postextubation laryngeal edema
   d. Application of noninvasive ventilation is not indicated

38. Hyperbaric oxygen is indicated as primary therapy in the following conditions:
   a. Decompression sickness
   b. Carbon monoxide poisoning
   c. Air or gas embolism
   d. Clostridial myositis and myonecrosis
   e. Healing of deep seated wounds

39. Which conditions would shift the oxygen dissociation curve (ODC) to the left?
   a. Hyperthermia
   b. Acidemia
   c. Decreased 2,3 DPG
   d. Methemoglobinemia

40. Which of the following findings is/are TRUE with acute pulmonary embolism occluding about 40% of the pulmonary vasculature?
   a. A right atrial pressure of 8 mm Hg
   b. A right pulmonary artery diameter of 35 cm on CT
   c. A mean pulmonary arterial pressure of 55 mm Hg
   d. A pulmonary capillary wedge pressure of 12 mm Hg

41. Which of the following in TRUE?
   a. Weaning is the process of liberation from mechanical ventilation
   b. No universal consensus exists for the process of weaning
   c. The on-going need for inotropes precludes weaning
   d. Synchronized intermittent mandatory ventilation (SIMV) alone is considered a poor weaning strategy
   e. Delay in weaning prolongs critical care stay, increases costs and is associated with a higher mortality

42. The following are recognized strategies in the prevention of VAP:
    a. Daily ventilator tubing changes
    b. Chlorhexidine mouth care
    c. Head-up positioning of 30 to 45°
    d. Daily sedation holds
    e. Prone positioning

43. PEEP:
    a. In severe ARDS, a PEEP >15 cm H_2O improves mortality
    b. PEEP increases FRC
    c. Hepatic and renal blood flow is increased with higher levels of PEEP
    d. PEEP application increases intrathoracic pressure, diminishing venous return to the right heart
    e. An observed increase in lung compliance suggests alveolar recruitment

44. A 54-Year-old male, known case of COPD was admitted in the ICU with acute respiratory acidosis and subsequently, intubated and ventilated. However, the repeat ABG post ventilation still showed hypercarbia, hence the resident changed the ventilator settings as follows: 1. Increased the respiratory rate from 12/ min to 20/min and reduced the I: E ratio to 1: 1. But within 30 mins the patient deteriorated further, developed sudden hypotension and an acute rise in both the peak and plateau pressures, more so the latter. What is/are the measures to be taken to correct the condition?
    a. Reduce the respiratory rate to 12/min
    b. Disconnect from the ventilator and wait for sometime
    c. Decrease the I:E ratio to 1:3
    d. Wait and watch

ANSWERS

A Type Answers

Q1. Answer a

PaO_2 and $PaCO_2$ in all alveolar units are determined by the ventilation/perfusion ratio (V/Q). In normal individuals this V/Q ratio is about 0.8. If this ratio is altered then gas exchange of oxygen and carbon dioxide is not optimal. This results in fall in PaO_2 which may or may not be accompanied by elevated $PaCO_2$. Oxygen content is 99% dependent on haemoglobin, and only 1% of oxygen transport is independent of hemoglobin. So once the haemoglobin is fully saturated with oxygen, increasing the PaO_2 will not significantly contribute to oxygen content.

$$O_2 \text{ Content} = Hb \times 1.39 \times SaO_2 + PaO_2 \times .003$$

In other words, the amount of oxygen carried in arterial blood is limited by the hemoglobin concentration and its ability to bind O_2. This is also the reason that high V/Q areas cannot compensate for hypoxia caused by low V/Q areas of the lung. On the other hand, doubling of alveolar ventilation can result in doubling of CO_2 elimination. Here the high V/Q areas can compensate for hypercapnia caused by low V/Q areas.

Murray JF. The Normal Lung: The basis for diagnosis and treatment of Pulmonary Disease. Philadelphia, WB Saunders, 1976.

Q2. Answer a

Normal PaO_2 varies significantly with age and body position. In supine position because of basal atelectasis PaO_2 falls. The normal reference range for PaO_2 is 80 to 100 mm Hg, thus having a significant standard deviation. $PaCO_2$ remains constant at 40 mm Hg throughout life. It is not affected by age and body position. Like the $PaCO_2$, pH does not change with age.

Carveri I, Zoia MC, Fanfulla F et al. Am J Respir Crit Care Med. 1995;152:934.

Q3. Answer d

Hypoventilation, low V/Q ratio, large right to left shunt can cause both hypoxemia and hypercapnia. High partial pressure of inspired carbon dioxide is usually not in the differential diagnosis of hypercapnia. It can however occur iatrogenically, when the patient is on T piece with extended tubings attached to the expiratory port, or on simple nasal mask with oxygen flow less than 6 L/min due to rebreathing. Diffusion impairment leads to hypoxia and not hypercapnia.

Demers RR, Irwin RS. Respir Care. 1979;24:328.

Q4. Answer d

Patient has typically presented with acute exacerbation of COPD (AECOPD). Treatment of choice is stepping up of bronchodilators and adding injectable steroids. There is no pneumonic patch on the X-ray but antibiotics can be decided based on the nature of sputum. Fever increases carbon dioxide production by 13% for each 1°C rise in temperature above normal. So treating fever is an important intervention here. Patient with AECOPD usually develop respiratory muscle fatigue and benefit from BIPAP support. High caloric diet or carbohydrate rich diet can increase CO_2 production. This puts an extra load on the already diseased lung; hence the total caloric load should be reduced. In addition to above, over oxygenation should be avoided as it blunts the hypoxic drive in these patients leading to CO_2 retention. Ketogenic diet has been tried in these patients.

Weinberger SE, Schwartz stein RM, Weiss JW. N Engl J Med.1989;321:1223.

Q5. Answer d

The first step in the management of acute hypercapnia is the calculation of alveolar-arterial oxygen gradient (A-aDO_2). Here the AaDO_2 is about 5 which rules out a V/Q mismatch or shunt as underlying process. In face of a normal A-aDO_2 drug overdose should be very high on our suspicion list. Naloxone can be administered to rule out a narcotic overdose. Sometimes acute status asthmaticus may also present in a fatigued state with high $PaCO_2$. But with no prior history of asthma and normal AaDO_2 it is unlikely. If the patient is stuporous then BIPAP should be avoided, and in fact this patient qualifies for an intubation. PE also results in widened AaDO_2.

Gray BA, Blalock JM. Interpretation of alveolar- arterial oxygen difference in patients with hypercapnia. Am Rev Respir Dis. 1991;143(1):4-8.

Q6. Answer c

Fatal PE accounts for 20% of all pregnancy related deaths in US. This is due to hypercoagulable state associated with pregnancy. In addition to this, various other factors also play an important role. Like caesarean section, has 10 times greater risk of fatal PE when compared to vaginal delivery. Bed rest, obesity, family history of thromboembolism further increase the risk. Surgical procedures during pregnancy and early puerperium, and lactation suppression with estrogen also put patient at an enhanced risk. Historically ventilation-perfusion (V/Q) scanning was recommended as the primary screening examination for PE during pregnancy. However helical CT has been found to be safe in all trimesters. The radiation dose is almost comparable to the dose exposure during V/Q scanning. Moreover, CT angiography also helps us in diagnosing or ruling out any other abnormalities. Fetal exposure to radiation during imaging studies should be minimized by use of brachial access and abdominal shield.

Schuster ME, Fishman JE, Copaland JF et al. Pulmonary embolism in pregnant patients. AJR. 2003;181:1495.

Q7. Answer a

Patient is still looking fatigued and this fatigue may itself start contributing towards hypercapnia now. Patient is not showing intolerance to BIPAP so changing to full face mask would not give any additional benefit.

Ebeof CT, Benotti PN, Byrd RP, et al. The effect of bi-level positive airway pressure on postoperative pulmonary function following gastric surgery for obesity. Respiratory Medicine. 2002;96(9):672-6.

Q8. Answer c

Patient usually remains asymptomatic until the trachea has been stenozed to about 30% of its original diameter. The classical loop during the spirometry is not obtained unless the diameter is narrowed to 8-10mm. Tracheal stenosis may be treated by laser resection, stenting, resection anastomosis or balloon dilatation.

De S, De S. Post intubation tracheal stenosis. Indian J Crit Care Med. 2008;12(4):194-7.

Q9. Answer b

In pure pulmonary disease VV ECMO usually suffices, and if there is associated hemodynamic instability VA ECMO is the procedure of choice. According to extracorporeal life support organization (ELSO) registry, the incidence of neurological injury in patients with respiratory failure alone is about 10%, which rises to about 50% if ECMO is started during CPR.

Brogan TV, Thiagarajan RR, Rycus PT et al. Intensive Care Med. 2009;35:2105.

Muralidharan R, Shinohara RT et al. Arch Neurol. 2011;68:1543.

Q10. Answer b

Sudden decrease in respiratory compliance is due to an acute event. Pleural effusion usually results over a period of time. A hemothorax also may first cause hemodynamic compromise before causing fall in respiratory compliance. Bronchospasm may cause dynamic hyperinflation resulting in reduced chest compliance.

James B, Haenel RRT, Jeffrey L. Johnson .Mechanical ventilation in critical illness. Anesthesia Secrets (Fourth Edition), 2011.

Q11. Answer b

In the face of refractory hypoxemia it is important to identify the bleeding side. Patient can then be placed with presumed bleeding lung in dependent position so as to prevent the spillage to the nonbleeding lung. Auscultation may not always be conclusive as conducted sounds may not allow the correct identification of side. CT chest and bronchoscopy usually take time and would be required at some point later once oxygenation stabilizes.

Q12. Answer b

Prone positioning has been shown to result in reducing duration of mechanical ventilation in the landmark PROSEVA trial. Recommendation is to do prone positioning in early ARDS. Intensivists have tried prone ventilation in cardiac surgery patients safely and successfully.

Guerin C, Reigneir J, Richard JC et al. Prone positioning in severe acute respiratory distress syndrome. N Engl J Med. 2013;368:2159.

Wardenburg CV, Wenzl M, Dell Aquila MA et al. Prone positioning in cardiac surgery: For many but not for everyone. Seminars in Thoracic and cardiovascular surgery. 2016;26(2):281-87.

Q13. Answer c

Proximal embolization of bronchial artery may result in anterior spinal cord infarction. In about 5% of the population, anterior spinal artery originates from a bronchial artery. There have been case reports of Guillain Barré syndrome in association with small cell lung carcinoma. But there was no presenting complaint of lower limb weakness and very unlikely it developed on its own over few hours of admission. Critical illness neuropathy is also not likely to develop so fast. In Eaton Lambert syndrome the onset is again insidious and it would result in generalized weakness.

> Kim MH, Sik M, Hwang et al. Paraneoplastic Guillain Barré syndrome in small cell lung cancer. Case report oncol. 2015;8(2): 295-300.

Q14. Answer d

McConnell's sign is an echocardiographic feature characterized by regional pattern of acute ventricular dysfunction, with mid free wall akinesia and sparing of the apex of right ventricle. It has been described as an early, and specific sign of acute PE but its specificity has been questioned. Sign of Leser-Trelat is a manifestation of paraneoplastic syndrome characterized by appearance of seborrheic keratosis with skin tags and acanthosis nigricans. Warburg effect forms the working principle of positron emission tomography (PET) scan. It refers to intracellular trapping of the 18 fluoro-2-deoxy glucose (FDG) within tumor cells because of high rate of glycolysis in them. Anton's syndrome is called visual anosognosia. It is a type of stroke which is commonly confused as delirium. Visual imagery is received but cannot be interpreted.

> Riddoch G. Dissocciation of visual perception due to occipital injuries with special reference to appreciation of movement. Brain. 1917;40:15-57.

Q15. Answer c

The diagnosis of acute cellular rejection is made by the identification of lymphocytic perivascular or peribronchial infiltrates in lung tissue. Many episodes of acute rejection are incidentally diagnosed on surveillance biopsies in asymptomatic patients.

> Martinni T, Chan DF, Palmer SM. Acute rejection and humoral sensitization in lung transplant recipients. Proc Am Thorac Soc. 2009;6:54-65.

Q16. Answer d

Chest pain has been found to be most frequently indicative of REPE. Cough is frequently present when patient undergoes thoracentesis, and not necessarily indicative of REPE. Hemoptysis is usually not present. Dyspnea is usually associated with REPE but not necessarily indicative of the same. It is advisable to limit the pleural fluid volume drainage to less than 1.5 liters in one sitting.

> Doelken P, Huggins JT, Pastis NJ, et al. Pleural manometry – techniques and clinical implication. Chest. 2004;126:1764.

Q17. Answer c

Many clinicians worldwide advocate that chest X-ray should not be relied upon to diagnose pneumothorax in critically ill patients. This is secondary to difficulty in interpreting films in supine position, in heterogeneous ARDS with potential loculated pneumothorax, or in patients with pleural adhesions. Although CT chest is considered as the gold standard for diagnosing pneumothorax, it is not always feasible in critically ill patients. Our patient was on ECMO so CT chest was not feasible. Lung ultrasonography (USG) in experienced hands can diagnose pneumothorax bed side. The "lung point" (absence of lung sliding next to lung sliding) has been found to have a specificity of 100% though the sensitivity is lower. Similarly, presence of B- lines has 100% negative predictive value for pneumothorax, at the point examined. Multiple areas have to be screened to rule out pneumothorax with confidence. Bronchoscopy has got no role in diagnosing pneumothorax.

> Sanchis J, Gich I, Pedersen S; Aerosol Drug Management Improvement Team (ADMIT). Systematic review of errors in inhaler use: Has patient technique improved over time? Chest 2016;150(6):e155-e157.

Q18. Answer b

Postoperative complications contribute significantly to prolonged hospitalizations, readmissions, admission to ICU, excessive healthcare expenditure and mortality. Reporting its prevalence is quite complicated due to lack of uniform definition. That is probably the reason why we see a large variation in prevalence rates

(2–40%) reported. Hospital length of stay increases as many as by 8 days, with about 2 to 12 fold increase in the hospital costs. About 26% of those who develop postoperative respiratory failure die within 30 days. It is also frequently the cause for hospital readmissions.

> Restrepo RD, Braverman J. Current challenges in the recognition, prevention and treatment of postoperative pulmonary atelectasis. Expert Review of Respiratory medicine. 2015;l 9:1.

Q19. Answer e

Usually the clinical impression and plain radiograph are sufficient to make the diagnosis of atelectasis. But sometimes in ICU with patient developing low grade fever, use of HRCT chest, MRI, lung ultrasound are useful in confirming the noninfective cause of fever in form of atelectasis. PFT tests are of benefit but not so in ICU patients who are in respiratory failure.

> Shander A, Fleisher LA, Baris PS et al. Clinical and economic burden of postoperative pulmonary complication: patient safety summit on definition, risk – reducing intervention and prevention strategies. Crit Care Med. 2011;39(9):2163-72.

Q20. Answer d

It is only in cystic fibrosis (CF) patients that the uses of some of mucoactive agents have shown some beneficial effect. In the non CF population, there is insufficient evidence presently for its routine use. While some patients may be benefitted, it cannot be recommended for general use in acutely ill patients at this time.

> Papacostas MF, Luckell P, Hupp S. The use of pulmonary clearance medications in the acutely ill patient. Expert review of respiratory medicine. 2017;11(10).

Q21. Answer d

Mepolizumab and Reslizumab are biologic agents targeting a Type 2 inflammatory pattern. These agents have broadened the scope of treatment options in severe asthma. But in some cases of refractory asthma this may not be so. In recent years we have realised that in this patient subset, there are two important key mechanisms causing respiratory system dysfunction—abnormal or maladaptive breathing pattern, i.e. dysfunctional breathing/ DB, and inappropriate, episodic closure of the larynx or inducible laryngeal obstruction (ILO). These findings are now being viewed as comorbid or contributing factors in disease status (i.e. asthma plus). Therefore, their early recognition and prompt targeted therapy in the form of specialist physiotherapy along with de-escalation or avoidance of deleterious therapies like steroids are essential. These asthma plus mechanisms may contribute to acute deterioration, usually refractory, in long standing asthmatic patient.

> Hull JH, Walsted ES, Backer V. The asthma- plus syndrome. Expert review of respiratory medicine. 2017;11(7):513-5.

Q22. Answer d

Patients with asthma experience acute upper and lower airway reactions on exposure to aspirin and cyclooxygenase-1-inhibitory drugs. Airway inflammation may still persist even in the absence of exposure to these medications. Aspirin exacerbated respiratory diseases is characterized by a history of aspirin sensitivity, asthma, nasal polyps and chronic rhinosinusitis. Aspirin desensitization is the definitive treatment. HRCT chest has no added benefit unless we are suspecting some alternative diagnosis. Peak flow rate measurements are best avoided in patients with acute asthma as it may precipitate bronchospasm. There is no consensus on the usefulness of mucolytic agent in patients with acute asthma so far.

> Cook KA, Steulnson DD. Current complications and treatment of aspirin-exacerbated respiratory disease. Expert eview of Respiratory Medicine. 2016;10(12).

Q23. Answer e

It is essential to first diagnose the disease with the help of histopathology. Since groin is the most accessible site in this patient, it is the preferred site for biopsy. Since he is not spiking fever and his WBC count is normal, it does not look like an infective process like staphylococcal infection. Empirical antitubercular therapy in an acutely sick patient is not warranted until all investigations have been exhausted. A patient who is comfortable on conventional oxygen delivery device does not need HFNC. It may however be started in case of worsening distress. Doing an endobronchial needle aspiration and biopsy would certainly have been an option if the patient did not have an alternative accessible site for tissue diagnosis.

> Rodeo A et al. Annals of the American thoracic society. 2016;13(6).

Respiratory

Q24. Answer c

When confronted by a patient in shock with evidence of right ventricular failure in a patient who is hospitalized without any DVT prophylaxis prompts one to think possibility of massive PE. However, ST-T changes in inferior leads and a raised troponin levels do not usually form part of this catastrophic presentation. A formal echocardiogram is essential in this situation to better characterize the abnormality and provide further information. Doing CTPA is also a possibility but patient has to be moved from the ICU for it. And since the patient is hemodynamically compromised, it should be done if formal echocardiography is inconclusive. A formal echocardiogram in this patient revealed a large ventricular septal defect with left to right shunt secondary to inferior myocardial infarction.

Steinbach TC, Luks AM. Ann Am Thorac Soc. 2015;12(4):599-603.

Q25. Answer c

Patient's rapidly deteriorating course especially bilateral diffuse lung opacities raises concerns about an infective pathology, interstitial lung disease (ILD) or lymphangitis carcinomatosis. A definitive diagnosis is essential not only for treatment of the current episode but also for the patient's candidacy for liver transplantation. Irreversible lung disease and metastatic disease would render the patient unfit for liver transplantation. Thus an extensive work up is warranted. Patient should be started on broad spectrum antibiotics but steroids and antitubercular therapy are best avoided till the diagnosis is biopsy proven. Patient should undergo a detailed bronchoscpy with transbronchial lung biopsy. An acute presentation and bilateral lung shadows make the possibility of hepatopulmonary syndrome less likely under the present circumstances.

Burke KE, Vanderlean PA, Folch E, et al. Ann Am Thorac Soc. 2014;11(7):1149-51.

Q26. Answer e

Primary alveolar hypoventilation is caused due to primary depression of respiratory center in the brain. Thoracoplasty leads to hypoventilation and respiratory failure secondary to restricted mobility of chest wall. Polymyositis leads to respiratory failure due to respiratory muscle weakness. Vocal cord tumor leads to increased airway resistance in the upper airways, and hypercapnia. It is sepsis and capillary leak syndrome where lung parenchyma is involved leading to respiratory failure, and that too type I respiratory failure.

Pratter MR, Irwin RS. Extrapulmonary causes of respiratory failure. J Int Care Med. 1986;1:197.

Q27. Answer e

Snoring is more indicative of upper airway obstruction and a possible underlying OSA more than OHS. In addition to above, sometimes facial plethora indicating polycythemia may also point towards it.

Piper A et al. Clinical manifestation and diagnosis of obesity hypoventilation syndrome. Uptodate Topic 7698 version 25.

Q28. Answer d

Vasoreactivity test should be positive before initiating patient on calcium channel blockers especially in group I PAH. Negative vasoactive test is an indicator for advanced therapy with a prostanoid endothelial receptor antagonist, phosphodiesterase (PDE) 5 inhibitor or guanylate cyclase stimulant (non CCBs). Ambrisentan (type A endothelial 1 receptor antagonist), and tadalafil (PDE 5 inhibitor) combination improves outcome in patients with WHO functional class II or III. Substituting with drugs within the same family may not produce similar benefits. Addition of inhaled treprostinil (or IV, subcutaneous) may be helpful in patients with progressive or rapid disease. Oral treprostinil is FDA approved for NYHA class II or III based on FREEDOM-M study. Selexipag is FDA approved for NYHA class II and III based on GRIPHON study. IV Epoprostenol and IV treprostinil are recommended in class IV pulmonary hypertension. PAH should be considered as a chronic disease and these patients should receive immunization and with influenza and pneumococcal vaccines.

William H, Lews RJ. Treatment of pulmonary hypertension in adults, Uptodate version 56, Topic 8250.

Q29. Answer a

Various studies have indicated that the pneumothorax can reduce in size at the rate of 1.25% per day. It is estimated that a large, nonrecurring spontaneous pneumothorax may resolve completely over 6 to 12 weeks time.

Montgomery S et al. Natural course of large spontaneous pneumothorax. Heart & Lung the journal of Acute & Critical Care, 2005;34(5):332-4.

Q30. Answer d

Circulatory arrest with electromechanical dissociation is an established and most dreaded complication seen in patients with severe asthma post intubation. It can result in severe cerebral ischemic injury if not tackled timely. This occurs secondary to development of excessive dynamic hyperinflation (DHI) during initial uncontrolled mechanical ventilation. DHI results in electromechanical dissociation. An unnecessary and prolonged CPR may be done if it is not recognized correctly. Once detected, immediate disconnection from the ventilator for 60-90 seconds should be done. Profoundly decreasing the minute ventilation may help in identifying and reversing this deadly complication. In case DHI is very high, use of heliox or ECMO may be needed. Pneumothoraces are most commonly related to insertion of lines but nevertheless may still occur if there has been a main stem bronchial intubation. Unlikely that this young patient may have had an acute coronary event. Aspiration would have resulted in hypoxia and would have been witnessed during intubation. Esophageal intubation would have resulted in cardiac arrest immediately after the process. And if end tidal CO_2 was being monitored it was less likely.

Kollef M. Lung hyperinflation caused by inappropriate ventilation resulting in electromechanical dissociation: a case report. Heart Lung. 1992;21:74-7.

Q31. Answer a

Patient is young non-smoker with a very small primary pneumothorax. He should be observed after putting him on supplemental oxygen. There is some evidence suggesting quicker resolution of pneumothorax after administration of oxygen. High flow oxygen (>28%) results in improving arterial oxygenation and this lowers the partial pressure of nitrogen, resulting in acceleration of the rate of resorption of air from the pleural cavity hastening lung expansion.

BTS guidelines for the management of spontaneous pneumothorax. Thorav. 2003;58:ii39.

Q32. Answer c

If the patient is getting physically fatigued it is always better to secure the tube and connect to ventilator. Moreover it is recommended to have a low threshold for intubation in patients requiring NIV after fresh gastric by bypass surgery. BiPAP results in aerophagia which may result in breakdown of suture and bowel perforation. There are many case reports showing potential complication associated with BIPAP use immediately after gastric bypass surgery.

A potential complication of bilevel positive airway pressure after gastric bypass surgery. Obes Surg. 2004;14(2):282-4.

Q33. Answer d

Hypophosphatemia is frequently observed in alcoholic patients due to various mechanisms, such as inappropriate phosphaturia, increased gastrointestinal loss of phosphate. Excessive antacid may worsen a pre-existing hypophosphatemia. Patients with severe and/or chronic hypophosphatemia are more likely to be symptomatic. Skeletal disorders like muscle weakness, bone pain, rhabdomyolysis, and altered mental status are the most common presenting features in chronic severe hypophosphatemia. Hypophosphatemia has been associated with acute respiratory failure. The mechanism is due to decreased high-energy substrate availability at the cellular level leading to respiratory muscle dysfunction. Folic acid, pyridoxine and thiamine should be administered to patients undergoing alcohol withdrawal.

Elisaf MS et al. Mechanisms of hypophosphatemia in alcoholic patients. Int J Clin Pract. 1997;51:501-3.

Q34. Answer d.

Admit to hospital, start empirical antibiotic therapy within 4 hours of admission

Pneumonia is classified according to the origin as community-acquired (CAP) or hospital-acquired [(nosocomial pneumonia (NP)]. According to the definition, CAP occurs in the absence of immune compromise or prior hospital admission within the previous 7 days. The decision regarding the most appropriate site of care is the first and single most important decision in the overall management of CAP. Various severity scoring systems and predictive models have been developed. The six-point CURB-65 score, one point for each of confusion, urea > 7 mmol/L, respiratory rate > 30 breaths per min, low systolic (< 90 mm Hg) or diastolic (≤ 60 mm Hg) blood pressure and age > 65 years, is based on information available at initial hospital assessment and enables patients to be stratified according to increasing risk of mortality (score 0: 0.7%; score 1: 2.1%; score 2: 9.2%; and scores 3–5: 15–40%). Patients who have a CURB-65 score of 3 or more (as the patient in this question, with a CURB-65 score of 3) are at high risk of death. These patients require urgent hospital admission. Patients with CURB-65 scores of 4 and 5 should be assessed with specific consideration to the need for transfer to a critical care unit (high dependency unit or intensive care unit). Microbiological tests (blood and sputum cultures) are recommended for patients with moderate and high severity CAP admitted to the hospital. All patients should receive antibiotics as soon as the diagnosis of CAP is confirmed. The objective for any service should be to confirm a diagnosis of pneumonia with chest radiography and initiate empirical antibiotic therapy within 4 hours of presentation to the hospital.

> Lim WS, et al. BTS guidelines for the management of community acquired pneumonia in adults: update 2009. Thorax 2009;64:Suppl. 3 iii1–iii55.
>
> Mandell LA, et al. Infectious Diseases Society of America/American Thoracic Society consensus guidelines on the management of community-acquired pneumonia in adults. Clin Infect Dis 2007; 44: Suppl. 2 S27–S72. Woodhead M. Pneumonia. In : Palange P, et al., eds.
>
> ERS Handbook of Respiratory Medicine. 2nd Edn. Sheffield, European Respiratory Society, 2013; pp. 199-202.

Q35. Answer a

Positive pressure ventilation carries an elevated risk of barotrauma. The rupture of the alveolar wall due to increased transpulmonary pressure results in air leakage that causes either a pneumothorax or a pneumomediastinum. ARDS is known to be an independent risk factor for pulmonary barotrauma. If pneumothorax develops in patients on positive pressure mechanical ventilation, it may rapidly progress to tension pneumothorax, causing cardiovascular compromise; therefore, pneumothorax should be drained as fast as possible. The insertion of a chest tube for pneumothorax developing during mechanical ventilation is recommended. A small-bore chest tube as the first choice because it has fewer complications than large-bore tubes. Manual aspiration with thoracentesis is not recommended because it does not allow continuous drainage of the air leak. In case persistent air leakage is observed for more than 5 days, surgical intervention is considered. Video-assisted thoracoscopic surgery is preferred to open thoracotomy. Increasing the inspiratory oxygen fraction and decreasing the positive end-expiratory pressure (PEEP) may slow down the further development of the pneumothorax but are insufficient measures to prevent a tension pneumothorax.

> Baumann MH et al. Management of spontaneous pneumothorax: an American College of Chest Physicians Delphi consensus statement. Chest. 2001;119:590–602.

Q36. Answer b

BIPAP should be used in exacerbations of COPD when pH is < 7.35 and $PaCO_2$ is > 6.0 kPa (> 45 mm Hg). Although the case presented here shows severe acidosis, a BIPAP trial is recommended in ICU under monitoring, as even a failed trial of NIV leading to a delayed endotracheal intubation does not lead to higher mortality. The efficacy of NIV in treating acute exacerbations of COPD was studied in a European, randomized, multicenter study conducted in 85 COPD patients assigned to receive conventional treatment (oxygen therapy plus drugs) or NIV. The group of patients treated with NIV had fewer intubations (26% versus 74%, p < 0.001), fewer complications (14% versus 45%, p < 0.01), shorter length of hospital stay (23 ± 17 versus 35 ± 33 days, p < 0.02) and lower mortality (9% versus 29%; p < 0.02). CPAP would not improve hypercapnia, hence, bilevel NIV is preferred. Morphine would not correct respiratory acidosis, could further worsen due to the respiratory depressant action of morphine.

> Plant PK, et al. Early use of non-invasive ventilation for acute exacerbations of chronic obstructive pulmonary disease on general respiratory wards: a multicentre randomised controlled trial. Lancet. 2010;355:1931-35.
>
> Roberts CM, et al. Acidosis, non-invasive ventilation and mortality in hospitalised COPD exacerbations. Thorax. 2011;66:43-8.

Q37. Answer a

10-mg bolus of recombinant tissue-type plasminogen activator intravenously, then 90 mg over 2 hours.

The patient has suffered massive PE with a subsequent cardiogenic shock. Thrombolysis with rTPA in hemodynamically unstable patients (systolic blood pressure < 90 mm Hg) has survival benefit over heparin.

Surgical embolectomy and selective intra-embolic thrombolysis through a pulmonary artery catheter are second-line options for massive PE when systemic thrombolysis is contraindicated.

>Konstantinides S, et al. Management of venous thrombo-embolism: an update. Eur Heart J. 2014;35:2855-63.
>
>Konstantinides S, et al. 2014 ESC guidelines on the diagnosis and management of acute pulmonary embolism. Eur Heart J. 2014;35:3033-69.
>
>Todd JL, et al. Thrombolytic therapy for acute pulmonary embolism. Chest. 2009;135:1321-29.

Q38. Answer a

The patient has severe community-acquired pneumonia (CURB-65 score 3) involving at least two lobes. He needs hospital admission, in ICU. The risk of pseudomonal infection should be assessed to guide empirical antibiotic therapy. The preferred regimen would be a non-antipseudomonal third-generation cephalosporin and a respiratory fluoroquinolone (moxifloxacin or levofloxacin) or a macrolide (a new macrolide (azithromycin). The patient is allergic to penicillin. Hence, the cephalosporin needs to be substituted with aztreonam, a monobactam, which is safe in patients with penicillin allergy. Oral antibiotics are not an option in severely ill patients.

>Mandel LA, et al. Infectious Diseases Society of America/American Thoracic Society consensus guidelines on the management of community-acquired pneumonia in adults. Clin Infect Dis. 2007;44:Suppl. 2,S27–S72.
>
>Woodhead M, et al. Guidelines for the management of adult lower respiratory tract infections – summary. Clin Microbiol Infect. 2011;17:Suppl. 6,1-24.

Q39. Answer c

DO_2 is the amount of oxygen that is transported to the tissues via the circulatory system. It depends on CaO_2 and CO.

Q40. Answer a

This patient has COPD and CAP. The Gram stain indicates that the patient is infected by Streptococcus pneumoniae. The patient has improved clinically with IV ceftriaxone and is able to take oral medication, hence there is no need to continue IV ceftriaxone. There is no need for a chest radiograph to be repeated prior to discharge in those who have made a satisfactory clinical recovery. A CT scan is not expected to give any further information, as radiological resolution lags behind clinical improvement. According to the 2009 British Thoracic Society guidelines: resolution of fever for > 24 hours; pulse rate < 100 beats per min; resolution of tachypnea; the patient is clinically hydrated and taking oral fluids; resolution of hypotension; absence of hypoxia; improvement in white cell count, no microbiological evidence of Legionella, staphylococcal or Gram-negative enteric bacilli infection; and no concerns over gastrointestinal absorption. There is no recommendation for a broader empiric antibiotic therapy with imipenem, in this scenario. The combination with erythromycin offers no clinical benefit in an empiric therapy. There is no need for bronchoscopy as patient is improving.

>Lim WS et al. BTS guidelines for the management of community acquired pneumonia in adults: update 2009. Thorax. 2009;64:Suppl. 3, iii1–iii55.

Q41. Answer a

Weaning failure is associated with severity of the underlying disease. The weaning failure of this patient is caused by neuromuscular weakness manifesting as tachypnea and hypercapnia during the trial. This patient most likely suffers from critical-illness neuromyopathy; mechanical ventilation, neuromuscular blocking agents and aminoglycoside antibiotics and steroid treatment, are the implicating factors. An electromyogram is the most appropriate diagnostic test to identify critical-illness neuromyopathy. Muscle biopsy is too invasive for this patient but would probably prove nonspecific changes of the myocytes.

>Kress JP, et al. ICU-acquired weakness and recovery from critical illness. N Engl J Med. 2014;370:1626-35.

Q42. Answer b

Despite advances in intensive care practice, mortality and morbidity of patients with severe ARDS remains high. The low-tidal-volume ventilation strategy (ARDS-Net protocol) has been shown to be effective in improving survival. However, some patients with severe ARDS cannot be managed with the ARDS-Net strategy. In these patients, rescue therapies, such as prone ventilation, nitric oxide and ECMO are considered. The CESAR

(Conventional Ventilation or ECMO for Severe Adult Respiratory Failure) trial has shown that an ECMO-based protocol improved survival without severe disability, compared with conventional ventilation. The recent severe respiratory failure due to the H1N1 influenza pandemic has led to an increased use of ECMO. Inhaled corticosteroids are ineffective in ARDS. There is no evidence in the described case of bacterial infection warranting vancomycin.

> Peek GJ, et al. Randomised controlled trial and parallel economic evaluation of conventional ventilatory support versus extracorporeal membrane oxygenation for severe adult respiratory failure (CESAR). Health Technol Assess. 2010;14:1-46.

Q43. Answer c

The evidence to support the use of CPAP and NIV is not as clear-cut in acute cardiogenic pulmonary edema. Interventions are oxygen therapy, diuretics, opioids and therapy directed to the primary cause. There have been a series of meta-analyses comparing the trials with CPAP and NIV show that there was no difference between these modalities and a subsequent large randomised clinical trial (3CPO) showed that while NIV produced an early reduction in breathlessness and improvement in physiological variables, but this did not cause an improvement in mortality. NIV reduced intubation rate in a hypercapnic respiratory failure. While an early small study suggested an increase in myocardial infarction rate in patients treated with NIV, this has not been significant in large 3CPO trial and meta-analyses.

> Gray AJ. Acute cardiogenic pulmonary edema. In: Elliott MW, et al. (eds). Non-Invasive Ventilation and Weaning: Principles and Practice. London, Hodder Arnold. 2010; pp. 298-306.
>
> Masip J, et al. Non-invasive ventilation in acute cardiogenic pulmonary oedema:systematic review and meta-analysis. JAMA. 2005;294:3124-30.
>
> Peter JV, et al. Effect of non-invasive positive pressure ventilation (NIPPV) on mortality in patients with acute cardiogenic pulmonary oedema: a meta-analysis. Lancet 2006;367:1155-63.
>
> Collins SP, et al. Noninvasive ventilation in acute cardiogenic pulmonary edema. N Engl J Med. 2008;359:24-33.

Q44. Answer c

Acute transfusion reactions present within 24 hours of a blood transfusion. Acute transfusion reactions are typically classified as:
- Transfusion-related acute lung injury (TRALI)
- Circulatory (volume) overload or Transfusion Associated Circulatory Overload (TACO)
- Endotoxemia through bacterial contamination
- Acute hemolytic reactions
- Nonhemolytic febrile reactions
- Allergic reactions

The case presented here fulfills the diagnostic criteria of TRALI, as established from a group of experts during the American-European Consensus Conference in 2004 (table). The main symptom of TRALI is dyspnea, which often co-occurs with tachypnea, tachycardia, cyanosis and frothy pulmonary secretions. Fever, hypotension or hypertension is also reported. The main cells involved in TRALI pathogenesis are neutrophils. The main pathology involves activation and sequestration of neutrophils, which damage the endothelial barrier. The closest differential is TACO. The clinical picture of which resembles that of cardiogenic pulmonary edema. Apart from dyspnea and tachypnea, the features of volume overload are jugular venous distension, S3 gallop and high systolic blood pressure. When symptoms of acute respiratory distress occur during transfusion, the procedure should immediately be discontinued and not resumed even if the symptoms diminish. Treatment of TRALI is symptomatic and based on oxygen therapy. Approximately 70% of patients require intubation. Diuretics are not indicated. There is also no role for corticosteroids or antihistamines.

> Transfusion-related acute lung injury: a clinical review. Lancet. 2013;382:984-94.
>
> Jaworski S, et al. Transfusion-related acute lung injury: a dangerous and underdiagnosed noncardiogenic pulmonary edema. Cardiol J. 2013;20:337-44.
>
> Kleinman S, et al. Toward an understanding of transfusion-related acute lung injury: statement of a consensus panel. Transfusion. 2004;44:1774-89.

Q45. Answer d

The patient is presently having all features suggestive of ARDS. She should be ventilated using a lung-protective strategy that involves volume-controlled ventilation with a tidal volume of 4–8 mL/kg of ideal body weight, a plateau pressure < 30 cmH$_2$O and a modest amount of PEEP. At the moment most important step would be to decrease the plateau pressure by decreasing tidal volume to 360 mL, the plateau pressure will also decrease, but decreasing the PEEP will probably deteriorate oxygenation. By decreasing the ventilator frequency, the patient will probably increase triggering of the ventilator.

> The Acute Respiratory Distress Syndrome Network. Ventilation with lower tidal volumes as compared with traditional tidal volumes for acute lung injury and the acute respiratory distress syndrome. N Engl J Med. 2000;342:1301-8.
>
> ARDS Definition Task Force. Acute respiratory distress syndrome: the Berlin definition. JAMA. 2012;307:2526-33.
>
> Esan A, et al. Severe hypoxaemic respiratory failure. Ventilatory Strategies. Chest. 2010;137:1203-16.

Q46. Answer c

Compression ultrasound of the lower limbs is the first-line diagnostic test that should be used in this pregnant woman with possible symptoms of DVT of her left calf because it is not associated with exposure to radiation. If the ultrasound examination is negative, chest radiography would be the next recommended test followed by ventilation/perfusion scintigraphy if the radiograph was normal. If the scintigraphy is nondiagnostic, CT angiography is recommended. D-dimer level increases in normal pregnancy and, therefore, the specificity and sensitivity of D-dimer during pregnancy are only 15% and 73%, respectively.

> Leung AN, et al. An official American Thoracic Society/Society of Thoracic Radiology Clinical Practice Guideline: evaluation of suspected pulmonary embolism in pregnancy. Am J Respir Crit Care Med. 2011;184:1200-08.
>
> Bourjeily G, et al. Pulmonary embolism in pregnancy. Lancet. 2010;375:500-12.

Q47. Answer a

This patient has CAP of low severity (CURB-65 score 0). According to current guidelines, she should be routinely managed with broad spectrum antibiotics as an outpatient and no further investigations are necessary in the primary care setting in this low-risk patient.

The CURB-65

Sign	Finding
C	Mental confusion
U	Blood urea concentration > 7 mmol/L
R	Respiratory rate ≥ 30 breaths/min
B	Systolic blood pressure < 90 mm Hg or diastolic blood pressure ≤ 60 mm Hg
65	Age ≥ 65 years

Using the CURB-65 index, pneumonia is considered mild (score 0-1, mortality 1.5%), moderate (score 2, mortality 9.2%), or severe (score 3-5, mortality 22%).

> Woodhead M et al. Guidelines for the management of adult lower respiratory tract infections: summary. Clin Microbiol Infect. 2011;17:Suppl.6,1-24.

Q48. Answer c

The patient suffers from a TRALI that occurs most often after platelet transfusion (one TRALI per 400 units platelets, one TRALI per 5000 units packed red blood cells). The treatment is supportive and consists of restriction of fluid and ventilatory support. In this case the hypoxemic respiratory failure has improved after 1 hour on NIV, there is no need to intubate and place the patient on invasive mechanical ventilation or increase pressure support (IPAP). TRALI is commonly transient and improves within hours, antibiotics and a cardiology work-up at this stage is not needed.

> Sihler KC, et al. Complications of massive transfusion. Chest. 2010;137:209-20.

Q49. Answer c

On the basis of her history, and clinical and laboratory data, this patient has late-onset (> 5 days in the hospital) ventilator-associated pneumonia (VAP) and has risk factors for multidrug-resistant (MDR) pathogens (history of steroid usage). If there is a low prevalence of MDR, Gram-negative bacteria locally, evidence suggests that antipseudomonal β-lactam monotherapy is sufficient. But, aminoglycosides should be added with the β-lactam antibiotic in the initial treatment of VAP. This patient showed signs of a clinical response as evidenced with lower temperature and less purulent sputum. Clinical improvement precedes radiological improvement. India being a high prevalence region of MDR and Extreme Drug Resistant (XDR) organisms both antibiotics need to be continued.

> Torres A, et al. Treatment guidelines and outcomes of hospital-acquired and ventilator-associated pneumonia. Clin Infect Dis. 2010;51:Suppl. 1, S48-S53.

Q50. Answer d

This patient suffers from acute exacerbation of COPD. He is on long-term oxygen treatment at 2 L/min. NIV improves mortality and respiratory symptoms in patients with acute COPD exacerbations with type 2 respiratory failure. Systemic steroids, dual bronchodilator inhalation and antibiotics are standard treatment for acute COPD exacerbations. Increasing the supplemental oxygen from 2 to 5 L/min may be dangerous as the hypercapnia will increase and the respiratory acidosis will worsen.

> Robinson TD, et al. The role of hypoventilation and ventilation–perfusion redistribution in oxygen-induced hypercapnia during acute exacerbations of chronic obstructive pulmonary disease. Am J Respir Crit Care Med. 2000;161:1524-9.

Q51. Answer a

The presence of a central venous catheter (CVC) is the most common risk factor for the occurrence of upper limb DVT—mainly caused by stasis, trauma to the endothelium of the vessel, thereby acting as a source of thrombus of thrombus formation and propagation. The diameter of the catheter relative to the vessel is the most important factor for DVT. The smaller the diameter relative to the vessel, lesser the chance of stasis. Catheter related infection also increases the risk of catheter related DVT. (OPTION B is incorrect). Increased duration of catheter usage is related to an increased risk of upper extremity DVT (option C IS INCORRECT). Peripherally Inserted Central Catheter (PICC) line inserted in the antecubital vein have a decreased incidence of pneumothorax, but a higher incidence of DVT as compared to the larger veins (subclavian, internal jugular).

However the thrombus formed rarely propagates to the larger vessels unlike those formed at the larger vessels. (option D is incorrect).

Q52. Answer d

Prone positioning has become an important strategy in the management of ARDS patients that has survival benefits. It causes redistribution of blood from dorsal to ventral regions as manifested by re-expansion of the dorsal region and collapse of the ventral regions. Following are the criteria for consideration of prone positioning:
1. PaO_2/FiO_2 ratio<150
2. Nonimprovement of saturation in spite of adequate recruitment maneuvers for at least 12–24 hours.
3. Patient is hemodynamically stable.
    Should be applied at least for 16 hrs with the use of lung protective ventilation maneuvers.
    Airway pressure release ventilation (APRV) involves prolonging the inspiratory time thereby increasing the airway pressure and keeping the alveoli recruited and thus improving the oxygenation. However it shows no survival benefit. (Option A INCORRECT)
    High frequency oscillatory ventilation (HFOV) is a lung protective ventilator mode. However a recent meta-analysis infers it may be harmful in certain settings. (Option B INCORRECT)
    Nitric Oxide cannot improve the oxygenation of a patient, can increase the treatment cost and deteriorate the renal functions. (Option C INCORRECT).

> Ferguson ND, Cook DJ, Guyatt GH et.al.; OSCILLATE Trial investigators; Canadian Critical Care Trials Group. High frequency oscillation in early acute respiratory distress syndrome. N Eng J Med. 2013;368(9):795-805.

Q53. Answer d

This strategy was first proposed in the ARDS NET study, but is becoming popular in patients with normal lungs also example undergoing surgery under general anesthesia. There was a trial on small versus large Tidal volume management in donor lungs prior to transplantation. In this study, the smaller Tidal volume strategy fared better for eventual transplantation.

An RCT in the perioperative settings involving 100 patients for elective lobectomy. 50 of these patients received a Tidal volume of 10 ml/kg with no PEEP, while the other 50 received 5 ml/kg Tidal volume and 5 cm H_2O PEEP. The incidence of postoperative complications was significantly lower in the low TV group (4% versus 22%, p value<.05).

Hemmes SN, Serpa Neto A, Schultz MJ. Intraoperative ventilatory strategies to prevent postoperative pulmonary complications: a meta-analysis. Curr Opin Anaesthesiol. 2013;26(2):126-33.

Q54. Answer b

There is an increase in the peak pressure with a marginal increase in the plateau pressure. This reflects an abrupt increase in airway resistance—may be due to a mucus plug in the tube or a major airway or a biting or kinking of the tube. So endotracheal tube suctioning would be the most appropriate step.

Pulmonary edema or pneumothorax would also increase the peak pressure but also would be accompanied by a rise in the plateau pressure also. Tube dislodgement would cause a leak alarm in the circuit and the pressures would decrease. Hence choices A, C and D are incorrect.

Q55. Answer d

VV ECMO involves pumping of the blood through oxygenator and then back to venous system, usually at right atrium. CO_2 clearance is dependent on the gas flow through the oxygenator, which can clear all of patients CO_2 produced.

However, because a significant portion of the cardiac output (CO) is bypassed in the oxygenator, need for supplemental oxygen and PEEP through ventilator remains.

The major aim of ECMO is lung protection by decreasing the plateau pressure and FiO_2 to less dangerous levels. However conventional ventilator strategy should be still employed. Because CO_2 can be managed by VV ECMO, higher tidal volumes are not required, neither is the need of 100% oxygen.

Schmidt M, Tachon G, Devilliers et al. Blood oxygenation and decarboxylation determinants during venovenous (ECMO for respiratory failure in adults). Int Care Med. 2013;39:838-46.

Q56. Answer c

In patients with critical illness, the volume of distribution is increased with tissue swelling, volume resuscitation and capillary leak. Hence, to reach the desired plasma levels quickly, loading dose is indicated thereby providing timely and adequate treatment for the infection. Secondly critically ill patients also have initial increased metabolism of antibiotics due to their hypermetabolic state. Thus antibiotics with a high volume of distribution need a loading dose also.

Q57. Answer a

Exacerbation of very severe COPD is a CRITICAL condition. The first-line treatment of these patients is ventilatory support. If tolerated, NIV is the preferred mode. In very severe COPD, the decision to start mechanical ventilation is based on the patient's wishes, his/her quality of life and consulting family members. Those patients who require mechanical ventilation due to COPD exacerbation have lower 5-year life expectancy than patients who do not need ventilation. Mechanical ventilation for acute respiratory failure in patients with COPD is associated with high rates of ICU mortality (37–64%) but, nevertheless, this treatment is not futile.

Global Initiative for Chronic Obstructive Lung Disease. Global Strategy for the Diagnosis, Management, and Prevention of Chronic Obstructive Pulmonary Disease.www.goldcopd.org/uploads/users/files/GOLD_Report_2015_Apr2.pdf

Q58. Answer a

Recruitment involves availability of larger number of alveoli for the same tidal volume. This results in lesser ventilation, perfusion mismatch, lesser plateau pressure and lesser peak airway pressure thus $ETCO_2$ is also improved. In a volume controlled mode, as per the tidal volume fixed peak airway pressure is set. Thus peak airway pressure depends on the ventilator settings and not on the lung mechanics.

K Type Answers

Q1. Answer TFTF

Two different classes of β_2 agonists are available. Effect of inhaled short acting β_2 agonists lasts for 3–5 hours like salbutamol, terbutaline, albuterol, etc. These are the mainstay of bronchodilator therapy for acute asthma. Long acting β_2 agonists have a bronchodilatory effect for about 12 hours. Examples are salmeterol and formeterol. Neither of these drugs are approved for management of status asthmaticus. Intravenous administration of B2 adrenergic agents is no longer recommended for the routine management of status asthmaticus. No evidence exists showing superiority of intravenous administration over inhalational route of administration. Various studies have shown that MDIs equipped with spacer devices are equally effective as small volume nebulizers in the management of acute asthma.

Lawford P, Jones BJM, Milledge JS:BMJ1:84,1978.

Idis AH, M Dermott MF, Raucci JC et al. Chest. 103:665,1993

Q2. Answer FTTF

Crazy paving pattern may indicate infectious and noninfectious pathology including neoplasia. Additional tests in the form of transbronchial lung biopsy and bronchoalveolar lavage (BAL) are needed to make the definitive diagnosis.

Ross SE et al. "Crazy-Paving" Pattern at Thin-Section CT of the Lungs: Radiologic-Pathologic Overview. Radiographics. 2003;23(6).

Q3. Answer TFTF

REPE is an iatrogenic complication due to rapid emptying of the pleural cavity. The incidence is less than 1% and mortality can be as high as 20%. Young individuals with large pneumothoraces are at particular risk. Chances of REPE increase with increase in the duration of lung collapse (>7 days). About 64% of patients develop symptoms in the first hour of pleural puncture. About 1800 mL of fluid can be removed in single sitting as per recommendation of the Pleural Group of physicians. The procedure should be stopped if the fluid stops draining spontaneously or if the patient experiences persistent cough or chest discomfort.

Clinics (Sao Paulo). 2010;65(12):1387-9.

Q4. Answer FFTT

IL2 receptor antagonists (daclizumab, basiliximab) and lymphocyte depleting agents (AT4, OKT3), if used during induction phase, have been shown to decrease the acute rejection episodes in various studies. Azithromycin has been found to be associated with improvement in FEV_1 by about 15%, and overall survival in a significant number of lung transplant recipients. In an RCT by Corris et al. azithromycin was found to improve FEV1 by 0.2 L in patients with established BOS post lung transplant. Azithromycin is the preferred neomacrolide on clarithromycin for both prevention and treatment of CR post Ltx. Montelukast (leukotriene receptor antagonist, LTRA) has anti- inflammatory properties affecting eosinophilic airway inflammation. Couple of studies have shown montelukast to attenuate decline in FEV_1 in patients with CR, unresponsive to azithromycin.

Herck AV et al. Prevention of chronic rejection after lung transplantation. J Thorac Dis. 2017;9(12):5472-88.

Q5. Answer TTFF

In a recent study, patients with COPD and coexistent bronchiectasis, were found to experience more severe exacerbations. In another recent meta-analysis, it was also associated with increase in the duration of ICU and hospital stay with increased risk for mortality. Bronchiectasis is compounded by colonisation of the airways with organisms such as *Pseudomonas aeruginosa*, *Hemophilus influenzae* and *Staphylococcus aureus*. These are difficult, and often impossible to eradicate. This is also associated with poor prognosis. There is no literature about the prevalence of MDR organisms so far. We have indirect evidence that bronchiectasis may complicate ICU stay.

Du Q, Liu JJX, Sun Y. Bronchiectasis as a comorbidity of chronic obstructive pulmonary disease: A systematic review and meta-analysis. PLOS One. 2016;11(3):e0150532.

Q6. Answer TTFFT

Various parameters determining VILI are 1) inspiratory stress 2) dynamic strain 3) static strain 4) driving pressure (DP). Stress is actually the force applied across the system, i.e. transpulmonary pressure. Strain is the linear deformation of lungs, which has been further divided into dynamic and static components. Dynamic strain is the ratio of tidal volume (Vt) and end expiratory lung volume. Static strain is the lung volume increase after the PEEP is applied. It is the dynamic strain which promotes VILI as the amount of distortion of pulmonary structure is determined by the initial lung volume. In other words, a large Vt may not be as deleterious as a fully expanded lung as compared to a collapsed lung. Static strain can be deleterious by causing overinflation. Driving pressure is the Pplat-PEEP, and it is the ratio of Vt and respiratory system compliance. Energy represents the area between the inspiratory limb of the pressure volume curve and the volume axis.

Pedro L. Silva, Paola Pelosi and Patricia R.M Rocco. Optimal mechanical ventilation strategies to minimise ventilator induced lung injury in non-injured and injured lungs. Expert review of Respiratory medicine. 2016;10(12): 1243-5.

Q7. Answer TTFTF

Chronic ILD, PE, and right to left shunt cause respiratory failure with elevated A-a oxygen gradient. Because of hypoxia, patient hyperventilates resulting in respiratory alkalosis. High altitude causes respiratory failure secondary to low FiO_2. Patient will have respiratory alkalosis but a normal A-a O_2 gradient. Hepatic failure can result in hypoxia due to associated pulmonary AV shunts. This is associated with increased A-a O_2 gradient. But in presence of normal lungs, the A-a O_2 gradient should be normal.

Conference Report. Mechanism of acute respiratory failure. Am Rev Respir Dis. 1977;115:1071.

Q8. Answer FFTTF

Despite mucosal edema and hyperemia of airways, spirometric studies have revealed no significant changes in FEV_1 during pregnancy suggesting normal airway function. FRC decreases by 15–25%, total lung capacity decreases by 4% to 6% and residual volume shows no change during pregnancy. During pregnancy, women develop chronic mild hyperventilation leading to $PaCO_2$ of 27 to 34 mm Hg. The minute ventilation increases by 20% to 40% near term due to an increase in tidal volume of 30 to 35%. Normal PaO_2 is between 100 to 110 mm Hg during pregnancy. Oxygen consumption is found to increase by 20 to 30% by the third trimester due to increased fetal demands.

Liberatore SM, Pistelli R, Patalano F et al. Respiratory function during pregnancy. Respiration. 1984;46:145.

Lim VS, Katz AI, Linheimer MD. Acid base regulation in pregnancy. Am J Physiol. 1976;231:1764.

Q9. Answer TTFFT

Risk factors associated with tocolytic induced pulmonary edema have been found to be longer duration of IV β adrenergic tocolytic therapy (up to 48 hours), pre-eclampsia, multiple gestation, concomitant sepsis and large volume of crystalloid infusion. IV β adrenergic tocolytic therapy should be restricted to 24 to 48 hours. It should be discontinued at the earliest sign of respiratory distress. Sodium intake should not be more than 4 to 6 gm per day. Steroids with low mineralocorticoid potency should be used during pregnancy. Clinical improvement usually occurs with 12 hours of discontinuation of tocolytic drug. Patient with cardiac disease especially with outflow obstruction should not receive tocolytic therapy.

Candian Preterm Labor Investgation group: Treatment of preterm labour with the beta adrenergic agonist ritodrine. N Engl J Med. 1992;327:308.

Q10. Answer TTFFT

Intracranial hemorrhage is the most devastating complication in patients' receiving thrombolytic therapy. Thrombolytic therapy is relatively contraindicated in pregnancy. It has been associated with maternal mortality of 1% and fetal loss of 6%. Uncontrolled severe hypertension is also a relative contraindication to thrombolytic therapy. Previous hemorrhagic stroke, active internal bleeding and intracranial surgery are absolute contraindications for thrombolytic therapy.

Kearon C, AKI EA, Omelas J et al. Antithrombotic therapy for VTE Disease: CHEST guideline and Expert Panel report. Chest. 2016;149:315-52.

Q11. Answer FTFTF

Definitive therapy for BPF in include surgical approaches which include bronchial stump stapling, thoracoplasty and decortication. However, there has been a trend towards conservative management of these patients. Pleurodesis may potentially close the BPF if the defect is small. It is likely to be ineffective if the BPF is large or multiple in number. With the chest tube in place about 25% of minute ventilation escapes via BPF in ARDS patients. About 20% of CO_2 excretion takes place via this route in 50% of patients. Application of negative pressure to chest drain can increase flows through BPF, leading to inappropriate cycling on ventilator, especially on the pressure support mode. It also delays the healing of BPF. So the minimum pressure required to keep the lung inflated should be applied to patients with BPF. A trial of HFV in patients with BPF and diffuse lung disease in ICU is warranted if they fail conventional ventilation.

Doelken P, Sahn SA. Pleural diseases in the critically ill patients. Irwin & Rippe's Intensive Care Medicine, sixth edition, p 625-42.

Q12. Answer TTTFT

Malnutrition, dyselectrolytemias like hypokalemia, hypomagnesemia, hypocalcemia, hypophosphatemia and hypothyroidism are associated with muscle weakness. Chronic renal failure and corticosteroids result in myopathy. Critical illness neuropathy is one of the most frequent causes of weaning failure in critically ill patients.

Richard S Irwin, Rolf D Hubmayr. Mechanical ventilation Part III: Discontinuation. Irwin & Rippe's Intensive care medicine, sixth edition, pp. 677-88.

Q13. Answer TFTFT

Duration of mechanical ventilation, ICU costs and ventilator related complications are decreased if protocol directed ventilatory management team handles the patient. No difference has been found between SBT or pressure support trial during weaning process. However, both have been found to be superior to SIMV mode for weaning. Esteban et al. had established that there is no difference between 30 minutes and 120 minutes SBTs. Unrecognized adrenal insufficiency can contribute to weaning failure. Various authors (Esteban et al. 1995, Meade M et al. 2001) found that there was no benefit of using twice daily SBT as compared to a single one.

Irwin RS, Hubmayr RD. Mechanical ventilation Part III: Discontinuation. Irwin & Rippe's Intensive care medicine, sixth edition, pp. 677-88.

Q14. Answer TTFFF

All asphyxiants lead to tissue hypoxia. Simple asphyxiants lead to decrease in ambient FiO_2 and chemical asphyxiants lead to cellular hypoxia by interfering with uptake, transport or utilization of oxygen. CO and CO_2 are the most common chemical and simple asphyxiants respectively. Symptoms worsen rapidly when ambient FiO_2 decreases to less than 0.15 due to increase in CO_2 levels in ambient air. Severity of CO poisoning correlates better with duration of exposure than the carboxyhemoglobin levels. Adult hemoglobin has a lesser affinity for CO than fetal hemoglobin making fetus more susceptible than mother to the effects of CO.

David J Prezant, Dorsett D. Smith, Lawrence C Mohr: Acute inhalational injury. Irwin & Rippe's Intensive Care Med, sixth edition, pp. 755-70.

Q15. Answer TFTFT

Viral pneumonia and CAP are most common pneumonias in pregnant patients. Pathogens responsible are *Streptococcus pneumoniae, Haemophilus influenzae* and atypical pathogens like mycoplasma pneumonia, legionella species, varicella and influenza A. Macrolide is the antibiotic of choice. This can however be replaced by a beta lactam against pneumonia if the local resistance to macrolide is higher than 25%. Risk of PE is increased by as much as 5 to 6 times during pregnancy. It is highest in the postpartum period. D-dimer is not reliable in pregnancy. Permissive hypercapnia with PCO_2 of 60 mm of Hg is tolerable without any adverse effect observed on the fetus, but higher CO_2 levels should be avoided during pregnancy. Recommended goal to be achieved remains at PaO_2 of 70 mm of Hg or higher to ensure adequate fetal oxygenation.

Schwaiberger D et al. Respiratory failure and mechanical ventilation in the pregnant patient. Crit Care Clin. 2016;32:85-95.

Q16. Answer TFFTT

The unique pathological finding in HPS is gross dilatation of pulmonary precapillary and capillary vessels. They are also increased in numbers. Less commonly there are associated pulmonary AV malformations and portopulmonary venous anastomosis. Both intrapulmonary shunting and diffusion impairments are responsible for hypoxia in HPS. Platypnea and orthodeoxia have been found to occur due to predominance of IPVD at the lung bases and the increase in blood flow through these dilated units when upright resulting in fall in oxygen saturation in the upright posture. Pulmonary function tests do not normalize after liver transplantation and may continue to show reduced diffusion capacity for carbon monoxide. Contrast enhanced transthoracic echocardiogram (CTTE) and radionuclide lung perfusion scan with technetium labeled macro aggregated albumin particles (MAA) are used to diagnose HPS. The presence of IPVD is indicated by appearance of micro bubbles in the left Atrium 3 to 6 cardiac cycle post injection. These bubbles pass rapidly through the abnormally dilated pulmonary vasculature.

Ramalingam VS et al. Respiratory complications in liver disease. Crit care clin. 2016;32:357-69.

Q17. Answer TFFTT

Current NHSN definition of VAE helps us in capturing possibility of noninfectious cause as a reason of deterioration. It is nonobjective. To qualify as a VAC, patient should have received 2 days of mechanical ventilation with either less or same level of FiO_2 requirements before the fresh increase in oxygen requirement develops. iVAC suggests a causal relationship between VAE and infection. The new definition or VAE criteria does not have any radiographic component. This is because radiographic studies are of adjunctive value in diagnosis of pneumonia but not essential, and so have been removed from VAE surveillance criteria.

Spalding M et al. Ventilator associated pneumonia: new definition: Crit Care Clin. 2017;33:277-92.

Q18. Answer TTFFT

The criteria for weaning as proposed by consensus conference of clinicians with experts are divided into required and optional criteria. The required criteria are that the cause of respiratory failure should have improved, pH should be more than 7.25, patient should have ability to initiate an inspiratory effort, PaO_2/FiO_2 of more than 150 or $SpO_2 > 90\%$ on FiO_2 of <0.4 and PEEP<5 cms of H_2O, hemodynamic stability (no or low dose vasopressor medication). Optional criteria are hemoglobin more than 8 to 10 mg/dL, mental status awake and alert or easily arousable, core temperature less than 38°C to 38.5°C.

The above criteria are based on observational studies and experience of the intensivists who attended the consensus conference. None of these have been validated in RCTs.

Macintyre NR et al. Evidence based guidelines for weaning and discontinuing ventilatory support: a collection task force facilitated by American college of chest physicians; The American association for respiratory care and American college of critical care medicine chest. 2001;120:375S.

Q19. Answer TTFTT

NIV should not be used in the following conditions: cardiorespiratory arrest, severe upper GI bleeding, poor bulbar function, severe encephalopathy, inability to protect airways, cardiorespiratory instability, hypotension with good inotropic dose, serious arrhythmias, uncooperative patient, recent facial esophageal or gastric injury, fixed anatomical abnormalities of nasopharynx.

Hess D. Noninvasive Positive Pressure Ventilation: Predictors of success and failure for adult acute care complications. Resp Care. 1997;97:424-30.

Q20. Answer FTTF

PCWP is most valuable in distinguishing between ARDS and cardiogenic pulmonary edema. PCWP is not indicative of capillary hydrostatic pressure but a value of less than 18 mm of Hg is helpful in excluding cardiogenic pulmonary edema. In healthy individuals neutrophils constitute 5% of the cells recovered from BAL fluid. In ARDS neutrophils makeup at least 80% of the recovered cells in lavage fluid. Due to inflammation there is exudation of proteinaceous material which is depicted as high protein (lavage/serum) ratio in ARDS patients. In early ARDS usually hypoxemia is out of proportionately worse than the chest X-ray findings. In early cardiogenic pulmonary edema chest X-ray abnormalities are more pronounced than the hypoxemia.

Aberle DR, Brown K. Radiological considerations in the adult respiratory distress syndrome. Clin chest Med. 1990;11:737-54.

Idell S, Cohen AB. Bronchoalveolar lavage in patients with adult respiratory distress syndrome. Clin chest med. 1985;6:459-71.

Q21. Answer TTFF

At the usual concentration of inhaled oxygen lungs innate antioxidant activity is sufficient to protect from oxygen toxicity. When this protective capacity is exceeded oxygen inhalation results in lung injury similar to ARDS. The toxic level of FiO_2 has been recognized to be 0.6. Exposure to a FiO_2 greater than 0.6 for periods greater than 48 hours is generally considered as toxic exposure to oxygen. Evaluation of adequacy of antioxidant

Respiratory

protection of lung is not yet possible, but 2 measures have been recommended to ensure the adequacy. A daily intake of Selenium (70 microgram per day for men and 55 microgram per day for women) has been recommended. The second is to correct vitamin E deficiency

>Halliwell B, Gutteridge JMC. Oxygen is a toxic gas: an introduction to oxygen toxicity and reactive oxygen species. In free radicals in biology and medicine. 3rd edition. Oxford: Oxford university Press, 1999:1-104.
>
>Fink M. Role of reactive oxygen and nitrogen species in acute respiratory distress syndrome. Curr Opin Crit Care. 8:6-11.

Q22. Answer TFTT

In normal circumstances the $ETCO_2$ is 2 to 3 mm of Hg lower than $PaCO_2$. As the gas exchange in lung is impaired this difference widens. It exceeds 3 mm of Hg due to various reasons like increased anatomic and physiological dead space (open ventilator circuit, shallow breathing, obstructive lung disease) and low cardiac output states (like PE, excessive auto PEEP). It is unusual for $ETCO_2$ to exceed $PaCO_2$ but is sometimes encountered in presence of high CO_2 production, high cardiac output and low inspired tidal volume in presence of high FiO_2.

>Stock MC. Capnography for adults. Crit Care Clin. 1995;11:219-32.
>
>Moorthy SS, Losasso AM, Wilcox J. End tidal PCO_2 greater than $PaCO_2$. Crit Care Med. 1984;12:534-5.

Q23. Answer TFTFT

Lambert beer law is based on the principle that absorption of light as it passes through a medium is dependent on the concentration of that substance that absorbs light, and the distance light has to travel. Oximetry is able to detect only two forms of hemoglobin oxygenation, Hb and HbO_2. In the red region (660 nm) oxygenated hemoglobin is found not to absorb light as much as deoxygenated hemoglobin, and in the infrared region (940 nm) the opposite holds true. Since the concentration of methemoglobin and carboxyhemoglobin is less than 5% in a healthy individual. It is not normally detected by oximetry. Percentage saturation is ratio of oxygenated hemoglobin to total hemoglobin so,

$$\%saturation = HbO_2/HbO_2 + Hb \times 100$$

One side of the finger probe has photo transmitter from where monochromatic light is emitted at 660 nm and 940 nm wavelengths. The opposite side of the finger probe has a photodetector which is able to amplify light of alternating intensity. That is why pulsatile flow in an artery will be amplified, and nonpulsatile flow related light will be blocked by the photodetector.

>Waher JA, Tremper KK. Noninvasive oxygen monitoring techniques. Crit Care Clin. 1995;11:199-217.

Q24. Answer TTTFF

$A-aDO_2$ is an indirect measure of ventilation perfusion abnormalities in the lung. It increases with age. It is calculated by difference between alveolar PO_2 and arterial PO_2. FiO_2 increase results is in increase in $A-aDO_2$ primarily due to loss of regional hypoxic vasoconstriction. The normal $A-aDO_2$ gradient is increased by approximately 5 to 7 mm of Hg for every 10% rise in FiO_2. Ratio of arterial to alveolar PO_2 (a/APO_2) is unaffected by FiO_2 unlike $A-aDO_2$. The normal a/APO_2 is 0.74 to 0.77 on room air, and increases to 0.8 to 0.82 while breathing 100% FiO_2. It is PaO_2/FiO_2 ratio which is indicative of shunt fraction. Normal RQ is about 0.8 ($RQ = VCO_2/VO_2$).

>Gammon RB Jefferson LS. Interpretation of arterial oxygen tension. Up-to-date website, 2006.
>
>Covelli HD, Nenan VJ, Tuttle WK. Oxygen-derived variables in acute respiratory failure. Crit care Med. 1983;11:646-9.

Q25. Answer TTFTT

Oxygen delivery (DO_2) is the amount of oxygen (in milliliters) that is delivered to the peripheral tissues per minute. It is determined by multiplying cardiac output to oxygen content. O_2 content is determined by:

$$O_2 \text{ content} = HB \times 1.34 \times \text{oxygen saturation} + PaO_2 \times 0.003$$

Normal value is 900 to 1100 ml per minute (absolute range) or 500–600 mL per minute per meter square (size adjusted range). Oxygen uptake (VO_2) is the volume of oxygen which is released at the peripheral tissue level. It is also referred to as oxygen consumption of the tissues. It is calculated by multiplying cardiac output to arteriovenous oxygen content difference. Normal value is 200-270 mL per minute (absolute range) or 110-160 mL per minute per meter square (size adjusted range) at rest. Ratio of VO_2 to DO_2 is referred to as oxygen extraction ratio (O_2ER). This ratio is generally multiplied by 100 and is then expressed as a percentage

$$O_2ER = VO_2/DO_2$$

Normal O_2ER is about 0.25 (0.2-0.3). This indicates that 25% of the total oxygen delivered to the capillaries is taken up by the tissues.

Carbon dioxide elimination (VCO_2) occurs at the level of lung. Similar to VO_2 it is the product of cardiac output and venoarterial CO_2 content difference. Normal VCO_2 in healthy adults is about 162-220 mL per minute (absolute range) or 90-130 mL per minute per meter square (size adjusted range).

Little RA, Edwards JD. Applied physiology. In ' Edwards JD, Shoemaker WC, Vincent JL, eds. Oxygen transport: principles and practice, London:WB Saunders, 1993:21-40.

Hameed SM, Aird WC, Cohn SM. Oxygen delivery. Crit Care Med. 2003;31(suppl):S658-67.

Nunn RF. Nunn's Applied respiratory physiology 4th ed. Oxford: Butterworth-Heinamann.

Q26. Answer TFFTT

End expiratory hold maneuver is normally used to detect DHI. It however may underestimate DHI in asthmatics who may have many noncommunicating alveoli with higher auto PEEP during the measuring maneuver. It is the plateau pressure which is a better estimate of the DHI. Clinically auto PEEP and plateau pressure are the two measurements followed to make any changes. DHI can be decreased by decreasing minute ventilation. It can be decreased by increasing expiratory time which may be achieved by lowering respiratory rate, increasing inspiratory flows and shifting to square pattern of flow. In COPD patient intrinsic PEEP should be lower than auto PEEP to assist in triggering the ventilator. Auto PEEP frequently results in ineffective triggering efforts.

Koh Y. Ventilatory management in patients with chronic airflow obstruction. Crit care Clin. 2007;23(2):169-81.

Q27. Answer TFTFF

In a critically ill patient pneumothorax can alter the prognosis of the patient, though the underlying disease remains the primary determinant of outcome. There is no role of needle aspiration of pneumothorax in critically ill patients especially those who are on mechanical ventilation, post-surgical patients and post chest trauma patients. There is a school of thought that the chest drain should be placed in the second intercostal space in the midclavicular line for drainage of pneumothorax in a supine ventilated patient. Another school of thought advocates that the insertion of chest drain in the fourth or fifth intercostal space in mid or anterior axillary line works equally well, and is perhaps safer. Previous guidelines had recommended use of large bore tubes for drainage of pneumothorax but currently small bore tubes are preferred as first line therapy. Large tube may be used if there is associated BPF, hemothorax or parapneumonic effusions. A recent study had found no difference in the post chest tube pneumothorax when it was removed during end inspiration (8% recurrence) or end expiration (6% recurrence).

Bell RL, Ovadia P, abdullah F et al. Chest tube removal: end inspiration or end expiration? J trauma. 2001;50:674-7.

Q28. Answer TFFTF

Patient is an immunocompromised host and likelihood of having infections with cytomegalovirus, pneumocystis carinii, aspergillus and mucor remain high. Aspergillus and mucor usually cause focal pneumonias. Patient can also be infected with normal community-acquired organisms like legionella and staphylococcus aureus. Staphylococcus aureus usually results in focal pneumonia.

Tamm M. The lung in the immunocompromised patient. Infection complications part 2. Respiration. 1999;66:199-207.

Charles D Gomersall. Pneumonia,Oh's Intensive care manual, sixth edition, Pg 415-28.

Q29. Answer FFTFF

All the DOAC's—apixaban, dabigatran, edoxaban or rivaroxaban are approved by FDA for treatment of venous thromboembolism (VTE). Rivaroxaban and apixaban do not require overlap therapy with heparin and can even be started in emergency department. DOAC's have been found to be associated with similar rates of recurrent PE as compared to long-term warfarin therapy. These are associated with lower rates of hemorrhage. None of the DOACs have been extensively studied in presence of active cancer. Unfractionated heparin is useful and indicated if patient requires embolectomy or thrombolysis or if there is a high-risk of bleeding. This is due to its short half-life. Unfractionated heparin and low molecular weight heparin are preferred over warfarin or DOACs in patients with venous thromboembolism and active cancer. Warfarin is teratogenic and is contraindicated in pregnancy. Mortality and hemodynamic stability have been found to improve with systemic thrombolysis in patients with massive and submassive that is (intermediate risk) PE. Only alteplase is approved by USFDA for the treatment of massive PE. Surgical thromboembolectomy is indicated if there is a contraindication to, or failed thrombolysis in patients with massive hemodynamically unstable PE. Since the procedure has significant mortality (about 20%), it should be performed before cardiogenic shock or end organ damage develops.

Corrigan D et al. Pulmonary embolism: the diagnosis, risk stratification, treatment and disposition of emergency department patients. Clin Exp Emerg Med. 2016;3(3):117-25.

Q30. Answer TFFFT

In addition to the prediction value for patients pre-test probability for PE (Wells score and revised Geneva score), pulmonary embolism rule out criteria (PERC) has been incorporated in the PE guidelines. A low pre-test probability and negative PERC confidently rules out PE with the false negative rate lower than the test threshold. Approximately 50% of patients with PE have a negative venous ultrasound, so it is not sufficient to rule out PE alone. About two thirds of patients may have a non-diagnostic VQ scan. CTPA is the first imaging modality and most sensitive for PE. A negative D dimer along with non-high pre-test probability has a post-test probability of PE less than 2% . Thus negative D dimer has a high production value for PE.

Corrigan D et al. Pulmonary embolism: the diagnosis, risk stratification, treatment and disposition of emergency department patients. Clin Exp Emerg Med. 2016;3(3):117-25.

Q31. Answer FTFFT

Cold water humidifiers are simple inexpensive and ineffective. Maximum water content achieved is 9 gram/m^3 (about 50% relative humidity (RH)at room temperature). They are no longer used. Hot water or heated humidifiers are considered as gold standard especially in the presence of thick or bloody secretions or high minute ventilation. However, micro droplet formation has been reported with their use which may be a potential source of infection. Modern HMEs have been found to have a small dead Space (30 to 95 mL). This may be counterproductive and impose respiratory load in a particular patient. The incidence of nosocomial pneumonia has been found to be similar with both HME and hot water humidifier during prolonged ventilation. Hygroscopic HMEs are more effective than hydrophobic HMEs because of its inherent design. These absorb moisture onto a paper like material that is chemically coated (calcium chloride or lithium chloride) which increases their efficiency. These are found to retain their ability to humidify for at least 4 days. In the latest guidelines published by American association of respiratory care (AARC) a temperature of 33 +/-2 degree centigrade with relative humidity of 100% and water vapor level of 44 mg/L are recommended. Heated humidifiers are classified as bubble, passover, counter flow and in line vaporizer.

Haithem SH, Modrykanien AM. Humidification during mechanical ventilation in the adult patient. Biomed Research International; volume 2014, Article ID 715434, 12 pgs

Q32. Answer TFTFF

Heating and humidification in normal person takes places in a nasopharyngeal space. The cilia present in sol layer pushes the overlying mucus layer towards the glottis which is then swallowed subconsciously. The cilia beat at the rate of 10 mm/minute at 37°C and 100% relative humidity. Humidification and heating of the dry inhaled gas occurs progressively down the airway and the boundary of isothermic saturation occurs just below the carina. The exact minimum moisture level required for optimal ciliary functioning and mucus clearance is not known. It has been observed that mucus flow reduces markedly if RH falls to 75% at 37°C (absolute humidity of 32 gm/m^3), and completely stops if RH falls to below 50% (absolute humidity of 22 gm/m^3). So the minimum RH of 75% or AH of 33 gm/m^3 is required to keep up with the normal function. It has been found that at absolute humidity level of 32 gm/m^3, the gas temperature does not matter unless excessive. In intubated patients the upper airway is bypassed, and relative humidity falls to below 50% which in turn has ill effects. It results in increased mucus viscosity, reduced ciliary function, mucosal ulceration, tracheal inflammation and sometimes necrotizing tracheobronchitis. High FiO_2 also is known to cause acute tracheobronchitis with significant reduction in tracheal mucus velocity within 3 hours.

Forbes AR. Humidification and mucus flow in the intubated trachea. Br J Anesthesia. 1973;45:874-8.

Chalon J, Patel C, Ali M et al. Humidity and the anesthetized patient. Anesthesiology. 1974;50:195-8.

Sacker MA, Landa J, Hirsch J et al. Pulmonary effects of oxygen breathing: a six hour study in normal man. Ann Intern Med. 1975;82:40-3.

Q33. Answer FTFTT

When constant PEEP is maintained in both inspiratory and expiratory phases of respiratory cycle the term 'continuous positive airway pressure (CPAP)' is used. The primary role of PEEP is to maintain the recruitment, increase FRC thereby decreasing intrapulmonary shunt by improving the V/Q ratio. PEEP can indirectly reduce extravascular lung water especially in patients with left ventricular failure by reducing the venous return and left ventricular afterload. It can also result in reduction in oxygen delivery as reduced venous return decreases the cardiac output. So PaO_2 may actually rise but net oxygen delivery may go down. In presence of severe airflow obstruction PEEP is used to decrease the triggering load. For this it is a must that extrinsic peep (PEEPe) should be less than intrinsic peep or auto peep (PEEPi). If PEEPe is more than PEEPi patient will have worsening hyperinflation.

Suter PM, Fairley B, Isenberg MD. Optimum end expiratory airway pressure in patients with acute pulmonary failure. N Engl J Med. 1975;292:284-9.

Vieira SRR, Puybasset L, Richecoeur J et al. A lung computed tomographic assessment of positive end expiratory pressure induced lung overdistension. Am J Respir Crit Care Med. 1998;158:1571-7.

Q34. Answer TFFFT

Bronchodilators and parenteral steroids are mainstay treatment of acute exacerbation of COPD. However, combination of both beta agonist and anticholinergic has been shown to be more effective in exacerbation than either agent alone. Albert et al. had shown methylprednisolone 0.5 mg/kg 6 hourly dose to be effective in controlling exacerbation of COPD. Although nebulized mucolytics have been proposed but have never been established in acute exacerbation of COPD. There is however reports of bronchospasm occurring with some inhaled mucolytics like mistabron. In fact oral mucolytic agents like ambroxol have been shown to decrease cough frequency and severity in a stable COPD patient. Uses of respiratory stimulants like acetazolamide, medroxyprogesterone, naloxone, doxapram and almitrine have been suggested during exacerbation of COPD. But this holds true when acute respiratory failure is attributed to a reduced respiratory drive and not due to increased respiratory load or decreased pump capacity. There have been some recent evidence that NIV may be useful in patients with low pH value (as low as 7.00) and severe hypercapnia (as highest 140 mm of Hg). Our patient is conscious so a noninvasive trial is definitely warranted. Intubation should be a standby plan.

Clavis F Vogelmeier et al. Global strategy for the diagnosis, management and prevention of chronic obstructive lung disease, 2017 Report. GOLD executive summary. Am J Respir Crit Care Med. 2017;195(5).

Petty T. The National Mucolytic Studt. Results of a randomized, double blind, placebo controlled study of iodinated glycerol in chronic obstructive bronchitis. Chest. 1990;97:75-83.

Crummy F, Buchan C, Miller B et al. The use of noninvasive ventilation in COPD with severe hypercapnic respiratory acidosis. Respir Med. 2007; 101:53-61.

Q35. Answer FTTFT

The clinical syndrome of radiation induced lung injury is similar regardless of the pulmonary or nonpulmonary origin of tumor. It correlates with the dose of radiation received and is usually monitored by V_{20}, i.e. the volume of normal lung receiving radiation of 20 Gy or more. V_{20} has been found to significantly predict the risk of development of radiation pneumonitis,

V_{20} < 20%–0% risk by 2 years

V_{20} 22–31%–7% risk for 2 years

V_{20} 32–40%–13% risk for 2 years

V_{20} > 40%–36% risk by 2 years

Various chemotherapeutic agents are known to increase the probability of developing radiation pneumonitis like taxim, cyclophosphamide, bleomycin, irinotecin, and doxorubicin to name a few. Radiation pneumonia is graded in various ways but most common is by common toxicology criteria for adverse events. High dose of oral steroids like prednisolone forms the mainstay of treatment. It is usually given for a period of 8 to 12 weeks. Patients should concurrently be given pneumocystis prophylaxis.

Bledsoe TJ et al. Radiation pneumonitis. Clin Chest Med. 2017;38:201-8.

Q36. Answer FTFT

The BLUE protocol (bedside lung ultrasound in emergency) has been designed for evaluation of respiratory failure. The FALLS protocol (fluid administration limited by lung sonography) rules out sequentially obstructive shock, cardiogenic shock then with fluid administration is able to differentiate between hypovolemic and distributive shock.

SESAME protocol (sequential emergency sonography assessing mechanism of origin of severe shock of indistinct cause). It is basically dependent on evaluation of pneumothorax, intra-abdominal bleeding, cardiac tamponade and myocardial infarction as the causes of cardiac arrest. RUSH protocol is a systemic algorithm for evaluation of shock. It basically looks at the pump (heart), the tank (IVC, peritonial and pleural fluid), and pipes (Aorta—aneurysm, dissection, venous Doppler to rule of DVT) for assessment of patients with shock.

Lichtenstein D, Malbrain M. Lung ultrasound in the critically ill (LUCI): A translational discipline. Anaesthesiology Intensive Therapy. 2017;49(5):430-6.

Jain S et al. Application of rapid ultrasound in shock in the ICU for management of shock. Indian J Crit Care Med. 2014;18(8): 550-51.

Q37. Answer FTFT

Postextubation laryngeal edema may result in respiratory failure with subsequent reintubation. Risk factors for postextubation laryngeal edema are larger endotracheal tube, prolonged intubation and female sex. Patients at low risk can be somewhat confidently identified by the laryngeal ultrasound or cuff leak test. But in high-risk patients no reliable test for prediction exist. Intravenous or nebulized steroids can prevent the episodes if applied timely. Use of noninvasive ventilation or a helium/ oxygen mixture have not been found to be helpful. These were associated with worst outcomes as they resulted in delay in intubation.

Wouter A Pluijms, Walther NKA et al. Postextubation laryngeal edema and stridor resulting in respiratory failure in critically ill adult patients. Updated review. Critical Care. 2015;19:295.

Q38. Answer TTTTF

Hyperbaric oxygen therapy is delivering 100% oxygen at 2 to 3 atmospheric pressure. It can be delivered either in a monoplace or a multiplace chamber. It serves to increase the amount of oxygen carried in the plasma rather than that bound to hemoglobin. Hyperbaric oxygen therapy may be used for enhancement of healing of problem wounds but it is not the primary treatment for deep seated wounds.

Tibbles PM, Edelsberg JS. Hyperbaric oxygen therapy. N Engl J Med. 1996;334:1642-8.

Q39. Answer FFTT

Hyperthermia and acidemia result in shift of ODC to the right and increase oxygen availability to the tissues. 2,3 DPG is a by product of glycolysis and therefore binds hemoglobin in hypoxic tissues predominantly facilitating release of oxygen, i.e. shifting the ODC to the right. Methemoglobin, carbon monoxide, fetal hemoglobin have higher affinity for oxygen, that is why effectively shift ODC to the left.

Q40. Answer TFFT

The diameter of the pulmonary artery of > 33 mm has a sensitivity of 93% and specificity of 95% for a chronically elevated pulmonary arterial pressure. With an obstruction of more than 50% pulmonary hypertension (i.e. a mean pulmonary artery pressure > 25 mm Hg) develops. An elevated mean pulmonary artery pressure of 50 mm Hg is not consistent with acute pulmonary embolisms but may be associated with chronic thromboembolic pulmonary hypertension (CTEPH). A slightly elevated right atrial pressure is compatible with acute pulmonary embolism. There is no left heart failure in acute pulmonary embolism and a normal pulmonary artery wedge pressure of 12 mm Hg is compatible with this diagnosis.

Alpert JS et al. Experimental pulmonary embolism; effect on pulmonary blood volume and vascular compliance. Circulation. 2010;49:152-7.

Q41. Answer TTFTT

There is no universal strategy or consensus currently for weaning critical care patients from mechanical ventilation. Further research and international collaboration is needed. Combining SIMV with spontaneous breathing/pressure support may improve efficiency. The use of synchronized intermittent mandatory ventilation (SIMV) alone from recent weaning trials is deemed the least efficient method for weaning. Delay in weaning prolongs critical care stay thereby increasing costs and associated with a higher mortality. The ongoing need for inotropes does not preclude weaning.

Lermitte J, Garfield MJ. Weaning from mechanical ventilation. Contin Educ Anaesth Crit Care Pain. 2005;5(4):113-7.

Waldmann C, Soni N, Rhodes A. Oxford Desk Reference eriticaf Care. Oxford, UK: Oxford University Press, 2008.

Q42. Answer FTTTF

Daily changes of ventilator tubing may increase the VAP risk due to cross-contamination from excess handling of equipment. Chlorhexidine mouth care has been demonstrated to reduce the incidence of VAP. Head-up positioning of 30 to 45° reduces micro-aspiration, and thus the incidence of VAP. Daily sedation holds have been demonstrated to reduce patient time spent on the ventilator, and thus reduce the incidence of VAP. Prone positioning improves mortality in severe ARDS, but its impact on VAP rates per se is as yet unclear.

Guerin C, Reignier J, Richard JC, et al. Prone positioning in severe acute respiratory distress syndrome. Now Engl J Med. 2013;368(2):159-68.

Hunter JD. Ventilator-associated pneumonia. Br Med J. 2012;344:e3325.

Q43. Answer FTFTT

In severe ARDS, high PEEP (>15 cm H_2O) does not improve mortality. Some PEEP (around 5-10 cm H_2O) is associated with improved oxygenation. Application of PEEP increases FRC. Decreased renal blood flow and reduced splanchnic and hepatic perfusion can occur with higher levels of PEEP. PEEP application increases intrathoracic pressure, diminishing venous return to the right heart. Following PEEP application, an observed increase in lung compliance is suggestive of alveolar recruitment.

The National Heart, Lung and Blood Institute ARDS Clinical Trials Network. Higher versus lower positive end-expiratory pressures in patients with the acute respiratory distress syndrome. New Engl J Med. 2004;351:327-36.

Waldmann C. Soni N, Rhodes A. Oxford Desk Reference Critical Care. Oxford, UK: Oxford University Press, 2008.

Q44. Answer TTTF

This patient due to inadequate time for exhalation has developed symptoms suggestive of auto-PEEP—this is giving rise to increased intrathoracic pressure, which in turn is pressing on the inferior vena-cava and causing hypotension and increased plateau pressure. This is a medical emergency; the most appropriate measure would be to disconnect the ventilator, which would release the accumulated air, thereby, reducing the intrathoracic pressure.

Reducing the respiratory rate would allow more time per breath, hence greater time to release the air, hence would improve exhalation.

Increasing the time for exhalation would allow a slower exhalation, which would help to release the air.

Laghi AF, Goyal A. Auto-PEEP in respiratory failure. Minerva anestheliol. 2012;78(2):201-21.

CHAPTER 3

Neurointensive Care

Harsh Sapra, Gaurav Kakkar

A Type Questions
(One best answer)

1. Following penetrating trauma to the lumbar spinal cord, a patient develops ipsilateral hemiplegia with contralateral pain and temperature sensory deficits. What is this syndrome of hemi-section of the spinal cord called?
   a. Brown-Séquard syndrome (BSS)
   b. Quadriplegia
   c. Post-polio syndrome
   d. Guillain-Barré syndrome (GBS)

2. The usual first sign of uncal herniation:
   a. Ipsilateral 3rd nerve palsy
   b. Contralateral 3rd nerve palsy
   c. Supraventricular tachycardia
   d. Tonic-clonic seizure
   e. Ipsilateral hemiparesis

3. A 51-year male with known atrial fibrillation, diabetes mellitus and hypertension presents with inability to balance, slurred speech and ataxia of 4 hours duration. The most appropriate treatment option for clinical suspicion of acute thrombotic stroke of a major intracranial vessel is:
   a. Immediate thrombolysis by paramedics or in triage
   b. Only thrombolysis once CT head confirms thrombotic stroke
   c. Bridging thrombolysis and thrombectomy after CT Head confirms thrombotic stroke
   d. Only mechanical thrombectomy once CT head confirms thrombotic stroke
   e. Blood alcohol levels, IV fluids and monitoring in HDU

4. A 34-year male recovered from a decompressive craniectomy after a road traffic accident (RTA). At his 12 months follow-up visit he is independent for his daily activities within the house but has not fully recovered to join back work. Which of the following best describes his Glasgow Outcome Scale (GOS):
   a. GOS 1
   b. GOS 2
   c. GOS 3
   d. GOS 4
   e. GOS 5

5. Which antibody is associated with the Miller Fisher variant of Guillain-Barré syndrome (GBS)?
   a. Anti-GQ1b ganglioside antibody
   b. Anti-GBM antibody
   c. Anti -La antibody
   d. Anti-Jo1 antibody
   e. Anti-Ro antibody

6. Which of the following is NOT a contraindication for organ donation?
   a. Hepatitis C
   b. Previous transplant with immunosuppressants
   c. Motor neuron disease (MND)
   d. Uncontrolled hypertension with end organ impairment
   e. Carcinoma prostate

7. All the following are correct brain stem tests *except*:

a. Corneal reflex mediated via Vth and VIIth cranial nerves
b. Gag reflex mediated via IXth cranial nerve
c. Cold caloric test mediated via VIIIth and IIIrd cranial nerves
d. Cough reflex mediated via Xth cranial nerve
e. Pupillary reflex to mediated via IVth cranial nerve

8. **What is the usual time for vasospasm to set-in after aneurysmal subarachnoid hemorrhage (SAH)?**
   a. 24 hours to 14 days
   b. 7 to 14 days
   c. 3 days to 14 days
   d. 10 days to 14 days
   e. None of the above

9. **In cold water caloric reflex test for an intact brain, the direction of tonic deviation of eyes is:**
   a. Away from the cold ear
   b. Towards the cold ear
   c. Nystagmus
   d. No movement
   e. None of the above

10. **Tubercular Meningitis (TBM) is termed Multi-Drug Resistant (MDR) in the following instance:**
    a. Proven resistance to any 1st line ATT drug
    b. Proven resistance to INH
    c. Proven resistance to Rifampicin
    d. Proven resistance to both INH and Rifampicin
    e. None of the above

11. **Which of the following is true for the location of intracranial aneurysms?**
    a. 70% anterior and 30% posterior circulation
    b. 80% anterior and 20% posterior circulation
    c. 85–90% anterior and 10–15% posterior circulation
    d. 70% posterior and 30% anterior circulation
    e. Equal distribution between anterior and posterior

12. **The following are poor outcome predictors after intracranial brain hemorrhage (ICH) except:**
    a. ICH volume > 30 mL
    b. Infratentorial bleed
    c. GCS < 8/15 at presentation
    d. Satellite sign
    e. Essential hypertension

13. **The presence of 'Plateau Wave' on the intracranial pressure (ICP) trace suggests:**
    a. Sudden surges in ICP to 50 to 80 mm Hg lasting 5–20 minutes
    b. Smaller surges in ICP to 20 mm Hg for 1 to 2 minutes
    c. Failing compliance of the brain to ICP and risk for ischemia
    d. Interference artefact
    e. None of the above

14. **The presence of 'B waves' on the ICP trace suggest:**
    a. Sudden surges in ICP to 50 to 80 mm Hg lasting 5–20 minutes
    b. Smaller surges in ICP to 20 mm Hg for 1 to 2 minutes
    c. Failing compliance of the brain to ICP and risk for ischemia
    d. Interference artefact
    e. None of the above

15. **The presence of 'A waves' on the ICP trace suggest:**
    a. Sudden surges in ICP to 50 to 80 mm Hg lasting 5–20 minutes
    b. Smaller surges in ICP to 20 mm Hg for 1–2 minutes
    c. Failing compliance of the brain to ICP and risk for ischemia
    d. Interference artefact
    e. None of the above

16. **All the following are true for 'Vein of Galen' arteriovenous malformation (AVM) except:**
    a. Cannot be diagnosed until after birth
    b. First presentation of the child may be as heart failure
    c. Cranial bruit and prominent facial veins are common signs
    d. Careful serial embolization is the treatment of choice
    e. Untreated cases have a very high mortality

17. **Which one of the following is not a contraindication of plasmapheresis?**
    a. Pseudohyponatremia
    b. Hypercalcemia
    c. Autonomic dysfunction
    d. Active bleeding
    e. Severe sepsis

18. **Vertebral artery is a direct branch of the:**
    a. Internal carotid artery
    b. Posterior cerebral artery

c. Basilar artery
d. Subclavian artery
e. None of the above

19. Which one of the following is not a sign of Spinal Cord Injury?
    a. Unexplained hypotension
    b. Bradycardia
    c. Priapism
    d. Diaphragmatic breathing
    e. Spastic areflexia

20. Which of the following intervention/drug has proven benefit in the management of Traumatic Brain Injury (TBI)?
    a. Therapeutic hypothermia
    b. ICP monitoring and its treatment
    c. Magnesium sulphate
    d. Erythropoietin
    e. Simvastatin

21. In Herpes Simplex Encephalitis (HSE) which is false?
    a. Bi-modal age distribution with peaks at < 20 years and > 50 years of age
    b. One third of HSE occurs in children
    c. Neonatal HSE is predominantly caused by HSV-2
    d. Adult HSE is predominantly caused by HSV-1
    e. Steroids along with Acyclovir are the mainstay of treatment

22. In Adult, Gram negative meningitis, all are true *except*:
    a. Mostly nosocomial in head trauma and rarely community acquired in adults
    b. E. coli and Klebsiella account for over half the cases of Gram negative meningitis
    c. CSF Lactate is useful in confirming bacterial meningitis
    d. Dexamethasone is not recommended routinely for Gram negative meningitis as adjuvant therapy
    e. Typical treatment lasts for 14 days

23. Which of the following drugs cannot be used intrathecally or intraventricularly in meningitis?
    a. Tigecycline
    b. Amikacin
    c. Gentamicin
    d. Colistin
    e. Polymyxin B

24. Which is true for Mean Arterial Pressure (MAP)?
    a. MAP = Diastolic + 2/3 (Systolic – Diastolic)
    b. MAP = Systolic + 1/3 (Systolic – Diastolic)
    c. MAP is overall a better parameter for brain perfusion
    d. In neurocritical care patients transducer for MAP measurement is placed at Mid-axillary line
    e. MAP = CO × PVR ; accurately predicts MAP in routine ICU practice

25. Regarding INTERACT-2 trial for choice of a target for the systolic blood-pressure level in acute intracranial hemorrhage (ICH); all are true Except:
    a. Lowering systolic blood-pressure target of 110 to 139 mm Hg or a target of 140 to 179 mm Hg was compared
    b. No effect on death or disability than standard reduction to a target of 140 to 179 mm Hg
    c. Modified Rankin Scale (mRS) at 90 days showed no improvement
    d. CT scan of the head without the use of contrast material was obtained at 24 hours
    e. Intracranial pressure monitoring was not a part of the intervention

26. For invasive rhinocerebral mucormycosis which is *False*:
    a. Ethmoidal sinusitis is the commonest air sinusitis causing cerebral infection
    b. Ophthalmoplegia and proptosis are the commonest early signs
    c. Hyperbaric oxygen treatment is fungistatic
    d. Immunosuppressants and diabetes are leading risk factors
    e. Amphotericin is the only anti-fungal used in its treatment

27. Regarding brain abscess; all are true *except*:
    a. Hematogenous spread is the most common cause
    b. Patent foramen ovale (PFO) is a risk factor
    c. The only brain infection where lumbar puncture is not recommended
    d. *Streptococcus* is the most common causative organism
    e. Hypodense lesion with ring enhancement is the usual CT finding

28. Which of the following occur as CNS manifestations in HIV?
    a. CNS lymphoma
    b. Kaposi sarcoma
    c. Progressive multifocal leuco-encephalopathy
    d. Cryptococcal meningitis
    e. All of the above

29. Nutrition in neurocritical care, which is not true?
    a. Early enteral nutrition improves outcome
    b. Low osmolarity parenteral nutrition can be given via peripheral lines
    c. Ketones provide energy more efficiently to the brain than glucose
    d. Monitoring residual volume achieves higher caloric goals
    e. Not monitoring residual volume does not increase the risk of VAP

30. In acute disseminated encephalomyelitis (ADEM), which is not true?
    a. Autoimmune disease with a usual precursor viral illness
    b. 50%–70% have a good prognosis and recover fully
    c. Steroids are the first line treatment
    d. Methylprednisolone is preferred over Dexamethasone
    e. Plasmapheresis has no role in its treatment

31. In the Lund concept of TBI management, all are true *except*:
    a. It's a volume targeted approach to TBI management
    b. If ICP is elevated, a cerebral perfusion pressure (CPP) of 50 is considered acceptable
    c. Based on preserving osmotic pressure and reducing hydrostatic pressure
    d. Contradicts traditional CPP-intracranial pressure (ICP) paradigm
    e. Diuretics are contraindicated

32. Medical conditions NOT predisposing to SAH:
    a. Ehlers-Danlos syndrome
    b. Marfans syndrome
    c. Coarctation of aorta
    d. Polycystic kidneys
    e. Liver cirrhosis

33. Percentage of patients requiring external ventricular drain (EVD) for hydrocephalus in SAH is:
    a. 50%
    b. 75%
    c. 25%
    d. 5%
    e. 15%

34. What is the most likely diagnosis from the magnetic resonance angiography (MRA) and digital subtraction angiography (DSA) image below?

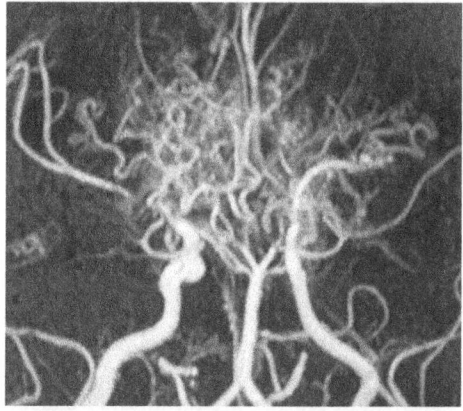

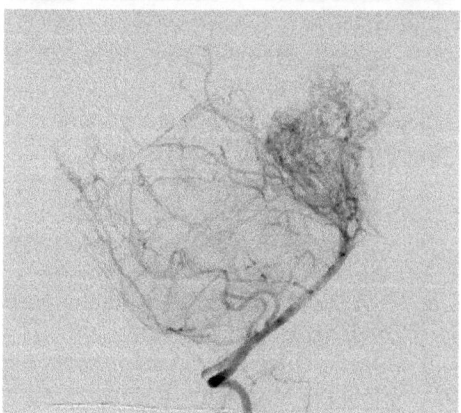

    a. Moyamoya disease
    b. Intracranial aneurysm
    c. TB vasculitis
    d. Meningitis
    e. None of the above

35. What is the most likely diagnosis from the following radiology image?

Neurointensive Care

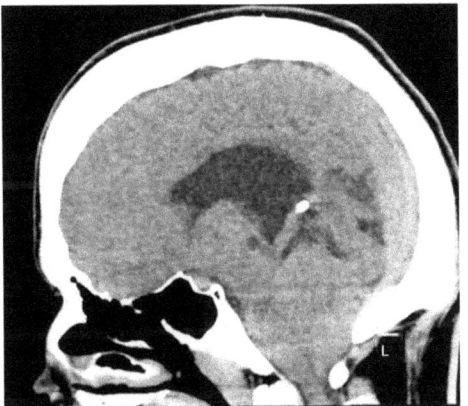

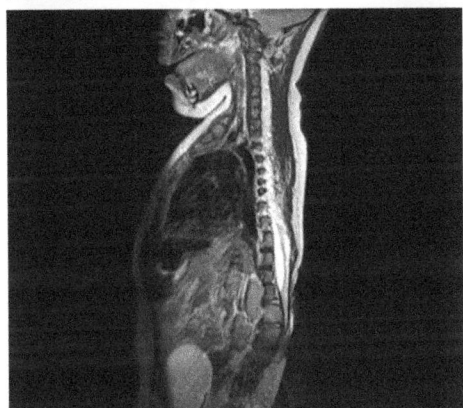

a. Arnold-Chiari malformation–Type 1
b. Moyamoya disease
c. Subarachnoid hemorrhage
d. Tumor
e. None of the above

36. Image EEG:

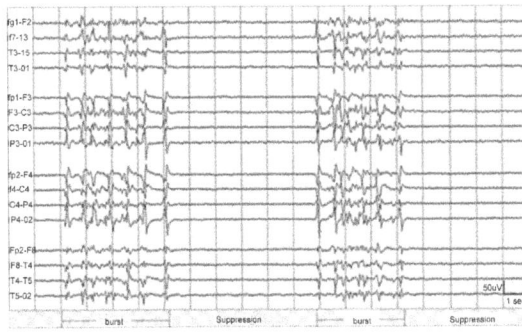

State the diagnosis from the EEG strip:
a. Status epilepticus
b. Brain dead
c. Burst suppression
d. Norma brain
e. None of the above

37. State the diagnosis from the EEG strip:

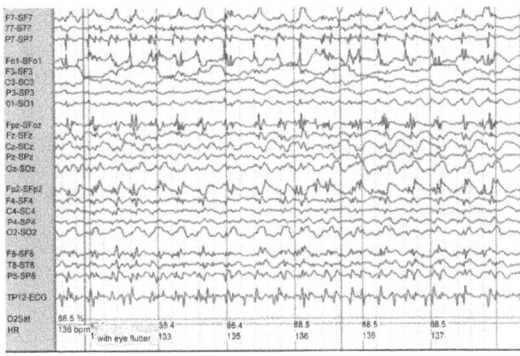

a. Status epilepticus
b. Brain dead
c. Burst suppression
d. Normal brain
e. None of the above

38. Consider TCD and DSA image and pick the correct statement:

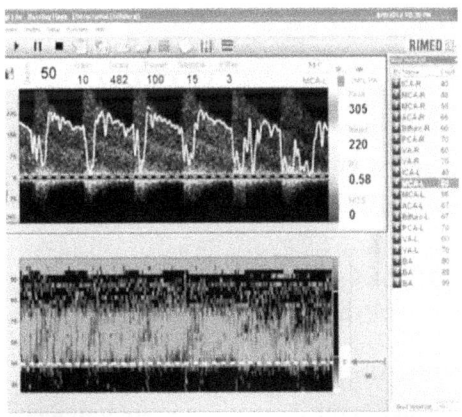

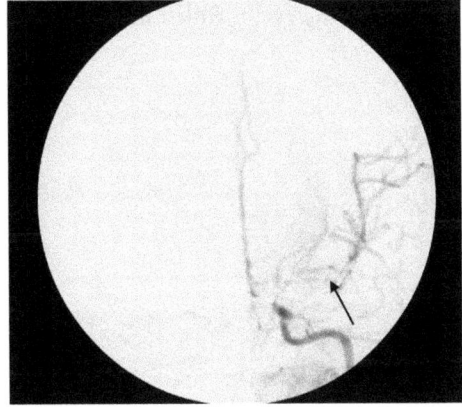

a. Image of DSA and TCD indicate MCA spasm
b. Milrinone is likely to be used for cerebral vasodilatation

c. Patient is likely to have right sided weakness
d. Nimodipine 60mg every 4 hours is indicated
e. All of the above

39. **Consider the following two images and answer the following statements:**

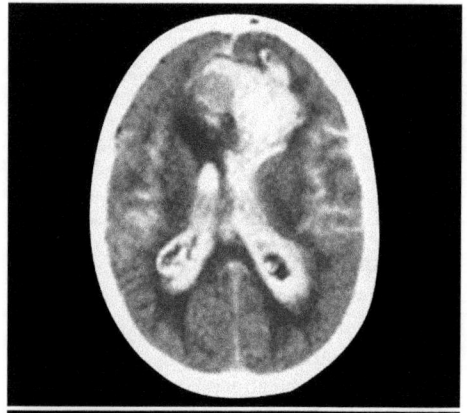

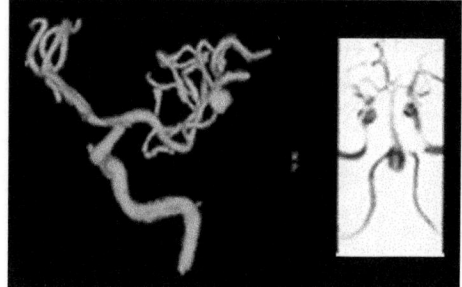

a. There is a basilar tip aneurysm on the DSA
b. There are multiple aneurysms on the DSA
c. Fischer Grade 4 on the CT head
d. Patient has WFNS Grade 4 SAH
e. All of the above

40. **Which is the most appropriate statement for the following graph which has ICP on the y axis?**

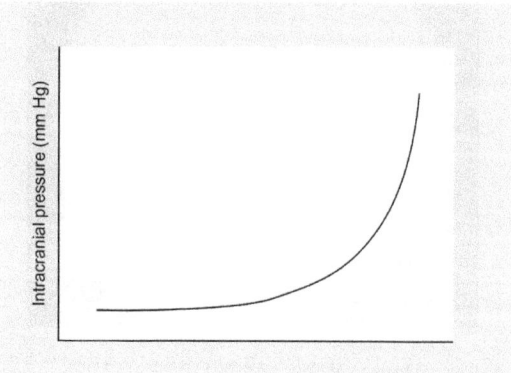

a. Depicts relation between cerebral blood flow arterial $paCO_2$
b. Depicts relation between ICP and cerebral volume
c. Depicts relation between cerebral blood flow and arterial pO_2
d. Depicts autoregulation of cerebral blood flow and MAP

41. **Which is the most appropriate statement for the following graph which has cerebral blood flow in mL/100 g/min on the y axis?**

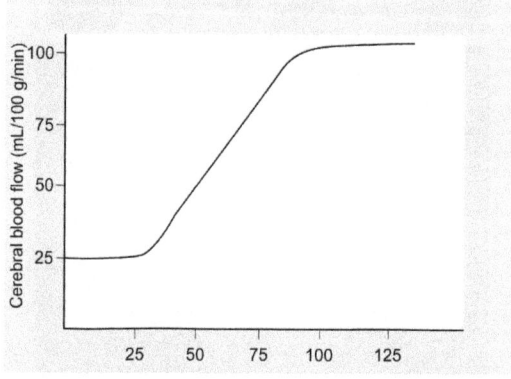

a. Depicts relation between cerebral blood flow arterial $paCO_2$
b. Depicts relation between intracranial pressure and cerebral volume
c. Depicts relation between cerebral blood flow and arterial pO_2
d. Depicts autoregulation of cerebral blood flow and MAP

42. **Which is the most appropriate statement for the following graph with cerebral blood flow in mL/100 g/min on the y axis?**

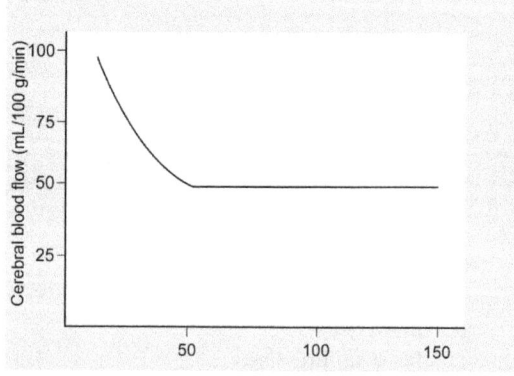

a. Depicts relation between cerebral blood flow arterial paCO₂
b. Depicts relation between intracranial pressure and cerebral volume
c. Depicts relation between cerebral blood flow and arterial pO₂
d. Depicts autoregulation of cerebral blood flow and MAP

43. Which is the most appropriate statement for the following graph?

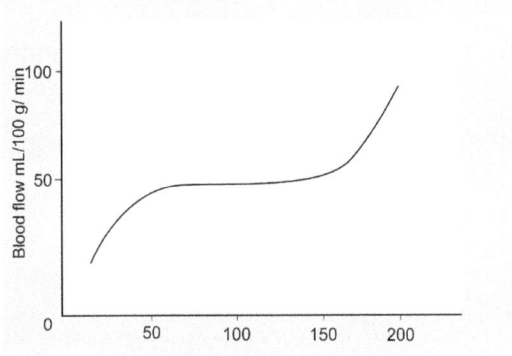

a. Depicts relation between cerebral blood flow and arterial paCO₂
b. Depicts relation between intracranial pressure and cerebral volume
c. Depicts relation between cerebral blood flow and arterial pO₂
d. Depicts autoregulation of cerebral blood flow and mean arterial pressure (MAP)

44. Regarding non-convulsive status epilepticus (NCSE), which one is not true?
a. Incidence can be as high as 48% in neuro ICU patients
b. Continuous EEG (cEEG) is better at diagnosing status than standard EEG
c. cEEG cannot diagnose brain ischemia
d. Cerebral blood flow and EEG are physiologically coupled together
e. Persistent lateral epileptiform discharges (PLEDs) are pathognomonic

45. A phenytoin loading dose was erroneously given as a bolus to a patient rather than an infusion. Which statement is most inappropriate?
a. Acute sodium channel blockade causes wide QRS complexes
b. Patient is prone to ventricular dysrhythmias
c. Calcium chloride is an antidote
d. Cerebellar features are seen in phenytoin toxicity
e. Intravenous phenytoin can be given faster than fosphenytoin

46. In syndrome of inappropriate antidiuretic hormone secretion (SIADH) all are true *except*:
a. Serum hyponatremia
b. Increased urinary sodium
c. Normal to low plasma osmolarity
d. Hypovolemic state requiring fluid boluses
e. Raised urinary osmolarity

47. In cerebral salt wasting syndrome, all are true *except*:
a. Serum hyponatremia
b. Increased urinary sodium
c. Hypovolemic state
d. Normal to high serum osmolarity
e. Low urinary osmolarity

48. Which statement holds true for cerebral microdialysis?
a. Can only be done in TBI to individualize CPP management
a. Gold tip of the probe must be sighted inside the injury site e.g. contusion
b. Lactate/pyruvate ration less than 25 indicate ischemia
c. Increase in glycerol is an indicator of neuronal cell membrane damage
d. Gives direct information for both glucose and oxygen in neuronal extracellular tissue

49. Which is FALSE about brain tissue oxygen (PbtO₂)?
a. Measures the partial pressure of oxygen in the intracellular neurons
b. Normal value ranges from 25–35 mm Hg
c. Less than 10 mm Hg for > 30 min correlates to high morbidity and mortality
d. Employs the Clark cell electrode to measure tissue oxygenation
e. The same probe can also measure the temperature in the affected brain

50. Regarding stress ulcer prophylaxis in neurocritical care, what is NOT TRUE?
a. All patients admitted in neurocritical care require stress ulcer prophylaxis
b. All patients ventilated in neurocritical care require stress ulcer prophylaxis

c. Incidence of upper GI bleeding in neuro-critical care unit is declining
d. Stress ulcer prophylaxis should be stopped as soon as enteral feed is established
e. H_2 receptor antagonists can cause encephalopathy

K Type Questions
[Marked True (T)/False (F)]

1. **Regarding diffuse axonal injury (DAI):**
   a. Decompressive craniectomy improves functional outcome as judged by Glasgow Outcome Scale (GOS) at 6 months
   a. Decompressive craniectomy improves survival as judged by GOS at 6 months
   b. Severity of clinical symptoms are disproportionate to the radiological findings
   c. DAI has got both a primary and a secondary component
   d. Microbleeds are a radiological marker for DAI

2. **Regarding deep vein thrombosis (DVT) prevention in TBI:**
   a. DVT risk increases with Traumatic Brain Injury (TBI) severity
   b. Nearly half the number of patients with TBI are at risk of developing DVT
   c. Sequential compression devices (SCD) significantly reduce the DVT risk in TBI
   d. Injury severity score > 15 is an independent risk predictor
   e. Low molecular weight heparin (LMWH) is contraindicated for treatment

3. **ICP based management in TBI:**
   a. Reduces in-hospital mortality
   b. Based on level 1 evidence
   c. Indicated for GCS 8 with abnormal CT scan
   d. Not indicated for GCS 8 with normal CT scan
   e. Is the mainstay for treatment of TBI patients

4. **Regarding hyperosmolar therapy with mannitol for raised ICP:**
   a. Mannitol is better than hypertonic saline (HTS)
   b. Mannitol increases the blood viscosity
   c. Can increase brain tissue oxygen ($PbtO_2$)
   d. Should not be used in hypovolemic patients
   e. Effective dose is 0.25–1 g/kg body weight

5. **Regarding hypertonic saline (HTS) for raised ICP:**
   a. HTS is the recommended drug/fluid of choice
   b. HTS causes a more intense and sustained reduction in ICP than an equivalent dose of mannitol
   c. Can increase brain tissue oxygen ($PbtO_2$)
   d. Contraindicated with serum sodium 145 meq/L
   e. Reduces extracellular glutamate and prevents neuronal damage

6. **Regarding cerebral perfusion pressure (CPP):**
   a. Recommended value for survival is 60–70 mm Hg
   b. Recommended value for favorable outcome is 60–70 mm Hg
   c. Higher CPP is required in patients with impaired auto-regulation
   d. Optimal CPP needs to be tailored to individual patients
   e. ARDS is a concern with aggressive CPP target > 75 mm Hg

7. **Post-traumatic epilepsy (PTE):**
   a. Is defined as recurrent seizures only after 7–14 days of injury
   b. Rate of sub-clinical seizures could be > 25%
   c. Vagus nerve stimulator is used for treatment
   d. Higher chances of developing epilepsy than the general population
   e. Can be diagnosed within 7 days of injury

8. **Risk factors for post-traumatic seizure (PTS) after head injury are:**
   a. Depressed skull fracture
   b. GCS < 10
   c. Immediate seizure or seizure at site
   d. Post-traumatic amnesia > 30 min
   e. Cortical contusions

9. **Regarding seizure prophylaxis in TBI:**
   a. Recommended only in severe head injury
   b. Levetiracetam is the recommended drug of choice
   c. Valproate is recommended for refractory seizures
   d. Ketamine is useful for refractory seizures
   e. Phenytoin is useful only in late post-traumatic seizures

10. **Tracheostomy in head injury:**
    a. Early tracheostomy improves outcome

b. Early tracheostomy reduces rate of VAP
c. Early tracheostomy increases the number of ventilator free days
d. Contraindicated in raised ICP
e. Aids neurological recovery

11. **Steroids in TBI:**
    a. Improve outcome if administered early
    b. Reduce ICP only if administered early
    c. Methylprednisolone is contraindicated in TBI
    d. Dexamethasone is better than methylprednisolone in reducing ICP
    e. Reduce brain edema by reducing vascular permeability

12. **Regarding external ventricular drain (EVD) in neuro ICU:**
    a. Does not accurately monitor ICP
    b. Zero mark should be at the mid axillary line
    c. Should never be clamped
    d. Is an uncommon cause of CNS infection
    e. Inserted in operating rooms have better outcomes than ICU insertions

13. **The following are risk factors for a poor outcome post aneurysmal subarachnoid hemorrhage (SAH):**
    a. Male sex
    b. Presence of comorbid conditions
    c. Posterior circulation aneurysm
    d. World Federation of Neurosurgeons (WFNS) grade IV
    e. Multiple aneurysms

14. **Proven therapies in the management of vasospasm include:**
    a. Triple H therapy
    b. Oral nimodipine
    c. Antifibrinolytics
    d. Balloon angioplasty
    e. IV Milrinone with intra-arterial vasodilation

15. **Regarding the following statements in SAH:**
    a. The ISAT study demonstrated a better outcome for coiled versus clipped aneurysms
    b. The overall case mortality for SAH is 10%
    c. Intraoperative hypothermia improves neurological outcome
    d. CT is 100% sensitive in detecting aneurysms
    e. Best results are at tertiary centers

16. **Regarding hyper acute thrombotic stroke service:**
    a. IV thrombolysis has better results than mechanical thrombectomy (MT)
    b. Combined IV thrombolysis and MT has best results
    c. MT has a higher procedural mortality than thrombolysis
    d. MT is only useful for distal clots
    e. IV thrombolysis is better for large vessel clots

17. **Regarding hyper acute thrombotic stroke service:**
    a. General anesthesia is contraindicated
    b. Sedation has better outcome
    c. Invasive monitoring is usually required intraoperatively
    d. Postoperative ventilation is a predictor of poor outcome
    e. Postoperative monitoring with TCD improves outcome

18. **Modified Rankin Scale (mRS):**
    a. Measures degree of disability in stroke patients
    b. Combines clinical and radiological parameters
    c. Lower score indicates a better outcome
    d. Score of 6 indicates a dead patient
    e. Most prevalent scoring system due to lack of any variability

19. **Using TCD in neuro ICU:**
    a. B Mode is the preferred mode to aid diagnosis of vasospasm
    b. The usual probe frequency emitted is in multiples of 2 MHz
    c. Most common insonation window used is the parietal region
    d. Only useful for middle cerebral artery analysis
    e. Less sensitive than cerebral angiography

20. **Guillain–Barré syndrome (GBS):**
    a. Central nervous system damage is mediated by the immune system
    b. Mortality is around 30%
    c. FVC < 15 mL/kg body weight is predictive of respiratory failure
    d. Anti-ganglioside antibodies is a typical diagnostic marker
    e. IV immunoglobulins and plasmapheresis are the mainstay of treatment

21. **In cavernous venous sinus thrombosis:**
    a. Most common causative agent is *Staphylococcus aureus*

b. MR venogram is the preferred imaging investigation
c. Steroids are contraindicated
d. Mortality can be around 30%
e. Anticoagulation with LMWH during acute illness improves outcome

22. **Consider the following for induced hypothermia to 33°C:**
    a. Decreases cardiac output
    b. Decreases metabolic rate
    c. Causes insulin resistance
    d. Can cause pancreatitis and raised serum amylase
    e. ABG samples corrected for temperature will show respiratory alkalosis

23. **In posterior reversible encephalopathy syndrome (PRES):**
    a. Most cases occur with hypertension or immunosuppression
    b. Common in preeclampsia
    c. Diagnosis is usually clinical
    d. Vasogenic parieto-occipital edema on MR is diagnostic
    e. Prompt treatment usually results in full recovery

24. **The following are usually suggestive of seizure activity in a comatose patient:**
    a. Tongue bite
    b. Incontinence
    c. Aspiration
    d. Pin point pupils
    e. Hypothermia

25. **The following investigations should be ordered in the management of a comatose patient:**
    a. Immediate blood glucose
    b. Serum ammonia
    c. Coagulation profile
    d. Electrolytes including Na, K, Ca, Mg
    e. Arterial blood gas analysis

26. **Supportive measures in the management of a comatose patient:**
    a. Recovery position
    b. Thiamine 50–100 mg
    c. 25 mL of 50% Dextrose
    d. Naloxone 400 mcg IV stat
    e. Flumazenil

27. **Regarding apnea test:**
    a. $PaCO_2$ is above 60 mm Hg with no spontaneous respirations is positive
    b. Chronic CO_2 retainers may have false positives
    c. Rate of increase of $PaCO_2$ in apneic patient is 3–6 mm Hg/min
    d. Core body temperature of at least 32°C is mandatory
    e. Euvolemia in the preceding 6 hours is a prerequisite

28. **Regarding extradural hematomas (EDH):**
    a. Usual cause is a dural venous bleed from bridging veins
    b. Usual cause is injury to the middle meningeal artery
    c. Common location is laterally over the cerebral hemispheres
    d. Can cause ipsilateral third nerve palsy
    e. Lucid interval can occur and causes higher mortality

29. **Regarding chronic subdural hematomas:**
    a. Usual cause is a dural venous bleed from bridging veins
    b. Usual cause is injury to the middle meningeal artery
    c. Appears biconvex on CT head image
    d. Burr hole evacuation of solid clot is the usual treatment
    e. Lower mortality than extradural haematomas

30. **Regarding autoregulation of cerebral blood flow (CBF):**
    a. Autoregulation maintains normal CBF between MAP of 50–150 mm Hg
    b. Curve is shifted to the left in chronic hypertension
    c. Ischemic threshold for cerebral blood flow = < 18 mL/100 g/min
    d. CBF is decreased by volatile anesthetic agents
    e. CBF is decreased by propofol

31. **Cerebral metabolic rate of oxygen consumption ($CMRO_2$):**
    a. Is 50 mL/min
    b. Is 3–3.8 mL/100 g/min
    c. 20% of total basal oxygen requirements
    d. Cerebral blood flow X arteriovenous oxygen content difference
    e. Is easily monitored in traumatic brain injury patients

32. **A 72-year-male with chronic AF on warfarin is presents with an acute subdural hematoma**

after a blunt head injury. Presenting GCS is E3V4M6 13/15 with stable vitals and normal blood test results except a raised INR = 4.1. The best options for treating the coagulopathy in ICU towards preparation for surgical evacuation are:
   a. 4 units of FFP stat if Prothrombin Complex Concentrate (PCC) is not available
   b. Appropriate dose of PCC if available
   c. Vitamin K 10 mg after 12 hours of presentation
   d. Point of care testing using Thromboelastography® (TEG®) and Thromboelastometry (ROTEM®)
   e. Wait upto 12 hrs for self-correction of INR for surgery

33. A 21-year-female presents in status epilepticus. Comment on the following statements:
   a. Lorazepam 4 mg IV over 1-2 minutes and repeat after 5 minutes if required
   b. Phenytoin loading if no response
   c. Intubate and ventilate if seizures continue
   d. Ketamine is useful in refractory seizures
   e. Inhalational sevoflurane for super-refractory seizures

34. Regarding Nimodipine:
   a. Level 1 evidence for treating post aneurysmal SAH vasospasm
   b. Best administered IV for vasospasm treatment
   c. Binds specifically to L type voltage gated calcium channels
   d. Beneficial effects cease after 7 days post ictus
   e. Should be administered after definitive treatment of the aneurysm

35. In Wernicke's encephalopathy:
   a. Most of the cases are diagnosed at postmortem
   b. Oral high dose Thiamine is life saving
   c. Hyperemesis gravidarum is a risk factor
   d. Untreated Wernicke's leads to Korsakoff's Psychosis
   e. No biological marker exists, diagnosis is usually clinical

36. For the International Subarachnoid Treatment (ISAT) study; 2003 and 2005:
   a. Landmark study revolutionizing the treatment of traumatic SAH
   b. Absolute risk reduction of 7.4% at 1 year mortality favoring coiled versus clipped aneurysms
   c. Intra procedural rupture greater in coiling than with clipping
   d. Post-procedure re-bleeding at first year greater with coiling than clipping
   e. Missing long-term follow-up was a shortcoming of this trial

37. In an ICP waveform of a compliant brain:
   a. P1 represents intracranial compliance
   b. P2 represents aortic valve closure
   c. P1 should have highest upstroke
   d. P1 is higher than P2 indicates intracranial hypertension
   e. P3 is called dicrotic wave

38. The following are usually seen in diabetes insipidus:
   a. High output of concentrated urine
   b. Urine output rate > 250 mL/hr
   c. Serum sodium > 150 mmol/L
   d. Urine osmolarity < 200 mosmol/L
   e. Uncommon after head injury

39. Regarding super refractory status epilepticus (SRSE):
   a. Status lasting is more than 24 hours or on withdrawal of anaesthetic
   b. Ketogenic diet is useful specially in pediatric patients
   c. Ketamine has shown beneficial results due to NMDA antagonism
   d. Magnesium infusion is useful adjuvant drug in treatment
   e. Immunotherapy with IV immunoglobulin has shown benefit

40. The following are true for burst suppression:
   a. Barbiturates can be used but propofol is ineffective
   b. Indicated in Refractory Status Epilepticus (RSE)
   c. Indicated in refractory raised ICP
   d. Indicated in intracranial aneurysmal clipping
   e. Hypertension is a common side effect

41. Burst Suppression Ratio (BSR):
   a. Measures the amount of time within an interval spent in the suppressed state
   b. BSR of 0 indicates that the brain is active
   c. BSR of 1 indicates that the brain has no electrical activity
   d. BSR and burst suppression probability are functionally the same
   e. A typical 'burst suppression' would have 5-10 bursts/minute

42. In tubercular meningitis:
    a. Cloudy CSF
    b. CSF glucose < 50
    c. CSF protein > 45
    d. CSF lymphocytes increased at a later stage
    e. CSF monocytes significantly increased

43. Regarding 'Terson Syndrome', consider the following:
    a. Is a condition of TBI with vitriolic intraocular hemorrhage
    b. Usually due to retinal venous hypertension
    c. Fundoscopic is the gold standard for diagnosis
    d. Predictor of higher mortality in SAH
    e. More associated with posterior circulation aneurysms

44. Autonomic dysreflexia from spinal cord injury:
    a. Develops with neurological spinal injury level at or above T6 level
    b. Most common cause of Bladder and Bowel dysfunction
    c. Sympathetic prevail above the level of injury
    d. Parasympathetic prevail below the level of injury
    e. Baroreceptor response is preserved in this condition

45. Following constitute a normal CSF analysis:
    a. CSF Lactate 3.5–8.0 mmol/L
    b. CSF Glucose 50–80 mg/dL
    c. CSF Protein 20–45 mg/dL
    d. CSF Lymphocytes 0–4
    e. CSF Chloride 80–90

46. What is true/false in the following statements regarding this microdialysis chart in a SAH patient?

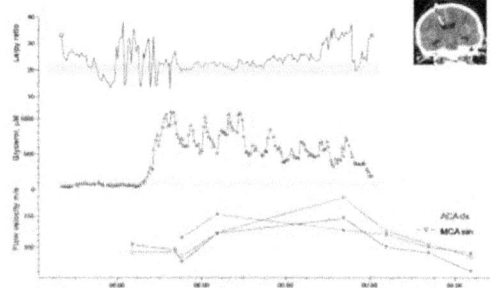

Microdialysis Graph: Lactate/pyruvate ratio; Glycerol and TCD Flow Velocity

   a. Indicates normal brain activity
   b. Indicates ischemia as seen by the suddenly rising lactate/pyruvate ratio above normal levels from initial downward trend
   c. Dramatic increase in glycerol indicates brain damage
   d. TCD flow velocity shows spasm much later than the biomarkers
   e. Tip of the EVD is seen in the ventricles in the CT

47. Regarding NIHSS Score:
    a. Tool to quantify the impairment caused by a brain space occupying lesion (SOL)
    b. About 11 items carrying a score of 0-4 for each
    c. Maximum possible score is 42
    d. Score of 0 indicates normal function
    e. Validated tool for predicting patient outcome

48. Consider the following statements regarding pituitary adenomas:
    a. Postoperative steroids are routinely required
    b. Hyponatremia is a common postoperative problem
    c. CSF leak is a risk factor for meningitis
    d. Transsphenoidal microsurgery is reserved for large tumours
    e. Diabetes insipidus is not a known complication

49. In pediatric neurosurgical patients:
    a. Location of majority of the tumors is infratentorial
    b. Increase in ICP is compensated by increase in size of the skull
    c. Posterior fossa tumors are least likely to have raised ICP
    d. Most common tumor is craniopharyngioma
    e. CMRO2 is higher in the pediatric age group

50. The following are used for the detection of venous air embolism:
    a. Transesophageal echocardiography
    b. Oesophageal stethoscope
    c. End tidal carbon dioxide sampling
    d. Pulmonary artery pressure monitoring
    e. Transcranial doppler (TCD)

51. A 25-year-old female presented with a history of fever, confusion, right sided weakness for 3 days duration. Except a cold sore on the lip, there is no other positive clinical finding:
    a. CT scan is useful as first investigation of choice
    b. Lumbar puncture should be done immediately in emergency department itself

c. Most likely diagnosis is Viral meningitis
d. Acyclovir and Cephalosporin should be empirically started
e. Most likely diagnosis is herpes simplex encephalitis (HSE)

52. A 24-year-old motorcyclist presented with a history of fall on the right side from his motorcycle after a RTA.

    Non-contrast CT head is shown in Figs. A and B.
    a. CT head is typical of an acute subdural hematoma (SDH)
    b. CT head is typical of an acute extradural hematoma (EDH)
    c. Ruptured dural venous vessels are likely to be responsible for the hematoma
    d. A 'Lucid interval' is quite possible in the above scenario
    e. A skull bone fracture is seen on the left side

53. A 74-year-old gentleman presented to the outpatients department with a 4 week history of generalized weakness, bouts of confusion and poor appetite. His GCS was 15/15 with grade 4 power in all 4 limbs. His comorbidities included hypertension, type-2 diabetes for which he was on an ace inhibitor, metformin, and aspirin. A CT/MR head is shown in Figs. A and B:
    a. His clinical and radiological findings do not match and this is an incorrect scan
    b. The scans show an acute SDH on the right side
    c. The scans show a chronic SDH on the right side
    d. The scans show an acute extradural hematoma on the right side
    e. The patent requires a craniotomy for hematoma evacuation

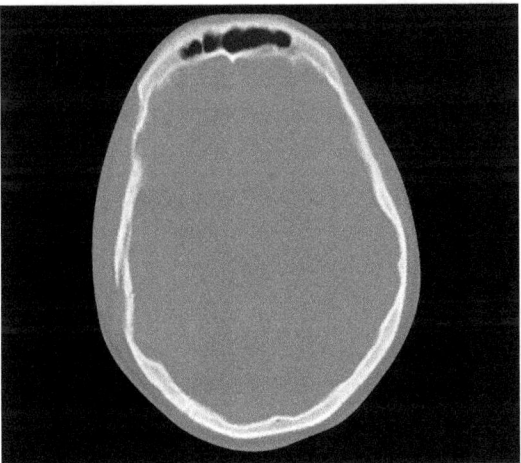

Fig. A

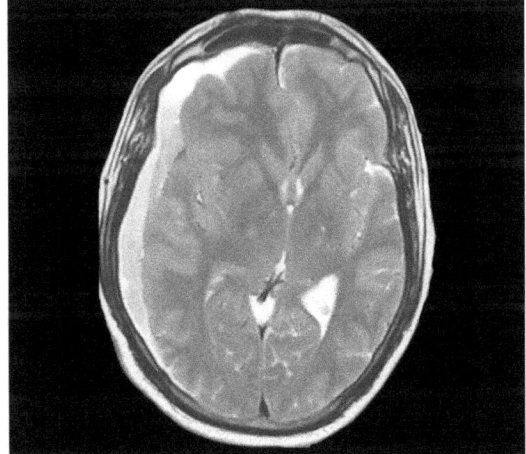

Fig. A

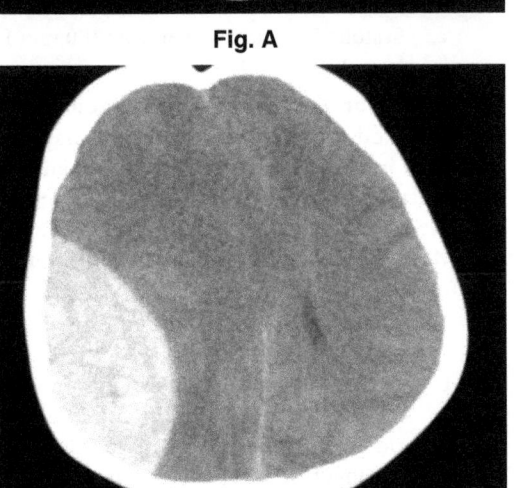

Fig. B

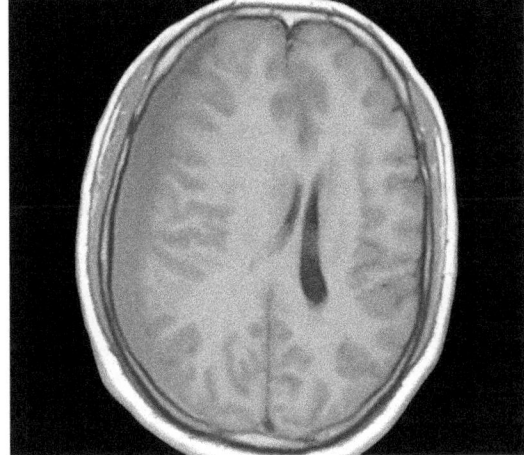

Fig. B

54. A 52-year-old female underwent an uneventful transsphenoidal resection of a pituitary macroadenoma. She was recovering appropriately in the postoperative setting when 2 hours post-surgery, she had a witnessed seizure.

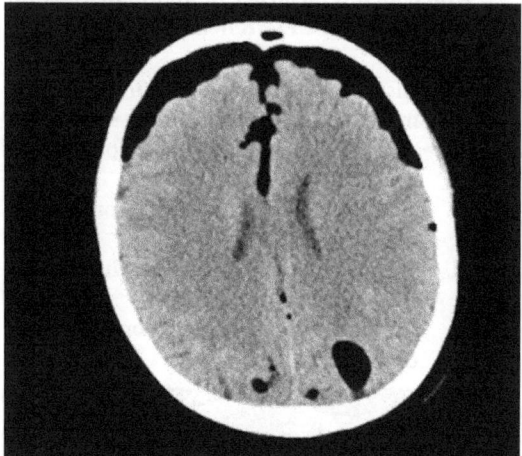

Fig. A

A non-contrast CT scan of the head revealed in Fig. A finding. Consider the following statements:
   a. The most likely cause for the seizure is pneumocephalus
   b. Risk factors for pneumocephalus include hyperventilation and intraoperative osmotherapy
   c. An urgent craniotomy to decompress the brain is an appropriate option
   d. High-flow nasal oxygen is a useful treatment option
   e. Mount Fuji sign is seen in tension pneumocephalus

55. A 64-year-old woman presented with a basal ganglia bleed with a presenting GCS of E3V3M5. Post 48 hours presentation she was intubated and ventilated in the ICU and was having episodic bradycardia.
   The following are true:
   a. The ICH score is invalid in this case due to intraventricular extension
   b. An EVD to drain CSF is urgently required
   c. Poor prognostication signs present on the CT scan
   d. Most likely cause is intracranial aneurysm rupture

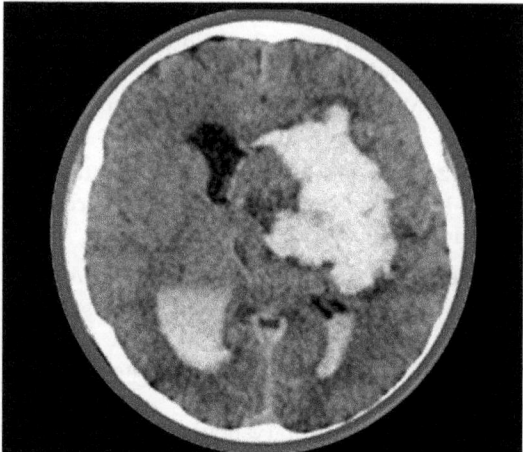

Fig. A

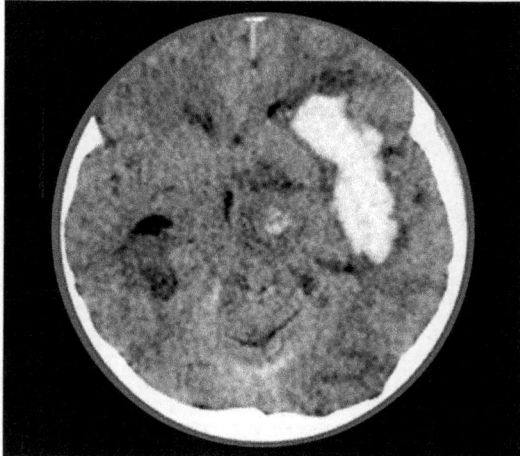

Fig. B

   e. Systolic BP should be at least 160 mm Hg to maintain CPP

56. A 29-year-woman had presented with a confused state after a sudden collapse at work in the last 6 hours. Her CT head non-contrast and DSA is shown in Figs. A and B. She is transferred to the neurointensive care with a GCS of E3V4M6 (13/15). Consider the following:
   a. The CT head is suspicious of a right MCA aneurysm bleed
   b. Tranexamic acid is useful in prevention of re-bleeding in early presenting cases
   c. Definitive treatment is surgical clipping of the aneurysm as endovascular treatment is not possible

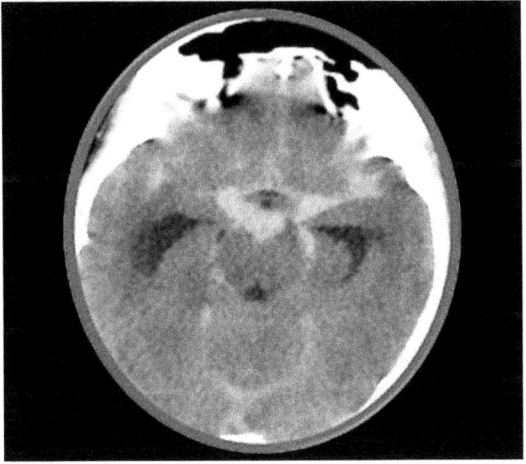

Fig. A

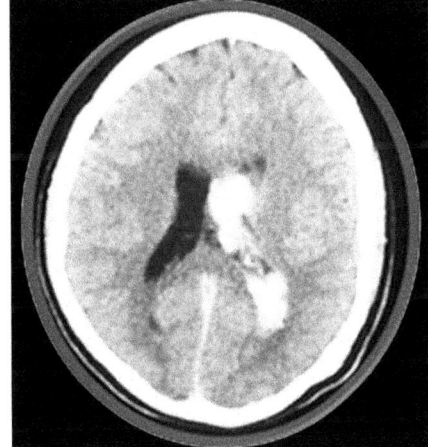

Fig. A

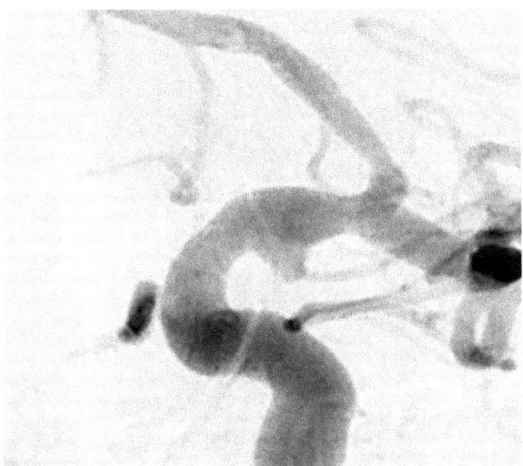

Fig. B

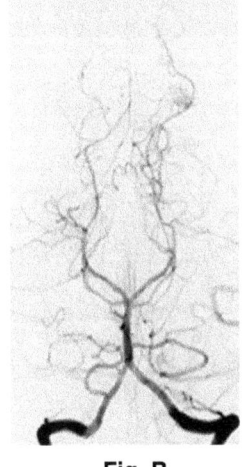

Fig. B

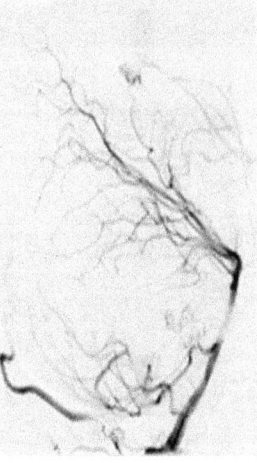

Fig. C

d. Nimodipine 60 mg every 4 hours per oral route must be started immediately
e. She could get delayed cerebral vasospasm until up to further 14 days

57. A 57-year-old male is ventilated in the neurointensive care with intraventricular hemorrhage from an AVM with a presenting GCS of 11/15.

The scans and DSA are shown in Figs. A to C. His ICH volume is 28 mL with no infratentorial extension.
   a. This patient's ICH score is 2
   b. ICH score is a validated clinical grading score and was not designed to prognosticate mortality
   c. Predicted mortality for this ICH score is less than 30%
   d. CT blood volume of more than 30 mL is a poor sign on ICH score
   e. Endovascular treatment to embolize the AVM should be attempted to prevent further bleeding

58. A 64-year-old is in ventilated in neuro ICU for 6 days-post-intracerebral hematoma. He has suffered two seizure episodes for which he is on appropriate anticonvulsants. His serum sodium is 118 mmol/L. The following are likely towards the diagnosis of SIADH.
   a. Urinary Na is less than 18 mmol/L
   b. Treatment by water restriction

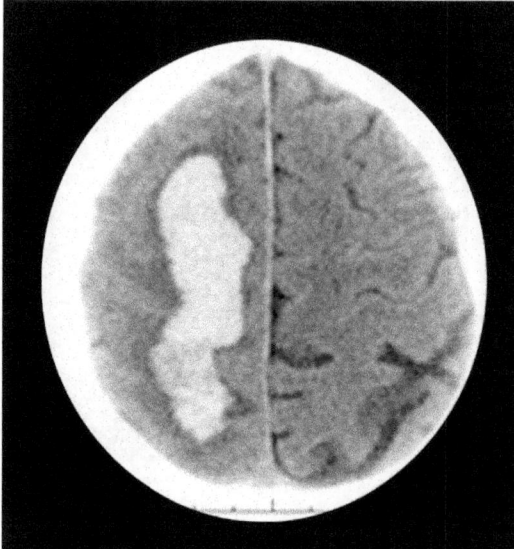

Fig. A

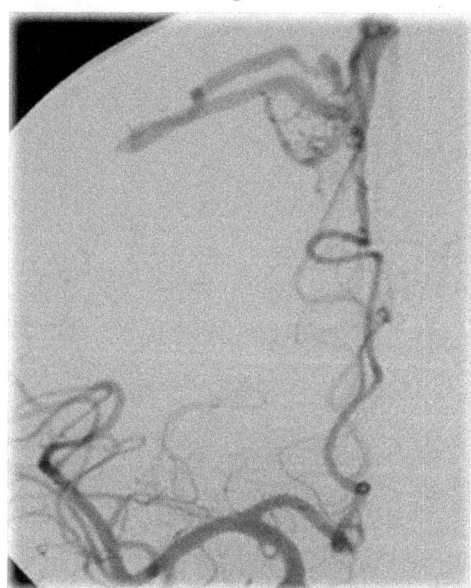

Fig. B

c. Plasma osmolality is greater than urinary osmolarity
d. Pitting oedema
e. Hypovolaemia is likely in this case

59. A 47-year-old woman with rheumatic heart disease presented with a 5-day history of headache, fever, lethargy and confusion. On examination she had right sided weakness and brisk reflexes. Her echocardiography was positive for mitral valve vegetations whilst her scans and DSA revealed a hemorrhage from a likely ruptured mycotic aneurysm.

The following are true:
a. Mycotic aneurysms are common complications of patients with infective endocarditis
b. Viridans streptococci and Staph aureus are common causative organisms
c. Endovascular therapy should be considered for ruptured mycotic aneurysms
d. IV antibiotic therapy alone for at least 6 weeks has shown benefit for unruptured mycotic aneurysms
e. Any cardiac corrective surgeries should await unless there is left heart failure from infective endocarditis

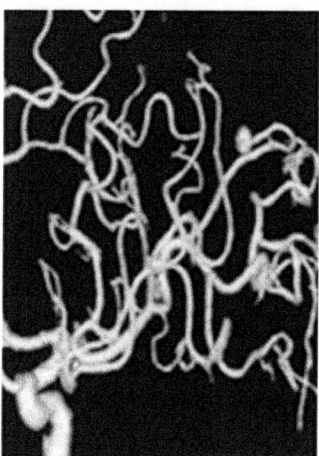

Fig. A

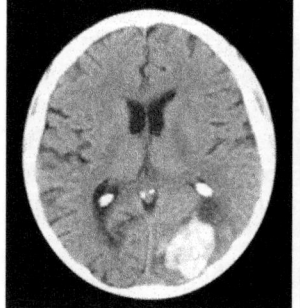 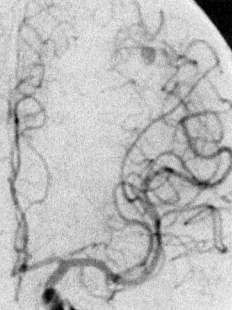

Fig. B Fig. C

60. A 58-year-old male presented to emergency with right sided weakness, headache and history of collapse. In the ED, he was conscious, oriented with right hemiparesis.

Blood pressure was elevated to 188/95 whilst other parameters were normal.

CT non-contrast head and CT angiography is shown in Figs. A to C. Consider the following in this patient's further treatment:
  a. IV thrombolysis is contraindicated due to intracerebral bleed seen on the CT
  b. Mechanical thrombectomy with bridging thrombolysis is most suited
  c. Scan shows a hyperdense MCA sign due to clot in the left MCA
  d. The above scan and finding is associate with poor outcome
  e. It would be prudent to lower the presenting blood pressure

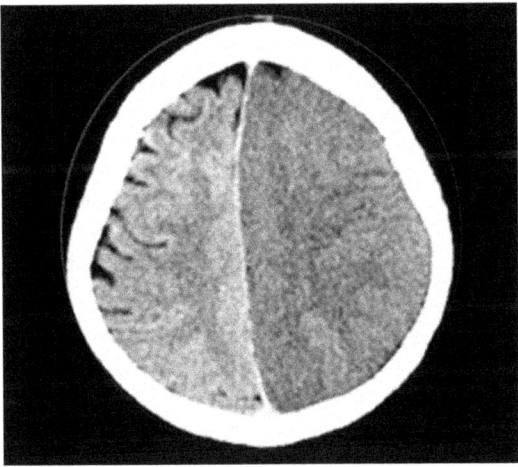

Fig. B

  a. CT shows a complete left internal carotid artery infarction
  b. There are signs of raised ICP
  c. An urgent decompressive craniectomy should be considered
  d. Decompressive craniectomy is likely to improve outcome
  e. Medical management with hypertonic saline is a better treatment option than decompressive craniectomy

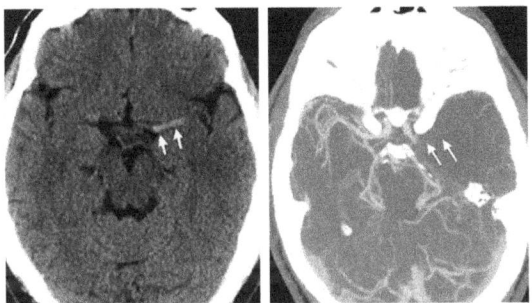

Fig. A   Fig. B

61. A 63-year-old female is 4 days post admission in the neurocritical care unit after presenting with a right sided stroke which was outside the window period. She is currently ventilated and the non-contrast CT head is shown in Figs. A and B:

62. A 42-year-old woman on oral contraceptive pill (OCP) presented with a fluctuating GCS and a history of preceding headache with vomiting of 2 weeks duration. All blood results were within normal limits.

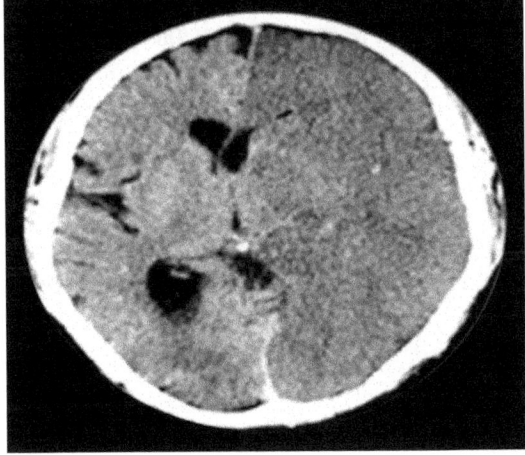

Fig. A

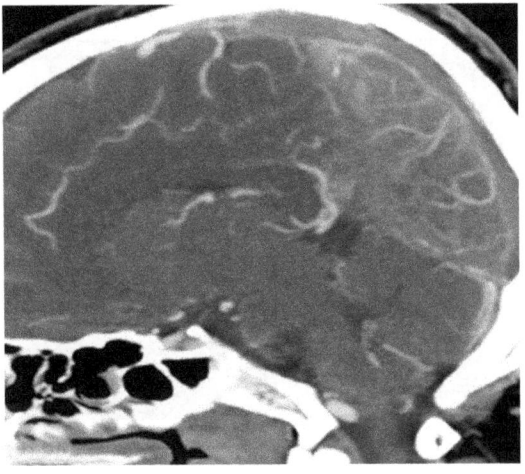

Fig. A

A CT venogram revealed a superior sagittal sinus thrombosis. The following are true:
a. OCP is a known risk factor for cerebral venous sinus thrombosis
b. Venous infarcts are present after some days unlike arterial infarcts and are present in at least 50% cases of cerebral venous sinus thrombosis
c. Heparin is the mainstay of the treatment
d. Endovascular heparin at the site of clot is a viable treatment option
e. Dural AV fistula is a known complication

63. A 48-year-old immunocompetent male presented in a confused and drowsy state with a history of right sided earache and ear discharge for 7 days with intermittent fever. All serum investigations were normal except a raised CRP and white cell counts.

A MRI brain revealed the above findings and a diagnosis of Brain Abscess was postulated. What are the next treatment options?
a. Conservative treatment with broad spectrum antibiotics only until ear discharge dries up
b. Surgical drainage of brain abscess along with broad spectrum antibiotics
c. Candida is the most common cause of Brain abscesses
d. Risk Factors for brain abscess include endocarditis, dental infections, patent foramen ovale (PFO)
e. Aureus *staphylococcus* is the common pathogen isolated in Brain abscess associated with Otitis Media or Dental infections

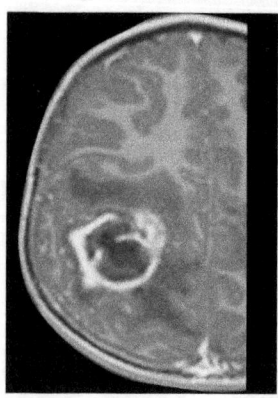
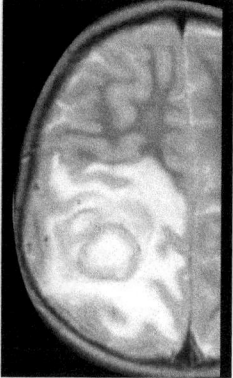

Fig. A   Fig. B

64. A 67-year-old hypertensive, diabetic female post on-pump prolonged CABG is admitted in the ICU and is failing to show any signs of neurological response.

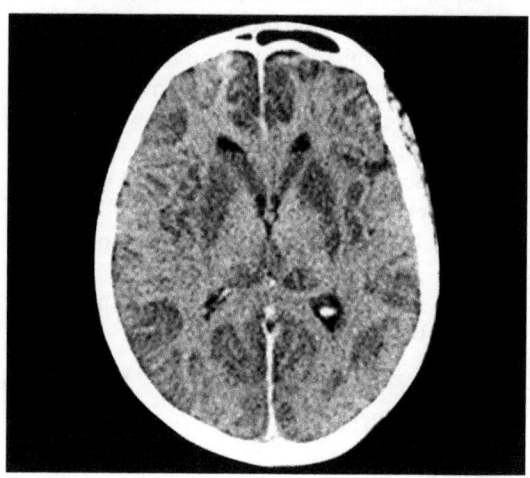

Fig. A

With the above scan findings, the most likely diagnosis is:
a. Nonconvulsive status epilepticus
b. Hypoxic-ischemic encephalopathy
c. Acute ischemic stroke
d. Infective endocarditis
e. Herpes simplex encephalitis

65. A 35-year-old female presenting with fever, confusion and agitation. No significant past history. Blood results show a marginally raised primarily lymphocytic white cell count. CSF from lumbar puncture did not show any growth on PCR yet. The MRI scan findings are as shown in Figs. A and B. The following are true:
a. MRI typical of Cerebral Venous Sinus Thrombosis
b. MRI typical of herpes Simplex Encephalitis
c. HSV encephalitis has high mortality
d. Usually presents with bilateral affection of the temporal lobes
e. Plasmapharesis is known to improve survival

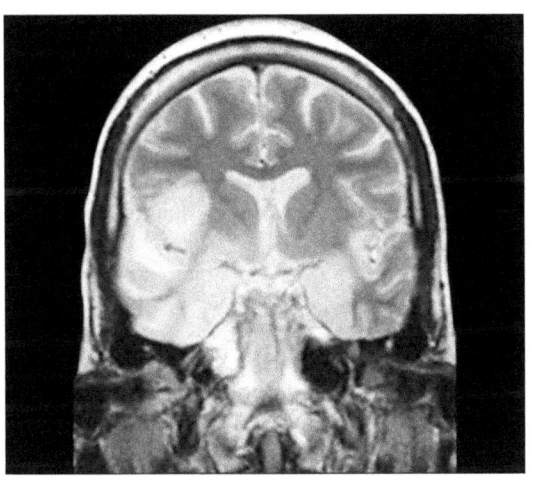
Fig. A

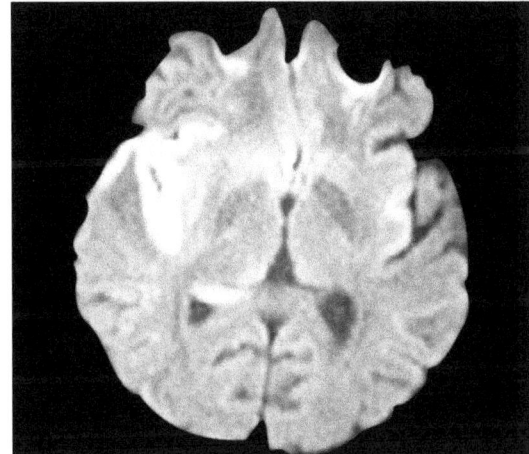
Fig. B

ANSWERS

A Type Answers

Q1. Answer a

This lateralization is not seen in any of the other syndromes. In BSS there is damage to one half of the spinal cord, resulting in paralysis and loss of proprioception on the ipsilateral side and loss of pain and temperature on the contralateral side of the lesion. It can be caused by trauma, tumors, infection or inflammation but by far the most common cause is penetrating injury to the spinal cord.

Ranga U, Aiyappan SK. Brown Séquard Syndrome. The Indian Journal of Medical Research. 2014;140(4):572-3.

Q2. Answer a

Uncal Herniation is the most common type of transtentorial herniation where the inner most part of the temporal lobe, the uncus, is compressed to an extent that it herniates towards the brainstem. The downward movement is across the tentorial incisura compressing the posterior cerebral arteries. It also squeezes the 3rd cranial nerve affecting the parasympathetic input of the eye causing pupillary dilatation. It can cause contralateral hemiparesis and not ipsilateral.

Stevens RD, Shoykhet M, Cadena R. Emergency Neurological Life Support: Intracranial Hypertension and Herniation. Neurocritical care. 2015; 23 (Suppl 2):S76-S82.

Q3. Answer c

Bridging thrombolysis and thrombectomy after CT head confirms thrombotic stroke. Once a hemorrhage is ruled out by the CT head and a thrombotic major vessel stroke identified with a CTA, bridging thrombolysis is started immediately and the patient is shifted to the intervention lab for a mechanical thrombectomy. If the thrombotic stroke is a small vessel distal stroke, then thrombolysis is still given and patient is reviewed for resolution of symptoms and considered for thrombectomy. Recent trials have confirmed that the best outcome after thrombotic stroke is via both a bridging thrombolysis and mechanical thrombectomy for major vessel strokes, rather than the two options practiced individually in isolation.

Muralidharan R. External ventricular drains: Management and complications. Surgical Neurology International. 2015;6(Suppl 6):S271-S274.

Q4. Answer e

GOS of 5 indicates full independence for in-house daily activities but not returned to work. GOS is a clinical tool used to categorize the outcome of patients after traumatic head injury as follows:
1. Death
2. Persistent vegetative state with minimal response
3. Severe disability
4. Moderate disability
5. Good recovery

Weir J, Steyerberg EW, Butcher I et al. Does the extended glasgow outcome scale add value to the conventional glasgow outcome scale? Journal of Neurotrauma. 2012;29(1):53-8.

Q5. Answer a

Miller Fischer (MF) syndrome is a clinically and serologically well-defined syndrome with a triad of ataxia, ophthalmoplegia and areflexia and is considered to be a variant of the GBS. The Anti-GQ1b ganglioside antibody is specifically associated with the MF syndrome whilst Anti GD3, Anti GM1 correlate more to GBS.

Winer JB. An update in Guillain-Barré syndrome. Autoimmune Diseases. 2014;2014:793024.

Q6. Answer e

Hepatitis C, previous transplant with immunosuppressants, MND, uncontrolled hypertension with end organ impairment are contraindications for organ transplantation. All of the above are contraindications to organ transplantation. However, there are some case reports of organ transplants with donors who have received previous immunosuppressants. It is likely that in the future there will be more relative contraindications than complete absolute ones. However, previous infective exposure to diseases like Hepatitis C, HIV or Hepatitis B remains absolute contraindications.

> Kumar L. Brain death and care of the organ donor. Journal of Anaesthesiology, Clinical Pharmacology. 2016;32(2):146-52.

Q7. Answer e

Brain stem reflexes are generated via the following cranial nerves: (1) Corneal reflex is mediated via Vth and VIIth cranial nerves; (2) Gag reflex of posterior pharyngeal valve via IXth cranial nerve; (3) Cold caloric testing via VIIIth and IIIrd cranial nerves; (4) Cough reflex from bronchial stimulation via Xth cranial nerve; (5) Pupillary reflex to incidental light via IIIrd cranial nerve and not the IVth cranial nerve.

> Dhanwate AD. Brainstem death: A comprehensive review in Indian perspective. Indian Journal of Critical Care Medicine : Peer-reviewed, Official Publication of Indian Society of Critical Care Medicine. 2014;18(9):596-605.

Q8. Answer c

Delayed cerebral vasospasm is a dreaded complication of SAH and is responsible for a significant proportion of comorbidity. It can set in from as early as the 3rd postictal day until 2 weeks postictal. There are case reports of vasospasm happening up to 21 days postictal. The most important intervention to prevent this is regular Nimodipine 60 mg every four hours as soon as possible from the time of the ictus to up to 4 weeks postictal. It is also important to keep the patients euvolemic and prevent dehydration. High-risk patients should undergo regular transcranial doppler (TCD) to identify radiological vasospasm early so that it can be treated and development of clinical vasospasm can be avoided.

> Connolly ES, Rabinstein AA et al. Guidelines for the management of aneurysmal subarachnoid hemorrhage stroke. 2012;STR.

Q9. Answer a

Caloric test is a test of the vestibulo-occular reflex that involves irrigating the auditory canal with either cold or warm water. This method was developed by Robert Bárány who won a Nobel Prize in 1914 for this discovery. Under normal conditions, the fast phase of the nystagmus to the cold water stimulus is to the opposite side while it is towards the same side on irrigation with warm water. In brain dead patients, the fast phase of the nystagmus will be absent as it is controlled by the cerebrum, hence the response to cold irrigation will be to the same side. Hot and cold water produce currents in opposite directions and therefore a horizontal nystagmus in opposite directions. One mnemonic used to remember the FAST direction of nystagmus is COWS. COWS: Cold Opposite, Warm Same. Cold water = FAST phase of nystagmus to the side opposite from the cold water filled ear. Warm water = FAST phase of nystagmus to the same side as the warm water filled ear. In other words: Contralateral when cold is applied and ipsilateral when warm is applied.

> Dhanwate AD. Brainstem death: A comprehensive review in Indian perspective. Indian Journal of Critical Care Medicine : Peer-reviewed, Official Publication of Indian Society of Critical Care Medicine. 2014;18(9):596-605.

Q10. Answer d

MDR TBM is applied when there is proven resistance to both INH and Rifampicin and not just either of the drugs. When the resistance pattern spreads to most first line drugs, it is called Extensive Drug resistance (XDR) TBM. There is increasing incidence of MDR & XDR TB meningitis cases in India and South East Asia and the trend requires revisiting of the public health policies surrounding its disease burden and management.

> Wang T, Feng GD, Pang Y et al. High rate of drug resistance among tuberculous meningitis cases in Shaanxi province, China. Scientific Reports. 2016;6:25251.

Q11. Answer c

Most of the intracranial aneurysms are located anteriorly in the circle of Willis, most commonly at the junction/bifurcation of the internal carotid, anterior cerebral, the middle cerebral or the anterior communicating. The remaining posterior ones are only 10-15% and are predominantly in the vertebral, basilar tip or the posterior cerebral arteries. The anterior ones are easier to treat whilst the posterior ones are difficult and carry a slightly higher morbidity and mortality.

> Diringer MN. Management of aneurysmal subarachnoid hemorrhage. Critical care medicine. 2009;37(2):432-40.

Q12. Answer e

ICH scoring is used to classify intracerebral hemorrhage and includes the following parameters: Poor GCS, Age > 80 years, Intraventricular extension, Infratentorial extension and volume of the clot > 30 mL all are poor indicators of a good outcome. "Satellite sign: Presence of high density starry dots around the hemorrhage" are a bad prognostic sign in ICH. Essential hypertension is a known cause but not an outcome predictor.

> Rathor MY, Rani MFA, Jamalludin AR, et al. Prediction of functional outcome in patients with primary intracerebral hemorrhage by clinical-computed tomographic correlations. Journal of Research in Medical Sciences: The Official Journal of Isfahan University of Medical Sciences. 2012;17(11):1056-62.

Q13. Answer a

Plateau Wave in ICP = Sudden surges in ICP to 50 to 80 mm Hg lasting 5–20 minutes
B wave in ICP = Smaller surges in ICP to 20 mm Hg for 1 to 2 minutes
A waves in ICU = Failing compliance of the brain to raised ICP with risk for ischemia.

> Pickard JD, Czosnyka M. Management of raised intracranial pressure. Journal of Neurology, Neurosurgery, and Psychiatry. 1993;56:845-58.

Q14. Answer b

Lundberg B waves are oscillations of ICP at a frequency of 0.5 to 2 waves/min and are associated with an unstable ICP. Lundberg B waves are possibly the result of cerebral vasospasm, because during the occurrence of these waves, increased velocity in the middle cerebral artery can be demonstrated on TDS.

> Pickard JD, Czosnyka M. Management of raised intracranial pressure. Journal of Neurology, Neurosurgery, and Psychiatry. 1993;56:845-58.

Q15. Answer c

Lundberg A waves "or plateau waves" are steep increases in ICP lasting for 5 to 10 minutes. They are always pathological and represent reduced compliance and intracranial hypertension indicative of early brain herniation.

> Pickard JD, Czosnyka M. Management of raised intracranial pressure. Journal of Neurology, Neurosurgery, and Psychiatry. 1993;56:845-58.

Q16. Answer a

Vein of Galen AVM can be diagnosed before birth in-vivo, as well; they have a high mortality and require careful serial embolizations. If left untreated it causes increased intracranial blood volume and flow leading to pressure symptoms and may cause cardiac failure in extreme cases due to severe shunting. They need a high index of suspicion and prompt treatment.

> Karanam LSP, Baddam SR, Joseph S. Endovascular management of vein of Galen aneurysm malformation: A series of two case reports. Journal of Pediatric Neurosciences. 2011;6(1):32-5.

Q17. Answer b

Hypocalcemia is a contraindication of plasmapheresis. It is a side effect of plasmapheresis. Sepsis, autonomic dysfunction, coagulopathy, hypo or pseudohyponatremia are all absolute contraindications.

> Nguyen TC, Kiss JE, Goldman JR, et al. The role of plasmapheresis in critical illness. Critical Care Clinics. 2012;28(3):453-68.

Q18. Answer d

Vertebral is a direct branch from the Subclavian artery on both sides. Each vessel courses superiorly along each side of the neck to merge inside the skull with the opposite vertebral to form the basilar artery. It is important to rule out vertebral artery dissection in severe or suspected neck trauma cases as this is one of the most common missed injuries of the vertebral arteries.

> Yuan SM. Aberrant origin of vertebral artery and its clinical implications. Braz J Cardiovasc Surg. 2016;31(1):52-9.

Q19. Answer e

Spinal Cord injury leads to flaccid areflexia, bradycardia, hypotension, priapism, and diaphragmatic breathing. It is important to recognize and treat spinal shock which leads to severe cardiovascular compromise due to temporary or permanent loss of sympathetic tone.

Van Middendorp JJ, Goss B, Urquhart S, et al. Diagnosis and prognosis of traumatic spinal cord injury. Global Spine Journal. 2011;1(1):1-8.

Q20. Answer b

Only ICP monitoring and its management is proven in TBI management. Rest all options have no evidence for support. We are yet to find a magic bullet to treat traumatic head injury Statins, Magnesium, Hypothermia, Erythropoietin have all had RCTs that provide no evidence to support use in TBI.

Carney N, Totten AM, O'Reilly C, et al. Guidelines for the Management of Severe Traumatic Brain Injury, 4th Edition. Neurosurgery, 2016.

Q21. Answer e

HSV encephalitis is a serious neurological disease caused by HSV-1 virus in adults and children. In neonates, usually the HSV-2 is responsible for the disease. There is a bi-modal age distribution and typical bilateral temporal lesions are seen on the MRI. Treatment primarily rests with prompt initiation of IV Acyclovir. Steroids have no proven role.

Chaudhuri A, Kennedy P. Diagnosis and treatment of viral encephalitis. Postgraduate Medical Journal. 2002;78(924):575-83.

Q22. Answer e

Most are caused by nosocomial infections from E. coli and Klebsiella in most cases. CSF lactate is a useful marker in diagnosing and initiating treatment. Steroids have no proven role yet and the duration of treatment must last at least 21 days, with a combination therapy of drugs like 4th generation cephalosporins, carbapenems and/or colistin as required.

Pomar V, Benito N, López-Contreras J, et al. Spontaneous gram-negative bacillary meningitis in adult patients: characteristics and outcome. BMC Infectious Diseases. 2013;13:451.

Q23. Answer a

Tigecycline is not licensed to be used intrathecally or intraventricularly. Tigecycline does not significantly pass through blood brain barrier (BBB). There are a scanty no of case reports of using intraventricular tigecycline but it cannot be recommended yet for intrathecal/intraventricular routes. The drugs that can be used are Gentamicin, Polymyxin, Colistin and Amikacin.

Fang YQ, Zhan RC, Jia W, et al. A case report of intraventricular tigecycline therapy for intracranial infection with extremely drug resistant Acinetobacter baumannii. Medicine (Baltimore). 2017;96(31):e7703.

Q24. Answer c

Mean Arterial Pressure (MAP) is defined as the average pressure in the arteries during a single cardiac cycle and is thought to be a better indicator of perfusion. It can be calculated in many ways and one of the ways is MAP = Diastolic + 1/3 of the Pulse pressure. Its normal range is between 70–110 mm Hg.

Prabhakar H, Sandhu K, Bhagat H, et al. Current concepts of optimal cerebral perfusion pressure in traumatic brain injury. J Anaesth Clin Pharmacol. 2014;30(3):318-27.

Q25. Answer c

An acute hypertensive response in patients with intracerebral hemorrhage is common and may be associated with hematoma expansion and increased mortality. The second Intensive Blood Pressure Reduction in Acute Cerebral Hemorrhage Trial (INTERACT2) included patients with spontaneous intracerebral hemorrhage who had a systolic blood pressure of 150 to 220 mm Hg within 6 hours after symptom onset. The rate of death or disability among patients randomly assigned to intensive reduction in the systolic blood-pressure level, with a target systolic blood pressure of less than 140 mm Hg within 1 hour, was nonsignificantly lower than the rate among those assigned to guideline-recommended treatment, with a target systolic blood pressure of less than 180 mm Hg, with the use of a variety of antihypertensive medications. However, ordinal analysis of the modified Rankin scores indicated improved functional outcomes with intensive lowering of blood pressure.

Hill MD, Muir KW. INTERACT-2: should blood pressure be aggressively lowered acutely after intracerebral hemorrhage? Stroke. 2013;44(10):2951-2.

Q26. Answer e

Rhinocerebral mucormycosis is a rare opportunistic infection of the sinuses and brain caused by saprophytic fungi. Ethmoidal sinusitis is the most common air sinus causing cerebral infection or mucormycosis. Ophthalmoplegia and Proptosis are the most common early signs. Hyperbaric Oxygen treatment is Fungistatic. Immunosuppression and diabetes are leading risk factors. Amphotericin B is the only reliable systemic antifungal agent approved for the treatment of mucormycosis, and the highest possible tissue levels should be achieved. But other antifungal such as Itraconazole, Isavuconazole, posaconazole, caspofungin etc. are also effective against it.

> Ibrahim AS, Spellberg B, Walsh TJ, et al. Pathogenesis of Mucormycosis. Clinical Infectious Diseases: An Official Publication of the Infectious Diseases Society of America. 2012;54(Suppl1).

Q27. Answer a

Brain abscess is a neurological emergency as soon as diagnosed warranting surgical evacuation and sampling for culture/sensitivity of the offending organisms. Usual organisms are Staph aureus but the ones resulting from dental infections are caused by Actinomyces, Hemophilus and Streptococci. Candida infection in the form of brain abscess is rare and is usually seen in immunocompromised or those on prolonged IV antibiotics. Risk factors include: Endocarditis, Nasal Sinus infections, dental infections and a PFO. Direct spread from infective structures is the leading cause, e.g. otitis media, dental abscess, chronic sinusitis etc. The two most common differential diagnosis of this lesion in clinical practice include neurocysticercosis (NCC) and tuberculomas. In brain abscess when a capsule forms, a round or ovoid area of hypoattenuation will be seen with ring enhancement that dissipates on delayed images.

> Miranda AH, Castellar-Leones SM, Elzain MA, et al. Brain abscess: Current management. Journal of Neurosciences in Rural Practice. 2013;4(Suppl1):S67-S81.

Q28. Answer e

HIV enters the central nervous system soon after infection. More than 40% of the HIV patients suffer with CNS complications and are the actual presenting complaints in 20% of the cases. They include Kaposi sarcoma, CNS Lymphoma, Cryptoccoccal meningitis myopathy and multifocal leukoencephalopathy. HIV associated neurocognitive disorder (HAND), Toxoplasmosis, Tubercular Meningitis, CMV encephalitis, Neurocysticercosis, Vacuolar Myelopathy. Neuro Immune Reconstitution syndrome (Neuro IRIS) is also a complication that arises actually when the patient responds to treatment and the immune system effectively wakes up.

> Spudich S, González-Scarano F. HIV-1-related central nervous system disease: Current issues in pathogenesis, diagnosis, and treatment. Cold spring harbor Perspectives in Medicine. 2012;2(6):a007120.

Q29. Answer d

It is known that early enteral nutrition improves outcome in critically ill patients. Low osmolarity parenteral nutrition can be given via peripheral lines. Ketones provide energy more efficiently to the brain than glucose. Not monitoring Residual volume does not increase the risk of VAP.

> Dionyssiotis Y, Papachristos A, Petropoulou K, et al. Nutritional alterations associated with neurological and neurosurgical diseases. The Open Neurology Journal. 2016;10:32-41.

Q30. Answer e

In ADEM, steroids and plasmapheresis both are treatment options and it has a good prognosis usually and about 50-70% of the patients have a full recovery. It is an autoimmune disease with a usual precursor viral illness. Steroids are the first line treatment with methylprednisolone preferred over dexamethasone.

> Alexander M, Murthy JMK. Acute disseminated encephalomyelitis: Treatment guidelines. Annals of Indian Academy of Neurology. 2011;14(Suppl1):S60-S64.

Q31. Answer e

In Lund Concept, there is a volume targeted approach to TBI management. If ICP elevated a CPP of 50 is considered acceptable. It is principally based on preserving osmotic pressure and reducing hydrostatic pressure, and it contradicts traditional CPP-ICP paradigm. Diuretics are often used in the Lund approach in the treatment of patients with severe traumatic brain injury.

Grände PO. Lund Concept. J Neurosurg Anesthesiol. 2011;23(4):358-62.

Q32. Answer e

Medical conditions which involve screening for SAH patients and their families are; Ehlers Danlos syndrome, Marfan's syndrome, Polycystic kidneys and Coarctation of the aorta. All of these conditions are known to be risk factors for SAH and in some countries active screening programs are run to rule out SAH in such patients and their close relatives.

Gijn JV, Rinkel GJE. Subarachnoid hemorrhage: diagnosis, causes and management. Brain. 2001;124(2):249-78.

Q33. Answer c

SAH is a disease with a huge burden of morbidity and mortality. Endovascular treatment has significantly reduced this burden but still one of the early complications of SAH is hydrocephalus for which an urgent EVD is routinely required. It provides a drainage passage for the blood stained CSF and also reduces the intracranial pressure at the same time. Up to about 25% of the patients require EVD in the initial stages of SAH.

Kirmani AR, Sarmast AH, Bhat AR. Role of external ventricular drainage in the management of intraventricular hemorrhage; its complications and management. Surg Neurol Int. 2015;6:188.

Q34. Answer a

Moyamoya is a rare CNS disease in which the CNS arteries are blocked at the base of the brain. This results in clusters of tiny vessels trying to compensate for the blockage giving it a typical "puff of smoke "appearance" which mean Moyamoya in Japanese. The patient presents with recurrent transient ischemic attack (TIA) and strokes. Whilst it cannot be cured, endovascular treatment or surgery provides good results, by providing alternate blood flow.

Tarasów E, Kułakowska A, Łukasiewicz A et al. Moyamoya disease: Diagnostic imaging. Polish Journal of Radiology. 2011;76(1):73-9.

Q35. Answer a

It is a spectrum of hind brain abnormalities affecting the structural relationship between the cerebellum, skull, upper cervical cord and the brain stem. It has types 1-4 wherein type 1 is the most common and least severe. In type-1, there is small herniation of the cerebellar tonsils below the foramen magnum without any syrinx formation. The formation of Syrinx is seen in more advanced types.

Schneider B, Birthi P, Salles S. Arnold-Chiari 1 malformation type 1 with syringohydromyelia presenting as acute tetraparesis: A case report. The Journal of Spinal Cord Medicine. 2013;36(2):161-5.

Q36. Answer c

EEG is typical of burst suppression with periods of high voltage activity alternating with periods of no activity in the brain. It might be seen in deep anesthesia, comatose states or hypothermia. It is sometimes deliberately achieved in states like refractory status or brain surgery where brain is at risk of hypoperfusion.

Bergey GK. Refractory Status Epilepticus: Is EEG burst suppression an appropriate treatment target during drug-induced coma? What is the holy grail? Epilepsy Curr. 2006;6(4):119-20.

Q37. Answer a

The EEG shows epileptiform activity with regular discharges. There is also evidence of biphasic waves with waxing and waning evolution.

Brenner RP. EEG in convulsive and nonconvulsive status epilepticus. J Clin Neurophysiol. 2004;21(5):319-31.

Q38. Answer e

The image is of DSA and TCD indicating MCA spasm. In the TCD there is increased peak velocity in the MCA segment whilst the MCA shows severe spasm on the actual DSA run. Milrinone is likely to be used for cerebral vasodilatation although there is no level-1 evidence for its use. It is common practice in some Canadian and

North American centers. The patient is likely to have right sided weakness. Nimodipine 60 mg every 4 hours is indicated and has level-1 evidence for its use, from as soon as the patient is admitted.

Connolly ES, Rabinstein AA et al. Guidelines for the Management of Aneurysmal Subarachnoid Hemorrhage. Stroke. 2012; STR.

Q39. Answer e

There is a basilar tip aneurysm on the DSA image and also seen are multiple aneurysms. The Fischer Grade on the CT Head is Grade 4 because there is extensive intraventricular blood from the SAH. The WFNS classification also has it as Grade 4 SAH as the patient is likely to be in a comatose state.

E. Sander Connolly, Alejandro A. Rabinstein et al. Guidelines for the Management of Aneurysmal Subarachnoid Hemorrhage Stroke. 2012;STR.0b013e3182587839.

Q40. Answer b

The ICP remains constant up to a certain limit or inflection point with increasing cerebral volume beyond which any further increase in cerebral volume has a tremendous increase in ICP. This is in reflection from the Monro Kellie doctrine which states the pressure-volume relationship between CSF, blood and brain tissue.

Raboel PH, Bartek J, Andresen M, et al. Intracranial pressure monitoring: invasive versus noninvasive methods—A review. Critical care Research and Practice. 2012; Article ID 950393.

Q41. Answer a

At normotension the relationship is linear between CBF and $PaCO_2$ and at a $PaCO_2$ of 80 mm Hg CBF is approximately doubled beyond which no further increase is possible. At a $PaCO_2$ of 20 mm Hg, flow is halved and no further reduction is possible due to maximal vasoconstriction of the arterioles.

Yoon SH, Zuccarello M, Rapoport RM. $PaCO_2$ and pH regulation of cerebral blood flow. Front Physiol. 2012;3:365.

Q42. Answer c

In the normoxemic range there is no effect on CBF. When there is reduction of paO_2 below 50 mm Hg, cerebral blood flow increases significantly thereby increasing the ICP if not corrected.

Borgström L, Jóhannsson H, Siesjö BK. The relationship between arterial pO_2 and cerebral blood flow in hypoxic hypoxia. Acta Physiol Scand. 1975;93(3):423-32.

Q43. Answer d

Due to autoregulation, the brain receives a constant supply of blood flow over a range of MAPs. This limit is roughly between 50-150 mm Hg of MAP. Above and below these limits, the flow could increase or decrease accordingly. In chronic hypertensives for instance, this curve would be shifted to the right.

Cipolla MJ. The Cerebral Circulation. San Rafael (CA): Morgan & Claypool Life Sciences; 2009.

Q44. Answer c

The incidence of NCSE can be as high as 48% in neuro ICU patients and continuous EEG (cEEG) is better at diagnosing status than standard EEG. cEEG can diagnose brain ischemia with changing pattern of waveforms. Cerebral blood flow and EEG are physiologically coupled together and PLEDs are pathognomonic.

Khawaja AM, Wang G, Cutter GR, et al. Continuous electroencephalography (cEEG) monitoring and outcomes of critically Ill patients. Medical Science Monitor: International Medical Journal of Experimental and Clinical Research. 2017;23:649-58.

Q45. Answer c

Phenytoin toxicity causes acute sodium channel blockade leading to wide QRS complexes. The patient gets prone to ventricular dysrhythmias and sodium bicarbonate is used in the treatment. Cerebellar features like ataxia are seen in phenytoin toxicity. There should be regular phenytoin levels on patients who are on the drug and repeat levels should be done in case of systemic illnesses where volume of distribution or polypharmacy is likely to affect the drug levels. Fosphenytoin preparation does not contain propylene glycol and was initially thought to provide a safer means for rapid intravenous infusion, although cardiac toxicity and deaths from fosphenytoin have been reported.

Robertson K, von Stempel CB, Arnold I. When less is more: a case of phenytoin toxicity. BMJ Case Reports. 2013;2013: bcr2012008023.

Q46. Answer d

In SIADH, there is hyponatremia with fluid retention and increased urinary sodium excretion. The serum osmolarity is normal to low while the urine osmolarity is raised. It is a volume loaded state and the treatment is fluid restriction. The only way to differentiate from cerebral salt wasting is clinically judging the volume status in each, as the latter is a volume depleted state.

> Liu BA, Mittmann N, Knowles SR, et al. Hyponatremia and the syndrome of inappropriate secretion of antidiuretic hormone associated with the use of selective serotonin reuptake inhibitors: a review of spontaneous reports. CMAJ. 1996;155:519.

Q47. Answer e

In Cerebral Salt Wasting syndrome, there is serum hyponatremia with Increased Urinary Sodium and a normal to high serum osmolarity. The urine osmolarity is high. It is a volume depleted state and requires fluid (saline) administration.

> Maesaka JK, Imbriano L, Mattana J, et al. Differentiating SIADH from Cerebral/Renal Salt Wasting: Failure of the volume approach and need for a new approach to hyponatremia. Journal of Clinical Medicine. 2014;3(4):1373-85.

Q48. Answer d

Cerebral microdialysis can be done in various cerebral pathologies like TBI, SAH and stroke. Its aim is to individualize CPP management by getting early warning signals from changes in extracellular fluid in the brain. The probe must be sighted in the 'Penumbra' of the injury site and not directly at the injury site. Lactate/Pyruvate ratio more than 25 indicates ischemia and an increase in Glycerol is an indicator of neuronal cell membrane damage. It does not give direct information about brain tissue oxygen.

> Darvesh AS, Carroll RT, Geldenhuys WJ, et al. In vivo brain microdialysis: advances in neuro psycho pharmacology and drug discovery. Expert opinion on drug discovery. 2011;6(2):109-27.

Q49. Answer a

$PbtO_2$ measures the partial pressure of oxygen in the extracellular neuronal space and not intracellularly. The normal value ranges from 25–35 mm Hg. A value of less than 10 mm Hg for > 30 min correlates to high morbidity and mortality. It employs the Clark cell electrode to measure tissue oxygenation and the same probe can also measure the temperature in the affected brain.

> Harutyunyan G, Mangoyan H, Mkhoyan G. Brain tissue oxygen reactivity: clinical implications and pathophysiology. Frontiers in Pharmacology. 2014;5:100.

Q50. Answer a

All patients admitted to neurocritical care do not require stress ulcer prophylaxis. Only patients at risk require gastric protection and they are patients on ventilation, renal support or the ones who are coagulopathic or with previous history of gastric ulcers. Also, the incidence of upper GI bleeding in neuro ICU patients is declining over the years due to better ICU care and better treatment of H. Pylori. Stress ulcer prophylaxis should be stopped as soon as enteral feed is established. The H_2 receptor antagonists can cause encephalopathy.

> Cook DJ, Griffith LE, Walter SD et al. The attributable mortality and length of intensive care unit stay of clinically important gastrointestinal bleeding in critically ill patients. Critical Care. 2001;5(6):368-75.

K Type Answers

Q1. Answer FTTTT

Classically, DAI has been considered a primary-type injury, with damage occurring at the time of the accident. Another component comprises the secondary factors (or delayed component), where swelling occurs forming retraction of the neuron bulbs. The degree of microscopic injury usually is considered to be greater than the diagnostic imaging which usually shows traumatic micro-bleeds. DAI is suggested in any patient who demonstrates clinical symptoms disproportionate to his or her CT-scan findings. DAI results in instantaneous loss of consciousness, and most patients (>90%) remain in a persistent vegetative state, since brainstem function typically remains unaffected. DAI rarely causes death. Decompressive Craniectomy to treat raised ICP has resulted in increased survival but not corresponding increase in functional outcome as shown by the DECRA and RESCUEicp trial.

Vieira R de CA, Paiva WS, de Oliveira DV, et al. Diffuse Axonal Injury: Epidemiology, Outcome and Associated Risk Factors. Frontiers in Neurology. 2016;7:178.

Q2. Answer TTTTF

Conventionally, patients with TBI, especially those with ICH have been left off pharmacoprophylaxis due to concerns of haematoma expansion. With increasing surveillance, the incidence of DVT in neurosurgical trauma patients is seen to be high and could go up to 50% by one estimate. The timing of starting pharmacoprophylaxis is controversial with most data concluding to start by day 4 and almost universal agreement to start by day 7. Injury Severity Score > 15 is an independent risk factor. Nonpharmacological treatment with SCD significantly reduces DVT incidence and so does LMWH which is the drug of choice.

Abdel-Aziz H, Dunham CM, Malik RJ, et al. Timing for deep vein thrombosis chemoprophylaxis in traumatic brain injury: an evidence-based review. Critical Care. 2015;19(1):96.

Q3. Answer TFTFF

ICP based management has been given a Level IIB status by the most recent BTF guidelines 2016. Head injury management by measuring ICP has shown to decrease the in-hospital and 2-week mortality. An ICP monitoring is indicated in severe head injury where GCS is 8 or below with an abnormal CT scan or with a normal CT scan and two out of three features (age>40, Systolic < 90, mm Hg, motor posturing.) However, non ICP models of managing head injury have shown similar outcomes.

Chesnut RM, Temkin N, Carney N et al. A trial of intracranial-pressure monitoring in traumatic brain injury. N Engl J Med. 2012;367:2471-81.

Q4. Answer FTFTT

Hyperosmolar therapy is one treatment intervention in the care of patients with severe head injury resulting in cerebral edema and intracranial hypertension. The effect of hyperosmolar solutions on brain tissue was first studied nearly 90 years ago. Since that time, mannitol has become the most widely used hyperosmolar solution to treat elevated ICP. Recent studies showing the superiority of HTS due to more favorable cerebral physiological effects. It acts by drawing water from the brain by raising the blood viscosity.

Knapp JM. Hyperosmolar therapy in the treatment of severe head injury in children: mannitol and hypertonic saline. AACN Clin Issues. 2005;16(2):199-211.

Q5. Answer FTTFT

Mannitol has been the traditionally used hyperosmolar agent although there is paucity of historical studies for it to be called the 'Gold Standard'. There are more recent studies showing the superiority of HTS due to more favorable cerebral physiological effects. However, this is yet to be translated to better patient outcome in any of the studies and hence the delay in HTS to be recommended as the better drug. It does decrease glutamate to protect brain, increases $PbtO_2$, and is used safely up to serum Na of 150 mmol/l. Mannitol increases the blood viscosity and has no effect on $PbtO_2$. It should not be used in Hypovolemic patients due to the risk of acute kidney injury and worsening hypovolemia due to its diuretic effects.

Boone MD, Oren-Grinberg A, Robinson TM, et al. Mannitol or hypertonic saline in the setting of traumatic brain injury: What have we learned? Surg Neurol Int. 2015;6:177.

Q6. Answer TTFTT

CPP of 60–70 mm Hg is recommended for achieving both better survival and also patient outcome. When cerebral autoregulation is completely disturbed pushing the CPP to higher levels can be counterproductive. Hence the need for an individualized optimal CPP which can be tailored with newer monitoring modalities like Pressure reactivity etc. Aggressively pushing CPP with inotropes can cause complications like ARDS.

Nancy Carney, Annette M. Totten, Cindy O'Reilly, et al. Guidelines for the management of severe traumatic brain injury, Fourth Edition. Neurosurgery. 2016;1.

Q7. Answer TTTTF

PTE is a syndrome of recurrent seizure disorders occurring at least after 7–14 days of TBI. Seizures happening within 7 days are termed reactive to head injury from organic causes and are not PTE. In significant no of PTE patients, seizures happen in a subclinical state and thus cEEG and video EEG are important investigations.

Apart from pharmacological agents, temporal lobectomy and vagal nerve stimulator are known treatments for drug resistant PTE.

> Verellen RM, Cavazos JE. Post-traumatic epilepsy: an overview. Therapy. 2010;7(5):527-31.
>
> Szaflarski JP, Nazzal Y, Dreer LE. Post-traumatic epilepsy: current and emerging treatment options. Neuropsychiatric Disease and Treatment. 2014;10:1469-77.

Q8. Answer TTTTT

Risk factor for seizures after TBI include penetrating injury, skull fracture, ICH, seizure at scene, brain contusions, Amnesia > 30 min, GCS < 10. Pharmacotherapy might be required in any category of head injury depending on the risks associated. Phenytoin is useful for seizure control in early stages within 7 days but if started late the efficacy is vastly reduced. Levetiracetam is equally effective and devoid of side effects but is yet to make it to guideline recommendations with current available evidence. Valproate is limited to its role in simple seizures whilst ketamine is known to be effective in refractory seizures.

> Nancy Carney, Annette M Totten, Cindy O'Reilly, et al. Guidelines for the Management of Severe Traumatic Brain Injury, Fourth Edition. Neurosurgery. 2016;1.

Q9. Answer FFFTF

The available literature supports the use of antiepileptics for early PTS prophylaxis during the first week after a TBI. Phenytoin has been extensively studied for this indication and is recommended by BTF guidelines for early PTS prophylaxis. Levetiracetam has demonstrated comparable efficacy to phenytoin for early PTS prophylaxis and may be a reasonable alternative to consider in this patient population.

> Torbic H, Forni AA, Anger KE et al. Use of antiepileptics for seizure prophylaxis after traumatic brain injury. Am J Health Syst Pharm. 2013;70(9):759-66.

Q10. Answer FFTFF

Tracheostomy in neurosurgical patients aids in respirator weaning and sedation control to assess neurological condition. It does not help per se in neurological recovery. Raised ICP is only a relative contraindication for tracheostomy. Early tracheostomy is proven to increase the number of ventilator free days in ICU but does not increase the outcome or reduce the incidence of VAP.

> Shirawi N, Arabi Y. Bench-to-bedside review: Early tracheostomy in critically ill trauma patients. Critical Care. 2006;10(1):201.

Q11. Answer FFTFF

The use of steroids is not recommended for improving outcome or reducing ICP. In patients with severe TBI, high dose of methylprednisolone was associated with increased mortality and is contraindicated. Dexamethasone also has no role in improving outcome or decreasing ICP.

> Hoshide R, Cheung V, Marshall L, et al. Do corticosteroids play a role in the management of traumatic brain injury? Surgical Neurology International. 2016;7:84.

Q12. Answer FFFFF

EVD insertion in neuro ICU is one of the most important interventions. It is also one of the most important measures to monitor ICP and reduce elevated ICP by CSF drainage. The EVD catheter should be zeroed and placed at the level of the Foramen of Monro which should be at the level of the external auditory meatus in supine position and in between the eyebrows in the lateral position. The EVD should always be clamped during transfer or patient movement to avoid over or under drainage of CSF which can cause catastrophic consequences. Infection is a common complication of EVD catheters and poses a continual challenge. The outcome of EVD insertion in ICU and OR is not known to be different; however complete sterility is the must irrespective of the place of the procedure.

> Muralidharan R. External ventricular drains: Management and complications. Surgical Neurology International. 2015;6(Suppl 6):S271-S274.

Q13. Answer FTTTT

The risk factors for poor outcome in SAH include Female sex, WFNS grade 4, multiple aneurysms, posterior circulation aneurysms, low presenting GCS, delayed presentation and presence of major comorbidities. SAH is a neurological condition with high morbidity and mortality and usually half of the patients do not reach hospital alive. Of the remaining at least 20% end up with complications especially from delayed cerebral vasospasm.

Connolly ES, Rabinstein AA et al. Guidelines for the Management of Aneurysmal Subarachnoid Hemorrhage Stroke. 2012; STR.0b013e3182587839.

Q14. Answer TTFFF

Triple therapy and oral nimodipine are proven therapies for SAH management and are recommended in the 2012 ASA/AHA guidelines. Angioplasty and IV Milrinone are performed for vasospasm treatment in some centers of the world but its benefit is not consistent and is currently not a universally recommended and acceptable treatment as per the international guidelines.

Connolly ES, Rabinstein AA et al . Guidelines for the Management of Aneurysmal Subarachnoid Hemorrhage Stroke. 2012; STR.0b013e3182587839.

Q15. Answer TFFFT

ISAT study was a landmark study which recommended coiling over clipping for aneurysmal SAH treatment. CT scan is not 100% sensitive and Digital Subtraction Angiography should be done to rule out an aneurysm. It is a condition with high mortality nearing about 50%. The proven therapies to improve outcome are Oral Nimodipine and HHH. Hypothermia has no benefit in treating SAH patients. Outcomes are better if these complex patients are managed at tertiary care centers.

Connolly ES, Rabinstein AA et al. Guidelines for the Management of Aneurysmal Subarachnoid Hemorrhage Stroke. 2012; STR.0b013e3182587839.

Q16. Answer FTFFF

In Hyper Acute Thrombotic Stroke the recommended treatment is bridging thrombolysis and clot evacuation by MT if presentation is within window period. Thrombolysis alone is only useful in small vessels and is unable to dissolve large vessel clots. MT is useful for large vessel clots and is unable for clot evacuation of very small distal vessels. Complications of MT are lesser with significantly better outcomes. During MT, no one anesthetic (GA or Sedation) is superior to another. Options need to be tailored for individual scenario. GA is recommended for posterior circulation strokes due to the risk of clot migration and brainstem stroke. TCD and invasive monitoring are usually not required as time is of the essence to minimize 'door to needle' time. Postoperative ventilation is a predictor of poor outcome.

Palaniswami M, Yan B. Mechanical thrombectomy is now the gold standard for acute ischemic stroke: Implications for routine clinical practice. Interventional Neurology. 2015;4(1-2):18-29.

Q17. Answer FFFTF

Q18. Answer TFTTF

mRS is a validated clinical scoring system to assess functional outcome after stroke or neurological injury. It runs from 0-6 with 0 being no disability and 6 being a dead patient. It suffers from inter-personnel variability and bias but still is one of the most acceptable scoring systems. It does not have any radiological parameters and is purely a clinical scoring system.

Harrison JK, McArthur KS, Quinn TJ. Assessment scales in stroke: clinimetric and clinical considerations. Clinical Interventions in Aging. 2013;8:201-11.

Q19. Answer FTFFT

TCD is used in neuro ICU to screen and diagnose vasospasm especially in patients with SAH. Its usual frequency is in the range of 2 MHz and it is performed through the temporal insonation window where the bony table is at its least thickness. It can be used to assess middle, anterior and posterior cerebral arteries. The probe is used in power M mode to diagnose vasospasm. It is less sensitive than the gold standard which is angiography.

Bathala L, Mehndiratta MM, Sharma VK. Transcranial Doppler: Technique and common findings (Part 1). Annals of Indian Academy of Neurology. 2013;16(2):174-9.

Q20. Answer FFTFT

GBS is an autoimmune condition affecting the peripheral nervous system and not the central nervous system. Although the recovery is usually prolonged, the mortality is low and usually less than 10%. FVC <15 mL/kg body weight is predictive of respiratory failure and need for ventilation. Diagnosis is clinical and no single laboratory or radiological parameter is diagnostic. Plasmapheresis and IV Immunoglobulins are the mainstay treatments.

Winer JB. An Update in Guillain-Barré Syndrome. Autoimmune Diseases. 2014;2014:793024.

Q21. Answer TTFTT

Cavernous venous sinus thrombosis is a difficult to diagnose neurological condition and carries a high mortality. The most common causative agent is *S. aureus* and MR venogram is the radiological investigation of choice. Steroids are used in the treatment and LMWH is recommended.

Alvis-Miranda HR, Castellar-Leones MS, Alcala-Cerra G, et al. Cerebral sinus venous thrombosis. Journal of Neurosciences in Rural Practice. 2013;4(4):427-38.

Q22. Answer TTTTT

Induced hypothermia below 33°C causes decrease in cardiac output, deranged clotting and decreases the metabolic rate. Insulin resistance happens at this level of hypothermia leading to hyperglycemia. Pancreatitis is also known to occur in induced hypothermia with increase in serum amylase levels. There is no consensus as to whether ABGs should be temperature corrected or not. When they are, respiratory alkalosis is the finding.

Song SS, Lyden PD. Overview of Therapeutic Hypothermia. Current treatment options in neurology. 2012;14(6):541-8.

Q23. Answer TFFTT

PRES is rare and occurs in hypertensive crisis and with history of recent or previous immunosuppressants. It can be seen in preeclampsia but is not common. Diagnosis is difficult and is based on radiological findings of vasogenic parieto-occipital edema at MRI, which can be bilateral. Once the condition is diagnosed and treated, patients make full recovery.

Hobson EV, Craven I, Blank SC. Posterior reversible encephalopathy syndrome: A truly treatable neurologic illness. Peritoneal dialysis international: Journal of the International Society for Peritoneal Dialysis. 2012;32(6):590-4.

Q24. Answer TTTFF

Tongue biting, particularly if it is lateral, is highly specific to generalized tonic-clonic seizures. Objective evidence for incontinence and aspiration is highly specific to convulsive epileptic seizures.

Benbadis SR, Wolgamuth BR, Goren H, et al. Value of tongue biting in the diagnosis of seizures. Arch Intern Med. 1995; 155(21):2346-9.

Q25. Answer TTTTT

Laboratory tests in coma: Blood samples will be taken to check for: Complete blood count, Electrolytes, glucose, thyroid, kidney and liver function, Carbon monoxide poisoning, Drug or alcohol overdose, Serum ammonia, Coagulation profile, Arterial Blood Gas analysis etc. Lumbar puncture can check for infections in the nervous system.

Gray JT, Gavin CM. Assessment and management of neurological problems. Emergency Medicine Journal. 2005;22(6).

Q26. Answer TTTTF

Q27. Answer TTTTT

Apnea test is done to confirm absence of spontaneous respiratory activity. Prerequisites are normothermia, normal electrolytes, euvolemia of last 6 hours (minimal), absence of any sedative drugs and normoglycemia. On stopping controlled ventilation, the rate of rise of paCO$_2$ is 3-6 mm Hg/min and a paCO$_2$ > 60 mm Hg with no spontaneous respiratory efforts is considered positive towards brain stem death.

Goila AK, Pawar M. The diagnosis of brain death. Indian Journal of Critical Care Medicine: Peer-reviewed, Official Publication of Indian Society of Critical Care Medicine. 2009;13(1):7-11.

Q28. Answer FTTTT

Acute EDH is usually an arterial bleed with middle meningeal artery as the usual culprit. The hematoma is parieto-temporal and appears bi-convex on CT Head. There can be a lucid interval delivering a false sense of hope which can lead to mortality. In contrast, chronic subdural hematomas are as a result from dural venous tears. The hematoma liquefies over time and hence it can be evacuated in a liquefied form through burr holes. They cause less acute pressure symptoms, giving the brain time acclimatize and hence lead to a lower mortality.

Q29. Answer TFFFT

Q30. Answer TFTFT

Cerebral autoregulation is maintained between MAP of 50-150 mm Hg in normal circumstances. This gets disturbed during trauma or disease of the brain. In chronic hypertensive the curve is shifted to the right. Cerebral blood flow is increased by volatiles beyond 1 minimum anesthetic concentration (MAC) and is usually decreased or unaffected by Propofol. The ischemic threshold for cerebral blood flow is <18 mL/dL.

Ainslie PN, Brassard P. Why is the neural control of cerebral autoregulation so controversial? F1000 Prime Reports. 2014;6:14.

Q31. Answer TTTTF

The brain receives a large amount of blood supply as compared to its weight. 20% of the cardiac output is received by the brain which equates to a $CMRO_2$ of 50 mL/min or 3-3.8 mL/100 gm/min or 20% of basal oxygen requirements. It can also be calculated from:

$CMRO_2$ = CBF X a-v oxygen content difference. It is however not easy to measure at the bedside in routine clinical practice.

Cruz J, Jaggi JL, Hoffstad OJ. Cerebral blood flow and oxygen consumption in acute brain injury with acute anemia: an alternative for the cerebral metabolic rate of oxygen consumption? Crit Care Med. 1993;21(8):1218-24.

Q32. Answer TTFTF

Deranged clotting due to coumarin derivatives is best corrected with PCC instead of FFPs. FFP is the most commonly used agent for the replacement of coagulation factors in absence of PCC. It contains vitamin K-dependent coagulation Factors II, VII, and X; however, it lacks sufficient levels of factor IX. Vitamin K is indicated and helps in replenishing vitamin K-dependent clotting factors. TEG or RoTEM help in dynamic assessment of the clot. With a decreasing GCS, this patient needs to be operated and cannot wait for the clotting's spontaneous correction.

Zareh M, Davis A, Henderson S. Reversal of warfarin-induced hemorrhage in the emergency department. West J Emerg Med. 2011;12(4):386-92.

Q33. Answer TTTTT

All are suitable treatment options. Volatile anesthetics are a mainstay in super refractory seizures where no other drug has been able to walk. In such cases patients are put on Sevoflurane via an anesthetic machine either in the ICU or with suitable scavenging options. Ketamine is also a suitable option for refractory and super-refractory seizures and has been underutilized so far.

Trinka E, Höfler J, Leitinger M, et al. Pharmacotherapy for Status Epilepticus. Drugs. 2015;75:1499-521.

Q34. Answer TFTFF

Nimodipine treatment should start as soon as the diagnosis of SAH is made with an oral dose of 60 mg every 4 hours. It has level I evidence and should be continued for at least 21 days post the day of the bleeding. It blocks L-type voltage gated calcium channels and is best given orally or via a nasogastric tube.

Yasuda SU, Tietze KJ. Nimodipine in the treatment of subarachnoid hemorrhage. DICP. 1989;23(6):451-5.

Q35. Answer TFTTT

Wernicke's encephalopathy is a clinical diagnosis and needs high index of suspicion. It is usually missed leading to high mortality. Treatment is with high dose IV Thiamine or oral thiamine is insufficient to treat it. No biological marker exists and the diagnosis is clinical. Chronic or Acute alcoholism is a risk factor.

McCormick LM, Buchanan JR, Onwuameze OE, et al. Beyond alcoholism: Wernicke-Korsakoff syndrome in patients with psychiatric disorders. Cognitive and behavioral neurology: Official journal of the Society for Behavioral and Cognitive Neurology. 2011;24(4):209-16.

Q36. Answer FTFTT

ISAT was a landmark study revolutionizing the treatment of aneurysmal SAH and not traumatic SAH. It demonstrated a 7.4 absolute risk reduction in death for coiling vs clipping. Intra- procedural rupture was less with coiling whilst postoperative rebleeding rates were more with coiling. Its critique was that long term follow-up in years was missing.

> Darsaut TE, Jack AS, Kerr RS, et al. International subarachnoid aneurysm trial – ISAT Part II: Study protocol for a randomized controlled trial. Trials. 2013;14:156.

Q37. Answer FFTFT

ICP waveforms show 3 upstrokes in one wave as shown in the picture.

P1 (Percussion wave or systolic upstroke) represents arterial pulsation, P2 (Tidal wave or intracranial compliance) represents intracranial compliance and P3 (Dicrotic wave or aortic valve recoil) represents venous pulsation. In normal ICP waveform P1 should have highest upstroke, P2 in between and P3 should show lowest upstroke. On eyeballing the monitor, if P2 is higher than P1, it indicates intracranial hypertension.

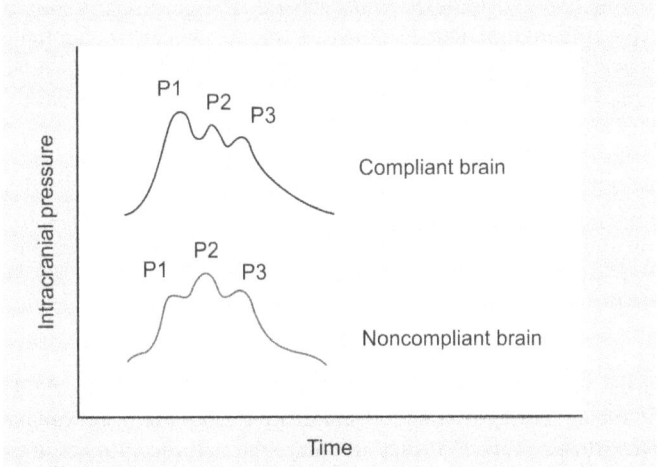

> Ragland J, Lee K. Brain edema and intracranial hypertension. J Neurocrit Care. 2016;9(2):105-12.

Q38. Answer FTTTF

Diabetes insipidus is common after head injury and pituitary surgery. There is raised serum sodium with high volume of dilute urine usually > 250 mL/hr. Serum osmolarity is high whilst urine osmolarity is low. Serum sodium > 150 mmol/L and the specific gravity of urine < 1.003.

> Kalra S, Zargar AH, Jain SM et al. Diabetes insipidus: The other diabetes. Indian Journal of Endocrinology and Metabolism. 2016;20(1):9-21.

Q39. Answer TTTTT

Status lasting more than 24 hours or on withdrawal of anesthetic is called super refractory. It is extremely difficult to treat and Ketamine has shown to be useful. There is new evidence for ketogenic diet to be beneficial especially in children. Magnesium infusion is useful adjuvant drug in treatment along with immunotherapy with IV immunoglobulin.

> Buchhalter J. Treatment of super-refractory status epilepticus: The sooner the better with less adverse effects. Epilepsy currents. 2013;13(5):217-18.

Q40. Answer FTTTF

The use of propofol, barbiturates or midazolam for burst suppression of RSE can be justified. When using propofol, the duration of high doses should be limited to 48 hours and the risk of propofol infusion syndrome should be kept in mind. High doses of barbiturates terminate seizures effectively but prolong ventilator treatment and intensive care. Burst suppression can be achieved with both barbiturates and propofol. It is indicated in RSE, refractory raised ICP, intracranial aneurysmal clipping. Due to the effect of the drugs, hypotension is a common side effect.

Parviainen I, Kälviäinen R, Ruokonen E. Propofol and barbiturates for the anesthesia of refractory convulsive status epilepticus: pros and cons. Neurol Res. 2007;29(7):667-71.

Q41. Answer TTTTT

BSR in EEG monitoring measures the amount of time within an interval spent in the suppressed state. A BSR of 0 indicates that the brain is active whilst a BSR of 1 indicates that the brain has no electrical activity. BSR and Burst suppression probability are functionally the same and a typical 'burst suppression' would have 5-10 bursts/minute.

Chemali JJ, Wong KF, Solt K, et al. A state-space model of the burst suppression ratio. Conf Proc IEEE Eng Med Biol Soc. 2011;2011:1431-4.

Q42. Answer TTTTF

In tubercular meningitis predominant findings are of decreased CSF glucose and normal to raised CSF protein. Presence of lymphocytes and not monocytes in the CSF is indicative of TB meningitis. The opening CSF is also cloudy in color. Newer test like tubercular DNA analysis can also be used to aid diagnosis.

Chin JH. Tuberculous meningitis-Diagnostic and therapeutic challenges. Neurol Clin Pract. 2014;4(3):199-205.

Q43. Answer FTTTF

Terson Syndrome is condition of SAH with accompanying vitreal hemorrhage. It occurs in the anterior circulation and is indicative of higher mortality. Pathophysiology is due to raised venous pressures from transmitted high ICP to optic nerve. Diagnosis is made at fundoscopy with typical images.

Lee SH, Seo JH, Park SH, et al. Terson syndrome in aneurysmal subarachnoid hemorrhage: A case report. Annals of rehabilitation medicine. 2015;39(4):640-4.

Q44. Answer TTFFT

Autonomic dysreflexia develops with neurological spinal injury level at or above the T6 level and is the most common cause of bladder and bowel dysfunction. Splanchnic sympathetic prevail below the level of injury whilst parasympathetic prevail above the level of injury. The baroreceptor response is preserved in this condition which sends the sympathetic crisis signal to the brain.

Milligan J, Lee J, McMillan C, et al. Autonomic dysreflexia: Recognizing a common serious condition in patients with spinal cord injury. Canadian Family Physician. 2012;58(8):831-5.

Q45. Answer FTTTF

Normal CSF sample would have a clear color with CSF glucose 50-80 mg/dL, CSF protein 20-45 mg/dL, CSF lymphocytes 0-4 and CSF chloride 116-122. A normal CSF lactate is less than 3 mmol/l.

Q46. Answer is FTTTT

The image depicting microdialysis and TCD is not that of a normal brain. The L/P ratio curve indicates ischemia as seen by the suddenly rising lactate/pyruvate ratio above normal levels from the initial downward trend. The dramatic increase in glycerol indicates brain damage whilst the TCD Flow velocity shows spasm much later than the actual rise in biomarkers. The Tip of the EVD is also seen in the ventricles in the CT Head image.

Darvesh AS, Carroll RT, Geldenhuys WJ et al. In vivo brain microdialysis: advances in neuropsychopharmacology and drug discovery. Expert opinion on drug discovery. 2011;6(2):109-27.

Q47. Answer FTTTT

NIHSS score is a validated tool to quantify the degree of impairment caused by Stroke. It has 11 items carrying a score of 0-4 for each. The maximum possible score is 42. A Score of 0 indicates normal function. It is also a validated tool for predicting patient outcome.

Sartor EA, Albright K, Boehme AK et al. The NIHSS Score and its components can predict cortical stroke. Journal of Neurological Disorders & Stroke. 2013;2(1):1026.

Q48. Answer FTTFF

Pituitary adenomas are now routinely operated via the trans-sphenoidal approach worldwide. On most occasions perioperative steroids are not routinely required. Postoperative hyponatremia is a common but treatable problem. Due to CSF leak there can be risk of meningitis. Diabetes insipidus is a known complication that can occur in the postoperative phase.

    Jane JA, Laws ER. Surgical Treatment of Pituitary Adenomas. Endotext; 2000.

Q49. Answer TTFTT

Most of the brain tumors in the pediatric age group are infratentorial. Craniopharyngioma is the most common and any increase in the ICP is compensated by the size of the skull. The posterior fossa tumors are notorious to have raised ICP and the $CMRO_2$ is higher in the pediatric age group.

    Garrè ML, Cama A. Craniopharyngioma: modern concepts in pathogenesis and treatment. Curr Opin Pediatr. 2007;19:471.

Q50. Answer TTTTF

Except the trans-cranial Doppler, all other listed devices are used to detect Venous Air Embolism. Most sensitive of them is the TOE followed by the esophageal stethoscope and then the $ETCO_2$.

    Bathala L, Mehndiratta MM, Sharma VK. Transcranial Doppler: Technique and common findings (Part 1). Annals of Indian Academy of Neurology. 2013;16(2):174-9.

Q51. Answer TFFTT

A lumbar puncture should only be done after a CT scan has ruled any major signs of raised ICP. A CT head in this case should be the initial investigation followed by a lumbar puncture and MRI. A cold sore on the lip gives a likely cause of Herpes Simplex encephalitis. A diagnosis of meningitis is unlikely due to lateralizing signs. Acyclovir and 3rd-4th generation cephalosporins are indicated immediately until diagnosis is confirmed to prevent long term sequelae. Untreated HSE has a mortality of 70% whilst treated one still has a mortality of around 20-25%.

    Polhill S, Soni M. Encephalitis in the ICU setting. Current Anesthesia and Critical Care. 2007;18:107-16.

Q52. Answer FTFTF

Scan typically shows a biconvex extradural hematoma on the right side with a skull fracture in the right temporal region. Acute Extradural hematoma is usually an arterial bleed with middle meningeal artery as the usual culprit. The hematoma is parieto-temporal and appears bi-convex on CT Head. There can be a lucid interval delivering a false sense of hope which can lead to mortality. In contrast, Chronic SDH are as a result from dural venous tears. The hematoma liquefies over time and hence it can be evacuated in a liquefied form through burr holes. They cause less acute pressure symptoms, giving the brain time acclimatize and hence lead to a lower mortality.

    Soon WC et al. Traumatic Acute Extradural Hematoma-Indications for surgery revisited. Br J Neurosurg. 2016;30(2):233-4.

Q53. Answer FFTFF

Findings are suggestive of a chronic SDH on the right side extending from the frontal region to parieto-temporal region.

    Chronic SDH are as a result from dural venous tears. The hematoma liquefies over time and hence it can be evacuated in a liquefied form through burr holes. They cause less acute pressure symptoms, giving the brain time to acclimatize and hence lead to a lower mortality. They usually happen in elderly who are on blood thinners and trivial traumas can lead to rupture of bridging veins especially when the actually brain volume has shrunk due to age effects.

    Adhiyaman V et al. Chronic subdural hematoma in the elderly. Postgraduate Medical Journal. 2002;78(916):71-75.

Q54. Answer TTFTT

Pneumocephalus is a common finding after neurosurgical operations especially those involving the base of skull, pituitary or chronic subdurals. Other risk factors include; hyperventilation, osmotherapy, barotrauma. Usually high flow oxygen is all that is required to denitrogenation the air and decompress the pneumocephalus. High Flow Nasal Oxygen is a useful recent machine for this purpose. Rarely, tension pneumocephalus might develop with a classical Mt Fuji sign that requires urgent open decompression.

    Schirmer CM, Heilman CB, Bhardwaj A. Pneumocephalus: Case Illustrations and Review. Neurocritical Care. 2010;13(1):152-8.

Q55. Answer FTTFF

Hypertensive basal are quite common and are commonly due to uncontrolled long standing hypertension. Bad prognostication signs include: Intraventricular hemorrhage, Infratentorial bleeding, Age > 80 years, Low GCS on presentation, and volume of bleed > 30 mL. EVD is a quick and easy way to drain CSF and decrease the ICP and can be lifesaving. There is growing evidence to suggest that lowering the blood pressure to below 160 mm Hg helps prevent hematoma expansion. ICH score goes up if there is intraventricular extension of the hematoma.

> Sahni R, Weinberger J. Management of intracerebral hemorrhage. Vasc Health Risk Manag. 2007;3(5):701-9.

Q56. Answer FFFTT

The risk factors for poor outcome in SAH include female sex, WFNS grade 4, multiple aneurysms, posterior circulation aneurysms, low presenting GCS, delayed presentation and presence of major comorbidities. SAH is a neurological condition with high morbidity and mortality and usually half of the patients do not reach alive to the hospital. Of the remaining at least 20% end up with complications especially from delayed cerebral vasospasm which can happen up to 2 weeks post ictus. Tranexamic acid has shown some benefit in prevention of rebleeding in aneurysms that are presenting late. Tranexamic acid has no role in preventing re-bleeding. Triple therapy and Oral Nimodipine are proven therapies for SAH management and are recommended in the 2012 ASA/AHA guidelines. Angioplasty and IV Milrinone for vasospasm treatment are used in some centers of the world but their benefit is not consistent and is currently not a universally recommended and acceptable treatment as per the international guidelines.

> Connolly ES, Rabinstein AA, et al. Guidelines for the management of aneurysmal subarachnoid hemorrhage stroke. 2012; STR.0b013e3182587839.

Q57. Answer TTTTT

ICH score is a clinically validated score to determine the grading of ICH. It was designed to grade the severity of the disease and not for routine prognostication as is sometimes used. However, high ICH scores do indicate a severe mortality. The ICH Score has the following parameters: Age, Presenting GCS, Volume of Blood, Intraventricular extension and Infratentorial lesion. Definitive treatment in the form of endovascular embolization helps in prevention of re-bleeding and is less risky than open surgery.

> Clarke JL, et al. External validation of ICH score. Neurocrit Care. 2004;1(1):53-60.

Q58. Answer FTFFF

In SIADH, there is hyponatremia with fluid retention and increased urinary sodium excretion. The serum osmolarity is normal to low while the urine osmolarity is raised. It is a volume loaded state and the treatment is fluid restriction. The only way to differentiate from cerebral salt wasting is clinically judging the volume status in each, as the latter is a volume depleted state.

> Bersten AD, Soni N. Oh's Intensive Care Manual. 5th Edition. 2003.

Q59. Answer FTTTT

Mycotic Cerebral Aneurysms are rare. They can present in patients with Infective Endocarditis and are difficult to diagnose unless a high index of suspicion is kept. Viridans Strep and Staph aureus are the usual causative organisms. Some studies report a good outcome with prolonged medical therapy with IV antibiotics for unruptured mycotic aneurysms. Ruptured mycotic aneurysms should be treated with endovascular surgery as well whilst any corrective cardiovascular surgery should wait for the cerebral disease to stabilize unless there is evidence of frank left heart failure from the endogenic cardiac disease.

> Kuo I et al. Ruptured intracranial mycotic aneurysm in infective endocarditis: A natural history. Case Reports I Medicine. 2010, Article ID 168408.

Q60. Answer FTTFF

The images show the classical Left MCA 'Dot Sign' due to the presence of a thrombus in the left MCA. Mechanical thrombectomy and bridging thrombolysis are the most effective treatment nowadays for acute ischemic stroke done as part of hyper acute stroke service. The clinical outcomes are getting better with good mRS scores of at least 40% in the best reported studies. The blood pressure should not be lowered to allow collaterals to flow until the offending vessel is restored.

Absolute Contraindications to thrombolysis (1) Intracranial hemorrhage on CT; (2) Clinical presentation suggests SAH; (3) Neurosurgery, head trauma, or stroke in past 3 months; (4) Uncontrolled hypertension (>185 mm Hg SBP or >110 mm Hg DBP); (5) History of ICH; (6) Known intracranial arteriovenous malformation, neoplasm, or aneurysm; (7) Active internal bleeding; (8) Suspected/confirmed endocarditis; (9) Known bleeding diathesis; (a) Platelet count < 100,000; (b) Patient has received heparin within 48 hours and has an elevated aPTT (greater than upper limit of normal for laboratory); (c) Current use of oral anticoagulants (ex: warfarin) and INR >1.7; (d) Current use of direct thrombin inhibitors or direct factor Xa inhibitors; (9) Abnormal blood glucose (<50 or >400 mg/dL)

Relative Contraindications/Warnings to tPA (1) Only minor or rapidly improving stroke symptoms; (2) Major surgery or serious non-head trauma in the previous 14 days; (3) History of gastrointestinal or urinary tract hemorrhage within 21 days; (4) Seizure at stroke onset; (5) Recent arterial puncture at a noncompressible site; (6) Recent lumbar puncture; (7) Post myocardial infarction pericarditis; (8) Pregnancy; (9) Additional Warnings to tPA >3 hr Onset; (10) Age >80 years; (11) History of prior stroke and diabetes; (12) Any active anticoagulant use (even with INR <1.7); (13) NIHSS >25; (14) CT shows multilobar infarction (hypodensity >1/3 cerebral hemisphere)

Palaniswami M, Yan B. Mechanical thrombectomy is now the gold standard for acute ischemic stroke: Implications for routine clinical practice. Interventional Neurology. 2015;4(1-2):18-29.

Q61. Answer TTTFF

CT shows malignant left ICA infarction and edema of the left side with midline shift. Malignant ischemic strokes presenting outside the window period may result in severe cerebral edema of the affected side. Hypertonic saline is increasingly being preferred over mannitol to reduce the pressure effects. However, in this case time has passed for any medical management due to signs of raised ICP. Decompressive craniectomy is required for the cerebral edema to resolve. It however has shown increased survival without increasing functional outcome in some of the latest reported studies.

Bansal H et al. Decompressive craniectomy in malignant middle cerebral artery infarct: An institutional experience. Asian J Neurosurg. 2015;10(3):203-06.

Q62. Answer TTTTT

Cerebral Sinus Thrombosis is a difficult to diagnose condition which can be fatal. OCPs area a known risk factor along with severe dehydration and habitual use of IV narcotic drugs. Venous infarcts usually present after some days on the scans unlike arterial infarcts. Treatment is IV Heparin and increasingly endovascular therapy directed at the site of the thrombus is being employed. Complication includes dural AV fistulas and hydrocephalus.

Saposnik G et al. Diagnosis and Management of Cerebral Venous Thrombosis. Stroke. 2011;42;1158-92.

Q63. Answer FTFTF

Brain abscess is a neurological emergency as soon as diagnosed warranting surgical evacuation and sampling for culture/sensitivity of the offending organisms. Usual organisms are Staph Aureus but the ones resulting from dental infections are caused by Actinomyces, hemophilus and Streptococci. Candida infection in the form of brain abscess is rare and is usually seen in immunocompromised or those on prolonged IV antibiotics.

Risk factors include: Endocarditis, Nasal Sinus infections, dental infections and a PFO.

Carlos M, Isada MD. Brain Abscess. 2010. Clevelandclinicmeded.com

Q64. Answer b

The scan shows complete loss of grey matter and hypoxic encephalopathy likely from ischemic insult. There are no features suggestive of Stroke or Herpes encephalitis. Status is unlikely to be the cause given the history and can be easily confirmed with an EEG that might show no electrical activity.

Heinz UE, Rollnik J. Outcome and prognosis of hypoxic brain damage patients undergoing neurological early rehabilitation. BMC Res Notes. 2015;8;243.

Q65. Answer FTTTF

Increased signal intensity in the temporal lobes is classical of HSV encephalitis. HSE is caused by HSV-1 in usually 95% of the cases. Mortality ranges from 50 to 70% and the mainstay of treatment is IV Antivirals. Diagnosis is confirmed with CSF PCR for HSV or with brain biopsy in cases with negative PCR. MR images usually show abnormal signal enhancement in the temporal and limbic systems usually bilaterally but can be asymmetrical.

Polhill S, Soni M. Encephalitis in the ICU setting. Current Anesthesia and Critical Care. 2007;18:107-16

CHAPTER 4

Gastrointestinal

Manoj Singh, Ashutosh Bhardwaj, Mehul Solanki

A Type Questions
(One best answer)

1. Standard supportive measures for patients with mild pancreatitis include the following:
   a. Intravenous fluid and electrolyte therapy
   b. Withholding of analgesics to allow serial abdominal examinations
   c. Subcutaneous octreotide therapy
   d. Nasogastric decompression
   e. Prophylactic antibiotics

2. Which of the following statements about the segmental anatomy of the liver is FALSE?
   a. Segments are subdivisions in both the French and American systems
   b. Segments are determined primarily by the hepatic venous drainage
   c. The French anatomic system is more applicable than the American system to clinical hepatic resection
   d. Segments are important to the understanding of the topographic anatomy of the liver

3. Which of the following statements most accurately describes the current therapy for pyogenic hepatic abscess?
   a. Antibiotics alone are adequate for the treatment of most cases
   b. All patients require open surgical drainage for optimal management
   c. Optimal treatment involves treatment of not only the abscess but the underlying source as well
   d. Percutaneous drainage is more successful for multiple lesions than for solitary ones

4. Which of the following statements is true about benign lesions of the liver?
   a. Adenomas are true neoplasms with a predisposition for complications and should usually be resected
   b. Focal nodular hyperplasia (FNH) is a neoplasm related to birth control pills (BCPs) and usually requires resection
   c. Hemangiomas are the most common benign lesions of the liver that come to the surgeon's attention
   d. Nodular regenerative hyperplasia does not usually accompany cirrhosis

5. Which of the following statements about malignant neoplasms of the liver is true?
   a. Hepatocellular carcinoma is probably the number 1 cause of death from cancers worldwide
   b. The most common resectable hepatic malignant neoplasm in the United States is colorectal metastasis
   c. Hepatoma has at least one variant that has a much more benign course than hepatomas in general
   d. Hepatomas are generally slower growing than was formerly believed
   e. Asymptomatic focal nodular hyperplasia must be resected to save conversion to malignant types

6. Which of the following statements is true about bile duct cancers?
   a. If resected, proximal lesions are usually curable

b. The more proximal the lesion, the more likely is resection to be curative
c. Radiation clearly prolongs survival
d. Transplantation is usually successful, if the lesion seems confined to the liver
e. None of the above is true

7. **Regarding Echinococcus liver disease caused by Echinococcus granulosus versus E multilocularis; all are true about the later *except*:**
   a. Is not a neoplasm
   b. Is endemic to parts of the United States
   c. Is usually incurable by resection since it is rarely resectable
   d. Is less deadly than Echinococcus granulosus
   e. Often present in adulthood due to the typical slow growth

8. **Which of the following statements about hemobilia is true?**
   a. Tumors are the most common cause
   b. The primary treatment of severe hemobilia is surgical
   c. Percutaneous cholangiographic hemobilia is usually minor
   d. Ultrasonography usually reveals a specific diagnosis

9. **Ligation of all of the following arteries usually causes significant hepatic enzyme abnormalities *except*:**
   a. Ligation of the right hepatic artery
   b. Ligation of the left hepatic artery
   c. Ligation of the hepatic artery distal to the gastroduodenal branch
   d. Ligation of the hepatic artery proximal to the gastroduodenal artery

10. **The most common acid-base disorder is in liver disease is:**
    a. Metabolic acidosis
    b. Respiratory alkalosis
    c. Metabolic alkalosis
    d. Respiratory acidosis

11. **Which of the following is the most effective definitive therapy for both prevention of recurrent variceal hemorrhage and control of ascites?**
    a. Endoscopic sclerotherapy
    b. Distal splenorenal shunt
    c. Esophagogastric devascularization (Sugiura procedure)
    d. Side-to-side portacaval shunt
    e. End-to-side portacaval shunt

12. **Which of the following complications of portal hypertension most commonly may require surgical intervention?**
    a. Hypersplenism
    b. Variceal hemorrhage
    c. Ascites
    d. Encephalopathy

13. **Which of the following clinical situations are considered good indications for portosystemic venous shunt (PVS)?**
    a. A 50-year-old cirrhotic man had an emergency portacaval shunt for bleeding varices and postoperatively had an ascites leak and mild superficial wound infection
    b. A 57-year-old woman with primary biliary cirrhosis (PBC) has difficult to control ascites and diuretic-induced encephalopathy
    c. A 46-year-old resistant alcoholic has chronic ascites uncontrolled by diuretics combined with repeat paracentesis
    d. A 34-year-old woman taking birth control pills (BCPs) had rapid onset of ascites and is found to have hepatic vein thrombosis causing the Budd-Chiari syndrome

14. **Which of the following are indications for cholecystectomy?**
    a. The presence of gallstones in a patient with intermittent episodes of right side upper quadrant pain
    b. The presence of gallstones in an asymptomatic patient
    c. The presence of symptomatic gallstones in a patient with angina pectoris
    d. The presence of asymptomatic gallstones in a patient who has insulin dependent diabetes

15. **Which of the following statement about cholangitis is INCORRECT?**
    a. Charcot's triad is always present
    b. Associated biliary tract disease is always present
    c. Chills and fever are due to the presence of bacteria in the bile duct system
    d. The most common cause of cholangitis is choledocholithiasis

16. **The initial goal of therapy for acute toxic cholangitis is to:**

a. Prevent cholangio-venous reflux by decompressing the duct system
b. Remove the obstructing stone, if one is present
c. Alleviate jaundice and prevent permanent liver damage
d. Prevent the development of gallstone pancreatitis

17. Which statement is true regarding endocrine and exocrine tissue of the pancreas?
    a. The islets of Langerhans total 1 million per gland and drain their secretions via intercalated duct cells through the ampulla of Vater
    b. Islet alpha cells produce glucagon
    c. Islet sigma cells produce somatostatin
    d. The acini and ductal systems constitute the endocrine portion of the pancreas

18. Pancreatic exocrine secretory products include a bicarbonate-rich electrolyte solution as well as digestive enzymes. Which of the following statement is false?
    a. Cholecystokinin (CCK) is the most potent endogenous stimulant of pancreatic enzyme secretion
    b. The chloride and bicarbonate concentrations of pancreatic juice vary and depend on the secretory flow rate
    c. Secretin is the most potent endogenous stimulant of pancreatic water and electrolyte secretion
    d. The peptidases synthesized by acinar cells are released into the pancreatic duct system in active form

19. Which of the following statements about adenocarcinoma of the pancreas is correct?
    a. Ductal adenocarcinoma is the most common histology type
    b. Most cases occur in the body and tail of the pancreas, making distal pancreatectomy the most commonly performed resectional therapy
    c. For cancers of the head of the pancreas resected by pancreatico-duodenectomy, prognosis appears to be independent of nodal status, margin status, or tumor diameter
    d. The most accurate screening test involves surveillance of stool for carbohydrate antigen (CA 19-9)

20. A 35-year-old woman presents with episodes of obtundation, somnolence, and tachycardia. An insulinoma is suspected based on a random serum glucose test value of 38 mg. per dL. Which of the following statements is/are true regarding diagnosis?
    a. The most important diagnostic study for insulinoma is an oral glucose tolerance test
    b. It may be helpful to perform ERCP in an effort to localize the tumor
    c. Most patients with insulinoma present with extensive disease, rendering them only rarely resectable or curable
    d. Elevated C-peptide or proinsulin levels and screening for anti-insulin antibodies

21. Which of the following statements about gastrinoma (Zollinger-Ellison syndrome) is incorrect?
    a. Most gastrinomas are malignant
    b. Extrapancreatic gastrinomas are common
    c. Diarrhea may be a prominent presenting feature of some patients with gastrinoma
    d. Acid-reducing medications, such as omeprazole have a role in medical management
    e. Diagnosis is based on an decreased fasting gastrin level

22. With regard to the control of pancreatic exocrine function, which of the following statement is incorrect?
    a. Cholecystokinin, a hormone released from the duodenal mucosa, is the predominant stimulus for pancreatic enzyme secretion
    b. Gastrin is a major stimulant for pancreatic bicarbonate secretion
    c. Secretin is released from the duodenum upon mucosal acidification and stimulates pancreatic bicarbonate secretion
    d. Acetylcholine, released from pancreatic nerves, stimulates enzyme secretion

23. A 50-year-old man develops acute pancreatitis due to alcohol abuse. Increase in serum amylase resolves by the third day after admission. By the eighth hospital day, the patient is noted to have recurrent fever (38.5°C), progressive leukocytosis (18,500 WBC/mm^3), and tachypnea. The most appropriate the next step is:
    a. Laparotomy with pancreatic debridement
    b. CT guided aspiration of peripancreatic fluid collections

- c. ERCP with sphincterotomy and placement of biliary stent
- d. Intravenous amphotericin B

24. The patient in the above question is treated by observation for 8 weeks. He continues to be symptomatic with epigastric pain. A repeat abdominal CT scan reveals a persistent 6 cm pseudocyst in the region of the body of the pancreas. The pseudocyst is unilocular and demonstrates a well-defined rim of fibrous tissue. The gastric antrum is displaced anteriorly. Using CT guidance, 300 mL of fluid is aspirated from the lesion which is shown to be collapsed radiographically. No further intervention is performed. What is the risk of pseudocyst recurrence after simple aspiration?
    - a. 80–85%
    - b. 60–65%
    - c. 40–45%
    - d. 20–25%

25. In prospective, randomized trials which of the following has been demonstrated to accelerate recovery from acute pancreatitis?
    - a. Peritoneal lavage
    - b. Anticholinergic blockade
    - c. Octreotide
    - d. H_2 receptor blockade
    - e. Ligustrazine

26. Which of the following medical procedures is not associated with an increased risk of post-procedure acute pancreatitis?
    - a. Common bile duct exploration
    - b. Endoscopic retrograde cholangio-pancreatography
    - c. Coronary bypass grafting
    - d. Distal gastrectomy
    - e. Upper GI endoscopy

27. A 42-year-old male develops acute pancreatitis in the setting of acute alcohol abuse. One week after onset of symptoms, computed tomography of the abdomen reveals a pseudocyst. Lower probability of spontaneous resolution may be expected in all of the following conditions *except*?
    - a. Size greater than 5 cm
    - b. Diffuse calcification of the pancreatic gland
    - c. Multilocularity
    - d. Location in the pancreatic tail
    - e. Duration more than 2 months

28. Appropriate timing of cholecystectomy in patients who present with moderate to severe gallstone associated acute pancreatitis with peripancreatic fluid collections is:
    - a. Cholecystectomy and intraoperative cholangiography after inflammation subsides
    - b. Elective cholecystectomy beyond 8 weeks
    - c. Endoscopic sphincterotomy before discharge followed by cholecystectomy at approximately 8 weeks
    - d. Observation
    - e. Cholecystectomy as soon as possible

29. Which of the following statement related to chronic pancreatitis is TRUE?
    - a. Alcohol abuse is the most common cause
    - b. Approximately 50% of chronic alcoholics develop chronic pancreatitis
    - c. Clinically significant chronic pancreatitis develops on average after five years of alcohol abuse in men
    - d. The risk of alcohol-induced chronic pancreatitis can be decreased by consumption of a high-protein diet
    - e. High fat diet with omega 3 fatty acids is also considered protective

30. Most appropriate test to confirm a clinical diagnosis of early chronic pancreatitis is?
    - a. Serum amylase determination
    - b. Calculation of urinary amylase clearance
    - c. Measurement of para-aminobenzoic acid absorption
    - d. Endoscopic retrograde cholangio-pancreatography

31. A 46-year-old male, admitted with the complaint of icteric skin color was earlier diagnosed with chronic pancreatitis. Which is the most common cause of obstructive jaundice in such cases?
    - a. Adenocarcinoma of the head of the pancreas
    - b. Choledocholithiasis
    - c. Fibrotic stricture of the common bile duct
    - d. Pancreatic pseudocyst formation
    - e. Intraductal hematoma

32. Which of the following is the most common clinical manifestation of chronic pancreatitis?
    - a. Epigastric pain with radiation to the hypogastrium

    b. Diabetes mellitus
    c. Steatorrhea
    d. Epigastric pain with radiation to the upper lumbar vertebrae
    e. Chronic constipation

33. **Which of the following statement is FALSE concerning treatment of pyogenic liver abscess?**
    a. Antibiotic therapy alone may be advisable in patients with multiple small abscesses
    b. Percutaneous drainage provides comparable results to surgical drainage in patients with unilocular large abscesses
    c. Sufficient antibiotic coverage for most hepatic abscesses includes coverage for gram-positive aerobic bacteria
    d. In patients with a primary biliary origin for the hepatic abscess, treatment must also be addressed at underlying biliary pathology, such as choledocholithiasis or biliary ductal obstruction
    e. Escherichia coli is isolated most frequently on culture

34. **A 67-year-old male presents with complaints of itching, dark urine, and epigastric pain. Physical examination reveals jaundice. Initial laboratory tests show total bilirubin of 6.5 mg/dL, alkaline phosphatase elevated at 3 the upper limit of normal and mild elevations in serum transaminases. Which one is the next diagnostic test?**
    a. Abdominal ultrasonography
    b. Computed tomography of the abdomen
    c. Magnetic resonance imaging of the abdomen
    d. Endoscopic retrograde cholangiography

35. **Commonest cause of death in the postoperative period following pancreaticoduodenectomy (Whipple procedure) is:**
    a. Myocardial infarction
    b. Intraperitoneal hemorrhage
    c. Pulmonary embolism
    d. Pneumonia

36. **The following statement is false concerning hepatic blood flow:**
    a. Although constituting only 2.5% of total body weight, the liver receives 25% of the cardiac output
    b. Hepatic blood flow is equally derived from the portal vein and hepatic artery
    c. The liver serves as a physiologic blood reservoir either releasing blood back into the systemic circulation at times of acute blood loss or in situations of volume overload serving as a site of extra blood storage
    d. An important function of the liver is to filter particulate debris which is performed by phagocytic Kupffer cells which line the hepatic sinusoidal endothelium

37. **The liver synthesizes key metabolites essential for the production of fuel substrates for other organs. These key metabolites *except*:**
    a. Glucose-6-phosphate (G6P)
    b. Acetyl CoA
    c. Pyruvate
    d. Oxaloacetate
    e. Creatinine phosphokinase

38. **The following statement(s) is/are true concerning the differential diagnosis between an amoebic and a pyogenic liver abscess:**
    a. The clinical presentation is often clearly distinguishable
    b. Routine liver chemistries frequently can distinguish pyogenic from amoebic liver abscess
    c. Serologic testing for the presence of antibody to entameba histolytica is the only specific and sensitive way to confirm the diagnosis of amoebic liver abscess
    d. Distinguishing pyogenic from hepatic abscesses preoperatively is not important since surgical drainage is imperative for both

39. **A patient is found to develop evidence of hepatitis approximately eight weeks after receiving blood transfusions during hysterectomy. Which of the following statement is true?**
    a. The virus responsible is most likely hepatitis C
    b. A chronic carrier state will ultimately develop in most patients
    c. There is no role for interferon in the treatment of chronic hepatitis C viral infection
    d. Chronic infection with hepatitis C is not associated with an increased risk of developing hepatocellular carcinoma

40. **A 20-year-old woman is admitted to the hospital with suspected acute gallstone**

pancreatitis based on clinical history and laboratory studies. What is the best initial imaging study in this situation?
a. Contrast-enhanced abdominal and pelvic computed tomography (CT) scan
b. Endoscopic ultrasound
c. Magnetic resonance imaging with magnetic resonance cholangio-pancreatography
d. Noncontrast abdominal and pelvic CT scan
e. Right upper quadrant ultrasound

41. A 45-year-old man develops acute pancreatitis several days after starting oral azathioprine for Crohn's disease. On presentation, his initial serum lipase level is 11,500 U/L. The offending drug is stopped, the patient is admitted to the hospital, and he is treated conservatively with intravenous (IV) fluids and analgesia. On hospital day 2, his serum lipase level is 6400 U/L, and on day 3 his serum lipase level is 5100 U/L, suggesting that the rate of decline has begun to slow. The patient begins to feel better clinically and is tolerating clear liquids by mouth. For what duration of time should daily serum lipase be monitored in this patient?
a. 2 more days
b. 1 week
c. 1 month
d. Until the value returns to normal
e. There is no further need to obtain daily serum lipase levels in this patient

42. A 50-year-old woman presents to the emergency department with epigastric abdominal pain radiating to her back with associated nausea and vomiting. Her serum lipase level is 8400 U/L, and the patient is diagnosed with acute pancreatitis. The patient is administered an IV analgesic. What is the next best step in caring for this patient?
a. Begin IV fluid resuscitation
b. Begin prophylactic antibiotics to minimize the risk of pancreatic infection
c. Change her diet to clear liquids by mouth only
d. Obtain a contrast-enhanced CT scan of the abdomen
e. Obtain a right upper quadrant ultrasound

43. Which of the following medications has been shown to definitively prevent the development of postendoscopic retrograde cholangio-pancreatography pancreatitis?

a. Allopurinol
b. Heparin
c. Octreotide
d. Prednisone
e. None of the above

44. A "sentinel loop" seen on an abdominal radiograph in a patient with acute pancreatitis suggests which of the following?
a. Gastric volvulus
b. A localized small or large bowel ileus
c. An obstructed common bile duct
d. An obstructed gallbladder
e. A pancreatic pseudocyst

45. A 48-year-old man had abdominal distension and obstipation. Computed tomography (CT) scan (abdomen) was performed which is shown below:

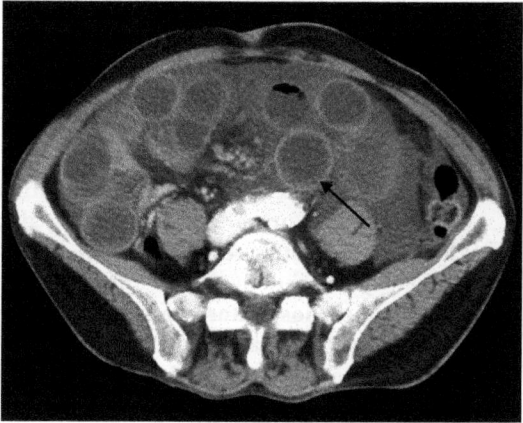

What is the likely diagnosis in this case?
a. Small intestinal perforation
b. Liver abscess
c. Mesenteric ischemia
d. Splenic abscess
e. Ascites

46. Which of the following statement is FALSE about Boerhaave syndrome?
a. Spontaneous perforation of the esophagus that results from a sudden increase in intraesophageal pressure combined with negative intrathoracic pressure
b. Associated with high morbidity and mortality
c. Upper GI endoscopy is the investigation of choice
d. ICU admission must be considered for patients with hemodynamic instability and in patients with comorbidities

47. A 65-year-old male patient with history of frequent abdominal pain and weight loss, presents with acute onset pain abdomen, severe in intensity associated with nausea and vomiting with one episode of tarry colored stool. On physical examination, he looks sick, is in respiratory distress and abdominal distension is noticed. An abdominal bruit was also noticed. HR and BP are 108/min and 90/65 mm Hg respectively. The radiologist reports significant findings in CT Angiography. Which of the following statement is FALSE?
    a. Diagnosis is acute on chronic thrombotic mesenteric ischemia
    b. Most common laboratory finding is metabolic acidosis with lactatemia
    c. Immediate resuscitation is recommended
    d. Antibiotics must be given as soon as possible

48. Which of the following is true statement regarding upper GI bleed?
    a. Use of tranexamic acid along with standard therapy is associated with decrease in mortality
    b. Patients with cirrhosis who present with acute upper GI bleeding should be given prophylactic antibiotics
    c. Emergency endoscopy (within 12 hours of presentation) is associated with increase in survival
    d. Upper GI barium studies may be done in the setting of acute upper GI bleeding

49. Which of the following statement is false for small bowel obstruction (SBO)?
    a. The most common causes of mechanical small bowel obstruction are postoperative adhesions
    b. Hallmark of small bowel obstruction is dehydration
    c. Nasogastric decompression is required in all patients
    d. Presence of free fluid and high-grade obstruction on CT scan as strong predictors for early surgery

50. A 28-year-old female underwent emergency lower segment cesarean section (LSCS) in view of thick meconium under spinal anesthesia uneventfully. On 2nd postoperative day, she had abdominal distension associated with pain abdomen and nausea. Patient also did not pass flatus or motion. On examination she was conscious, oriented but restless with pulse rate 110/min, BP: 110/78 mm Hg, RR: 35/min, SpO$_2$-98% on 40% venturi mask. Abdomen was grossly distended with diffuse mild tenderness and absent bowel sounds. Laboratory values were, Hb 12.9, TLC 19,200, Urea 15.9, Creat 0.4, Sodium 143, Potassium 3.6, Urine microscopy 10–20 pus cells. CT findings were suggestive of marked dilation of small bowel loops showing multiple air fluid levels, massive dilation of ascending colon, max diameter 9 cm. Which of the following is FALSE?
    a. Excessive parasympathetic suppression or sympathetic stimulation is the underlying cause
    b. The risk of colonic perforation increases when cecal diameter exceeds 10 to 12 cm and when the distension has been present for greater than six days
    c. Success rate of conservative management is approximately 20%
    d. Neostigmine is indicated in patients with acute colonic pseudo-obstruction and cecal diameter >12 cm or in patients who fail 24 to 48 hours of conservative therapy
    e. Endoscopy is contraindicated

K Type Questions
[Marked True (T)/False (F)]

1. The clinical picture of gallstone ileus includes which of the following?
    a. Air in the biliary tree
    b. Small bowel obstruction
    c. A stone at the site of obstruction
    d. Acholic stools
    e. Associated bouts of cholangitis

2. Which of the following parameters is/are included in the Ranson's prognostic signs useful in the early evaluation of a patient with acute pancreatitis?
    a. Elevated blood glucose
    b. Leukocytosis
    c. Amylase value greater than 1000 U per dL
    d. Serum lactic dehydrogenase (LDH) greater than 350 IU per dL
    e. Alanine aminotransferase greater than 250 U per dL

3. Which of the following statements about pancreatic ascites is/are correct?

a. Patients typically present with painful ascites, reflecting the release of toxic pancreatic enzymes into the peritoneal cavity
b. The standard evaluation of a patient with new-onset ascites includes abdominal paracentesis. In cases of pancreatic ascites, the peritoneal fluid contains high concentrations of both amylase and protein
c. Pancreatic ascites can follow an episode of acute pancreatitis
d. Patients with pancreatic ascites may fail to improve with nonoperative therapy and require surgical procedures. At abdominal exploration an acceptable approach to the pancreatic duct disruption involves suture ligation with omental patching

4. Which of the following statements about pyogenic abscess of the liver are true?
   a. The right lobe is more commonly involved than the left lobe
   b. Appendicitis with perforation and abscess is the most common underlying cause of hepatic abscess
   c. Mortality is largely determined by the underlying disease
   d. Mortality from hepatic abscess is currently greater than 40%

5. Which of the following statements characterize amebic abscess?
   a. Mortality is higher than that for similarly located pyogenic abscesses
   b. The diagnosis of amebic abscess may be based on serologic tests and resolution of symptoms
   c. In contrast to pyogenic abscess, the treatment of amebic abscess is primarily medical
   d. Patients with amebic abscess tend to be older than those with pyogenic abscess

6. A portal venous pressure of 30 mm Hg (elevated) and a hepatic venous wedge pressure of 5 mm Hg (normal) may be associated with which of the following causes of portal hypertension?
   a. Portal vein thrombosis
   b. Alcoholic cirrhosis
   c. Schistosomiasis
   d. Alcoholic hepatitis

7. Which of the following effects are advantages of combined vasopressin and nitroglycerin intravenous infusion, as compared with vasopressin infusion alone, in controlling acute variceal bleeding?

   a. Lower frequency of encephalopathy
   b. Lower incidence of vasopressin side effects
   c. More effective control of bleeding
   d. Less "rebound effect" when discontinuing the infusion

8. Which of the following statements about the peritoneovenous shunt (PVS) is/are correct?
   a. For cirrhotic patients with intractable ascites, the LeVeen shunt is an effective "bridge" to liver transplantation
   b. Replacement of ascites with saline or lactated Ringer's solution reduces the coagulopathy following PVS
   c. For patients with cirrhotic ascites, the survival using repeated paracentesis with 5% albumin infusion is equivalent to that with the PVS
   d. Oliguria (less than 25 mL per hour) in the immediate postoperative period following PVS should be treated with a 5% albumin infusion
   e. The transjugular intrahepatic portacaval shunt with stent (TIPSS) works on the same principle as the PVS

9. Which of the following explanations account(s) for the fact that hepatitis C is the most common cause of post-transfusion hepatitis?
   a. There are more carriers of hepatitis C virus (HCV) in the normal population who serve as blood donors
   b. Blood infected with hepatitis B virus (HBV) is eliminated through routine testing, leaving only HCV as the other blood-borne pathogen
   c. Current serologic tests for HCV antigen do not exclude carriers
   d. Questions designed to eliminate risk groups for HCV from the normal donor population may not be as specific as would be desirable
   e. Hepatitis C is a more virulent form of viral hepatitis, so it is expected that more cases of post transfusion hepatitis would occur

10. About HBV infections select TRUE or FALSE:
    a. Are usually asymptomatic
    b. May not be clinically recognized but may lead to chronic hepatitis
    c. Reliably protect against subsequent HBV infection regardless of the measured antibody titer to hepatitis B surface antigen (HBsAg)

d. Are completely prevented by postexposure administration of HBIg hepatitis B immunoglobulin (HBIg)
e. Preclude subsequent infection with HDV

11. Which of the following statements about the diagnosis of acute calculous cholecystitis are true?
    a. Pain is so frequent that its absence almost precludes the diagnosis
    b. Jaundice is present in a majority of patients
    c. Ultrasonography is the definitive diagnostic test
    d. Cholescintigraphy is the definitive diagnostic test

12. Which statements about acute acalculous cholecystitis are correct?
    a. The disease is often accompanied by or associated with other conditions
    b. The diagnosis is often difficult
    c. The mortality rate is higher than that for acute calculous cholecystitis
    d. The disease has been treated successfully by percutaneous cholecystostomy

13. Recurrent episodes of cholangitis:
    a. Suggest the presence of undetected or overlooked bile duct pathology
    b. Occur frequently in patients who have indwelling biliary tubes or stents
    c. May be ameliorated by long-term administration of antibiotics
    d. May be associated with the development of secondary biliary cirrhosis

14. Which of the following is/are prognostic signs reported by Ranson to predict outcomes associated with acute pancreatitis?
    a. Age greater than 60 years
    b. Hematocrit decrease of 105 within 48 hours of hospital admission
    c. Serum amylase value greater than 4 times upper limit of normal
    d. Serum glucose greater than 200 mg/dL on admission
    e. Ca^{2+} level less than 8 mg/dL within 48 hours of hospital admission

15. With regard to acute pancreatitis, which of the following statements is/are correct?
    a. The majority of patients presenting with acute pancreatitis of biliary type are female
    b. The majority of patients presenting with acute pancreatitis of alcoholic type are female
    c. The most common cause of acute pancreatitis in the United States is alcohol use
    d. Patients with alcohol-induced pancreatitis tend to be older than those with biliary-induced disease

16. A surgeon is suspected of having contacted hepatitis B virus via needle stick. Which of the following statement(s) is/are true concerning his diagnosis and outcome?
    a. Incubation of hepatitis B virus is about two weeks
    b. Jaundice is the first serologic indicator of hepatitis B infection
    c. The patient has about a 10% chance of developing a chronic carrier state
    d. All susceptible household or sexual contacts of the surgeon should receive hepatitis B viral vaccine
    e. The surgeon should receive hepatitis B immunoglobulin as soon as possible after the accidental needle stick

17. The following statement(s) is/are true concerning the diagnosis and treatment of hydatid cysts:
    a. Percutaneous aspiration is an important aspect of diagnosis and treatment of a hydatid cyst
    b. CT scan will often times show the classic findings of a cystic liver lesion with a calcific rim
    c. At operation, care must be taken to protect the operative field from spillage of the cyst fluid
    d. The use of a scoleocide has become obsolete with current surgical techniques

18. A 58-year-old man presents to the emergency department after several episodes of forceful vomiting of blood following periods of forceful retching. He had been binge drinking alcohol over the preceding 3 days. Mallory Weiss syndrome was diagnosed. Which of the following is/are true about diagnosis and management of this patient?
    a. Glasgow-Blatchford bleeding score (preendoscopy) of "6 or more" is associated with >50% risk of needing an intervention
    b. Characterized by a tear or laceration at or near the gastroesophageal junction
    c. Surgery is usually required
    d. Octreotide may be used

e. Flexible esophagogastroduodenoscopy is the investigation of choice

19. **Regarding acute mesenteric ischemia:**
    a. Mean arterial pressure less than 45 mm Hg leads to non-occlusive mesenteric ischemia
    b. Most common site of involvement is the origin of superior mesenteric artery (SMA) in thrombotic mesenteric ischemia
    c. Major blood supply of small intestine is by coeliac trunk
    d. Splanchnic circulation receives 25–30% of cardiac output
    e. For Nonocclusive mesenteric ischemia; blood supply must be reduced to < 50%

20. **A 60-year-old female patient, known case of osteoarthritis with history of frequent use of NSAIDS presented with complaints of maroon color stools and giddiness. On examination, orthostatic hypotension and altered sensorium is noticed. Which of the following statement/s is/are true?**
    a. Stool color is a reliable indicator of the location of the bleeding
    b. Nasogastric lavage is associated with decrease in mortality
    c. IV Erythromycin is associated with significant decrease in the need for second look endoscopy
    d. Octreotide is not primarily indicated in nonvariceal bleeding
    e. Restricted transfusion therapy is associated with significantly increased mortality in ischemic heart disease patients with GI tract bleed

21. **A 50-year-old woman presents to the emergency department with a 3-day history of watery diarrhea, fevers, and worsening abdominal pain. Her significant past medical history includes sinusitis, for which she has been taking antibiotics for the past 3 weeks. On physical examination, she is tachycardic and febrile, and her abdominal examination reveals diffuse abdominal tenderness and distention. Which of the following is TRUE?**
    a. CT scan of the abdomen and pelvis is diagnostic
    b. The use of loperamide in amoebic colitis may precipitate toxic megacolon
    c. Mucosal inflammation leading to the release of inflammatory mediators and bacterial products and colonic dilatation is the probable mechanism
    d. Characteristic pathologic features include diffuse ulcerations, raised mucosal nodules, yellowish-white superficial plaques with normal intervening mucosa and extensive denudation
    e. Colectomy is reserved for patients who do not improve within 48 to 72 hours, or who show evidence of perforation

22. **Which of the following statement/s is/are true in postoperative paralytic ileus (POI)?**
    a. "Normal" physiologic POI to postoperative gut dysmotility lasts from 0 to 24 hours (maximum 3 days) in the small intestine
    b. Routine placement of nasogastric tube in gut surgery is a risk factor
    c. Gastrografin can be used in the treatment of prolonged POI
    d. Opioid sparing analgesia is recommended
    e. Prolonged abdominal or pelvic surgery, lower gastrointestinal surgery and open surgery are known surgical risk factors

23. **An 80-year-old man presented with complaints of "black stools", increasing shortness of breath, chest tightness and epigastric pain. Which of the following class of drugs may be considered initially on suspicion of variceal bleeding along with myocardial ischemia?**
    a. Intravenous proton pump inhibitor (PPI)
    b. Fluids and blood products
    c. Anticoagulants and antiplatelet agents
    d. Prophylactic antibiotics
    e. Tranexamic acid

24. **Examples of medicines that can cause a paralytic ileus include:**
    a. Hydromorphone
    b. Hyperkalemia
    c. Hypokalemia
    d. Tricyclic antidepressants
    e. Dexmedetomidine (DEX)

25. **Regarding POI:**
    a. Lower gastrointestinal surgery poses more risk than upper gastrointestinal surgery
    b. Plain radiographs demonstrating air in the colon and rectum, with a clear transition zone or free air support a diagnosis of POI
    c. POI up to day 3 may be absolutely normal response to abdominal surgery
    d. CT is not required for the diagnosis since plain abdominal X ray is diagnostic
    e. Inj. Neostigmine 2.5 mg IV may be given on postoperative day-2

ANSWERS

A Type Answers

Q1. Answer a

Standard therapy for all patients with mild acute pancreatitis should include intravenous fluid resuscitation, electrolyte replacement, and analgesics. Nasogastric decompression is typically reserved for patients with significant ileus who are at risk for vomiting and aspiration. Subcutaneous therapy with octreotide, the octapeptide analog of somatostatin, has not been proven to influence the outcome in patients with mild pancreatitis. Prophylactic antibiotics are not used for mild pancreatitis. Antibiotics are reserved for patients with severe pancreatitis (defined as greater than three Ranson's prognostic signs with associated CT evidence of pancreatic or peripancreatic necrosis).

> Banks PA, Conwell DL, Toskes PP. The management of acute and chronic pancreatitis. Gastroenterol Hepatol (NY). 2010;6(2 Suppl 5):1-16.

Q2. Answer d

Segments are the major subdivision of the right and left lobes of the liver. In either the classic lobar (American) or the segmental (French) system, the most variable aspect is the biliary system. Therefore, the hepatic venous or portal system defines most segments. The French system depicts eight segments, with the caudate lobe as segment I and the other seven segments defined primarily by the hepatic venous system. Segments are not well-depicted by topography.

> Majno P, Mentha G, Toso C, et al. Anatomy of the liver: an outline with three levels of complexity: a further step towards tailored territorial liver resections. J Hepatol. 2014;60:654-62.

Q3. Answer c

The development of ultrasonography and computed tomography (CT) in the past two decades has enabled earlier diagnosis and advances in treatment of hepatic abscess. Formerly, open surgical drainage was considered necessary in essentially all cases of pyogenic abscess. Numerous recent series, however, have reported high success rates and low mortality from the percutaneous catheter drainage of abscesses under CT or ultrasonographic guidance. Optimal management of pyogenic abscess, however, involves not only treatment of the abscess, whether by percutaneous or surgical methods, but correction of the underlying source as well. All modes of therapy are more successful in treating solitary lesions than multiple ones.

> Holzheimer RG, Mannick JA (Eds). Surgical Treatment: Evidence-based and Problem-Oriented. Munich: Zuckschwerdt; 2001.

Q4. Answer a

Adenomas typically enlarge and cause symptoms, may rupture, and have a definite malignant potential. Therefore they should generally be resected when found. FNH is not a true neoplasm and generally has an uneventful course. Both are related to BCPs, although the relationship of adenoma is more firmly established. While small bile duct hamartomas are much more common, hemangiomas are the most common lesion to come to the attention of surgeons. They should not generally be biopsied because of possible hemorrhage. By definition, nodular regenerative hyperplasia occurs in the absence of cirrhosis.

> Colombo M, FornerA, Ijzermans J, et al. EASL clinical practice guidelines on the management of benign liver tumours. J Hepatol.2016;65(2):386-98.

Q5. Answer e

Although exact comparisons are impossible, hepatoma seems to be the most common cause of cancer death worldwide, despite its relative infrequency in the United States. Colorectal metastasis is a more common indication for surgical treatment in the United States. The fibrolamellar variant and possibly the very well-differentiated tumor probably have a better prognosis than hepatomas in general. Previous studies from Africa in which there was a high incidence of rupture account for the poor prognosis that was generally attributed to hepatoma. Recent studies from Europe and the United States have shown that survival after presentation is usually measured in years. Hemangioma and focal nodular hyperplasia usually do not need treatment, while adenoma requires hepatic resection due to the risk of malignant transformation and bleeding.

> Coelho JCU, Claus CMP, Balbinot P, et al. Indication and treatment of benign hepatic tumors. ABCD Arq Bras Cir Dig. 2011;24(4):318-23.

Q6. Answer e

Most bile duct cancers are discovered after they are incurable, and only a tiny subset of resected proximal lesions are cured. The more distal the lesion, the more likely is resection to achieve cure (e.g. approximately 30% 5-year survival for periampullary lesions as compared with 0% to 10% for hilar lesions). The use of adjuvant or primary radiation remains controversial because of the heterogeneity of the patient populations on which this modality has been used. Because of the localized nature of this disease it would seem that transplantation would produce favorable results; however, this has not been the case.

Treating Bile Duct Cancer. American Cancer Society. Available from: https://www.cancer.org/content/dam/CRC/PDF/Public/8555.00.pdf (Accessed 11 November, 2017).

Q7. Answer d

The parasitic infection is fairly common in certain parts of Europe but very rare in the United States. Resection without peritoneal soilage is the treatment of choice. The E. multilocularis form, which is endemic to parts of the United States, is more likely to be fatal because as it is rarely resectable. This form is more likely to resemble a malignancy than E. granulosus, although the natural course of the disease usually spans many years. Due to the typical slow growth, these often present in adulthood. Their symptoms include right upper quadrant abdominal pain, chlorosis, cholangitis, and anaphylaxis due to cyst rupture.

Mihmanli M, Idiz UO, Kaya C, et al. Current status of diagnosis and treatment of hepatic Echinococcosis. World J Hepatol. 2016;8(28):1169-81.

Q8. Answer c

By far the most common cause of hemobilia is trauma. Tumors also may cause the syndrome but are relatively uncommon causes. For severe hemobilia the best therapy is arteriographic embolization. Usually the site of bleeding or a false aneurysm can be identified. Operation should be reserved as a last resort or when the condition is recognized intraoperatively. Percutaneous cholangiography associated intrabiliary hemorrhage is usually, but not always, minor and self-limiting. Ultrasonography is a very nonspecific diagnostic technique for hemobilia. Arteriography remains the best diagnostic method.

Merrell SW, Schneider PD. Hemobilia-evolution of current diagnosis and treatment. West J Med. 1991;155(6):621-5.

Q9. Answer d

Ligation of the right or left hepatic artery frequently causes enzyme elevation but is usually tolerated by the patient, particularly when this is a life-saving maneuver. Ligation of the hepatic artery distal to the gastroduodenal branch is more risky but is also usually tolerated. Ligation of the hepatic artery proximal to the gastroduodenal one does not normally cause enzyme abnormalities because of abundant collateral flow through that branch.

Lee YT. Liver function tests after ligation of hepatic artery. J Surg Oncol. 1978;10(4):305-20.

Q10. Answer b

Metabolic alkalosis and hypokalemia are common in patients with cirrhosis because they often have associated secondary hyperaldosteronism (especially those with ascites), diarrhea, and frequent emesis. Hyperaldosteronism enhances H^+ and K^+ exchange for Na^+ in the distal tubule of the kidney. The cause of diarrhea in patients with cirrhosis is unknown, but malabsorption secondary to splanchnic venous hypertension may be a contributing factor. Emesis is common in alcoholic cirrhotics and patients with tense ascites. Deleterious effects of metabolic alkalosis include impaired tissue oxygen delivery secondary to shift of the oxyhemoglobin dissociation curve to the left and conversion of ammonium chloride to ammonia, which may contribute to encephalopathy.

Ahya SN, José Soler M, Levitsky J, et al. Acid-base and potassium disorders in liver disease. Semin Nephrol. 2006;26(6):466-70.

Q11. Answer d

Shunt operations are the most effective means of preventing recurrent variceal hemorrhage. Rebleeding rates after endoscopic sclerotherapy range from 40% to 60%. Although extensive esophagogastric devascularization has effectively prevented recurrent bleeding in Japanese series, these operations have been followed by rebleeding rates in excess of 25% in most Western series. Although one controlled trial has shown more frequent recurrent hemorrhage following the distal splenorenal shunt than after the portacaval shunt, most series have reported rebleeding rates of less than 10% for both of these operations. Both the liver and the splanchnic viscera are important sites of ascites formation. Since the distal splenorenal shunt maintains sinusoidal and mesenteric venous hypertension and requires interruption of important retroperitoneal lymphatics, it tends to aggravate rather than relieve ascites. Hepatic sinusoidal pressure may be unchanged or even increased after an end-to-side portacaval shunt. Only side-to-side portal-systemic shunts, such as the side-to-side portacaval shunt, reliably decompress both the liver and splanchnic viscera, thus preventing ascites formation.

Krige JEJ, Kotze UK, Bornman PC, et al. Variceal recurrence, rebleeding, and survival after endoscopic injection sclerotherapy in 287 alcoholic cirrhotic patients with bleeding esophageal varices. Ann Surg. 2006;244(5):764-70.

Q12. Answer b

While many patients with portal hypertension develop hypersplenism, it is rarely clinically significant. A splenectomy should not be performed unless platelet counts are persistently less than 20,000 per cu. mm. or white blood cell counts are less than 1200 per cu. mm. Unfortunately, splenectomy is sometimes done for clinically insignificant hypersplenism, thus obviating a distal splenorenal shunt, if the patient should subsequently bleed from varices. The initial treatment for most patients with bleeding esophageal varices should be endoscopic sclerotherapy; however, operation is required for the approximately one third of patients who fail sclerotherapy and for noncompliant persons, those living in remote geographic locations, and patients bleeding from gastric varices. Ascites can be controlled by a medical regimen of dietary salt restriction and diuretic therapy in more than 95% of patients. When ascites is intractable to medical management, either intermittent large volume paracenteses or a surgical peritoneovenous shunt should be done. With rare exceptions, encephalopathy should be treated medically. Most important is elimination of any precipitating factors that led to the neuropsychological disturbance. Lactulose, neomycin, and dietary protein restriction may also be components of the medical treatment regimen.

Collins JC, Sarfeh IJ. Surgical management of portal hypertension. West J Med. 1995;162(6):527-35.

Q13. Answer c

Because of the high complication rate and the long-term failure rate, the PVS is used only when other, more lasting options for therapy either are not available or are contraindicated. The chronic alcoholic patient may benefit from a peritoneovenous shunt because his ascites is the dominant problem related to his chronic liver disease, and persistent alcoholism is a contraindication to liver replacement in most centers. PVS may be quite effective for the temporary management of acute intractable postoperative ascites, such as in patient A; however, it is absolutely contraindicated in the presence of infection. Patient B has ascites as her dominant problem as well; however, with PBC as the underlying liver disease, she is an excellent candidate for transplantation. Patient D also has ascites as the major problem; however, the side-to-side portosystemic shunt is a far better long-term treatment option than PVS.

Collins JC, Sarfeh IJ. Surgical management of portal hypertension. West J Med. 1995;162(6):527-35.

Q14. Answer a

Cholecystectomy (and concomitant operative cholangiography) are indicated for symptomatic patients to relieve pain and to prevent the development of acute cholecystitis and its complications. Morbidity and expenses are less for elective cholecystectomy for acute cholelithiasis. The risk of the development of symptoms in patients who have asymptomatic stones is approximately 2% per year, a rate associated with mortality and morbidity that do not exceed those of elective cholecystectomy. Therefore, cholecystectomy is not indicated for asymptomatic patients. Patients who have angina pectoris should not have cholecystectomy until their coronary artery disease has been treated adequately, even if this requires a coronary artery bypass procedure. Heart disease is the most frequent cause of death after cholecystectomy. Prophylactic cholecystectomy, formerly recommended for insulin-dependent diabetics, is not indicated because several studies have shown that the mortality rate from acute cholecystitis is no higher for diabetics than for nondiabetics.

Lamberts MP, Özdemir C, Drenth JPH. Cost-effectiveness of a new strategy to identify uncomplicated gallstone disease patients that will benefit from a cholecystectomy. Surgical Endoscopy. 2017;31(6):2534-40.

Q15. Answer a

Although Charcot's triad (pain, chills and fever, jaundice) is diagnostic of cholangitis, the complete triad occurs only in 50% to 70% of patients. Fever is the most common symptom; therefore, cholangitis should be considered in all patients who have unexplained fever. Episodes of pain, chills, and fever are often so brief as not to concern the patient. Cholangitis does not occur in the absence of partial or complete bile duct obstruction. All patients diagnosed as having cholangitis should have appropriate diagnostic studies to determine the cause. This usually involves cholangiography. The presence of bacteria in bile does not produce symptoms in the absence of partial or complete obstruction of the bile duct system. When obstruction is present, pressure within the system increases, giving rise to efflux of bacteria or their toxic products into the hepatic venous circulation. This cholangio-venous reflux produces chills, fever, and the hemodynamic changes of sepsis. Death may ensue, if treatment is not instituted promptly. Choledocholithiasis, the most commonly associated problem, may produce partial or complete obstruction. When bacteria are not present in the bile duct system, choledocholithiasis may go undetected unless the degree of obstruction is sufficient to cause jaundice. Other causes of cholangitis are benign and malignant strictures, biliary-enteric anastomoses, invasive procedures, foreign bodies, and parasitic infestation of the bile ducts.

Afdhal NH. Acute cholangitis. Available from: https://www.uptodate.com/contents/acute-cholangitis?source=search_result&search=Charcot%27s%20triad&selectedTitle=1~5 (Accessed 11 November 2017).

Q16. Answer a

Uncontrolled sepsis and the consequent multisystem organ failure are the life-threatening sequelae of acute toxic cholangitis. Thus, the initial goal of treatment is to decompress the biliary duct system to prevent reflux of bacteria and their toxic products into the circulation. This can be done by intubating the duct system through the percutaneous, transhepatic, or the endoscopic route or by insertion of a T tube in the common duct at operation. Removal of the stone causing the obstruction is not necessary to stabilize the patient. Only after the duct is decompressed should the cause of the obstruction be addressed. When transhepatic biliary drainage has been used, endoscopic or surgical removal of the stone can be carried out after the patient has recovered completely. When initial therapy is sphincterotomy, the stone should be removed as part of the procedure. Often the stone falls out without manipulation. If surgical placement of a T tube is the initial treatment, the stone should be removed only if it is convenient to do so. The long-term goal of treatment of patients with bile duct obstruction is to prevent cirrhosis, ascites, portal hypertension, and hemorrhage from esophageal varices; however, death from sepsis is the immediate threat in acute toxic cholangitis. Gallstone pancreatitis may occur in patients who have an impacted stone in the distal duct, independent of the presence or absence of acute toxic cholangitis; however, gallstone pancreatitis is more often associated with the passage of a stone into the duodenum.

Timothy M Scott, DO Acute Cholangitis. Available from: https://emedicine.medscape.com/article/774245-overview (Accessed 11 November 2017).

Q17. Answer b

The endocrine portion of the pancreas is served by the islets of Langerhans, which number 1 million islets per gland. The islets of Langerhans drain their endocrine secretions into the bloodstream. Insulin-producing beta cells comprise the majority of the islet population. Alpha cells produce glucagon and constitute approximately 20% to 25% of the total islet cell number. Delta cells of the islets produce somatostatin. The acini and ductal systems constitute the exocrine portion of the pancreas. The acinar cells contain zymogen granules in their narrow, centrally located apical portion. The pancreatic duct system includes intercalated duct cells along the ductal pathway, terminating in the main excretory duct of the pancreas.

Chakraborty PP, Chowdhury S. A Look Inside the pancreas: The endocrine-exocrine cross-talk. Endocrinol Metab Synd. 2015;4:1.

Q18. Answer d

CCK is the most potent endogenous stimulant of pancreatic enzyme secretion. The pancreatic acinar cells respond to CCK with release of their zymogen granules into the ductal system. Peptidases are released in inactive form, later to be activated by contact with duodenal enterokinase and activated trypsin. Secretin is the most potent endogenous stimulant of pancreatic water and electrolyte secretion. The concentrations of the anions bicarbonate and chloride vary and are largely dependent on the secretory flow rate stimulated by secretin.

Chakraborty PP, Chowdhury S. A look inside the pancreas: the endocrine-exocrine cross-talk. Endocrinol Metab Synd. 2015;4:1.

Q19. Answer a

Adenocarcinoma of the pancreas is newly diagnosed in approximately 28,000 patients in the United States every year. It is the fifth most common cause of cancer death in the United States, exceeded only by lung, colorectal, breast, and prostate cancer. The majority of cases of adenocarcinoma of the pancreas occur in the head of the gland, and if resectable, are treated via pancreatico-duodenectomy. Recent studies have shown that factors favoring long-term survival after pancreatico-duodenectomy for adenocarcinoma of the head of the pancreas include negative nodal status, negative margin status, small tumor diameter, and diploid DNA content. No accurate screening tests for adenocarcinoma of the pancreas are currently available. The best serologic test appears to be the CA 19-9, which is elevated in the majority of patients with adenocarcinoma of the head of the pancreas. Unfortunately, the test is not sufficiently sensitive or specific, and further screening tests are needed.

Fernandez-del Castillo C. Clinical manifestations, diagnosis, and staging of exocrine pancreatic cancer. Available from: https://www.uptodate.com/contents/clinical-manifestations-diagnosis-and-staging-of-exocrine-pancreatic-cancer?source=search_result&search=adenocarcinoma%20of%20the%20pancreas&selectedTitle=1~150(Accessed 11 November, 2017).

Q20. Answer d

Insulinoma is the most common endocrine tumor of the pancreas. Insulinoma is associated with Whipple's triad, which consists of (1) symptoms of hypoglycemia at fasting; (2) documentation of blood glucose levels of less than 50 mg per dL; and (3) relief of symptoms following administration of glucose. The most reliable method for diagnosing insulinomas is a monitored fast. Neither an oral or an intravenous glucose tolerance test is indicated in the majority of patients being evaluated for insulinoma. Support for the diagnosis of insulinoma can come from documenting elevated C peptide and proinsulin levels. Screening for anti-insulin antibodies is indicated to rule out the possibility of surreptitious insulin administration. Tumor localization is typically performed with CT, endoscopic ultrasonography, or angiography. ERCP is not indicated for evaluation of most pancreatic endocrine tumors, as the tumors only rarely communicate with the main pancreatic duct system. As many as 90% of patients with insulinoma have benign solitary pancreatic adenomas amenable to surgical cure.

Kinova MK. Diagnostics and treatment of insulinoma. Neoplasma. 2015;62(5):692-704.

Q21. Answer e

Gastrinoma patients typically present with peptic ulceration of the upper gastrointestinal tract and abdominal pain. As many as 50% of patients may have diarrhea, which may be a prominent feature in some cases. Approximately 25% of gastrinoma patients have the disease associated with the MEN-1 syndrome, whereas 75% have a sporadic variety of the disease. Recent evidence indicates that extrapancreatic gastrinomas are common. Careful attention must be paid to the duodenum and peripancreatic lymph nodes at the time of abdominal exploration. Before elective operation it is imperative that the gastric acid hyper secretion be controlled. The control of gastric hyper secretion is best performed by the administration of one of the substituted benzimidazoles, such as omeprazole or lansoprazole. Diagnosis is based on an elevated fasting gastrin level in the presence of elevated basal gastric acid output.

Liang X, Ou Y, Jetal H. The clinical experience of surgical treating 9 cases of gastrinoma. Pancreatology. 2016;16(1):S36-S37.

Q22. Answer b

Enzyme secretion is regulated primarily through hormonal and neural factors. The enteric hormone cholecystokinin, released from endocrine cells in the duodenal mucosa, is the predominant regulator and stimulates acinar cells through specific membrane-bound receptors. Acetylcholine strongly stimulates acinar cells when released from postganglionic fibers of the pancreatic plexus and acts in synergy with CCK to potentiate enzyme secretion. Secretin weakly stimulates acinar cell secretion and potentiates the effect of cholecystokinin on the acinar cells. Bicarbonate is formed from carbonic acid by the enzyme carbonic anhydrase. Secretin, the major stimulant for bicarbonate secretion, is released from the duodenal mucosa in response to a duodenal luminal pH of less than 3.0. Cholecystokinin only weakly stimulates bicarbonate secretion, whereas it potentiates secretin-stimulated bicarbonate secretion. Gastrin and acetylcholine are weak stimulants of bicarbonate secretion.

> DiMagno EP, et al. Relationships among canine fasting pancreatic and biliary secretions, pancreatic duct pressure, and duodenal phase III motor activity—Boldyreff revisited. Dig Dis Sci. 1979;24(9):689-93.

Q23. Answer b

The common causes of pancreatic abscesses are infected pancreatic pseudocysts and necrotizing pancreatitis. The diagnosis is suggested by persistent fever, leukocytosis, and a palpable abdominal mass. Bacteremia and systemic toxicity are late clinical features. Percutaneous aspiration with positive cultures is the definitive preoperative test, facilitated by CT scanning or ultrasound-guidance to suspicious peripancreatic fluid collections. When diagnosed, the treatment of choice is wide surgical debridement with removal of all infected and revitalized tissues. Generous drainage is mandatory. One of the major sources of morbidity and mortality in this situation is the late development of mycotic visceral pseudoaneurysms, particularly involving the splenic circulation. These may be complex management problems, requiring angiographic embolization or other innovative treatment strategies.

> Ang TL, Teo EK, Fock KM. EUS-guided drainage of infected pancreatic pseudocyst: use of a 10F Soehendra dilator to facilitate a double-wire technique for initial transgastric access. Gastrointestinal Endoscopy. 2008;68(1):192-4.

Q24. Answer d

Generally, a pancreatic pseudocyst can be observed for a period of weeks or months in an effort to allow for spontaneous resolution. Percutaneous ultrasound-or CT-directed aspiration or drainage catheter placement is an initial treatment option. Simple aspiration is performed, if the initial aspirate is sterile; if the aspirate is infected, a catheter or open drainage procedure is appropriate. Determination of pancreatic ductal anatomy is important. Contrast injection into the pseudocyst at the time of aspiration should be considered to assess the possibility of pancreatic ductal communication and obstruction, or multiple cysts. The pseudocyst recurrence rate after simple aspiration is about 20% to 25%.

> Ang TL, Teo EK, Fock KM. EUS-guided drainage of infected pancreatic pseudocyst: use of a 10F Soehendra dilator to facilitate a double-wire technique for initial transgastric access. Gastrointestinal Endoscopy. 2008;68(1):192-4.

Q25. Answer e

A variety of pharmacologic agents that directly or indirectly reduce acinar cell enzyme release or ductal secretion have undergone clinical evaluation for the treatment of acute pancreatitis—generally with unimpressive results. Among the first were anticholinergic drugs. Despite extensive experience over many years, no objective data have emerged to support their use. Clinical trials of glucagon and calcitonin based on the same principle have produced a similar lack of supportive data. More recently, a somatostatin analog has been subjected to clinical trials for patients with acute pancreatitis. Somatostatin inhibits pancreatic enzyme and bicarbonate secretion by preventing the normal release of cholecystokinin, secretin, and other gut peptides. Despite the theoretical appeal, it has not been possible to demonstrate that somatostatin alters the natural history or prognosis of simple acute pancreatitis, although it does diminish pancreatic secretion.

Peritoneal lavage as a specific therapy for acute pancreatitis was proposed after experimental studies demonstrated improved survival in animals with fulminant pancreatitis. The concept was appealing in that activated proteases and other vasoactive substances identifiable in peritoneal aspirates from patients with pancreatitis would be removed, rather than systemically absorbed. Unfortunately, clinical trials using this approach have produced disappointing results, and the eventual overall mortality rate appears unchanged. Ligustrazine alleviates acute pancreatitis by accelerating acinar cell apoptosis at early phase via the suppression on p38 and Erk MAPK pathways. It is capable of attenuating the severity of acute pancreatitis and may have a therapeutic effect on patients with acute pancreatitis.

> Chen J, Chen J, Wang X, et al. Ligustrazine alleviates acute pancreatitis by accelerating acinar cell apoptosis at early phase via the suppression of p38 and Erk MAPK pathways. Biomed Pharmacother. 2016;82:1-7.

Q26. Answer e

Many surgical procedures in the upper abdomen are associated with postoperative pancreatitis. The incidence of acute pancreatitis after gastric resection ranges from 0.6% to 1.23%. After biliary tract surgery, particularly after common bile duct exploration itself, acute pancreatitis occurs with an incidence of 0.5% to 3%. Direct manipulation or retraction of the pancreas or pancreatic duct appears to be the most common cause. About 1% of patients develop acute pancreatitis after endoscopic retrograde.

Cholangio-pancreatography (ERCP). This is a predictable event, and the risk can be minimized by limiting the pressure used for contrast injection of the pancreatic duct. Acute pancreatitis also occurs in patients after coronary artery bypass surgery and a variety of other procedures remote from the pancreas. Although pancreatitis in this circumstance is thought to result from ischemia, hypotension is not always noted. The systemic consequences of activation of the inflammatory system may contribute to changes in microvascular blood flow.

>   Al-Bahrani AZ, Holt A, Hamade AM, et al. Acute pancreatitis: an under-recognized risk of percutaneous transhepatic distal biliary intervention HPB (Oxford). 2006;8(6):446-50.

Q27. Answer d

Initial management of pancreatic pseudocysts is based on symptoms. If the patient is asymptomatic and the cyst is small (< 5.0 cm) it can be safely observed as many of these will resolve over a period of weeks. Concurrent chronic alcoholic pancreatitis (by history or as indicated by pancreatic calcification), pseudocyst size greater than 5 cm, the presence of a multilocular or debris-filled pseudocyst cavity, and chronicity (longer than 6 weeks) are all factors that are associated with a lower probability of spontaneous resolution.

>   Pan G, Wan MH, Xie KL, et al. Classification and management of pancreatic pseudocysts. Medicine (Baltimore). 2015;94(24):e960.

Q28. Answer a

A patient who has simple cholelithiasis and an episode of acute pancreatitis is usually treated nonoperatively until clinical resolution of the pancreatitis occurs. The rate of recurrent biliary pancreatitis is as high as 34% to 56% within 6 weeks; therefore, an aggressive operative approach is appropriate. Cholecystectomy is often performed after the resolution of acute pancreatitis but before hospital discharge. Common bile duct instrumentation in this setting has a substantially increased risk of recurrent acute pancreatitis.

>   Nealon WH, Bawduniak J, Walser EM. Appropriate timing of cholecystectomy in patients who present with moderate to severe gallstone-associated acute pancreatitis with peripancreatic fuid collections. Ann Surg. 2004;239(6):741-51.

Q29. Answer a

In the United States, alcohol consumption is the major cause of chronic pancreatitis with approximately 70% of cases attributable to this factor. Most patients with symptomatic chronic pancreatitis have consumed large volumes of alcohol daily for a prolonged period of time. The average daily intake of alcohol is 150 to 175 g with the mean duration of alcoholism before recognition of pancreatitis being 18 years for men and 11 years for women. The incidence of chronic pancreatitis on autopsy studies of chronic alcoholics is 50 times the rate of nondrinking controls. Only 10% of alcoholics develop chronic pancreatitis, suggesting that factors other than long-term alcohol exposure may also influence susceptibility. In both experimental and clinical studies, the risk of alcohol-induced chronic pancreatitis is increased by a high-protein, high-fat diet.

>   Steven D Freedman, Patient education: Chronic pancreatitis (Beyond the Basics). Available from: https://www.uptodate.com/contents/chronic-pancreatitis-beyond-the-basics (Accessed 1 January 2018).

Q30. Answer d

Routine tests of blood or serum are not helpful in making a diagnosis of chronic pancreatitis. Although serum amylase levels are almost always elevated in acute pancreatitis, amylase levels may be normal, elevated, or subnormal in chronic pancreatitis. Determination of urinary amylase secretion and calculation of urinary amylase clearance does not improve sensitivity or specificity. Indirect tests of pancreatic function which measure absorption of nutrients that first require pancreatic digestion are not helpful in early cases of chronic pancreatitis. Clinically detectable malabsorption is absent until 90% of exocrine function is lost. Because of this, indirect tests of pancreatic function do not detect early disease. In addition, false positive tests may occur in other disease states associated with malabsorption (Crohn's disease, sprue, postgastrectomy states, or in association with diabetes mellitus, cirrhosis, or renal disease. ERCP has become widely recognized as the most sensitive and reliable method for diagnosing chronic pancreatitis. Sensitivity approaches 90% with equal specificity.

Duggan SN, Chonchubhair HM, Lawal O, et al. Chronic pancreatitis: a diagnostic dilemma. World J Gastroenterol. 2016;22(7): 2304-13.

Q31. Answer c

Biliary complications involving the common bile duct can occur in chronic pancreatitis because of the intimate association of that structure with the head of the pancreas. In two-thirds of individuals, the common bile duct traverses the pancreatic parenchyma and in an additional 25%, the common bile duct lies within a groove along the posterior surface of the pancreas. Fibrosis associated with chronic pancreatitis can encase and compress the common bile duct. Common bile duct stenosis is relatively common in chronic pancreatitis, occurring in approximately 10% of cases observed long-term. Cholangiography typically reveals a long, gradually tapering stricture conforming to the intrapancreatic portion of the common bile duct. In contrast, malignant strictures usually result in abrupt termination of the biliary duct. The proximal suprapancreatic portion of the bile duct is variably dilated.

Cho HG, Min HY, Jang DS, et al. Two cases of chronic pancreatitis with pseudocyst complicated by obstructive jaundice. Yonsei Med J. 2000;41(4):522-7.

Q32. Answer d

Abdominal pain is a dominant feature of chronic pancreatitis. The pain is typically epigastric, often radiates to the back, is occasionally associated with nausea and vomiting, and may be partially relieved by sitting upright or leaning forward. The pain is often worse 15 to 30 minutes after eating. Early in the course of chronic pancreatitis, the pain may occur in discrete attacks; as the condition progresses, the pain tends to become more continuous.

Freedman SD. Clinical manifestations and diagnosis of chronic pancreatitis in adults. Available from: https://www.uptodate.com/contents/clinical-manifestations-and-diagnosis-of-chronic-pancreatitis-in-adults?source=search_result&search=chronic%20pancreatitis&selectedTitle=1~150 (Accessed 1 January 2018).

Q33. Answer c

The preferred treatment of most patients with hepatic abscesses is broad-spectrum antibiotic coverage and drainage. A number of studies have demonstrated for most patients with large unilocular abscesses that percutaneous catheter drainage is as effective as surgical drainage. Bacteria that predominate in pyogenic liver abscesses are gram-negative aerobes, streptococcal species, and anaerobes. Therefore, broad-spectrum antibiotic coverage is necessary. Antibiotic coverage alone may be advisable in occasional patients who have multiple small abscesses not accessible to percutaneous or surgical drainage. Since many of these patients have an underlying biliary pathology as the source of the hepatic abscess, correcting this underlying pathology, for example, establishing biliary drainage surgically or nonoperatively is important.

Singh S, Chaudhary P, Saxena N, et al. Treatment of liver abscess: prospective randomized comparison of catheter drainage and needle aspiration. Annals of Gastroenterology. 2013;26:1-8.

Q34. Answer a

Standard transcutaneous ultrasonography is the appropriate first test in the evaluation of the patient with jaundice, because the presence of a dilated common bile duct or intrahepatic bile ducts is essentially diagnostic of extrahepatic biliary obstruction. This finding directs the physician to a search for the cause of the obstruction. If the bile ducts are not dilated, mechanical obstruction is unlikely and the diagnostic thrust should move toward hepatocellular disease. Ultrasonography is also the best test to determine whether gallstones are present; this is extremely important because choledocholithiasis is one of the conditions most likely to cause jaundice in the elderly population.

Bhargava SK, Usha T, Bhatt S, et al. Imaging in obstructive jaundice: a review with our experience. JIMSA. 2013;26(1):43.

Q35. Answer b

Pancreaticoduodenectomy is a formidable operation, and until recently, average operative mortality was reported to approximate 20%. In the past few years, several centers have reported large series with operative mortalities lower than 5%. The most dreaded complication of pancreaticoduodenectomy is disruption of the pancreaticoduodenectomy, which occurs in about 10% of patients. Anastomotic breakdown may lead to the development of an upper abdominal abscess or may present as a external pancreatic fistula. In its most virulent form, disruption leads to necrotizing retroperitoneal infection which may erode major arteries and veins of the upper abdomen, including the portal vein or its branches or the stump of the gastroduodenal artery. Impending catastrophe is often preceded by a small herald bleed from the drain site. Such an event is an indication to return to the operating room to widely drain the pancreatico-jejunostomy and to repair the involved blood vessel. Open packing of the wound may be necessary in controlling diffuse necrosis and infection. On rare occasions, completion pancreatectomy is required to control sepsis. Intraperitoneal hemorrhage is the most common cause of death from pancreaticoduodenectomy.

Gouma DJ, Geenen RC. Rates of complications and death after pancreatico-duodenectomy: Risk factors and the impact of hospital volume. Ann Surg. 2000;232(6):786-95.

Q36. Answer b

The liver constitutes about 2.5% of the total body weight but receives 25% of the cardiac output. Total hepatic blood flow is 100 to 130 mL/min/kg. About two-thirds of total hepatic blood flow is derived from the portal vein and one third from the hepatic artery. The liver also serves as a physiologic blood reservoir. About 25% to 30% of the liver volume is accounted for by blood, and in cases of acute blood loss up to 30%, or as much as 300 mL of the hepatic blood volume can be released into the systemic circulation without adverse effects on liver function. Conversely, in the case of right heart failure or other causes of systemic volume overload, as much as one liter of extra blood can be stored in the liver before passive congestion and liver injury occur. The hepatic sinusoids are lined by an endothelium punctuated with pores that allow proteins and other particles to diffuse out of the vascular tree and into proximity with hepatocytes. This extreme permeability of the liver allows rapid exchange of a diverse number of nutrients, hormones and environmental agents between the blood and the hepatocyte. The liver also acts as a filter for particulate debris, which enters the portal circulation through intestinal capillaries. Particles, such as bacteria are ingested by Kupffer cells by the process of phagocytosis. Kupffer cells line the hepatic sinusoidal endothelium where formed blood elements and matter may be in direct contact with these phagocytic cells.

Eipel C, Abshagen K, Vollmar B. Regulation of hepatic blood flow: The hepatic arterial buffer response revisited. World J Gastroenterol. 2010;16(48):6046-57.

Q37. Answer e

Hepatic processes in the liver are essential for the production of fuel substrates for other organs. The liver, by virtue of its terminal position in the portal system, is the organ that must regulate intestinally absorbed nutrients for tissue consumption or storage. The liver accomplishes its task by synthesizing three key metabolites: -glucose-6-phosphate, pyruvate and acetyl CoA. G6P can be stored as glycogen or converted into glucose, pyruvate, or ribose-5phosphate (a nucleotide precursor). Pyruvate can be converted into lactate, alanine (and other amino acids), and acetyl CoA, or it can enter the tricarboxylic acid cycle. Acetyl CoA is converted to HMG-CoA (a cholesterol and ketone body precursor) or citrate (for fatty acid and triglyceride synthesis), or it is degraded to carbon dioxide and water for energy.

Rui L. Energy metabolism in the liver. Compr Physiol. 2014;4(1):77-197.

Q38. Answer c

Distinguishing amoebic from pyogenic liver abscess can be a diagnostic challenge. It is of major importance, however, because effective medical therapy with metronidazole can obviate the need for either percutaneous or surgical drainage in most cases of amoebic abscess. The clinical presentation for both conditions with acute onset of fever, abdominal pain, and altered liver function tests are almost identical. Routine liver chemistries and radiographic studies can rarely distinguish between amoebic and pyogenic liver abscesses.

Specific serologic tests for the presence of antibody to E histolytica are specific and sensitive for amoebic hepatic abscess being positive in 95% of the cases, and therefore, are key in distinguishing the two infections.

Ahsan T, Jehangir MU, Mahmood T, et al. Amoebic versus pyogenic liver abscess. J Pak Med Assoc. 2002;52(11):497-501.

Q39. Answer a

Hepatitis C virus is a virus that is responsible for more than 90% of transfusion-associated hepatitis (TAH) and most sporadic non-A, non-B hepatitis throughout the world. The most common identifiable sources of acquisition of hepatitis C virus are prior transfusion of blood or blood-derived products or a history of intravenous illicit drug use. The usual incubation period of post-transfusion hepatitis C viral infection is 5 to 10 weeks. An initial elevation of liver enzymes may be associated with little or no clinical disturbance. In some patients, acute hepatitis C viral infection does not progress to chronic infection, however, chronic hepatitis C develops in up to 70% of patients with post transfusion hepatitis C infection with many progressing to cirrhosis. Hepatitis C does not appear to alter life expectancy at least in the first 15 years of infection. However, once cirrhosis and end stage liver disease develop, the clinical syndrome is indistinguishable from other forms of chronic liver disease with a predisposition to the development of hepatoma. Interferon alpha is the only FDA approved therapy for chronic hepatitis C viral infection. There is some evidence that early administration of interferon in acute hepatitis C viral infection may reduce the risk of progression to the chronic state. As yet, there is no evidence that interferon alters the natural history of chronic hepatitis C viral infection or changes the incidence.

Silverman AL, Gordon SC. Clinical epidemiology and molecular biology of hepatitis C. Laboratory Medicine. 1993;24(10):656-9.

Engle RE, Bukh J, Alter HJ. Transfusion-associated hepatitis before the screening of blood for hepatitis risk factors.Transfusion. 2014;54(11):2833-41.

Engle RE, Bukh J, Alter HJ. Transfusion-associated hepatitis before the screening of blood for hepatitis risk factors.Transfusion. 2014;54(11):2833-41.

Q40. Answer e

The diagnosis of gallstone pancreatitis should be suspected, if the patient has a prior history of biliary colic. Although gallstone pancreatitis is the most common cause of pancreatitis, other etiologies must be considered, prior to initiating treatment, like alcohol consumption over a period of years. Other causes include medication, genetic diseases, infectious agents, postoperative states, endoscopic procedure involving pancreatic and bile ducts and other types of injury to pancreas. Careful physical examination and laboratory tests are done initially. Right upper quadrant ultrasound is a best initial imaging study. The finding of gallstones and dilatation of the extra hepatic biliary tree on cross-sectional abdominal imaging lends further support to the diagnosis of gallstone pancreatitis. However, the sensitivity for detection of dilated bile ducts from biliary obstruction ranges in various studies from 55 to 91%. Trans abdominal ultrasonography seldom visualizes the pancreas in patients with acute pancreatitis due to air in the distended loops of the small bowel. Comparison of imaging techniques for acute pancreatitis Helical computerized tomography (CT) is one choice for accurate imaging diagnosis and staging of pancreatitis. A CT allows identification of pancreatic edema, fluid or cysts, and the severity of pancreatitis to be graded, detects complications including development of pseudocysts, abscess, necrosis, hemorrhage, and vascular occlusion.

Hazem ZM. Acute biliary pancreatitis: diagnosis and treatment. Saudi J Gastroenterol. 2009;15(3):147-55.

Q41. Answer e

In general, repeating serum amylase and lipase levels has no value once the diagnosis of acute pancreatitis has been made. In gallstone-related acute pancreatitis (i.e. in most cases), delaying surgery for several days for the pancreas to 'cool down' is common practice, but repeating serum pancreatic enzyme levels daily during this period is of no prognostic value, as the levels do not correlate with the severity, course, or outcome of the acute pancreatitis. The decision to proceed with treatment should be based on clinical measures, such as improvement of pain or increasing appetite.

Repeated pancreatic enzyme tests have diagnostic value, though. For example, in mild acute pancreatitis, symptoms tend to resolve in less than 1 week, whereas in severe cases, not only do symptoms persist beyond 1 week, but complications (new symptoms) also develop after the first week. In such cases, serum amylase and lipase levels may be repeated when the patient has signs and symptoms of persisting pancreatic or peripancreatic inflammation, blockage of the pancreatic duct, or development of a pseudocyst, but the purpose of retesting the levels is to diagnose complications, not to monitor the status of the pancreas. However, imaging tests generally have a higher sensitivity than serum amylase and lipase levels for diagnosing complications of acute pancreatitis. The diagnosis of pancreatitis requires two of the following three features: abdominal pain characteristic of acute pancreatitis, a serum amylase or lipase level at least three times the upper limit of normal and characteristic findings of acute pancreatitis on computed tomography (CT). In most patients, initial CT is not clinically warranted. It is warranted for patients who are transferred from other institutions after a few days of care, when the diagnosis of acute pancreatitis is in doubt, or when traumatic pancreatitis is suspected. Contrast-enhanced CT may be required at intervals during the hospitalization to detect and monitor the course of intra-abdominal complications of acute pancreatitis, such as the development of necrosis, fluid collections, and vascular complications. A serum amylase or lipase level greater than three times the upper limit of normal is characteristic of acute pancreatitis and almost excludes other conditions associated with elevated nonpancreatic enzyme levels.

> Yegneswaran B, Pitchumoni CS. When should serum amylase and lipase levels be repeated in a patient with acute pancreatitis? Cleveland Cli J Med. 2010;77(4):230-1.

Q42. Answer a

Acute Pancreatitis (initial management recommendations): (1) Aggressive hydration, defined as 250–500 mL per hour of isotonic crystalloid solution should be provided to all patients, unless cardiovascular, renal, or other related co morbid factors exist. Early aggressive intravenous hydration is most beneficial during the first 12–24 h, and may have little benefit beyond this time period (strong recommendation, moderate quality of evidence). (2) In a patient with severe volume depletion, manifest as hypotension and tachycardia, more rapid repletion (bolus) may be needed (conditional recommendation, moderate quality of evidence). (3) Lactated Ringer's solution may be the preferred isotonic crystalloid replacement fluid (conditional recommendation, moderate quality of evidence). (4) Fluid requirements should be reassessed at frequent intervals within 6 h of admission and for the next 24–48 h. The goal of aggressive hydration should be to decrease the BUN (strong recommendation, moderate quality of evidence).

> Tenner S, Baillie J, Witt J, et al. American College of Gastroenterology Guideline: Management of Acute Pancreatitis. Am J Gastroenterol. 2013.

Q43. Answer e

Despite advances in knowledge behind the mechanisms and risk factors for post-ERCP pancreatitis, the incidence of this condition is still high and is the most common complication of ERCP. The primary approach to prevention is through careful patient selection, sound endoscopic technique, and evidence-based medical management. Ongoing identification and special attention to risk factors for post-ERCP pancreatitis is vital, in order to optimize patient selection and to guide specific procedure techniques and other prophylactic measures. There are several mechanisms that contribute to the development of pancreatitis and that can be targeted for protective endoscopic or medical therapies. Preventive measures include procedural techniques such as the use of a guide wire cannulation, minimizing the total number of cannulation attempts, and avoiding contrast injections or trauma to the pancreatic duct. The placement of temporary pancreatic stents and administration of rectal NSAIDs in high-risk patients remain the interventions with proven efficacy and thus should be incorporated into clinical practice. High-quality studies are still needed to better evaluate other medical therapies.

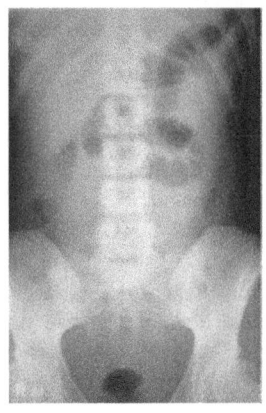

Q44. Answer b

A sentinel loop is a sign seen on a radiograph that indicates localized ileus from nearby inflammation. An isolated distended loop of bowel is seen near the site of injured viscus or inflamed organ. This loop is called a "sentinel loop." It arises from the body's efforts to localize traumatic or inflammatory lesions. The local distention of that intestinal loop is due to local paralysis and accumulation of gas in the intestinal loop.

Site of dilated loops	Cause
Right upper quadrant	Cholecystitis
Left upper quadrant	Pancreatitis
Right lower quadrant	Appendicitis
Left lower quadrant	Diverticulitis
Mid-abdomen	Ulcer or kidney/ureteric calculi

    Loo JT, Duddalwar V, Chen FK, et al. Abdominal radiograph pearls and pitfalls for the emergency department radiologist: a pictorial review. Abdominal Radiology. 2017;42(4):987-1019.

Q45. Answer c

CT shows dilated loops of small bowel with thickened walls (black arrow). CT is the primary imaging modality and it has been proven to be highly accurate in the diagnosis of mesenteric ischemia; scans sometimes depict the underlying etiology. Typically, CT scans show mesenteric edema with irregular thickening of the wall of the small or large bowel that is greater than 3 mm. Large-vessel disease (superior mesenteric artery/vein [SMA/SMV]; inferior mesenteric artery/vein [IMA/IMV]) is diffuse, whereas small-vessel arterial or venous disease is more likely to be focal. The best method of diagnosis is angiography, with CT being used when that is not available. Mesenteric ischemia is a medical condition in which injury of the small intestine occurs due to reduced blood supply. It can come on suddenly, known as acute mesenteric ischemia, or gradually, known as chronic mesenteric ischemia. Acute disease often presents with sudden severe pain. Symptoms may come on more slowly in those with acute on chronic disease. Signs and symptoms of chronic disease include abdominal pain after eating, unintentional weight loss, vomiting, and being afraid of eating. Risk factors include atrial fibrillation, heart failure, chronic renal failure, being prone to forming blood clots, and previous myocardial infarction. There are four mechanisms by which poor blood flow occurs: a blood clot from elsewhere getting lodged in an artery, a new blood clot forming in an artery, a blood clot forming in the superior mesenteric vein, and insufficient blood flow due to low blood pressure or spasms of arteries. Chronic disease is a risk factor for acute disease.

    Bobadilla JL. Mesenteric ischemia. The surgical clinics of North America. 2013;93(4):925-40.

Q46. Answer c

Boerhaave's syndrome is spontaneous esophageal perforation (full thickness tear) following forceful vomiting. If appropriate treatment is not given on time, it is fraught with early complications, leading to a very high mortality rate. This is a characteristic feature of this syndrome. Patient survival is in days. Preexisting esophageal disease is not a prerequisite for esophageal perforation but it contributes to increased mortality. Endoscopy has no role in the diagnosis of spontaneous esophageal perforation. Diagnosis is established by abdominal X-ray, esophagography and CT scanning. Both the endoscope and insufflation of air can extend the perforation and introduce air into the mediastinum. A related condition is Mallory-Weiss syndrome which is only a mucosal tear.

    Tamatey MN, Sereboe LA, Tettey MM, et al. Boerhaave's syndrome: diagnosis and successful primary repair one month after the oesophageal perforation. Ghana Med J. 2013;47(1):53-5.

Q47. Answer b

Physical examination in cases of mesenteric ischemia shows signs of malnutrition, pain that is disproportionate to examination findings—usually, diffuse mild abdominal tenderness, with no rebound or guarding, abdominal bruit, signs of peripheral vascular disease (e.g. carotid bruits, decreased pulses, and ischemic feet). CT angiography (CTA) has a sensitivity of 96% and a specificity of 94% for detecting CMI. An elevated lactate level is sensitive for mesenteric ischemia. However, the lactate has low specificity and is only elevated late in the disease course after bowel has infarcted. D-dimer testing has higher sensitivity for mesenteric ischemia than lactate. However, like lactate, it has a low specificity. In chronic mesenteric ischemia when the bowel has infarcted rise of lactate has less diagnostic value. An elevated lactate level is sensitive for mesenteric ischemia. However lactate has low specificity and is only elevated late in the disease course after bowel has infarcted.

The lactate levels may not be elevated in chronic mesenteric ischemia. D-dimer testing has higher sensitivity for mesenteric ischemia than lactate. However, like lactate, it has a low specificity. Classically, patients with mesenteric ischemia have leukocytosis, metabolic acidosis, elevated D-dimer and serum lactate. Although profound leukocytosis with peripheral white blood cell counts exceeding $20 \times 10^9/L$ have been reported, this finding is not useful to distinguish AMI from other diagnoses.

    Heijkant TC, Aerts BA, Teijink JA, et al. Challenges in diagnosing mesenteric ischemia. World J Gastroenterol. 2013;19(9):1338-41.

Q48. Answer b

Bacterial infections are common in cirrhotic patients with acute variceal bleeding, occurring in 20% within 48 h. Outcomes including early rebleeding and failure to control bleeding are strongly associated with bacterial infection. Mortality from variceal bleeding is largely determined by the severity of liver disease. Besides a higher child-pugh score, patients with hepatocellular carcinoma are particularly susceptible to infections. Despite several hypotheses that include increased use of instruments, greater risk of aspiration pneumonia and higher bacterial translocation, it remains debatable whether variceal bleeding results in infection or vice versa but studies suggest that antibiotic prophylaxis prior to endoscopy and up to 8 h is useful in reducing bacteremia and spontaneous bacterial peritonitis. Aerobic gram negative bacilli of enteric origin are most commonly isolated from cultures, but more recently, gram positives and quinolone-resistant organisms are increasingly seen, even though their clinical significance is unclear. Fluoroquinolones (including ciprofloxacin and norfloxacin) used for short term (7 d) have the most robust evidence and are recommended in most expert guidelines. Short term intravenous cephalosporin (especially ceftriaxone/cefotaxime), given in a hospital setting with prevalent quinolone-resistant organisms, has been shown in studies to be beneficial, particularly in high risk patients with advanced cirrhosis.

    Lee YY, Tee HP, Mahadeva S. Role of prophylactic antibiotics in cirrhotic patients with variceal bleeding. World J Gastroenterol. 2014;20(7):1790-6.

Q49. Answer c

Bowel rest, nasogastric decompression, and intravenous hydration are used to treat SBO; however, there are no data to support nasogastric tube (NGT) use in patients without active emesis. Patients with NG decompression have a significantly increased risk of pneumonia and respiratory failure as well as increased time to resolution and hospital length of stay.

    Fonseca AL, Schuster KM, Maung AA, et al. Routine nasogastric decompression in small bowel obstruction: is it really necessary? Am Surg. 2013;79(4):422-8.

Q50. Answer c

Primary findings suggest functional bowel obstruction. Ogilvie syndrome (OS) is the acute dilation of the colon in the absence of any mechanical obstruction in severely ill patients. Colonic pseudo-obstruction is characterized by massive dilatation of the cecum (diameter > 10 cm) and right colon on abdominal X-ray. Conservative therapy achieves resolution in 83% to 96% of patients within 2 to 6 days of initiating therapy. Conservative therapy is not appropriate for patients exhibiting peritoneal signs or with radiographic evidence of perforation. Conservative management requires close surveillance of patients with serial examinations, plain film X-rays, and laboratory studies. In general, conservative therapy should be employed for 48 to 72 hours unless the patient demonstrates clinical deterioration or increasing cecal distension beyond 12 cm.

    It is a type of megacolon, sometimes referred to as "acute megacolon", to distinguish it from toxic megacolon.

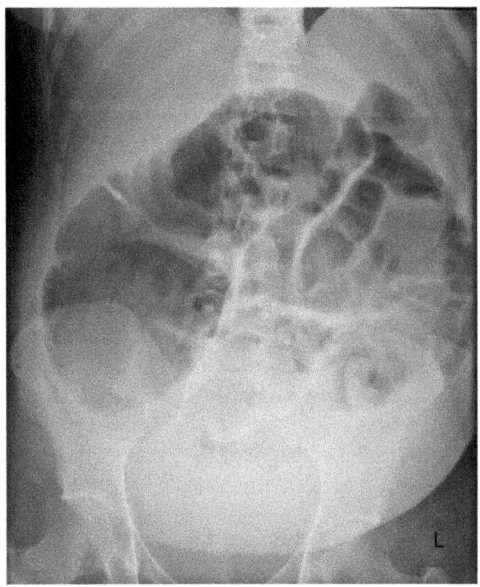

Conservative treatment is effective in 53 to 96% of cases with a risk of colonic perforation less than 2.5% and a mortality of 0 to 14%. The pathogenesis of OS is not completely understood. Its association with trauma, spinal anesthesia and metabolic or pharmacological factors suggests impairment of the autonomic nervous system, leading to excessive parasympathetic suppression or sympathetic stimulation. Cecal dilation greater than 10 cm can result in rupture or ischemic perforation of the bowel, which carries a mortality rate of up to 72%.

Colonoscopic decompression of the colon is effective, causing decreased cecal diameter in 73% to 100% of cases.

Alam HB, Fricchione GL, Guimaraes AS, et al. Case records of the Massachusetts General Hospital. Case 31-2009. A 26-year-old man with abdominal distention and shock. N Engl J Med. 2009;361(15):1487-96.

K Type Answers

Q1. Answer TTTFT

An antecedent biliary-enteric fistula is necessary to allow stone migration into the intestinal tract, and these results in air entering the biliary tree (pneumobilia). It also allows contamination of the bile ducts with intestinal bacteria, which in fact occurs in only a minority of such cases. The stone obstructs the narrower distal bowel, producing small bowel obstruction. Such a stone, if opaque, can be seen on plain radiography and, if not, can be appreciated by sonography. Stools are not alcoholic, since the cholecystoenteric fistula allows bile access to the intestinal lumen.

Nuño-Guzmán CM, Marín-Contreras ME, Figueroa-Sánchez M, et al. Gallstone ileus, clinical presentation, diagnostic and treatment approach. World J Gastrointest Surg. 2016;8(1):65-76.

Q2. Answer TTFTF

Several prognostic systems have been demonstrated to predict the severity of pancreatitis. Two Ranson prognostic criteria have been developed: One not due to gallstones and the other due to gall-stones. The systems have minor differences. In both of the Ranson systems elevated blood glucose, leukocytosis, and elevations of serum LDH have proved to have prognostic importance. Aspartate Aminotransferase (AST) Test (aka SGOT) and not Alanine aminotransferase (ALT) is included. Amylase elevation is not included.
- WBC > $16 \times 10^3/\mu L$. Yes. +1.
- Age > 55. Yes. +1.
- Glucose >200 mg/dL (>10 mmol/L). Yes. +1.
- AST > 250. Yes. +1.
- LDH > 350. Yes. +1.
- Hct drop >10% from admission. Yes. +1.
- BUN increase >5 mg/dL (>1.79 mmol/L) from admission. Yes. +1.
- Ca <8 mg/dL (<2 mmol/L) within 48 hours. Yes. +1.

Otsuki M, Takeda K, Matsuno S. Criteria for the diagnosis and severity stratification of acute pancreatitis. World J Gastroenterol. 2013;19(35):5798-805.

Q3. Answer FTTF

Pancreatic ascites typically occurs because of a pancreatic duct disruption, most commonly involving alcohol abuse and resultant acute pancreatitis. In pancreatic ascites, pancreatic exocrine secretions exit a pancreatic duct disruption and drain anteriorly into the peritoneal cavity. Patients typically present with painless massive ascites, as the pancreatic enzymes that extravasate into the peritoneal cavity are typically nonactivated. The diagnosis of pancreatic ascites is best made by paracentesis, in which the analysis of the ascites fluid reveals it to be high in amylase (more than 1000 U per dL) and high in albumin (more than 3 gm per dL). Nonoperative treatment is initially indicated in most patients with pancreatic ascites. Should nonoperative therapy fail, surgical therapy is directed to closure of the pancreatic duct disruption. Preoperative pancreatography is useful in directing surgical therapy. Distal pancreatic duct disruption may be treated with distal pancreatectomy or with Roux-en-Y pancreatico-jejunostomy. Pancreatic leaks in the more proximal aspects of the gland are treated with Roux-en-Y pancreatico-jejunostomy. Suture ligation of the pancreatic duct with omental patching is not considered appropriate therapy for pancreatic duct disruptions.

    Kozarek RA. Management of pancreatic ascites. Gastroenterol Hepatol (N Y). 2007;3(5):362-4.

Q4. Answer TFTF

Involvement of the right lobe with abscess formation approximates 70% of pyogenic abscesses. This is thought to be due to the streaming effect of superior mesenteric venous inflow to the right lobe. In addition, the greater volume of the right lobe predisposes more tissue to seeding by bacterial organisms. While appendicitis comprised 25% to 40% of cases in early series, early recognition and operative therapy for appendicitis have reduced its importance significantly. In current series, malignant or benign biliary obstruction is the underlying cause of 35% to 50% of cases. Recent studies have shown that the underlying disease or an immunocompromised host is more important prognostically than solitary versus multiple abscesses.

    Davis J, McDonald M. Pyogenic liver abscess. Available at: https://www.uptodate.com/contents/pyogenic-liver-abscess (Accessed 1 January 2018).

Q5. Answer FTTF

Mortality for uncomplicated amebic abscess should be less than 5%, in contrast to the 15% to 20% rate for pyogenic abscess. After the demonstration by radiologic examination of an abscess, appropriate serologic tests and resolution of symptoms after a course of treatment with an antiamebic agent, such as metronidazole constitute presumptive diagnosis of amebic abscess. Aspiration of abscess contents rarely yields amebic organisms. In contrast to pyogenic abscess, amebic abscess rarely requires surgical or percutaneous drainage, except in the case of an extremely large abscess or bacterial super infection. Amebic abscess affects males in a 9:1 to 10:1 ratio and generally affects a younger population than pyogenic abscess.

    Wuerz T, Kane JB, Boggild AK. A review of amoebic liver abscess for clinicians in a nonendemic setting. Can J Gastroenterol. 2012;26(10):729-33.

Q6. Answer TFTF

Pressure measured by wedging a catheter into a hepatic vein (hepatic venous wedge pressure) closely correlates with directly measured portal venous pressure in patients with portal hypertension when the site of elevated resistance is at the sinusoidal or postsinusoidal level. Such is the case in alcoholic cirrhosis and alcoholic hepatitis. When the site of increased resistance is at the presinusoidal level, either within (schistosomiasis) or outside (portal vein thrombosis) the liver, the hepatic venous wedge pressure is normal despite markedly elevated portal vein pressure. Although schistosomiasis is one of the more frequent causes of portal hypertension worldwide, in North America presinusoidal portal hypertension is considerably less common than alcoholic liver disease. A normal hepatic venous wedge pressure in a patient who has bled from varices should lead one to suspect a presinusoidal cause. A specific diagnosis can often be made by visceral angiography or liver biopsy.

    Bleibel W, Chopra S, Curry MP. Portal hypertension in adults. Available from: https://www.uptodate.com/contents/portal-hypertension-in-adults (Accessed 1 January 2018).

Q7. Answer FTTF

Vasopressin acts through vasoconstriction of splanchnic arterioles. Both portal venous inflow and portal venous pressure are reduced, resulting in control of acute variceal bleeding in approximately 50% of patients. However, the adverse side effects of systemic hypertension, bradycardia, decreased cardiac output, and coronary vasoconstriction are quite common during vasopressin infusion. Simultaneous administration of nitroglycerin or nitroprusside eliminates these side effects—and in one controlled trial enhanced therapeutic effectiveness. Although the mechanism of action of this combined infusion is not clear, vasodilatation of portal-systemic collaterals, resulting in a further reduction in portal pressure, may be responsible.

    Gin-HoLo. Management of acute esophageal variceal hemorrhage. Available from: https://doi.org/10.1016/S1607-551X(10)70009-7Get rights and content (Accessed 1 January 2018).

Q8. Answer FTTF

The PVS is a palliative procedure that does not prolong life. In comparing the early risks of the procedure with those of repeated paracentesis, the shunt cannot be justified as a temporizing procedure to facilitate ascites control in the patient awaiting liver transplantation. Oliguria is common in the first 24 hours after shunt insertion. A correctly placed PVS (patency confirmed using an intraoperative "shuntogram") expands the intravascular volume with a continuous reinfusion of ascites. Inspection should identify elevation of the jugular venous pressure, and a diuretic (usually furosemide) is needed. The mechanisms of action of the two shunts are very different. TIPSS reduces portal pressure and controls ascites by reducing the rate of ascites formation. PVS reinfuses the ascites fluid, thereby reducing the pre renal stimulus to sodium retention and making the patient more responsive to diuretic therapy.

Martin LG. Percutaneous placement and management of peritoneovenous shunts. Semin Intervent Radiol. 2012;29(2):129-34.

Q9. Answer FTFTF

The ability to specifically identify persons infected with HCV has only recently become available. Therefore, data about epidemiology are less than complete. It is very likely not true that more blood donors carry HCV because of the large preponderance of HBV in the United States. It is true; however, that successful elimination of most of the HBV carriers occurs through routine testing. Although serologic tests are available for HCV, they are tests, not of antigen, but of antibody. Therefore, this test alone may not screen out persons who are infected but have not yet developed or may never develop antibody. Risk groups for the relatively newly defined HCV may well not be comprehensively established, and therefore this explanation may be a contributor. There are no differences in virulence between these classes of hepatitis virus.

Engle RE, Bukh J, Alter HJ, et al. Transfusion-associated hepatitis before the screening of blood for hepatitis risk factors. Transfusion. 2014;54(11):2833-41.

Q10. Answer FTTFF

Although some types of hepatitis are more often asymptomatic than symptomatic, that is not the case for hepatitis B. Further, even if the HBV infection is asymptomatic, serious long-term side effects may occur. A prior infection with hepatitis B confers lifelong immunity even if the antibody titer wanes below the protective level of 10 mIU. HBIg is useful in reducing the incidence of postexposure HBV infection from around 30% with no intervention, to 15% with standard immune globulin, to about 5% to 7% with HBIg. HBV infection is required for infection with HDV and is therefore an essential step toward, rather than preventive of, HBV infection.

Viral Hepatitis. CDC. Available from: https://www.cdc.gov/hepatitis/hbv/index.htm (Accessed 1 January 2018).

Q11. Answer TFFT

The presence of pain is the essential symptom of acute calculous cholecystitis. Chronic cholecystitis associated with cholelithiasis may develop in the absence of pain, and in critically ill patients pain may not be a prominent feature of acalculous cholecystitis. Only about 10% of patients with acute cholecystitis have jaundice. Although an occasional patient may have concomitant bile duct obstruction, the jaundice associated with acute cholecystitis is probably due to absorption of bile pigments from the diseased gallbladder. The presence of jaundice in a patient with right-side upper quadrant pain should also suggest the possibility of acute cholangitis secondary to bile duct obstruction. Ultrasonography is very accurate in the detection of gallstones, but stones may be present in the absence of acute cholecystitis. Thickening of the gallbladder wall and a collection of fluid around the gallbladder are ultrasonographic findings in some patients with acute cholecystitis, but they are not always present and are not specific. Ultrasonography may be useful when the diagnosis is obscure because other conditions in the liver, pancreas, and kidney can be detected; however, it is not the definitive test for acute cholecystitis. Cholescintigraphy is specific for the diagnosis of acute calculous cholecystitis (accuracy over 95% in experienced hands). The rapidity, simplicity, and accuracy make cholescintigraphy the definitive diagnostic test in acute calculous cholecystitis; however, it must be interpreted cautiously in the context of another critical illness or recent surgery or trauma, because false-positives are not unusual in these situations.

Vollmer CM, Zakko SF, Afdhal NH. Treatment of acute calculous cholecystitis. Available from: https://www.uptodate.com/contents/treatment-of-acute-calculous-cholecystitis (Accessed 1 January 2018).

Q12. Answer TTTT

About half of the cases of acute acalculous cholecystitis are associated with other conditions, including sepsis, sarcoidosis, polyarteritis nodosa, and systemic lupus erythematosus. A majority of cases occur after trauma, burns, or major surgical procedures performed for other conditions. The precise pathogenesis has not been determined. The diagnosis of acute acalculous cholecystitis is often difficult because symptoms may be masked by another illness, injury, or the postoperative state. Unlike acute calculous cholecystitis, in which pain is always present, pain occurs in only about 70% of cases.

In addition, cholescintigraphy is sometimes inaccurate. These factors make the diagnosis difficult, and a high index of suspicion is necessary, especially in patients who have had operations or trauma. Unexplained abdominal pain, sepsis, and ileus should prompt a thorough investigation. The mortality rate for acute acalculous cholecystitis is higher than that of the calculous type. The incidence of gangrene and perforation of the gallbladder is higher. The accompanying illnesses and conditions and the frequent delays in diagnosis undoubtedly contribute to the higher death rate. Percutaneous cholecystostomy has been used as a diagnostic and therapeutic maneuver in patients who are thought to have acute acalculous cholecystitis. Aspiration and culture of bile assist in confirming the diagnosis, and continuous drainage successfully treats the acute condition.

Yesilbag Z, Karadeniz A, Kaya FO. Acute Acalculous Cholecystitis: A Rare Presentation of Primary Epstein-Barr Virus Infection in Adults-Case Report and Review of the Literature. 2017.

Q13. Answer TTTT

Cholangitis does not occur in the presence of a normal bile duct system, and all patients with cholangitis have an abnormality. Thus, recurrent episodes of cholangitis signal the need for diagnostic studies. Cholangiography usually will be necessary. The presence of any foreign body in the biliary tract is frequently associated with bactibilia and recurrent episodes of cholangitis. Even a silk suture exposed to the lumen of a bile duct has been known to cause cholangitis. Pigment stone and sludge formation may result from the bacterial deconjugation of bilirubin diglucuronide to bilirubin monoglucuronide, which precipitates as calcium bilirubinate. This material can occlude indwelling tubes and predispose to more frequent episodes of cholangitis. Long-term administration of an oral antibiotic may reduce the frequency and severity of attacks of cholangitis; however, this method of management should not be routine. Correction of the underlying problem is essential. Chronic obstruction and recurrent infection eventually lead to secondary biliary cirrhosis and its complications of portal hypertension, ascites, and bleeding esophageal varices. Once this stage of the disease is reached, correction of the underlying biliary tract problem does not reverse the changes in the liver. Once again, every effort should be made to eliminate the cause of the cholangitis early in the course of disease. The only effective treatment for end-stage liver disease is hepatic transplantation.

Koh YX, Chiow AKH, Chok AY, et al. Recurrent Pyogenic Cholangitis: Disease Characteristics and Patterns of Recurrence. 2013. Available from: https://www.hindawi.com/journals/isrn/2013/536081/ (Accessed 1 January 2018).

Q14. Answer FTFTT

Ranson prognostic signs include:

On Admission:
Age above 55 years.
White blood cell count above 16,000/μL
Glucose level above 200 mg/dL
Lactase dehydrogenate level above 350 IU/L
SGOT value above 250 IU/L

After 48 hours:
Hematocrit decrease of 10%
Blood urea nitrogen level increase of 5 mg/dL
Ca^{2+} level below 8 mg/dL
PaO_2 level below 60 mm Hg

Base deficit value above 4 mEq/L
Fluid sequestration greater than 6 L

>Carroll JK, Herrick B, Gipson T, et al. Acute pancreatitis: diagnosis, prognosis, and treatment. Fam Physician. 2007;75(10): 1513-20.

Q15. Answer TFTF

In autopsy series, the evidence for past acute pancreatitis averages 0.31%. Variations among populations are highly dependent on social factors, such as alcohol use and on environmental and hereditary determinants, such as the incidence of gallstones. Acute pancreatitis may occur at any age but is most common in adults between 30 and 70 years of age. In general, patients with gallstone-induced pancreatitis are older (age 40 to 60 years), whereas those with alcohol-associated pancreatitis are younger (age 30 to 40 years). The sex distribution of acute pancreatitis depends on the clinical cause of the disease, with women representing 68% of patients with gallstone-associated pancreatitis. Conversely, when alcohol is the primary association, men account for most patients. Clinical associations with acute pancreatitis can be divided into three broad categories-biliary stones, ethanol, and others. Biliary tract stone disease and ethanol-induced pancreatitis account for most cases of acute pancreatitis reported worldwide.

>Tang JCF. Acute Pancreatitis. Available from: https://emedicine.medscape.com/article/181364-overview (Accesed 1 January 2018).

Q16. Answer FFTTT

Hepatitis B viral infection is insidious. The incubation period of the virus is about eight weeks. The first serum indicator of infection by hepatitis B virus is detection of the serum hepatitis B surface antigen (HBsAg) which may proceed the onset of jaundice. In most cases, hepatitis B infection is self-limited and does not progress to chronic hepatitis. However, some 10% of patients with acute hepatitis B viral infection, whether it is clinical or subclinical, will develop a chronic carrier state. The carrier state is defined by the presence of HBsAg in serum for longer than six months. The best method of treatment of hepatitis B viral infection is primary prevention by vaccination. All susceptible household or sexual contacts of a person with a positive serum test for HBsAg should be advised to receive a full course of hepatitis B viral vaccine. Passive prophylaxis with hepatitis B immunoglobulin should be provided to any susceptible contact in whom there is recent potential parenteral exposure, such as an accidental needle stick.

>Olatosi JO, Anaegbu JO. Hepatitis B vaccination status and needle stick injury exposure among operating room staff in lagos, Nigeria. J West Afr Coll Surg. 2016;6(1):88-99.

Q17. Answer FTTF

Hydatid cysts are most commonly the result of infection with the tape worm, *Echinococcus granulosus*. Routine laboratory tests in patients with hydatid cysts are normal or nonspecifically abnormal. Although routine chest or abdominal radiographs may show a mass with a calcific rim, sonography and CT scan are the favored means of imaging hydatid cysts. The presence of calcifications and daughter cysts within the parent cyst suggests Echinococcus. Percutaneous needling of a hydatid cyst is unwise unless precautions against anaphylaxis are undertaken. A cyst's fluid is often under pressure, and needling may precipitate rupture with the potential for anaphylaxis or intraperitoneal seating. The classic treatment of hydatid cysts is operative. The surgical aim is to remove the cyst or cysts without dissemination of the organism. At operation, the cyst is drained of fluid through a cannula after carefully protecting the operative field from fluid leakage. If the aspirate is clear a parasiticidal fluid (ethyl alcohol or 20% sterile saline) is injected into the cyst to kill any adherent scoleces. The cyst contents and the pericystic wall is then removed with careful surgical dissection.

>Regev A, Reddy KR. Diagnosis and management of cystic lesions of the liver. Available from: https://www.uptodate.com/contents/diagnosis-and-management-of-cystic-lesions-of-the-liver?source=search_result&search=treatment%20of%20hydatid%20cysts&selectedTitle=2~28 (Accessed 1 January 2018).

Q18. Answer TTFFT

Mallory-Weiss syndrome or gastroesophageal laceration syndrome refers to bleeding from a laceration in the mucosa at the junction of the stomach and esophagus. This is usually caused by severe vomiting because of alcoholism or bulimia, but can be caused by any conditions which cause violent vomiting and retching such as food poisoning. The syndrome presents with hematemesis. The laceration is sometimes referred to as a Mallory-Weiss tear. Eighty percent of the cases resolve on its own whereas few cases may require laparoscopic surgery to sew the tear.

Modified Glasgow—Blatchford Score

Risk Factor	Score
Blood Urea (mmol/dL)	
≥ 18.2 to < 22.4	2
≥ 22.4 to < 28.0	3
≥ 28.0 to < 70.0	4
≥ 70.0	6
Hemoglobin (g/dL) for men	
> 12.0 to <13.0	1
≥ 10.0 to < 12.0	3
< 10.0	6
Hemoglobin (g/dL) for women	
≥ 10.0 to < 12.0	1
< 10.0	6
Systolic blood pressure (mm Hg)	
100–109	1
90–99	2
< 90	3
Other markers	
Heart rate ≥ 100 bpm	1
Maximum score	16

Gawrieh S, Shaker R. Treatment of actively bleeding Mallory-Weiss syndrome: epinephrine injection or band ligation?. Current gastroenterology reports. 2005;7(3):175.

Q19. Answer TTFTT

Clinical manifestation, risk factors, and classification of acute mesenteric ischemia (I) Arterial occlusive—sudden occlusion of the SMA by an embolus or thrombus in patients with pre-existing wall pathology. Predisposition: cardiac arrhythmia, particularly atrial fibrillation, coronary heart disease, clinical status following myocardial infarction, peripheral arterial occlusive disease. Clinical manifestations: Sudden-onset abdominal pain, pain-free interval approximately 6 to 12 hours after symptom onset, subsequent gangrene of the intestine with peritonitis (II) Arterial nonocclusive: Ischemia caused by reduction in cardiac output with reactive vessel spasm mesenterically. Predisposition: clinical status following heart surgery with extracorporeal circulation, particularly with complicated disease course, long-term hemodialysis, digitalis medication. Clinical manifestations: in responsive patients-increasing abdominal pain. In intubated patients: abdominal distension, increase in inflammatory parameters, signs of sepsis. Predisposition: paraneoplasia, pancreatitis, pancreatic carcinoma, congenital thrombophilia (e.g. AT III deficiency, protein C deficiency, protein S deficiency), hepatocellular carcinoma (HCC) with macrovascular invasion. Clinical manifestations: depends on severity of thrombosis, often nonspecific abdominal complaints lasting several days, venous infarction with peritonitis in a minority of cases. The superior mesenteric artery branches from the abdominal aorta inferior to the celiac trunk and provides oxygenated blood to most of the small intestine and the proximal large intestine. The splanchnic organs receive ~25–30% of the cardiac output under normal conditions. Basal blood flow to the splanchnic region far exceeds that required by tissue oxygen utilization, thus total flow is not determined primarily by metabolic needs. Flow increases substantially, however, during feeding and digestion.

Klar E, Rahmanian PB, Bücker A. Acute mesenteric ischemia: a vascular emergency. Dtsch Arztebl Int. 2012;109(14):249-56.

Q20. Answer FFTTF

Foul-smelling black stool may be caused by upper intestinal bleeding (stomach or upper small intestine), ulcers, or tumors. It is not specific to blood and may also be caused by iron supplements or bismuth. According to a study by Witting, the strongest predictors of an upper GI bleed are black stool, age <50 years, and blood urea nitrogen/creatinine ratio 30 or more. Out of 325 persons studied, seven (5%) of 151 with none of these factors had an upper GI tract bleed, versus 63 (93%) of 68 with 2 or 3 factors. Black stool, age less than 50 years, and blood urea nitrogen/creatinine ratio of 30 or greater, independently predict an upper GI tract bleeding source. Patients should not routinely undergo nasogastric lavage as part the management in acute upper gastrointestinal bleeding. Both erythromycin and metoclopramide have been studied in patients with acute upper GI bleeding. The goal of using a prokinetic agent is to improve gastric visualization at the time of endoscopy by clearing the stomach of blood, clots, and food residue. Erythromycin is considered in patients who are likely to have a large amount of blood in their stomach, such as those with severe bleeding. A reasonable dose is 3 mg/kg intravenously over 20 to 30 minutes, 30 to 90 minutes prior to endoscopy. Somatostatin, its analog octreotide, and terlipressin are used in the treatment of variceal bleeding and may also reduce the risk of bleeding due to nonvariceal causes. In patients with suspected variceal bleeding, octreotide is given as an intravenous bolus of 20 to 50 mcg, followed by a continuous infusion at a rate of 25 to 50 mcg per hour.

British Society of Gastroenterology Endoscopy Committee. Nonvariceal upper gastrointestinal haemorrhage: guidelines. Gut. 2002;51(Suppl 4):iv1-6.

Q21. Answer TTTTT

Pseudomembranous colitis (PMC) is a manifestation of severe colonic disease that is usually associated with Clostridium difficile infection, but can be caused by a number of different etiologies. Prior to the use of broad-spectrum antibiotics, PMC was more frequently related with ischemic disease, obstruction, sepsis, uremia, and heavy metal poisoning. The list of associated etiologies is vast, although Clostridium difficile infection (CDI) is still the most common cause. CT is more commonly used given the lower sensitivity of plain radiography. CT findings in CDI include colonic wall thickening and nodularity, bowel wall stranding and edema, ascites, the "accordion" sign (ingested oral contrast becomes trapped between thickened haustral folds), and the "double-halo" sign (submucosal edema indicated by two or three concentric rings in the large bowel seen on transverse imaging). Management of PMC usually entails discontinuation of offending agents, such as NSAIDs and diarrhea-promoting agents, likely caffeine, alcohol, and dairy products. Antidiarrheal medications like loperamide and diphenoxylate/atropine can be effective in symptomatic management and are often first-line agents for milder cases of PMC. A multitude of other treatments have been utilized in the management of PMC in particular, although only a few appear to be effective in randomized clinical trials. A Cochrane review published in 2009 for treatment of PMC found that budesonide was effective in the induction and maintenance of symptom and histologic resolution, as well as improving quality of life. In particular, budesonide is preferred over other corticosteroids because its rapid hepatic metabolism minimizes systemic effects. Evidence for the use of bismuth salicylate and mesalamine (with or without cholestyramine) was weaker, but was overall promising and favored utilizing these agents in active CC. Other agents, like Boswellia serrata extract, prednisolone, and probiotics, did not show any evidence of symptom improvement or cure. Subtotal colectomy with ileostomy remains the standard of care when toxic megacolon, perforation, or an acute surgical abdomen is present, but mortality rates are high. Recognition of risk factors for fulminant CDI and earlier surgical intervention may decrease mortality from this highly lethal disease.

Farooq PD, Urrunaga NH, Tang DM, et al. Pseudomembranous Colitis. Dis Mon. 2015;61(5):181-206.

Q22. Answer TTFTT

POI is a frequent, frustrating occurrence for patients and surgeons after abdominal surgery. Despite significant research investigating how to reduce this multifactorial phenomenon, a single strategy has not been shown to reduce POI's significant effects on length of stay (LOS) and hospital costs. Perhaps the most significant cause of POI is the use of narcotics for analgesia. Strategies that target inflammation and pain reduction, such as NSAID use, epidural analgesia, and laparoscopic techniques will reduce POI and are also accompanied by a simultaneous reduction in opioid use. Pharmacologic means of stimulating gut motility have not shown a positive effect, and the routine use of nasogastric tubes only increases morbidity. Alvimopan, a peripherally acting mu-antagonist, has shown significant reductions in POI and LOS by 12 and 16 hours, respectively, by blunting the effects of narcotics on gut motility while sparing centrally mediated analgesia. Use of alvimopan, along with a multimodal postoperative treatment plan involving early ambulation, feeding, and avoiding nasogastric tubes, will likely be the crux of POI treatment and prevention.

Lubawski J, Saclarides T. Postoperative ileus: strategies for reduction. Ther Clin Risk Manag. 2008;4(5):913-7.

Q23. Answer TTFTF

General management of upper gastrointestinal bleeding in adults: Triage, General support, Fluid resuscitation, Blood product transfusions, Medications-Acid suppression, Prokinetics, Vasoactive medications, Antibiotics for patients with cirrhosis, Tranexamic acid, Anticoagulants and antiplatelet agents. Tranexamic acid is an antifibrinolytic agent that has been studied in patients with upper GI bleeding. A meta-analysis that included eight randomized trials of tranexamic acid in patients with upper GI bleeding found a benefit with regard to mortality but not with regard to bleeding, surgery, or transfusion requirements. It can lead to thrombosis in coronary artery or can aggravate recent MI. This suggests that there is no role for tranexamic acid in the treatment of upper GI bleeding, since the current standard of care is to treat patients with PPI and endoscopic therapy (if indicated).

Mandal A, Missouris CG. Tranexamic acid and acute myocardial infarction. Br J Cardiol. 2005;12:306-7.

Hayat U, Lee PJ, Ullah H, et al. Association of prophylactic endotracheal intubation in critically ill patients with upper GI bleeding and cardiopulmonary unplanned events. Gastrointest Endosc. 2017;86(3):500.

Q24. Answer TTTF

Drugs that can cause a paralytic ileus include: hydromorphone, morphine, oxycodone, tricyclic antidepressants, such as amitriptyline and imipramine. Other causes include: intestinal cancer, Crohn's disease, diverticulitis, Parkinson's disease, which affects muscles and nerves in the intestines. These are the most common ileus causes in adults. Intussusception is the most common cause for an ileus in children. This is when a part of the intestine "telescopes" or slides into itself. Risk factors include: electrolyte imbalance, such as those involving potassium and calcium, history of intestinal injury or trauma, history of intestinal disorder, such as Crohn's disease and diverticulitis, sepsis, history of irradiation of or near the abdomen, peripheral artery disease, and rapid weight loss. Aging also naturally slows down how fast the intestines move. An older adult is at greater risk for ileus, especially since they tend to take more medications that could potentially slow movement of material through the intestines. DEX facilitates bowel movements and reduces the length of hospital stay in surgical patients. This may be attributed to the sympatholytic and opioid-sparing effects of DEX.

Ramirez JA, McIntosh AG, Strehlow R, et al. Definition, incidence, risk factors, and prevention of paralytic ileus following radical cystectomy: a systematic review. Eur Urol. 2013;64:588.

Q25. Answer TFTFF

POI refers to obstipation and intolerance of oral intake following abdominal or nonabdominal surgery. It is due to nonmechanical factors, primarily inflammation of the intestinal smooth muscle, leading to disruption of the normal coordinated propulsive motor activity of the gastrointestinal tract. The incidence of POI varies widely and depends upon the definition of postoperative ileus that is used and the type of surgery. The most important risk factors for prolonged POI include: prolonged abdominal or pelvic surgery, lower gastrointestinal surgery, open surgery, delayed enteral nutrition/nasogastric tube placement, intra-abdominal inflammation, postoperative complications, and possibly increased body mass index. Some degree of POI is a normal obligatory and physiologic response to abdominal surgery. It can also occur following non-abdominal surgery. The duration of postoperative gastrointestinal dysmotility appears to be shorter than historically reported with gastric and small intestinal activity returning within hours of surgery, and colonic activity returning by postoperative day 2 to 3. Physiologic POI is generally a benign condition that resolves without serious sequelae. Prolonged POI is said to occur when one or more of the following symptoms or signs persists for more than three to five days: Abdominal distention, bloating, and "gassiness", diffuse, persistent abdominal pain, nausea and/or vomiting, delayed passage of or inability to pass flatus, inability to tolerate an oral diet. The evaluation of the patient with suspected POI includes history and physical, plain radiography, and laboratory studies including CBC, electrolyte panel including magnesium, BUN, liver function tests, amylase and lipase. This work-up seeks to exclude other causes of ileus, and surgical entities that can lead to postoperative abdominal distention and decreased bowel activity that may require surgical management or other intervention, such as small bowel obstruction, bowel perforation, intra-abdominal abscess, or retroperitoneal bleeding. Plain radiographs demonstrating air in the colon and rectum, with no transition zone or free air support a diagnosis of postoperative ileus and may be adequate for distinguishing postoperative ileus from small bowel obstruction. However, if there remains any suspicion for small bowel obstruction or another diagnosis, we suggest CT of the abdomen. No studies have identified any specific therapy, other than supportive care, to resolve prolonged postoperative ileus. Supportive care includes pain control that minimizes opioid use, intravenous fluid and electrolyte therapy, dietary restriction, and selective placement of a nasogastric tube for gastrointestinal decompression for those with persistent nausea/vomiting. The patient should be closely monitored with serial abdominal examinations for improvement or worsening of their condition. Additional imaging studies are warranted, if conservative measures do not improve the patient's condition in 48 to 72 hours.

Holte K, Kehlet H. Postoperative ileus: a preventable event. Br J Surg. 2000;87:1480.

Lubawski J, Saclarides T. Postoperative ileus: strategies for reduction. Ther Clin Risk Manag. 2008;4(5):913-7.

CHAPTER 5

Nutrition in Critical Care

Abdul Ansari, Rajiv Jitendra Shah

A Type Questions
(One best answer)

1. What is the recommended daily protein intake in acute renal failure patients on dialysis?
   a. 2-3 (gm/kg Ideal body weight/day)
   b. 1-2 (gm/kg Ideal body weight/day)
   c. 0.5-1.5 (gm/kg Ideal body weight/day)
   d. 1.2-1.5 (gm/kg Ideal body weight/day)
   e. 1.5-2.5 (gm/kg Ideal body weight/day)

2. During stress which amino acid is labeled as "conditionally Essential" amino acid:
   a. Glutamine
   b. Arginine
   c. Leucine
   d. Isoleucine
   e. Valine

3. Deficiency of which element causes fatal cardiomyopathy?
   a. Iron
   b. Selenium
   c. Copper
   d. Iodine
   e. Manganese

4. Which vitamin is degraded by sulfite ion?
   a. Vitamin-A
   b. Vitamin-K
   c. Riboflavin
   d. Thiamine
   e. Vitamin-C

5. A 60 years old male comes with weight loss of 10% in last 6 months, with reduced functional capacity, decreased muscle mass and slight dependent edema. This patient falls in which criteria of Subjective Global Assessment (SGA):
   a. Criteria A (well malnourished)
   b. Criteria B (moderately malnourished)
   c. Criteria C (severely malnourished)
   d. Criteria D (critically malnourished)

6. According to ASPEN '16 guidelines, which of the following statement is true regarding nutritional assessment in the critically ill?
   a. Initial nutritional assessment of all hospitalized patients should be done within 48 hrs of admission
   b. Initial nutritional assessment of all hospitalized patients should be done within 24 hrs of admission
   c. Nutritional assessment done every 24 hrs
   d. Critically ill patients in ICU setting do not require full nutrition assessment

7. In non-protein caloric sources minimum amount of carbohydrate required to avoid ketosis is:
   a. 50–100 gm/day
   b. 50 gm/day
   c. >100 gm/day
   d. >400 gm/day

8. Which of the following should not be calculated as a caloric source?
   a. Carbohydrate
   b. Trace elements
   c. Proteins
   d. Fat soluble vitamins

9. **Deficiency of which of the following in critically ill patients is associated with lactic acidosis:**
   a. Vit-K
   b. Vit-B1
   c. Vit-C
   d. Vit-B12
   e. Vit-A

10. **Which of following is "Gold Standard" for caloric assessment?**
    a. Calculation of BMI
    b. Harris-Benedict formula
    c. Indirect calorimetry
    d. Ideal body weight
    e. Curreri formula

11. **Patient on TPN should be assessed for renal, liver profile:**
    a. Every 48 hrs
    b. Weekly
    c. Every 15 days
    d. As need arises
    e. Not routinely monitored

12. **EN is indicated in patients who are not expected to be on a full oral diet within:**
    a. 2 days
    b. 3 days
    c. 4 days
    d. 7 days
    e. None of the above

13. **A 48 years old female DM, Hypothyroidism, admitted in ICU post bariatric surgery, is hemodynamically stable with central venous catheter in situ. Which statement is true?**
    a. 30–35 kcal/kg Ideal body weight/day for pt with BMI>50
    b. Should receive supplemental thiamine prior to initiating dextrose containing IV fluids or nutrition therapy
    c. Protein should be provided in range of 2.0 gm/kg Ideal body weight/day for patient with BMI>40
    d. Early enteral nutrition is not recommended post-surgery

14. **Most accurate method to calculate energy expenditure in mechanically ventilated patients is with:**
    a. Harris-Benedict formula
    b. Faisy equation
    c. Holliday-Segar formula
    d. Parkland formula
    e. Curreri formula

15. **Which of the following biomarkers has the shortest half-life?**
    a. Albumin
    b. Transferrin
    c. Transthyretin
    d. Prealbumin
    e. Fibronectin

16. **Which of the following is absolute contraindication to EN?**
    a. Severe septic shock
    b. Abdominal distension
    c. High output fistula
    d. Upper GI bleed
    e. Mechanical ventilation

17. **Binary parenteral nutrition bags are useful in patients:**
    a. Receiving high dose of propofol
    b. With chronic renal failure
    c. With septic shock
    d. On hemodialysis
    e. Patients with ARDS

18. **Protein content of a solution of TPN can be calculated by multiplying nitrogen content with:**
    a. 6.0
    b. 5.45
    c. 7.25
    d. 6.25
    e. 6.5

19. **According to ESPEN guidelines, severe nutritional risk is defined by which of the following criteria?**
    a. Wt loss of 10–20% in 6 months
    b. Subjective global assessment (SGA) Grade-C
    c. BMI less than 15 kg/m^2
    d. SGA Grade D
    e. Serum albumin less than 20 gm/L (with no evidence of hepatic or renal dysfunction)

20. **According to ASPEN which statement is true?**
    a. Target of >50–65% of goal calories to be achieved in first week of hospitalization
    b. Target of >60% of goal calories in 48 hrs of hospitalization
    c. At least 85% of goal calories within first week of hospitalization

d. Enteral nutrition via tube feeding is not the preferred way of feeding in critically ill patients

21. **What is the recommended protein intake for the patients who are on Continuous Renal Replacement Therapy (CRRT)?**
    a. Less than 1.0 gm/kg body weight/day
    b. 1–5 gm/kg body weight/day
    c. 1.5–2.0 gm/kg body weight/day
    d. 2.0–2.5 gm/kg body weight/day
    e. More than 2.5 gm/kg body weight/day

K Type Questions
[Marked True (T)/False (F)]

1. **What is true regarding branched chained amino acids (BCAA)?**
    a. BCAA are synthesized by liver
    b. Are oxidized in skeletal muscles and adipose tissues
    c. Do not contribute to hepatic urea production
    d. BCAA decrease the passage of aromatic acids across blood brain barrier
    e. 50% of AA are provided by leucine, isoleucine and valine

2. **What is true regarding Glutamine?**
    a. Glutamine level is decreased in critically ill patients
    b. Not essential for cell proliferation
    c. It is primary source of fuel for rapidly growing tissues like intestinal mucosa & lymphocytes during stress, sparing glucose for other tissues
    d. Increases permeability of gut
    e. Useful in catabolic states

3. **Recommended dietary allowances (RDA) of fat soluble vitamins are:**
    a. Vitamin-A 900 µg
    b. Vitamin-D 10 µg
    c. Biotin- 30 µg
    d. Vitamin-K 120 µg
    e. Vitamin-E 15.0 mg

4. **What is true regarding vitamins?**
    a. Parenteral requirements of vitamins are higher than enteral requirements
    b. Vitamin-K is degraded by sulfite ions
    c. Vitamin-A, Riboflavin, folic acid and B12 are degraded by light
    d. Vitamin-K is degraded by light

5. **What is true regarding refeeding syndrome?**
    a. Only 1/3 of estimated basal energy needs should be given in first 24 hrs
    b. Fluid should be given liberally on the higher target
    c. Hypokalemia, hypocalcemia, hypomagnesemia, are its hallmark
    d. Changes lead to a deficit in intracellular as well as extracellular phosphorus
    e. Severe muscular weakness and risk of respiratory failure is due to hypokalemia and hypophosphatemia

6. **Immunomodulating diet formula can be given in which patients?**
    a. Trauma
    b. Burns
    c. Upper GI surgical patients
    d. Septic Shock
    e. ARDS

7. **Which statements regarding NUTRIC Score is true?**
    a. NUTRIC Score ranges from 0 to 20
    b. IL-6 level were not included
    c. APACHE II Score was taken into consideration
    d. High NUTRIC score patients had no benefit from nutrition
    e. Low NUTRIC score was associated with increased mortality

8. **Which statement is true according to ESPEN guidelines?**
    a. Undernutrition is more likely to develop in critical illness than in uncomplicated starvation
    b. Studies investigating the maximum time ICU patients can survive without nutrition support would be considered unethical and therefore not available
    c. All patients who are not expected to be on a full oral diet within 3 days should receive enteral nutrition (EN)
    d. Hemodynamically stable ICU patients with a functioning gut not tolerating target amount by 24 hours should be given supplementary parenteral nutrition

9. **Which of the following statements are true?**
    a. No significant difference in efficiency of jejunal versus gastric feeding in critically ill patients

b. Even if jejunal feeding can be devised easily, it should not be the first choice
   c. Jejunal feeding should be initiated in patients only after they prove that patient is intolerant to gastric feeding
   d. Gastric feeding is the choice in stable ICU patients

10. **Which statement is true regarding ESPEN guidelines?**
    a. No clinical advantage of peptide based formula over whole protein formula
    b. Routine use of peptide based formula is recommended
    c. Whole protein formula are appropriate in most patients
    d. Whole protein formula is recommended in all conditions

11. **Which statement is true regarding Immune modulating formula according to ESPEN guidelines?**
    a. Are enriched with arginine, nucleotides and omega-3 FA
    b. Superior in patients with trauma
    c. Not recommended in burns patient
    d. Not recommended in patients with severe illness who do not tolerate greater than 700 mL enteral formula per day

12. **Which statement is true regarding vitamins in ESPEN guidelines?**
    a. Thiamine & Vitamin-C deficiency pose special risks
    b. Thiamine supplements (100–300 mg/day) should be provided during 1st three days in ICU in at risk patients
    c. In patients with major burns & CRRT it is not recommended to give additional Vitamin-C supplementation
    d. Vitamin-K supplements is required in CRRT

13. **Which of the following statement are true?**
    a. Measurement of albumin, prealbumin and anthropometry is not validated in critical care
    b. Indirect calorimetry is not recommended
    c. In absence of indirect calorimetry, weight based equations are used to determine energy requirements
    d. Evidence of bowel function is not required for initiation of enteral nutrition

14. **Which statement is true regarding nutrition in acute respiratory failure (ARF)?**
    a. High fat low carbohydrate formulations are not recommended
    b. Fluid restricted energy dense formulations should be considered for patients with acute respiratory failure
    c. Routine monitoring of serum phosphate levels are not recommended
    d. In ARF, trophic enteral feeding was associated with less gastrointestinal intolerance

15. **Which statement is true regarding renal failure patients?**
    a. All patients with AKI should be on standard parenteral formulation when required
    b. Salt restricted diet in all ARF patients
    c. All patients require renal formulae typically caloric dense with low protein and modified electrolytes
    d. Renal formulae have no beneficial role in pre dialysis CRF patients

16. **Which statement is true regarding nutrition in hepatic failure patients?**
    a. Ideal weight is recommended instead of actual weight in predicted equations
    b. Restricted protein formulation is recommended
    c. TPN is the preferred route of nutrition therapy
    d. No evidence of benefit of branched chain amino acids (BCAA) in hepatic encephalopathy

17. **Which statements are true regarding nutrition in Acute Pancreatitis?**
    a. Patients with severe acute pancreatitis should be initiated EN with standard polymeric formula
    b. Immune enhancing formulations reduce mortality in severe acute pancreatitis
    c. In patients with severe acute pancreatitis EN at trophic rate
    d. TPN is considered within 1 week from onset of pancreatitis when EN is not feasible

18. **Which statements are true regarding nutrition in traumatic brain injury (TBI)?**
    a. Early EN feeding is recommended within 24–48 hrs

- b. Immune modulating formulae are recommended
- c. Eicosapentaenoic Acid/ Docosahexaenoic acid (EPA/DHA) formulations are not recommended in TBI
- d. Early enteral feeding is recommended immediately after neurosurgery

19. **Which statements are true regarding nutrition in open abdomen?**
    - a. Early EN (24-48 hrs post injury) should be considered in presence of open abdomen
    - b. Additional 15-30 grams of proteins/L of exudates lost should be replaced
    - c. Immune-modulating formulas is strongly recommended
    - d. Omega 3 Fatty Acids enriched formulas are strongly recommended
    - e. EN distends the abdomen and should not be started in open abdomen

20. **Which statements are true regarding nutrition in burn victims?**
    - a. Burn injury patient should receive protein in range of 1.5-2 gm/kg/day
    - b. Very early initiation of EN (4-6 hrs of injury) is recommended
    - c. According to Curreri formula for estimating caloric requirement for a patient for age>60 yrs, caloric requirement is 25 kcal/kg/day + 65 kcal/percent/day
    - d. 5% dextrose is fluid of choice

ANSWERS

A Type Answers

Q1. Answer c

Patients with renal disease should undergo formal nutrition assessment, including evaluation of inflammation, with development of a nutrition care plan. Patients with renal failure who require nutrition support therapy should receive enteral nutrition (EN) if intestinal function permits. Standard amino acid in total parenteral nutrition (TPN) formulations should be used in acute kidney injury. Energy requirements in patients with renal disease should be evaluated using indirect calorimetry when possible. If indirect calorimetry is not possible, individualized assessment of energy intake goals, as with other nutrition support patients, is recommended. To promote positive nitrogen balance in patients with acute kidney injury, protein intake should be adjusted according to catabolic rate, renal function, and dialysis losses. Protein intake for patients who receive maintenance HD is 1.2 g/kg/d. Several studies suggest and it is widely accepted that the protein intake during continuous renal replacement therapy (CRRT) should range between 1.8 and 2.5 g/kg/d.

> Brown RO et. al. A.S.P.E.N. Clinical Guidelines: Nutrition Support in Adult Acute and Chronic Renal Failure. A.S.P.E.N. Clinical Guidelines: Adult Renal Failure. Available from: http://www.sbnpe.com.br/wp-content/uploads/2016/07/JPEN-J-Parenter-Enteral-Nutr-2010-Brown-366-77.pdf (Accessed 1 January 2018).

Q2. Answer a

Conditional amino acids are usually not essential, except in times of illness and stress. Conditional amino acids include: arginine, cysteine, glutamine, tyrosine, glycine, ornithine, proline, and serine. However glutamine has been the focus of extensive scientific interest because of its importance in cell and tissue cultures and its physiologic role in animals and humans. Glutamine appears to be a unique amino acid, serving as a preferred respiratory fuel for rapidly proliferating cells, such as enterocytes and lymphocytes; a regulator of acid-base balance through the production of urinary ammonia; a carrier of nitrogen between tissues; and an important precursor of nucleic acids, nucleotides, amino sugars, and proteins. Abundant evidence suggests that glutamine may become a "conditionally essential" amino acid in the critically ill. During stress the body's requirements for glutamine appear to exceed the individual's ability to produce sufficient amounts of this amino acid. Provision of supplemental glutamine in specialized enteral or parenteral feeding may enhance nutritional management and augment recovery of the seriously ill while minimizing hospital stay. One best choice in this list is choice a. glutamine.

> Lacey JM, Wilmore DW. Is glutamine a conditionally essential amino acid? Nutr Rev. 1990;48(8):297-309.

Q3. Answer b

Because of risk of fatal cardiomyopathy caused by selenium deficiency, selenium supplementation is recommended for patients receiving long term PN. Selenium deficiency is a however an uncommon cause of cardiomyopathy, myopathy and osteoarthropathy. In Asia and Africa, dietary selenium deficiency is associated with a cardiomyopathy known as Keshan disease and an osteoarthropathy called Kashin-Beck disease. Chronic selenium deficiency may also occur in individuals with malabsorption and long term selenium-deficient parenteral nutrition. Selenium deficiency causes myopathy as a result of the depletion of selenium-associated enzymes which protect cell membranes from damage by free radicals.

> Burke MP, Opeskin K. Fulminant heart failure due to selenium deficiency cardiomyopathy (Keshan disease). Med Sci Law. 2002;42(1):10-3.
> Pandya S. Practical guidelines on fluid therapy. 2012. p. 339.

Q4. Answer d

Vitamins get degraded during preparations and storage. Such as Vitamin A, Riboflavin and Vitamin K are degraded by light and thiamine is degraded by sulfite ions used as preservative for amino acid solutions. The degradation effect of light exposure is greater for the solutions stored in plastic than in glass. Infusion solutions containing bisulfite are unsuitable vehicles for the administration of vitamin formulations containing thiamine. If a patient must receive multivitamins in infusion solutions with bisulfite, the solutions should be used immediately after their preparation, and the patient should be monitored for signs of thiamine deficiency.

Scheiner JM, Araujo MM, DeRitter E. Thiamine destruction by sodium bisulfite in infusion solutions. Am J Hosp Pharm. 1981; 38(12):1911-3.

Pandya S. Practical guidelines on fluid therapy. 2012. p. 340.

Q5. Answer b

SGA is an inexpensive and quick nutritional assessment method conducted at the bedside. It is a reliable tool for predicting outcomes in critically ill patients. It has broadly three groups- A (well nourished), B (moderately nourished) and C (severely malnourished).

Fontes D, Generoso Sde V, Toulson Davisson Correia MI. Subjective global assessment: a reliable nutritional assessment tool to predict outcomes in critically ill patients. Clin Nutr. 2014;33(2):291-5.

Q6. Answer a

Identifying patients who are at risk of adverse events because of their nutrition status is a core competency of nutrition practitioners. Patients at high risk are more likely to benefit from nutritional therapeutic interventions than those at low risk. Initial nutritional assessment of all hospitalized patients should be done within 48 hrs of admission.

Stephen A. McClave, Beth E. Taylor, Robert G. Martindale. Guidelines for the Provision and Assessment of Nutrition Support Therapy in the Adult Critically Ill Patient. ASPEN. 2016;40(2):159-211.

Q7. Answer c

Low carbohydrate diet or starvation lead to reduction in the circulating levels of insulin along with increased levels of glucagon. This activates phosphoenol pyruvate carboxykinase, fructose 1,6-biphosphatase, and glucose 6-phosphatase and also inhibits pyruvate kinase, 6-phosphofructo-1-kinase, and glucokinase. These changes indeed favor gluconeogenesis. However, the body limits glucose utilization to reduce the need for gluconeogenesis. In the liver in the well-fed state, acetyl CoA formed during the β-oxidation of fatty acids is oxidized to CO_2 and H_2O in the citric acid cycle. However, when the rate of mobilization of fatty acids from adipose tissue is accelerated, as, for example, during very low carbohydrate intake, the liver converts acetyl CoA into ketone bodies: Acetoacetate and 3-hydroxybutyrate. The liver cannot utilize ketone bodies because it lacks the mitochondrial enzyme succinyl-CoA:3-ketoacid CoA transferase required for activation of acetoacetate to acetoacetyl-CoA. Therefore, ketone bodies flow from the liver to extra-hepatic tissues (e.g. brain) for use as a fuel; this spares glucose metabolism via a mechanism similar to the sparing of glucose by oxidation of fatty acids as an alternative fuel. Indeed, the use of ketone bodies replaces most of the glucose required by the brain. Not all amino acid carbon will yield glucose; on average, 1.6 g of amino acids is required to synthesize 1 g of glucose. Thus, to keep the brain supplied with glucose at rate of 110 to 120 g/day (daily requirement), the breakdown of 160 to 200 g of protein (close to 1 kg of muscle tissue) would be required.

Anssi H Manninen. Metabolic Effects of the Very-Low-Carbohydrate Diets: Misunderstood "Villains" of Human Metabolism. J Int Soc Sports Nutr. 2004;1(2):7-11.

Q8. Answer c

Non protein calorie sources are carbohydrates providing 65-75% of total energy and fats providing 25-35% of total energy. Protein is generally used as anabolic source and is not used for energy production unless starvation is there.

Pandya S. Practical guidelines on fluid therapy. 2012. p. 340.

Q9. Answer b

Thiamine plays a critical role in energy metabolism. Critically ill children and adults may develop thiamine deficiency with ultimately increased mortality due to potentially irreversible consequences of severe type B lactic acidosis.

In cases of lactic acidosis with nutritional depletion a possible cause of thiamine deficiency must be considered.

Teagarden AM, Leland BD, Rowan CM, Lutfi R. Thiamine Deficiency Leading to Refractory Lactic Acidosis in a Pediatric Patient. Case Reports in Critical Care. 2017; Article ID 5121032.

Q10. Answer c

A computerized "metabolic cart" is used to collect the patient's expired gases to determine CO_2 production and O_2 consumption, which are used to calculate the Resting Energy Expenditure (REE) using Weir Equation:

> REE=[VO2(3.941) + VCO2(1.11)] 1440 min/day
>
> REF: JPEN 2012

Q11. Answer b

TPN associated liver dysfunction can be progressive and irreversible, particularly in children and patients with long-term treatment. The incidence of altered liver function tests is high in adult hospitalized patients treated with short-term TPN. However, the effect of nutritional factors in this alteration is low. Oral/ EN and reduction of soybean lipid supply can reduce increases in some liver function tests such as gamma-glutamyl-transferase and total bilirubin. The high association between all liver function tests and clinical systemic-hypermetabolic variables suggest the importance of specific nutritional strategies for this condition. A retrospective review was made of results of conventional liver function tests in adult patients who received fat-free total TPN for two weeks or longer and who did not have other obvious causes for liver function abnormalities. A "meaningful" increase (≥50% increase above baseline pre-TPN value) in SGOT levels was noted in 68% of patients, in alkaline phosphatase levels in 54%, and in serum bilirubin levels in 21% of patients. The median peak values for SGOT, alkaline phosphatase, and bilirubin were 3-, 1.9-, and 0.25-fold above the upper limit of normal, respectively. The median time interval of peak increase for each of the three tests was between 9 and 12 days after TPN was started. Liver biopsy specimens from four patients, taken when liver function values were abnormal, showed pronounced steatosis in three patients and mild periportal cholestasis in the fourth patient. The cause(s) of the elevated liver values is unknown, but possibilities include cellular damage, such as steatosis, and an "overshoot" of enzymes when starved patients are refed.

> Lindor KD, Fleming CR, Abrams A et al. Liver Function Values in Adults Receiving Total Parenteral Nutrition. JAMA.1979; 241(22):2398-2400.

Q12. Answer b

EN is indicated in patients who are not expected to be on a full oral diet within 3 days. EN is preferred over TPN. In addition to its digestive, absorptive, endocrine and metabolic functions, the intestine is also an effective barrier against bacteria and intraluminal toxins. Intestinal dysfunction is common in critically ill patients, but there is no objective definition for it. Fasting causes the disruption of intestinal integrity, through atrophy and a decrease in the size of microvilli, of the depth of the crypts, of the intestinal weight and cellular mass, resulting in a decrease in the number of cellular mitoses.

> Stephen A. McClave, Beth E. Taylor, Robert G. Martindale. Guidelines for the Provision and Assessment of Nutrition Support Therapy in the Adult Critically Ill Patient. ASPEN. 2016;40(2):159-211.

Q13. Answer b

Bariatric surgeries, such as sleeve gastrectomy and gastric banding, are treatments that are applied to patients with morbid obesity. However, gastric surgery can cause surgical or metabolic complications, such as thiamine deficiency. This metabolic complication presents with typical symptoms of confusion, ophthalmoplegia, nystagmus, and ataxia. Thiamin is a coenzyme of pyruvate dehydrogenase (PDH), which is a mitochondrial enzyme for oxidation of carbohydrate-derived substrate to generate ATP. In a thiamin deficiency, oxidation of carbohydrate is decreased due to the reduced activity of PDH. Thus a supplement of thiamin is reasonable for carbohydrate metabolism in such cases.

> Jeong HJ, Park JW, Kim YJ, Lee YG, Jang YW, Seo JW. Wernicke's Encephalopathy after Sleeve Gastrectomy for Morbid Obesity- A Case Report. Ann Rehabil Med. 2011;35(4):583-6.

Q14. Answer b

When indirect calorimetry is not available, Faisy equation is more accurate in mechanically ventilated patients. Faisy equation uses four variables namely height, weight, temperature and minute ventilation.

EE (kJ/day) = 8X W + 15 X H + 32 X MV + 94 X BT − 4834

> Walker RN, Heuberger RA. Predictive equations for energy needs for the critically ill. Respir Care. 2009;54(4):509-21.

Q15. Answer e

Fibronectin has the shortest half-life of about 15 hours followed by Prealbumin (2 days), Transthyretin (1.9 days), Transferrin (10 days) and Albumin 20 days. The current consensus is that laboratory markers are not reliable by themselves but could be used as a complement to a thorough physical examination.

Sungurtekin H, Sungertekin U. Nutrition assessment in critically ill patients. Nutri Clin Prac. 2008;23(6):635-41.

Q16. Answer a

Absolute contraindication to enteral feeding is patients with severe septic shock, gut perforation, generalized peritonitis, gut ischemia and gut obstruction.

Seron-Arbeloa C, Zamora-Elson M, Labarta-Monzon L, Mallor-Bonet T. Enteral Nutrition in Critical Care. J Clin Med Res. 2013;5(1):1-11.

Q17. Answer a

The use of commercially premixed 1- or 2-binary chamber bags has improved the quality of care because it avoids the prescription of individualized formulation by physicians. Moreover, the availability of commercially premixed bags may improve nutritional management when individualized TPN formulations may not be prepared in optimal conditions. However, prescription of 1- or 2-chamber bags is often associated with the failure to administer lipids or inadequate prescription of lipids (wrong dose or choice of lipid emulsion). The availability of premixed 3-chamber bags may improve nutritional care because it will help to add or avoid lipid intake. Binary bags are helpful in conditions like liver steatosis, increased serum triglycerides, patients on high dose propofol infusion etc.

Colomb V. Commercially Premixed 3-Chamber Bags for Pediatric Parenteral Nutrition Are Available for Hospitalized Children. J. Nutr. 2013;143(12):2071S-2076S.

Q18. Answer d

The protein content in foodstuffs is estimated by multiplying the determined nitrogen content by a nitrogen-to-protein conversion factor. Jones' factors for a series of foodstuffs, including 6.25 as the standard, default conversion factor, has now been used for 75 years. When however, 6.25 is used irrespective of the foodstuff, "protein" is simply nitrogen expressed using a different unit and says little about protein. This is oversimplification of complex metabolic needs of the body. Scientists fear opening the Pandora's Box when conversion factors of each food are debated. Application of this conversion factor is retained for simplification. Otherwise we may not find anything which may be applied clinically and we remain debating on accuracy alone.

Mariotti F, Tomé D, Mirand PP. Converting nitrogen into protein--beyond 6.25 and Jones' factors.Crit Rev Food Sci Nutr. 2008; 48(2):177-84.

Q19. Answer b

Fontes D, Generoso Sde V, Toulson Davisson Correia MI. Subjective global assessment: a reliable nutritional assessment tool to predict outcomes in critically ill patients. Clin Nutr. 2014;33(2):291-5.

Q20. Answer a

Keeping the intake closer to the target calorie intake and immediate use of Supplemental parenteral nutrition (SPN) whenever full EN fails to achieve the target calorie intake is desirable in the early phase of critical illness for improving the adequacy of clinical nutrition. The EN and EN+SPN groups were found to be similar in terms of rates of target achievement, mortality, and discharge, while a lower mortality rate and improved nutritional status were evident in achievers than in non-achievers of the target calorie intake regardless of the type of nutrition.

Stephen A. McClave, Beth E. Taylor, Robert G. Martindale. Guidelines for the Provision and Assessment of Nutrition Support Therapy in the Adult Critically Ill Patient. ASPEN. 2016;40(2):159-211.

Q21. Answer c

According to KDIGO guidelines administration of 0.8–1.0 g/kg/d of protein was recommended in noncatabolic AKI patients without need for dialysis, 1.0–1.5 g/kg/d in patients with AKI on RRT, and up to a maximum of 1.7 g/kg/d in patients on CRRT and in hypercatabolic patients. Although clinical research related to the metabolic implications of AKI and CRRT are still lacking, several key studies have helped guide nutrition therapy. Scheinkestel et al. measured energy and protein needs in 50 critically ill patients requiring CRRT in order to assess compliance of actual feeding with target feeding, correlate predictive energy requirements with the actual energy expenditure and determine if feeding regimens affect outcome. Patients were given protein 2 g/kg/day for six days vs. protein 1.5, 2, 2.5 g /kg/day, escalated every two days. The authors found that nitrogen equilibrium was attained only at a protein dose of 2.5 g/kg/day, and the probability of survival increased by 21% (P = 0.03) for each 1 g/day increase in nitrogen balance. The authors concluded that nitrogen balance was directly associated with hospital outcome (P=0.03) and ICU outcome (P=0.02), and that enteral feeding benefits patient outcome (P=0.04).

In this question choice is best as per the KDIGO guidelines.

Scheinkestel CD, Kar L, Marshall K, Bailey M, Davies A, Nyulasi I, Tuxen DV.

Prospective randomized trial to assess caloric and protein needs of critically Ill, anuric, ventilated patients requiring continuous renal replacement therapy. Nutrition. 2003;19(11-12):909-16.

KDIGO Clinical Practice Guideline for Acute Kidney Injury. 2012:2(1). Available from: http://www.kdigo.org/clinical_practice_guidelines/pdf/KDIGO%20AKI%20Guideline.pdf (Accessed 23 November 2017).

K Type Answers

Q1. Answer FTFTT

BCAAs have been shown to affect gene expression, protein metabolism, apoptosis and regeneration of hepatocytes, and insulin resistance. They have also been shown to inhibit the proliferation of liver cancer cells in vitro, and are essential for lymphocyte proliferation and dendritic cell maturation. In patients with advanced chronic liver disease, BCAA concentrations are low, whereas the concentrations of aromatic amino acids such as phenylalanine and tyrosine are high, conditions that may be closely associated with hepatic encephalopathy and the prognosis of these patients. BCAA supplements have been shown to reduce passage of aromatic amino acids into the brain. Based on these basic observations, patients with advanced chronic liver disease have been treated clinically with BCAA-rich medicines, with positive effects. BCCA are essential amino acids that cannot be synthesized in the body. BCAAs leucine, isoleucine, and valine, are three of the nine essential amino acids and are relatively abundant in the food supply accounting for approximately 20% of total protein intake. Adipose tissue is second only to skeletal muscle in its capacity to catabolize BCAAs, and that the capacities of skeletal muscle and adipose tissue are 6–7-fold larger than liver taking into account the relative masses of different tissues.

Tajiri K, Shimizu Y. Branched-chain amino acids in liver diseases. World J Gastroenterol. 2013;19(43):7620-29.

Q2. Answer TFTFT

Glutamine is the most abundant free amino acid in the human body and is necessary to modulate the inflammatory and oxidative stress responses in patients. Systemic glutamine availability is determined by the balance of endogenous glutamine production (mainly in muscular tissue) and its use by glutamine consuming organs (gut, kidney, liver and the immune system).

Several studies show that in catabolic ICU patients, the endogenous production of muscular glutamine is increased while the plasma levels of glutamine are decreased, indicating elevated glutamine needs.

The plasma levels of glutamine are extremely variable in the ICU population and are not always associated with increased mortality. The glutamine supplementation does not stop the glutamine efflux from muscle because the endogenous muscular production and plasma levels of glutamine are related to the severity of the illness. The REDOX study is a well conducted, large, multicenter trial illustrating the fact that early administration of glutamine in high doses (much higher than recommended) can have adverse effects. This was reflected by increased mortality in the group supplemented with glutamine in patients with multiorgan failure (including kidney dysfunction), some of whom had high basal serum levels of glutamine.

Martins P. Glutamine in critically ill patients: is it a fundamental nutritional supplement? Rev Bras Ter Intensiva. 2016;28(2):100-3.

Q3. Answer TTFTT

A vitamin is an organic compound and an essential nutrient that organism cannot synthesize the compound in sufficient quantities, and it must be obtained through the diet. Thus, the term 'vitamin' is conditional upon the circumstances and the particular organism. For example, Vitamin C is a vitamin for humans, but not for most other animals. Vitamin D is essential only for people who do not have adequate skin exposure to sunlight, as ultraviolet light promotes synthesis in skin cells. Supplementation is important for the treatment of certain health problems, but there is little evidence of nutritional benefit when used by otherwise healthy people.

Biotin is a water-soluble B-vitamin, also called vitamin B_7 and formerly known as vitamin H or coenzyme R. RDA quoted as Biotin- 30 μg is correct.

Lowry SF, Goodgame JT, Maher MM, Brennan MF. Parenteral vitamin requirements during intravenous feeding. Am J Clin Nutr. 1978;31(12): 2149-58.

Q4. Answer TFTT

Sulfite ion is a strong nucleophile and readily binds to thiamine (to the positively charged nitrogen in the thiazole ring), leading to secondary deficits of vitamin B1. Many vitamins are known to be specifically vulnerable to degradation by UV light, including vitamin A, B2 (riboflavin), B6, B12 and folic acid. Light also accelerates the destructive interaction between vitamins. Vitamin K is moderately stable to *heat*, but unstable to light, acid, and alkali.

Nutrition support for adults: oral nutrition support, enteral tube feeding and parenteral nutrition. NICE Guidelines. Available from: https://www.nice.org.uk/guidance/cg32/chapter/1-guidance (Accessed 1 January 2018).

Q5. Answer TFTTT

Refeeding syndrome can be defined as the potentially fatal shifts in fluids and electrolytes that may occur in malnourished patients receiving artificial refeeding (whether enterally or parenterally). With the change to anabolism on refeeding, potassium is taken up into cells as they increase in volume and number and as a direct result of insulin secretion. This results in severe hypokalemia. Hypokalemia, hypocalcemia, hypomagnesemia, are its hallmark. Rehydration and correction of potassium (give 2-4 mmol/kg/day), phosphate (0.3-0.6 mmol/kg/day), calcium, and magnesium (0.2 mmol/kg/day intravenously or 0.4 mmol/kg/day orally) are recommended carefully. For patients at high risk of developing refeeding syndrome, nutritional repletion of energy should be started slowly (maximum 0.042 MJ/kg/24 hours) and should be tailored to each patient. Changes in carbohydrate metabolism have a profound effect on sodium and water balance. The introduction of carbohydrate to a diet leads to a rapid decrease in renal excretion of sodium and water. If fluid repletion is then instituted to maintain a normal urine output, patients may rapidly develop fluid overload. This can lead to congestive cardiac failure, pulmonary edema, and cardiac arrhythmia. In refeeding syndrome, chronic whole body depletion of phosphorus occurs. Also, the insulin surge causes a greatly increased uptake and use of phosphate in the cells. These changes lead to deficit in intracellular as well as extracellular phosphorus. In this environment, even small decreases in serum phosphorus may lead to widespread dysfunction of cellular processes affecting almost every physiological system.

Mehanna HM, Moledina J, Travis J. Refeeding syndrome: what it is, and how to prevent and treat it. BMJ. 2008;336(7659): 1495-8.

Q6. Answer TFTFT

Immunomodulating diets have been claimed to be associated with a statistically significant reduction of secondary infections compared to control. The use of fish oil immunomodulating diets in intensive care unit patients was associated with a significant reduction in mortality secondary infections and length of hospital stay. However this is debated. No recommendation regarding supplementation with Omega-3 fatty acids, arginine, glutamine or nucleotides can be given for burned patients due to insufficient data. Patients with ARDS should receive EN enriched with Omega-3 fatty acids and antioxidants. Patients with a mild sepsis (APACHE II less than 15) should receive immune modulating EN with such a formula. No benefit could be established in patients with severe sepsis, in whom immune-modulating formula may be harmful and is therefore not recommended. ICU patients with very severe illness and who do not tolerate more than 700 mL

EN/day should not receive a formula enriched with arginine, nucleotides and Omega-3 fatty acids. In elective upper GI surgical patients immune-modulating formula enriched with arginine, nucleotides and Omega-3 fatty acids is superior to a standard enteral formula. Glutamine should be added to a standard enteral formula in burned patients and trauma patients.

> Kreymann KG, Berger MM, Deutz NEP, Hiesmayr M et al. ESPEN Guidelines on Enteral Nutrition: Intensive care. ESPN Guidelines.Clinical Nutrition. 2006;25:210-23.

Q7. Answer FFTFF

The NUTRIC Score is designed to quantify the risk of critically ill patients developing adverse events that may be modified by aggressive nutrition therapy. The score, of 1-10, is based on 6 variables.

Variable	Range	Points
Age	<50	0
	50 – <75	1
	>75	2
APACHE	<15	0
	15 – <20	1
	20 – 28	2
	>28	3
SOFA	<6	0
	6 – <10	1
	>10	2
Number of Co-morbidities	0-1	0
	>2	1
Days from hospital to ICU admission	0 – <1	0
	>1	1
IL-6	0 – <400	0
	> 400	1

High score associated with worse clinical outcomes (mortality, ventilation). These patients are the most likely to benefit from aggressive nutrition therapy.

> Kalaiselvan MS, Renuka MK, Arunkumar AS. Use of Nutrition Risk in Critically ill (NUTRIC) Score to Assess Nutritional Risk in Mechanically Ventilated Patients: A Prospective Observational Study. Indian J Crit Care Med. 2017;21(5):253-6.

Q8. Answer TTTF

The insufficient provision of nutrients is likely to result in undernutrition within 8-12 days following surgery and/or ICU admission. In order to prevent undernutrition and related adverse effects, all ICU patients who are not expected to be on a full oral diet within three days should receive EN. Undernutrition is more likely to develop in critical illness than in uncomplicated starvation. EN is accordingly recommended as the first choice route for nutrition support in ICU patients. The use of PN is however reported to lie between 12% and 71% and of EN between 33% and 92%, of critically ill patients who receive nutritional support. All patients receiving less than their targeted enteral feeding after 2 days should be considered for supplementary PN.

> Kreymann KG, Berger MM, Deutz NEP, Hiesmayr M et al. ESPEN Guidelines on Enteral Nutrition: Intensive care. ESPN Guidelines.Clinical Nutrition. 2006;25:210-23.

Q9. Answer FTTT

Enteral tube feeding is nutrition therapy given via a tube or stoma into the intestinal tract distal to the oral cavity. The tube could be inserted via the nose; i.e. nasogastric, nasojejunal or naso-post pyloric tube feeding; or via a stoma that is inserted endoscopically into the stomach; i.e. percutaneous endoscopic gastrostomy (PEG) or with a jejunal extension (PEG-J) or into the jejunum [percutaneous endoscopic jejunostomy (PEJ)].

Finally, the tube may also be placed surgically; i.e. surgical gastrostomy or jejunostomy. In Cochrane meta-analysis it was found that post-pyloric feeding appeared to reduce the rate of pneumonia and increase the amount of nutrition delivered to the patient. Its use did not result in fewer days on a ventilator nor in fewer deaths. The target amount of feeding for a person fed with a post-pyloric tube was reached without delay. Insertion of a post-pyloric feeding tube appears safe and did not increase the likelihood of complications. Recommendation for post-pyloric feeding was made for ICU patients, when this approach is feasible.

Alkhawaja S, Martin C, Butler RJ, Gwadry-Sridhar F. Post-pyloric versus gastric tube feeding for critically ill adult patients. Cochrane Review. Available from: http://www.cochrane.org/CD008875/ANAESTH_post-pyloric-versus-gastric-tube-feeding-critically-ill-adult-patient(Accessed 22 November 2017).

Q10. Answer TFTF

Formulas containing peptides and medium chain triglycerides can facilitate absorption in case of e.g. malabsorption or short bowel syndrome. Whole protein formulae are appropriate in most patients because no clinical advantage of peptide based formulae could be shown.

Kreymann KG, Berger MM, Deutz NEP, Hiesmayr M et al. ESPEN Guidelines on Enteral Nutrition: Intensive care. ESPN Guidelines.Clinical Nutrition. 2006;25:210-23.

Q11. Answer TTTT

Immune-modulating formulae (formulae enriched with arginine, nucleotides and Omega-3 fatty acids) are superior to standard enteral formulae in elective upper GI surgical patients, patients with a mild sepsis (APACHE II less than 15) and in patients with severe sepsis. No recommendation for immune-modulating formulae can be given for burn patients due to insufficient data.

In burned patients trace elements (Cu, Se and Zn) should be supplemented in a higher than standard dose. ICU patients with very severe illness who do not tolerate more than 700 ml enteral formulae per day should not receive an immune-modulating formula enriched with arginine, nucleotides and Omega -3 fatty acids. Glutamine should be added to standard enteral formula in burn patients and trauma patients.

Kreymann KG, Berger MM, Deutz NEP, Hiesmayr M et al. ESPEN Guidelines on Enteral Nutrition: Intensive care. ESPN Guidelines. Clinical Nutrition. 2006;25:210-23.

Q12. Answer TTFT

Symptoms and signs associated with thiamine deficiency lack sensitivity and specificity in critically ill patients. Consequently, depletion is frequently unrecognized and underdiagnosed by clinicians. Potentially deleterious consequences of thiamine depletion should be avoided by early and appropriate supplementation. Patients should be given a loading dose of 50–250 mg thiamine on admission to the Intensive Care Unit. Iron, Zinc, Vitamin C, Copper, Selenium and Vitamin A also decrease in critical illness.

Ascorbic acid (Vitamin C) infusion (66 mg/kg/hr for 24 hours) among burn patients sustaining injury >30% total body surface area (TBSA) has been considered due its anti-oxidative effects. Patients with AKI are prone to depletion of trace elements and vitamin. Reasons are multifactorial and include variable protein binding, redistribution between plasma and tissues, acute loss of biological fluids, dilution, varying concentrations of trace elements in dialysis/hemofiltration fluids, nutrient intake, and removal from plasma by CRRT. Water-soluble vitamin and trace element losses and requirements during CRRT remain the subject of debate and research. In general, water-soluble vitamins are highly removed by CRRT (e.g. 68 mg vitamin C and 290 μg folic acid per day). Proposed recommendations for daily supplementation of water-soluble vitamins are: 100 mg vitamin B1, 2 mg vitamin B2, 20 mg vitamin B3, 10 mg vitamin B5, 200 mg biotin, 1 mg folic acid, 4 μg vitamin B12, and 250 mg vitamin C. Vitamin C intake in patients with AKI should not exceed the recommended dose because of the potential risk of nephrotoxic secondary oxalosis. Thiamine loss may largely exceed the daily provision of this vitamin by standard TPN. Therefore, recommended supplements may vary accordingly. The fat-soluble vitamins E and K also need to be supplemented (10 IU/day and 4 mg/week), respectively but vitamin A must be reduced to compensate for deficient retinol degradation. Daily parenteral supplementation with standard doses of trace elements is supposed to compensate for CRRT removal.

Honoré PM, De Waele E, Jacobs R et al. Nutritional and Metabolic Alterations during Continuous Renal Replacement Therapy. Blood Purif. 2013;35:279-84.

Q13. Answer TFTT

Laboratory markers are not reliable by themselves but could be used as complement to a thorough physical examination. Indirect calorimetry is the method by which metabolic rate and substrate utilization are estimated in human beings starting from respiratory gas exchange measurements and urinary nitrogen excretion. This method is based on some models and assumptions that must be known and taken into consideration to correctly interpret the results obtained. Recent advances in technology and the availability of precise and portable metabolic carts have made this technique practical at the bedside even in critically ill patients. Predictive equations such as the Harris-Benedict equation multiplied by a stress factor of 1.6 and the Swinamer equation may be accurate enough for short-term nutrition support of critically ill patients when IC is unavailable. Bowel sounds are only indicative of contractility and may not relate to mucosal integrity, barrier function, or absorptive capacity. Bowel sounds and evidence of bowel function (i.e., passing flatus or stool) are not required for initiation of enteral feeding.

Ramprasad R, Kapoor MC. Nutrition in intensive care. J Anaesthesiol Clin Pharmacol. 2012;28(1):1-3.

Hejazi N, Mazloom Z, Zand F, Rezaianzadeh A, Amini A. Nutritional Assessment in Critically Ill PatientsIran. J Med Sci. 2016; 41(3):171-9.

Q14. Answer FTFT

Optimization of nutrition remains a significant challenge in ARF patients. There is conflicting evidence regarding the target caloric intake in ARF. The use of predictive equations for the estimation of resting energy expenditure remains inadequate. The gold standard of indirect calorimetry is costly and labor intensive, and may not be as accurate in intubated patients with high oxygen requirements. Whilst overfeeding should be avoided, early enteral feeding should be encouraged. There is no evidence of benefit in early commencement of parenteral nutrition. Cai et al. in 2003 demonstrated a significant improvement in pulmonary function in COPD patients with a high-fat, low carbohydrate diet as compared with the traditional high carbohydrate diet. Fluid restricted, calorically dense formulations could be considered for patients with acute respiratory failure without evidence of hypernatremia. High lipid, low carbohydrate specialty formulae designed to manipulate the respiratory quotient may be utilized in the CO_2 retaining patients who are difficult to wean from mechanical ventilation, but should not be routinely used. Hypophosphatemia may increase the need to mechanical ventilation. Therefore, monitoring serum phosphate level is a good prognostic factor to predict the need to ventilation. Initial trophic enteral feeding did not improve ventilator-free days, 60-day mortality, or infectious complications but was associated with less gastrointestinal intolerance.

Cai B, Zhu Y, Ma Yi, Xu Z, Zao Yi, Wang J, Comer GM, et al. Effect of supplementing a high-fat, low-carbohydrate enteral formula in COPD patients. Nutrition. 2003;19:229-32

Initial Trophic vs Full Enteral Feeding in Patients With Acute Lung Injury

The EDEN Randomized Trial. The National Heart, Lung, and Blood Institute Acute Respiratory Distress Syndrome (ARDS) Clinical Trials Network. JAMA. 2012;307(8):795-803.

Loi M, Wang J, Ong C, Lee JH. Metrics P. Nutritional support of critically ill adults and children with acute respiratory distress syndrome: A clinical review. 2017;19:1-8.

Q15. Answer TFFF

Patients with renal disease should undergo formal nutrition assessment, including evaluation of inflammation, with development of a nutrition care plan. Standard amino acid TPN formulations should be used in AKI. There is inadequate evidence at this time to support the use of essential amino acid (EAA) PN formulations with AKI. Formulation with EAA alone and combination with non-essential amino acids (NEAA) were debated. Dietary sodium intake is an important consideration in patients with all stages of chronic kidney disease, including those receiving dialysis therapy or those who have received a kidney transplant. In AKI however the salt restriction should be individualized carefully. Standard formulae are adequate for the majority of patients. However, requirements can differ and have to be assessed individually. When there are electrolyte derangements, formulae specific for CRF patients can be advantageous.

Brown RO, Compher C et al. A.S.P.E.N. Clinical Guidelines: Nutrition Support in Adult Acute and Chronic Renal Failure. Journal of Parenteral and Enteral Nutrition. 2010;34(4):366-377.

Q16. Answer TFFT

Ideally energy expenditure should be measured by indirect calorimetry. Predictive equations are equally good with a mean deviation of 11% from measured values. It remains controversial, however, whether actual, ideal or 'dry' body weight should be used for calculation, since ascites apparently is not an inert compartment regarding energy expenditure. Both, actual weight in severe hydropic decompensation or errors in estimates of 'dry' weight may lead to erroneous values deviating to the extremes and therefore, ideal body weight may be accepted as a safe approach. Nutritional support is a vital component in the treatment of acute liver failure and should be initiated early. It is required to prevent catabolism of body stores of proteins and it may decrease the risk of gastrointestinal bleeding from stress ulceration in critically ill patients. To prevent protein catabolism, severe protein restrictions should be avoided; a daily intake of 60 grams of protein is reasonable for most patients with acute liver failure. In recently published Cochrane review BCAA was shown to have a beneficial effect on hepatic encephalopathy. However there was no effect on mortality, quality of life, or nutritional parameters.

>Goldberg E, Chopra S. Acute liver failure in adults: Management and prognosis. Available from: https://www.uptodate.com/contents/acute-liver-failure-in-adults-management-and-prognosis?source=search_result&search=nutrition%20support%20in%20liver%20failure&selectedTitle=1~150 (Accessed 23 November 2017).

>Branched-chain amino acids improve symptoms of hepatic encephalopathy. Cchrane review. 2017. Available from: http://www.cochrane.org/CD001939/LIVER_branched-chain-amino-acids-improve-symptoms-hepatic-encephalopathy (Accessed 23 November 2017)

Q17. Answer FFTF

Feeding in acute pancreatitis depends on the severity and stage of the disease. In mild cases low residue, low fat, soft diet is used, provided there is no evidence of ileus or significant nausea and/or vomiting. Diet is increased cautiously as tolerated. Traditionally, patients have been advanced from a clear liquid diet to solid food as tolerated. Patients may require enteral or parenteral feeding if caloric and protein needs are not met. Low fat, semi-elemental feeding formulae (e.g. Peptamen AF) because of a reduction in pancreatic digestive enzymes are tolerated better. Start at 25 cc per hour and advance as tolerated to at least 30% of the calculated daily requirement (25 kcal/kg ideal body weight), even in the presence of ileus. Signs that the formula is not tolerated include increased abdominal pain, vomiting (with nasogastric feeding), bloating, or diarrhea (>5 watery stools or >500 mL per 24 hours with exclusion of Clostridium difficile toxin and medication-induced diarrhea) that resolves if the feeding is held. Although immunonutrition has no effect on mortality rate, there is a significant reduction in infection rates, ventilator duration and length of hospital stay in these patients. At present, there are no available reports on the clinical effects of immune-enhancing diets on these patients. Polymeric immune-enhancing diet may be safe to administer patients with acute pancreatitis. Considering the advantages, polymeric diets, particularly those containing glutamine, arginine, ω-3 fatty acids, nucleotides, and fiber, may be used in them, but the beneficial effects require further study. Randomized, controlled studies reported that patients who received immune-enhancing enteral feeds containing arginine, nucleotides and ω-3 fatty acids (fish oil) after operation and trauma had a lower rate of postoperative infections and wound complications compared with patients receiving isocaloric, isonitrogenous control feed.

>Vege SS. Management of acute pancreatitis. Available from: https://www.uptodate.com/contents/management-of-acute-pancreatitis?source=search_result&search=nutrition%20in%20Acute%20Pancreatitis&selectedTitle=1~150 (Accessed 23 November 2017).

Q18. Answer TTFF

Q19. Answer TTFFF

Early provision of EN in critically ill and injured patients has become standard practice in surgical intensive care units (ICUs) due to its proven role in reducing septic complications. Patients with an open abdomen after damage control surgery are common and the recognition of the abdominal compartment syndrome; the role and timing of EN in these challenging patients continue to be debated. Patients with an open abdomen are often among the sickest in the ICU and hence could benefit from early nutrition support. However, the exposed abdominal viscera can understandably create anxiety regarding the initiation of EN; there is theoretic concern over exacerbation of bowel distention with resultant inability to close the abdomen and an increased aspiration risk due to paralytic ileus. They advise that full EN to meet goal metabolic needs be initiated within 24 to 48 hours when feasible. This has been shown to maintain gut integrity, modulate the systemic inflammatory response, and reduce both mortality and infectious morbidity. Patient with open abdomen will have increased fluid, electrolyte, and protein requirements because of large volume losses of these substrates through their abdominal wound. Failure to recognize these losses in calculations of nitrogen balance and caloric needs will lead to underfeeding. It is estimated that 2 g to 4.6 g of nitrogen are lost per liter of abdominal fluid output depending on the type of temporary abdominal closure. Measurements of peritoneal fluid also demonstrate a significant amount of potassium, phosphorus, magnesium, and calcium, a finding that must be taken into account when providing electrolyte replacements. Nutritional formulae containing immune-modulating agents (glutamine, arginine, n-3 fatty acids, and ribonucleic acids) have been studied but the evidence is weak for strong recommendation.

Moore SM, Burlew CC. Nutrition Support in the Open Abdomen. Nutr Clin Pract. 2016;31(1):9-13.

Chabot E, Nirula R. Open abdomen critical care management principles: resuscitation, fluid balance, nutrition, and ventilator management. Trauma Surg Acute Care Open. 2017;2:1-9.

Q20. Answer TTTF

Proteolysis is greatly increased after severe burn and can exceed a half pound of skeletal muscle daily. Protein supplementation is needed to meet ongoing demands and supply substrate for wound healing, immune function, and to minimize the loss of lean body mass. Protein is used as an energy source when calories are limited. Currently, protein requirements are estimated as 1.5–2.0 g/kg/day for burned adults and 2.5–4.0 g/kg/day for burned children. Non-protein calorie to nitrogen ratio should be maintained between 150:1. There is no consensus regarding the optimal timing, route, amount, and composition of nutritional support for burn patients, but most clinicians advocate for early EN with high-carbohydrate formulas.

Nutritional support must be individualized, monitored, and adjusted throughout recovery. Further investigation is needed regarding optimal nutritional support and accurate nutritional endpoints and goals.

Curreri formula was proposed in 1972 and created by studying 9 patients and computing backwards to approximate the calories that would have been needed to compensate for the patients' weight loss.

The Curreri formula and many other older formulae overestimate current metabolic requirements, and more sophisticated formulae with different variables have been proposed.

Energy expenditure does fluctuate after burn, and fixed formulae often lead to underfeeding during periods of highest energy utilization and to overfeeding late in the treatment course. The ideal burn resuscitation is the one that effectively restores plasma volume, with no adverse effects. Isotonic crystalloids, hypertonic solutions and colloids have been used for this purpose, but every solution has its advantages and disadvantages. None of them is ideal, and none is superior to any of the others.

Hartmann solution (a solution similar to ringer lactate (RL) solution) and normal saline are commonly used. There are some adverse effects of the crystalloids: high volume administration of normal saline produces hyperchloremic acidosis, RL increases the neutrophil activation after resuscitation for hemorrhage or after infusion without hemorrhage. D-lactate in RL solution containing a racemic mixture of the D-lactate and L-lactate isomers has been found to be responsible for increased production of reactive oxygen species (ROS). RL used in the majority of hospitals contains this mixture. Another adverse effect that has been demonstrated is that crystalloids have a substantial influence on coagulation. Recent studies have demonstrated that in vivo dilution with crystalloids (independent of the type of the crystalloid) resulted in a hypercoagulable state.

Clark A, Imran J, Madni T, Steven E. Wolf. Nutrition and metabolism in burn patients. Burns Trauma. 2017;5:11.

CHAPTER

6

Renal

Manish Jain, Ashish Nandwani, Gaurav Kochar

A Type Questions
(One best answer)

1. Which of the following definition of Acute Kidney Injury (AKI) have been validated from epidemiological studies of AKI?
   a. Acute kidney injury network (AKIN) classification
   b. RIFLE (Risk, Injury, Failure, Loss, ESRD) classification
   c. KDIGO (Kidney disease improving global outcomes) classification
   d. All of the Above
   e. None of the above

2. As per KDIGO staging of Acute Kidney Injury (AKI), which is right?
   a. Stage 1- Urine Output <0.5 mL/kg/h for 3-6 hrs
   b. Stage 1- S. Creatinine 1.0 to 1.5 times baseline
   c. Stage 2- S. Creatinine 2.0 to 2.9 times baseline
   d. Stage 3- Anuria for >6 hrs
   e. Stage 4- Recent AKI currently polyuric phase

3. Regarding dialysis which of the following is false?
   a. Recommendation is Kt/V of 1.2-1.4 per session
   b. 3 times per week is recommended rather than 6 times per week
   c. Higher the Kt/V better the survival
   d. Large molecular weight solutes do not primarily depend on convection for removal
   e. Intradialytic hypotension (IDH) is defined as a decrease in systolic blood pressure by ≥20 mm Hg or a decrease in MAP by 10 mm Hg during dialysis

4. In case of AKI, a Blood Urea Nitrogen (BUN): Creatinine Ratio <10 is suggestive of:
   a. Pre renal AKI
   b. Post renal AKI
   c. Acute tubular necrosis
   d. Gastrointestinal hemorrhage
   e. Early stage of shock

5. Which of the following are unlikely in a case of acute kidney injury?
   a. Hyperkalemia
   b. Loss of Corticomedullary differentiation (CMD) on Ultrasonography (USG)
   c. Metabolic acidosis
   d. Anuria
   e. Hypocalcemia

6. Which is the best site to place a temporary hemodialysis catheter?
   a. Left internal jugular vein (LIJV)
   b. Right internal jugular vein (RIJV)
   c. Right subclavian vein
   d. Femoral vein
   e. Left Subclavian vein

7. For continuous veno-venous hemodiafiltration (CVVHDF), what is the recommended dose of replacement fluid?
   a. 40 mL/kg/hr

b. 30 mL/kg/hr
   c. 35 mL/kg/hr
   d. 20–25 mL/kg/hr
   e. 70 mL/kg/hr
8. **A patient on citrate anticoagulation on Continuous Renal Replacement Therapy (CRRT) develops cardiac arrhythmia. Which is the most likely cause?**
   a. Excessive ultrafiltration
   b. Inappropriate free serum calcium level
   c. Hyperkalemia
   d. Inadequate anticoagulation
   e. Hypokalemia
9. **A 70 years old male developed AKI following cardiac surgery and antibiotic use. He became oliguric and serum Cystatin C was 2.0 mg/L.**

   Which of the following is an indication for Renal Replacement Therapy (RRT)?
   a. Serum K⁺ 5.3 meq /L
   b. Serum PH 7.25
   c. Anuria for 3 hours
   d. Na⁺ 160 mmol/L
   e. Cystatin C 2.0 mg/L
10. **RRT modality of choice in a patient with intracranial hypertension is:**
    a. Intermittent hemodialysis
    b. CVVHD
    c. SLED
    d. Peritoneal dialysis
    e. Continuous arteriovenous techniques
11. **A patient of decompensated chronic liver disease (CLD) with ascites was found to have serum creatinine of 3.0 mg/dL from a baseline of 0.8 mg/dL over 4 days. His urine protein creatinine ratio was 0.4, total leukocyte count was 9.5 x 10⁹/L and USG suggestive of bilateral normal kidneys. What is the most likely diagnosis?**
    a. Hepatorenal syndrome (HRS) type 1
    b. HRS type 2
    c. HRS type 3
    d. Diabetic nephropathy
    e. Sepsis associated acute kidney injury (SAKI)
12. **In a 49-year-old patient with type 2 DM for 10 years and decompensated CLD, which of following is against diagnosis of Hepatorenal syndrome (HRS)?**
    a. Rise of S. Creatinine from 0.5 to 2.6 in 24 hrs
    b. Proteinuria of 30 mg/day
    c. Urine routine showing 3 to 5 RBCs per HPF
    d. Bilateral normal kidney on USG
    e. Urea Creatinine ratio > 20
13. **A 40-year-old nondiabetic patient presented with acute left ventricular failure (LVF) with Ejection Fraction of 20% due to ACS. On admission his S. Creatinine was 0.7 mg% which increased to 2.4 mg/dL after 3 days. His CVP was elevated and he had significant edema feet. MAP was 65 to 70 mm Hg. Urine routine examination was normal and Urine protein creatinine ratio was 0.03. What is the diagnosis?**
    a. Cardio Renal Syndrome (CRS) type 1
    b. CRS type 2
    c. CRS type 3
    d. Acute interstitial nephritis
    e. CRS type 4
14. **In obstructive uropathy with unilateral renal stone, which of following is least likely?**
    a. Oliguric renal failure
    b. Hydroureteronephrosis
    c. Unilateral Flank pain
    d. Microscopic hematuria
    e. pain radiating to the T11 to T12 dermatomes
15. **Which of following is a major risk factor for contrast induced nephropathy (CIN)?**
    a. Hypertension
    b. Use of fluconazole
    c. CHF
    d. Angiotensin-converting enzyme inhibitors (ACEI)
    e. Diabetes mellitus
16. **Which of following is false for contrast nephropathy?**
    a. Serum creatinine begins to rise within 24 hr of contrast administration
    b. Irreversible
    c. Nonoliguric renal failure
    d. Tubular injury
    e. Dehydration is a common risk factor
17. **All are true about renal physiology in normal pregnancy except:**
    a. Increase in renal bipolar diameter
    b. Increase in hematocrit
    c. Increase in glomerular filtration rate
    d. Decreased serum protein
    e. Decrease in serum creatinine

18. Renal abnormalities in preeclampsia (PE) are all *except*:
    a. Decreased renal blood flow and decreased GFR
    b. Proteinuria and endotheliosis
    c. Decreased renin release
    d. Decreased uric acid reabsorption
    e. Risk factor for the development of chronic kidney disease (CKD)

19. Which organism represents contamination of urine specimen in healthy non-pregnant women?
    a. E Coli
    b. Staphylococcus saprophyticus
    c. Pseudomonas aeruginosa
    d. Enterococci
    e. Proteus

20. Which of the following is the strongest single predictor of End Stage Renal Disease (ESRD) in Type 2 Diabetes Mellitus?
    a. Serum creatinine
    b. Serum albumin
    c. Albuminuria
    d. Hemoglobin
    e. Serum uric acid

21. Which of following is initial dose of Erythropoietin (EPO) in ESRD patients with anemia?
    a. 5 to 10 units/kg/week
    b. 10 to 20 units/kg/week
    c. 40 units/kg/week
    d. 50 to 100 units/kg/week
    e. More than 100 units/kg/week

22. What stage of CKD is a patient, with eGFR of 42 mL/min, and albuminuria 30–300 mg/g?
    a. G2A2
    b. G3A2
    c. G2A3
    d. G3A3
    e. G4A1

23. Which of following is not a type of AV fistula used in dialysis?
    a. Brachiobasilic
    b. Brachiocephalic
    c. Radiocephalic
    d. Radiobasilic

24. Oral Calcium Acetate is used in ESRD patient to treat:
    a. Hyperkalemia
    b. Hyperparathyroidism
    c. Metabolic acidosis
    d. Mild hyperkalemia
    e. All of the above

25. Type of anemia in CKD patients:
    a. Normocytic normochromic
    b. Microcytic hypochromic
    c. Aplastic anemia
    d. Hemolytic
    e. Macrocytic

26. Which of following in ESRD patient is said to cause nephrogenic fibrosing cholangitis?
    a. Gadolinium
    b. Arsenic
    c. Diclofenac
    d. Aluminium
    e. Calcium carbonate

27. A 52-year-old male is admitted with complaints of headache and dizziness. His BP is 220/120 mm Hg and PR 86/min. CT showed acute ischemic infarct. Which is the appropriate drug to lower the BP in this patient?
    a. Nifedipine
    b. Nicardipine
    c. Nitroglycerine
    d. Esmolol
    e. Amlodepine

28. Aminoglycoside with least nephrotoxicity is:
    a. Gentamycin
    b. Tobramycin
    c. Amikacin
    d. Netilmicin
    e. Streptomycin

29. Serum sodium 117 meq/L, plasma osmolality of 290 is suggestive of:
    a. Beer potomania
    b. SIADH
    c. Salt loosing nephropathy
    d. Cirrhosis complicated by hyponatremia
    e. Hyperlipidemia

K Type Questions
[Marked True (T)/False (F)]

1. **Regarding Contrast Induced Nephropathy (CIN):**
    a. Most of the cases show decline in urine output within 12 hours

b. Presence of Muddy brown granular and epithelial cell casts exclude the diagnosis
c. Pathologic changes of acute tubular necrosis are seen
d. FeNa <1 is usually seen
e. Creatinine usually rises between 3 and 7 days

2. **Regarding CIN:**
   a. In patients with diabetes and CKD, the reported risk following coronary angiography with or without intervention is 10-30%
   b. Higher risk when contrast is administered in artery than in veins
   c. Risk of CIN in patients with no history of CKD is 1-2%
   d. GFR <60 mL/min alone is sufficient to identify patient at risk of CIN
   e. Iohexol should be contrast agents of choice

3. **Choose correct statement:**
   a. Immediate dialysis after IV contrast administration helps preserve residual renal function
   b. 2012 KDIGO guidelines suggest administration of IV acetylcysteine for reducing risk of CIN
   c. Fluid administration 0.5 mL/kg/hr is recommended for prevention of CIN
   d. Creatinine usually recovers in 5-10 days
   e. Isotonic soda bicarb is the fluid of choice for prophylactic treatment of CIN

4. **Which statement is true regarding definition of AKI?**
   a. Increase in serum creatinine by ≥0.3 mg/dL (27 micromol/L) within 24 hours
   b. Creatinine increase ≥1.5 times the presumed baseline value that is known or presumed to have occurred within the prior seven days
   c. Decrease in urine volume to <3 mL/kg over six hours
   d. Assessment and optimization of fluid status should be done before diagnosis and classification
   e. KDIGO Stage 2 is - Increase in serum creatinine to 2.0 to 2.9 times baseline, **or** reduction in urine output to <0.5 mL/kg/hour for ≥12 hours

5. **Consider the following statements:**
   a. Oliguria is defined as <0.3 mL/kg per hour or <500 mL/day of urine output

   b. Urinary Angiotensinogen is one of the newer diagnostic markers of AKI
   c. Neutrophil Gelatinase Associated Lipocalin (NGAL) can differentiate prerenal disease from ATN
   d. Urine osmolality above 500 mosmol/kg is highly suggestive of prerenal disease
   e. BUN/serum creatinine ratio is often greater than 20:1 in prerenal disease.

6. **Regarding Hepatorenal Syndrome (HRS):**
   a. Usually associated with chronic liver disease with portal hypertension
   b. Not associated with acute liver failure
   c. Low incidence in primary biliary cirrhosis
   d. Urine sodium is usually less than 10 meq/L
   e. Presence of granular cast in urine rules out the diagnosis

7. **Mark true/false:**
   a. Type 1 HRS is defined as at least a twofold increase in serum creatinine to a level greater than .5 mg/dL (221 micromol/L) during a period of less than 1 weeks
   b. Lack of improvement in renal function after volume expansion with intravenous albumin (1 g/kg of body weight per day up to 100 g/day) for at least two days and withdrawal of diuretics
   c. Terlipressin is initial choice of treatment in critically sick patients
   d. In patients with Spontaneous Bacterial Peritonitis (SBP), the administration of intravenous albumin reduces the incidence of both renal impairment and mortality
   e. Pentoxifylline has been conclusively shown to be of benefit in preventing hepatorenal syndrome in patients having cirrhosis with ascites

8. **Regarding urine analysis:**
   a. Pink color urine may be seen during propofol administration
   b. Bacteruria may be associated with purple urine
   c. Whitish urine may be seen in pyuria
   d. Propofol is associated with green color urine
   e. Black color urine may be seen in myoglobinuria

9. **Mark true/false:**
   a. Leukocyte esterase by dipstick test may be falsely negative in concentrated urine

b. Nitrite positive urine indicates bacteriuria
c. Nitrite may be negative despite presence of Enterococcus
d. Positive sulfosalicylic acid test with negative dipstick for proteinuria suggests possibility of gammopathy
e. Granular cast mainly consist of degenerated granulocytes

10. **Mark true or false:**
    a. Approximately 5% of nondiabetic kidney transplant recipients develop New-onset diabetes after transplant (NODAT) by six months post transplantation
    b. Criteria for NODAT is similar to American Diabetes Association (ADA) criteria for the diagnosis of diabetes mellitus and impaired glucose tolerance
    c. Azathioprine increases risk for NODAT
    d. Oral hypoglycemic agents have no role in NODAT management
    e. Thiazolidinediones are drug of choice in NODAT

11. **Regarding loop diuretics:**
    a. Site of action is descending limb of loop of henle
    b. Site of action is ascending limb of loop of henle
    c. Furosemide belong to sulfonamide group
    d. Furosemide should be avoided in patients with allergy to sulfonamides
    e. Ethacrynic acid is not a loop diuretic

12. **Following commonly used antibiotics need renal dose adjustment:**
    a. Piperacillin + tazobactam
    b. Meropenem
    c. Levofloxacin
    d. Tigecycline
    e. Trimethoprim sulfamethoxazol

13. **All are indication for urgent dialysis**
    a. Fluid overload
    b. Hyperkalemia (serum potassium >5.5 mEq/L) or a rapidly increasing serum potassium
    c. Signs of uremia, such as pericarditis, or an otherwise unexplained decline in mental status
    d. Severe metabolic acidosis (pH <7.1)
    e. Creatinine >5.0 mg/dL

14. **Regarding diuretics:**
    a. Thiazide act on proximal tubule
    b. Thiazides are effective when loop diuretics fail
    c. Thiazide act on Na-K-Cl channel
    d. Thiazide act on Na-Cl cotransporter
    e. Thiazide cause hypocalciuria

15. **In patients with renal impairment:**
    a. Initial loading dose of vancomycin depends on creatinine level
    b. For patient on vancomycin and intermittent dialysis 5–10 mg/kg should be given after each session in general
    c. In a 90 kg obese patient with GFR of 30, dose of vancomycin is 1000 mg twice a day
    d. In a patient with GFR of <15 mL/min / 1.73 m^2 vancomycin dose is given as per the weight and vancomycin level 24 hrs after first dose
    e. Oral dose also requires adjustment

16. **Regarding aminoglycoside nephrotoxicity:**
    a. Acute kidney injury from aminoglycoside exposure typically manifests after five to seven days of therapy
    b. Intracellular accumulation of aminoglycosides occur in distal tubule
    c. Utilizing a once-daily dosing regimen may reduce the risk
    d. Hypomagnesemia is very common in aminoglycoside toxicity
    e. Nephrotoxicity usually results in oliguria

17. **Regarding Amphotericin B nephrotoxicity:**
    a. Volume expansion with intravenous sodium chloride may ameliorate the decline in GFR
    b. Proximal tubular dysfunction is prominent in amphotericin induced nephrotoxicity
    c. Amphotericin B with fat emulsion has been conclusively shown to be less nephrotoxic than amphotericin deoxycholate
    d. Intravenous administration of the total daily dose of Amphotericin B given as a continuous infusion over 24 hours has been associated with less nephrotoxicity compared with administration over four hours
    e. Continuous infusion of amphotericin B over 24 hours is an approved method

18. **Regarding Kt/V:**
    a. Not suitable measure if high flux membrane is used

b. Pre and post dialysis urea concentration is required for calculation
c. Post dialysis urea should be measured from sample taken as soon as possible after dialysis
d. May be overestimated in malnourished patient
e. Kt/V also disregards a possible effect of total body water on patient outcomes independent of its effect on urea

19. **Regarding hypokalemia:**
    a. QT interval progressively increase as hypokalemia worsens
    b. May be caused by proximal Renal Tubular Acidosis (RTA)
    c. May be caused by barter's syndrome
    d. For every 1 mEq/L that the plasma potassium is below 4.0, there is a total body deficit of 2000–4000 meq
    e. Trimethoprim may cause hypokalemia

20. **Consider 'Insulin with glucose' therapy for hyperkalemia:**
    a. It is ineffective in patients who already have hyperglycemia
    b. Insulin acts by blocking the activity of the Na-K-ATPase pump in skeletal muscle
    c. Glucose without insulin is equally effective in patients who have hypoglycemia due to exaggerated release of endogenous insulin
    d. The effect of insulin is immediate but lasts for 10 to 20 minutes
    e. This therapy should never be repeated due to risk of rebound hyperglycemia

ANSWER

A Type Answers

Q1. Answer d

Based on rise in serum creatinine and decrease in urine output various classifications have been proposed. KDIGO is universally accepted for AKI classification.

> KDIGO: Acute kidney injury work group. KDIGO clinical practice guideline for AKI. Kidney Int. (suppl.) 2:1-138, 2012.

Q2. Answer c

STAGING CRITERIA — Using the Kidney Disease: Improving Global Outcomes (KDIGO) criteria, AKI is staged as follows:

- Stage 1–Increase in serum creatinine to 1.5 to 1.9 times baseline, or increase in serum creatinine by ≥0.3 mg/dL (≥26.5 micromol/L), or reduction in urine output to <0.5 mL/kg/hour for 6 to 12 hours.
- Stage 2 – Increase in serum creatinine to 2.0 to 2.9 times baseline, or reduction in urine output to <0.5 mL/kg/hour for ≥12 hours.
- Stage 3 – Increase in serum creatinine to 3.0 times baseline, or increase in serum creatinine to ≥4.0 mg/dL (≥353.6 micromol/L), or reduction in urine output to <0.3 mL/kg/hour for ≥24 hours, or anuria for ≥12 hours, or the initiation of renal replacement therapy, or, in patients <18 years, decrease in estimated glomerular filtration rate (eGFR) to <35 mL/min/1.73 m^2.

The KDIGO criteria differ from the RIFLE classification in that the KDIGO criteria only utilize changes in serum creatinine and urine output, not changes in GFR for staging, with the exception of children under the age of 18 years, for whom an acute decrease in eGFR to <35 mL/min/1.73 m^2 is included in the criteria for stage 3 AKI.

As with the RIFLE and Acute Kidney Injury Network (AKIN) staging systems, KDIGO suggested that patients be classified according to criteria that result in the highest (i.e. most severe) stage of injury.

> Palevsky PM. Definition and staging criteria of acute kidney injury in adults. Available from: https://www.uptodate.com/contents/definition-and-staging-criteria-of-acute-kidney-injury-in-adults?source=search_result&search=kdigo%20aki&selectedTitle=1~150 (Accessed 8 September 2017).

Q3. Answer d

IDH is defined as a decrease in systolic blood pressure by ≥20 mm Hg or a decrease in MAP by 10 mm Hg associated with symptoms that include: abdominal discomfort; yawning; sighing; nausea; vomiting; muscle cramps; restlessness; dizziness or fainting; and anxiety. It impairs patient's well-being, can induce cardiac arrhythmias, and predisposes to coronary and/or cerebral ischemic events. In addition, IDH precludes the delivery of an adequate dose of dialysis, as hypotension episodes lead to the compartment effect and result in suboptimal Kt/V_{urea}.

> KDOQI Clinical Practice Guidelines for Cardiovascular Disease in Dialysis Patients. Available at: https://www2.kidney.org/professionals/kdoqi/guidelines_cvd/intradialytic.htm (Accessed 13 September 2017).

Q4. Answer c

- Prerenal (BUN:Cr >20:1) - BUN reabsorption is increased. BUN is disproportionately elevated relative to creatinine in serum. Likely causes are dehydration or hypoperfusion.
- Normal or Postrenal (BUN:Cr-10-20:1)- Normal range/ postrenal disease. BUN reabsorption is within normal limits.
- Renal (BUN:Cr <10:1)- Renal damage causes reduced reabsorption of BUN, therefore lowering the BUN:Cr ratio.

> Eric J, et al. Diagnosis and clinical evaluation of acute kidney injury. Comprehensive Clinical Nephrology. 5th Edition 2015:827-35.

Q5. Answer b

Hyperkalemia, Metabolic acidosis and anuria are common complication of AKI, while loss of CMD on USG is suggestive of chronic kidney disease. Hypocalcemia is common among such patients and is primarily related to increases in serum phosphorus levels caused by reduced GFR. Other contributors to hypocalcemia include skeletal resistance to parathyroid hormone and decreased synthesis of $1,25(OH)_2D3$.

> Ashley J, et al. Pathophysiology and Etiology of Acute Kidney injury. Comprehensive Clinical Nephrology. 5th Edition 2015; 802-18.

Q6. Answer b

1st choice - RIJV
2nd choice - Femoral vein
3rd choice - LIJV
4th choice - Subclavian vein

> KIDGO: Acute kidney injury work group. KIDGO clinical practice guideline for AKI. Kidney Int(Suppl) 2:1-138,2012.

Q7. Answer d

ATN and RENAL trials have shown no survival benefit above 25 mL/kg/hr, so 20–25 mL/kg/hr is the optimum dose.

> Ronco C, Bellomo R, Homel P. Effect of different dose in CVVHDF an outcome of ARF, a prospective randomized trial. LANCET 2000; 350:26-30.

Q8. Answer b

In CRRT, if citrate is used for anticoagulation it can cause hypocalcemia due to chelation.

> Miet S, Andrew D. Continuous renal replacement therapy. Oxford Textbook of nephrology, 4th edition 2016: p 1982.

Q9. Answer d

Absolute indication for RRT are Encephalopathy, Pericarditis, Bleeding, Neuropathy, Myopathy and metabolic acidosis, hyperkalemia, fluid overload resistant to medical management.

Non-renal indications are:
- Toxins/drugs-small, non-protein bound agents such as toxic alcohols, lithium, salicylate, theophylline, valproate
- Na^+ 160 mmol/L
- Temperature control hyperthermia
- Other controversial indications
  - Prevention of contrast nephropathy (no evidence)
  - Sepsis—removal of cytokines by high volume hemofiltration (HVHF) remains controversial
  - Rhabdomyolysis (usually RRT is only used when renal impairment occurs)

> Ricci Z, Ronco C. Timing, dose and mode of dialysis in acute kidney injury. Curr opin crit care. 2011;17:558-61.

Q10. Answer b

CVVHD or CRRT is better tolerated in such patient as risk of dialysis disequilibrium and increased intracranial pressure is decreased.

> Davenpart A. Continuous renal replacement therapies in patient with acute neurological injury. Semin Dial. 2009;22:165-68.

Q11. Answer a

HRS type 1 is diagnosed as cause of AKI in a case of decompensated CLD after excluding other causes of AKI (Sepsis, Hypotension, Medication, CKD, and Glomerular disease). There is rapid rise in Serum Creatinine with other causes unlikely in this patient making the possibility of HRS type 1.

> Andres C, Pere G. The Patient with Hepatorenal Syndrome. In: Oxford Textbook of nephrology, 4th edition 2016: p 1433.

Q12. Answer c

Diagnosis of HRS needs exclusion of other causes of AKI. Microscopic hematuria suggest some form of Glomerular disease and needs further evaluation.

> Andres C, Pere G. The patient with hepatorenal syndrome. Oxford Textbook of nephrology, 4th edition 2016: p1433.

Q13. Answer a

CRS type 1 is acute heart failure causing AKI. It is seen commonly in Acute LVF and congestive cardiac failure (CCF) cases. Urine examination and renal imaging is used to rule out other causes of AKI.

David J. Cardiovascular disease and chronic kidney disease–overview. Oxford Textbook of nephrology, 4th edition 2016: 777-79.

Q14. Answer a

Patients with urinary calculi may report pain, infection, or hematuria. Patients with small, nonobstructing stones or those with staghorn calculi may be asymptomatic or experience moderate and easily controlled symptoms.
- Stones within ureter: Abrupt, severe, colicky pain in the flank and ipsilateral lower abdomen; radiation to testicles or vulvar area; intense nausea with or without vomiting
- Stones obstructing ureteropelvic junction: Mild to severe deep flank pain without radiation to the groin; irritative voiding symptoms (e.g. frequency, dysuria); suprapubic pain, urinary frequency/urgency, dysuria, stranguria, bowel symptoms
- Midureteral calculi: Radiate anteriorly and caudally
- Distal ureteral stones: Radiate into groin or testicle or labia majora
- Stones passed into bladder: Mostly asymptomatic; rarely, positional urinary retention
- Upper ureteral stones: Radiate to flank or lumbar areas
Unilateral renal stone is unlikely to cause oliguria, as the opposite kidney continues to produce urine.

David A et al. Nephrolithiasis and Nephrocalcinosis. Comprehensive Clinical Nephrology. 5th Edition 2015:688-700.

Q15. Answer e

Top 3 risk factors for CIN are:
- pre-existing renal disease (especially Cr >120)
- diabetes mellitus
- age >75 yrs

Dehydration is associated with increased risk of contrast induced tubular injury and contrast nephropathy due to high osmolarity in renal tubules. Routinely holding medications such as ACEIs or diuretics is not recommended. However, one should try to hold any medication that could be nephrotoxic, such as nonsteroidal anti-inflammatory drugs (NSAIDs). Hypertension is a risk factor due to already developed hypertensive nephropathy which can be assessed by serum creatinine.

Douglas S, et al. Contrast induced acute kidney injury. In Oxford Textbook of Nephrology, 4th edition 2016; p. 2084-88.

Q16. Answer b

CIN is generally reversible over time. It causes AKI with bridging hemodialysis only needed in a few cases until renal function returns to normal. Serum creatinine usually peaks between 3 and 6 days following contrast exposure and slowly decreases afterwards. The most important determinant of the peak serum creatinine and the creatinine trajectory is the baseline creatinine clearance. It has been demonstrated that the change in serum creatinine between baseline and 12 hours after the administration of the contrast media is the best predictor of CIN. The Prevention of Radiocontrast Induced Nephropathy Clinical Evaluation (PRINCE) trial demonstrated that the first 24 hours after exposure to contrast media are the most crucial in determining renal failure outcome. In 80% of patients with CIN, serum creatinine increase became apparent in the first 24 hours.

Ashley J et al. Pathophysiology and Etiology of Acute Kidney injury. Comprehensive Clinical Nephrology. 5th Edition 2015:802-18.

Q17. Answer b

The plasma volume expansion has hemodilutional effect, causing decrease in hematocrit, i.e. the physiological anemia of normal pregnancy. The GFR increases 50% with subsequent decrease in serum creatinine, urea, and uric acid values. The kidneys increase in length and volume, and physiologic hydronephrosis occurs in up to 80% of women.

Baylis C, Davison J. Renal physiology in normal pregnancy. Comprehensive clinical nephrology. Chapter 43. 5th Edition 2015:498-505.

Q18. Answer d

There in increased uric acid reabsorption with hyperuricemia in preeclampsia due to uric acid production by placenta. Several studies have shown increased risk of cardiovascular disease (CVD) and CKD in patients with a history of PE. The cause-effect relationship of this association has not been fully elucidated, but these diseases are known to share the same risk factors, probably related to endothelial dysfunction. Maternal immunologically mediated endothelial damage is possible cause of generalized vasospasm and coagulation activation.

> Martin A, Brown M. Renal complications in normal pregnancy. Comprehensive clinical. 2015:512-13.

Q19. Answer d

Enterococci most often represent contamination in healthy non pregnant woman. It is considered as a causative agent in symptomatic patients. *Escherichia coli* is the most common infecting organism in patients with uncomplicated UTI. It causes around 85% of community-acquired infections and approximately 50% of nosocomial infections. Other gram-negative microorganisms causing UTI include *Proteus*, *Klebsiella*, *Citrobacter*, *Enterobacter*, and *Pseudomonas* spp. Gram-positive pathogens, such as *Enterococcus fecalis*, *Staphylococcus saprophyticus*, and group B streptococci, can also infect the urinary tract. Anaerobic microorganisms are frequently found in suppurative infections of the genitourinary tract (e.g., periurethral abscess and Fournier gangrene).

> Hooton T. Bacterial urinary tract infection. Comprehensive clinical nephrology. 2015;632-43.

Q20. Answer c

Reduction of end point in NIDDM with the angiotensin II antagonist losartan (RENAAL) study has shown that albuminuria remains the strongest predictor of ESRD.

> Keane WF et al. Risk scores for predicting the outcome in patients without type 2 diabetes and nephropathy: the RENAL study. Jasn. 2006;1:761-67.

Q21. Answer d

EPO is available as a therapeutic agent produced by recombinant DNA technology in mammalian cell culture. It is used in treating anemia resulting from CKD and myelodysplasia, from the treatment of cancer (chemotherapy and radiation). The initial dose is approximately 50 to 100 units/kg/week. Weekly or even less frequent dosing regimens have been shown to be effective and safe, although long-term studies are lacking. It may be administered every two to four weeks with equal efficacy.

> Iain C, Kai U. Anemia in chronic Kidney disease. Comprehensive Clinical Nephrology, 5th Edition 2015:967-974.

Q22. Answer b

CKD is defined as abnormalities of kidney structure or function, present for > 3 months, with implications for health and CKD is classified based on cause, GFR category, and albuminuria category (CGA).

GFR categories (mL/min/1.73 m^2) description and range:

G1	Normal or high	>90
G2	Mildly decreased	60–89
G3a	Mild to moderately decreased	45–59
G3b	Moderate to severely decreased	30–44
G4	Severely decreased	15–29
G5	Kidney failure	<15

Persistent albuminuria categories: description and range:

A1	A2	A3
Normal to mildly increased	Moderately increased	Severely increased
<30 mg/g <3 mg/mmol	30–300 mg/g 3–30 mg/mmol	>300 mg/g >30 mg/mmol

> KDIGO 2012 Clinical Practice Guideline for the Evaluation and Management of Chronic Kidney Disease. Available at: http://www.kdigo.org/clinical_practice_guidelines/pdf/CKD/KDIGO_2012_CKD_GL.pdf (Accessed 10 September 2017).

Q23. Answer d

Brachiobasilic, Brachiocephalic and Radiocephalic are three common types of AV fistula used as hemodialysis access.

>Jan H. Vascular access for dialysis therapy. Comprehensive Clinical Nephrology. 5th Edition. 2015:1045-55.

Q24. Answer b

Calcium acetate is used orally as a phosphorus binder, to control hyperphosphatemia and hyperparathyroidism. For hyperphosphatemia treatment, calcium acetate showed better efficacy and with a higher incidence of intolerance compared with calcium carbonate. There are insufficient data to establish the comparative superiority of the two calcium-based phosphate binders on all-cause mortality and cardiovascular end-points in hemodialysis patients.

>Kevin J, Jurgen F. Bone and Mineral metabolism in chronic kidney disease. Comprehensive Clinical Nephrology, 5th Edition 2015:984-99.

Q25. Answer a

Anemia of chronic disease, like anemia in ESRD, is normocytic normochromic.

>Iain C et al. Anaemia in chronic Kidney disease. Comprehensive Clinical Nephrology, 5th Edition 2015:967-74.

Q26. Answer a

A Gadolinium contrast used in MRI is said to be associated with Nephrogenic Fibrosing Dermopathy, when used in CKD patients.

>Kazuhiro K et al. Chapter 15 Magnetic resonance Imaging, Oxford Textbook of Nephrology, 4th edition. 2016:109-16.

Q27. Answer b

The American heart association recommends nicardipine in patients with acute ischemic stroke with BP >220/120 mm Hg. It has been proven to be better than labetalol in reducing the BP in first 30 min.

>Drozda J Jr et al. ACCF/AHA/AMA-PCPI 2011.J Am Coll Cardiol. 2011;58:316-36.

Q28. Answer e

Acute kidney injury (AKI) due to acute tubular necrosis is a relatively common complication of aminoglycoside therapy, with a rise in the serum creatinine concentration of more than 0.5 to 1 mg/dL (44 to 88 micromol/L) or a 50% increase in serum creatinine concentration from baseline occurring in 10 to 20% of patients. Aminoglycosides are freely filtered across the glomerulus; almost the entire drug is then excreted, with 5 to 10% of a parenteral dose being taken up and sequestered by the proximal tubule cells (PTCs), where the aminoglycoside can achieve concentrations vastly exceeding the concurrent serum concentration. Streptomycin, which has the least affinity for the PTCs binding site, has the least nephrotoxicity.

>Decker BS, Molitoris PA. Pathogenesis and prevention of aminoglycoside nephrotoxicity and ototoxicity. Available at: http://www.uptodate.com/contents/pathogenesis-and-prevention-of-aminoglycoside-nephrotoxicity-and-ototoxicity?source=see_link (Accessed 6th August 2017).

Q29. Answer e

This is Isotonic hyponatremia - hyperlipidemia fits the answer.

Isotonic hyponatremia is a form of hyponatremia with mOsm measured between 280 and 295. It can be associated with pseudohyponatremia, or with isotonic infusion of glucose or mannitol. Certain conditions, such as extraordinarily high blood levels of lipid (hyperlipidemia/hypertriglyceridemia) or protein (hyperparaproteinemia), magnify the electrolyte exclusion effect. This interferes with the measurement of serum sodium concentration by certain methods, leading to an erroneously low *measurement* of sodium, or pseudohyponatremia. The methods affected are the flame-photometric and indirect (but not direct) ion-selective electrode assays. This is distinct from a true dilutional hyponatremia that can be caused by an osmotic shift of water from cells to the bloodstream after large infusions of mannitol or intravenous immunoglobulin.

It is associated with hyperlipidemia more frequently than with elevated protein.

>Weisberg LS. Pseudohyponatremia: a reappraisal. The American Journal of Medicine. 1989;86(3):315-8.

K Type Answers

Q1. Answer FFTTF

Most patients with CIN are nonoliguric. In CIN urinary sediments may show classic findings of acute tubular necrosis (ATN), including muddy brown granular and epithelial cell casts and free renal tubular epithelial cells. However, the absence of these urinary findings does not exclude the diagnosis. The best data related to the pathogenesis of CIN are from animal models which show evidence of ATN. The fractional sodium excretion (FENa) is often <1% in patients with CIN in contrast to that in patients who develop AKI due to ischemic or toxin-induced ATN, when it is usually >1%. Creatinine generally increases within 24 to 48 hours after contrast exposure and usually starts to decline within three to seven days.

Schwab SJ, Hlatky MA, Pieper KS, et al. Contrast nephrotoxicity: a randomized controlled trial of a non-ionic and an ionic radiographic contrast agent. N Engl J Med. 1989;320:149.

Q2. Answer TTFFF

Reported risk of CIN In high risk patients following coronary angiography with or without intervention is 10 to 30%. Interventional rather than diagnostic coronary angiography is associated with higher risk of CIN. In patients who have no risk factors (particularly no CKD), the risk of CIN include all patients with estimated glomerular filtration rate <60 mL/min/1.73 m^2 with significant proteinuria (defined as albuminuria >300 mg/day) or co morbidities including diabetes, heart failure, liver failure, or multiple myeloma. Iodixanol is the only available non ionic iso-osmolal agent.

Iohexol a low osmolal agent carries higher risk of CIN than other non-iohexol low osmolal agents. American College of Cardiology/American Heart Association (ACC/AHA) guidelines suggest the use of either an iso-osmolal contrast agent or a low-molecular-weight contrast agent other than iohexol or the ionic low-osmolal agent, ioxaglate. The 2012 KDIGO guidelines recommended low-osmolal or iso-osmolal rather than high-osmolal contrast agents.

Aspelin P, Aubry P, Fransson SG et al. Nephrotoxic effects in high-risk patients undergoing angiography. N Engl J Med. 2003; 348:491.

Q3. Answer FTFTF

A 2012 meta-analysis that included eight studies of hemodialysis and three studies of hemofiltration/hemodiafiltration showed no benefit of post contrast exposure renal replacement therapy (RRT). There are no studies that support immediate dialysis after intravascular contrast media administration in order to preserve residual renal function or limit the risk of allergic reaction in hemodialysis patients. 2012 KDIGO guidelines suggest administration of acetylcystiene to prevent contrast nephropathy. Despite an absence of adequately designed randomized trials demonstrating benefit. Intravenous volume administration prior to intravascular contrast administration for patients at risk for contrast-induced nephropathy is the standard of care. In most cases of CIN creatinine usually starts to decline within three to seven days, and the patient returns to, or close to, baseline renal function. The 2012 KDIGO guideline work group did not make a specific recommendation for the use of bicarbonate preferentially to saline.

Cruz DN, Goh CY, Marenzi G, et al. Renal replacement therapies for prevention of radiocontrast-induced nephropathy: a systematic review. Am J Med. 2012;125:66.

Q4. Answer FTTTT

The KDIGO guidelines define AKI as follows:
- Increase in serum creatinine by ≥0.3 mg/dL (≥26.5 micromol/L) within 48 hours, or
- Increase in serum creatinine to ≥1.5 times baseline, which is known or presumed to have occurred within the prior seven days, or
- Urine volume <0.5 mL/kg/hour for six hours

The KDIGO criteria allow for correction of volume status and obstructive causes of AKI prior to classification.

KDIGO Clinical Practice Guideline for Acute Kidney Injury. Kidney Int. (Suppl) 2012;2:8.

Renal

Q5. Answer TFTTT

Measurement of urinary angiotensinogen may allow the prediction of severe AKI and other adverse outcomes. In ATN usually BUN/serum creatinine ratio is 10 to 15:1 in ATN (measured in mg/dL). In prerenal disease BUN/Cr ratio is often greater than 20:1. Urine osmolality above 500 mosmol/kg is highly suggestive of prerenal disease. NGAL may potentially be useful in differentiating prerenal disease from ATN.

Miller TR, Anderson RJ, Linas SL et al. Urinary diagnostic indices in acute renal failure: a prospective study. Ann Intern Med. 1978; 89:47.

Q6. Answer TFTTF

The HRS is one of many potential causes of AKI in patients with acute or chronic liver disease. Affected patients usually have portal hypertension due to cirrhosis, severe alcoholic hepatitis, or (less often) metastatic tumors, but can also have fulminant hepatic failure from any cause. Although hepatorenal syndrome can be seen in most forms of severe hepatic disease, patients with primary biliary cholangitis appear relatively protected. The decline in renal perfusion in this setting is associated with reductions in glomerular filtration rate (GFR) and sodium excretion (often to less than 10 meq/day in advanced cirrhosis). The urine sediment may show granular casts due to hyperbilirubinemia.

Ginès P, Schrier RW. Renal failure in cirrhosis. N Engl J Med. 2009;361:1279.

Q7. Answer FTFTF

Type 1 HRS is defined as at least a twofold increase in serum creatinine to a level greater than 2.5 mg/dL (221 micromol/L) during a period of less than two weeks. Also in the absence of other apparent causes of renal disease also there should be lack of improvement in renal function after volume expansion with intravenous albumin (1 g/kg of body weight per day up to 100 g/day) for at least two days and withdrawal of diuretics. A meta-analysis of four open-label trials including 154 patients with type 1 HRS revealed similar efficacy of terlipressin and norepinephrine but significantly more adverse events (mostly abdominal pain, chest pain, or arrhythmia) with terlipressin (28 versus 8%). Moreover Terlipressin therapy is more costly than norepinephrine therapy. A meta-analysis of four controlled trials found that Albumin infusion was associated with a significant decrease in the incidence of renal impairment (8 versus 31%) and a significant reduction in mortality (16 versus 35%) in patients with SBP.

Arroyo V, Ginès P, Gerbes AL, et al. Definition and diagnostic criteria of refractory ascites and hepatorenal syndrome in cirrhosis. International Ascites Club Hepatology. 1996;23:164.

Q8. Answer TTTTT

Pink urine may be seen in propofol infusion presumably due to uric acid crystals. White urine may be caused by pyuria, phosphate crystals, chyluria etc. Propofol can cause green or pink color of urine. Black urine may be due to hemoglobinuria, myoglobulinuria or ochronosis.

Atalla CS, Palka J. 11 Causes of Discolored Urine. Available at: http://reference.medscape.com/slideshow/discolored-urine-6008332 (Accessed 11 September 2017).

Q9. Answer TTTTF

False negative test for leukocyte esterase may be seen in concentrated urine due to impairment of cell lyses. Nitrite-positive urine indicates underlying bacteriuria. The most common cause of UTI enterobacteriaceae species produce the enzyme nitrate reductase, which converts urinary nitrate to nitrite. Enterococcus however express low levels of nitrate reductase and therefore nitrite may be negative in urine despite enterococcal infection. Nitrite may also be negative if urine dwell time in the bladder is short. The dipstick cannot detect nephrotoxic immunoglobulin light chains. Sulfosalicylic acid (SSA) detects all proteins in urine. A positive SSA test in conjunction with a negative dipstick usually indicates the presence of non-albumin proteins in the urine, most often immunoglobulin light chains. Granular casts represent degenerated cellular casts or the aggregation of proteins within a cast matrix.

Graff L. A Handbook of Routine Urinalysis. Lippincott, Williams and Wilkins, Philadelphia 1983.

Q10. Answer FTFFF

Recommendations of international consensus meeting for diagnosis of diabetes published in 2014:
Symptoms of diabetes plus random plasma glucose ≥200 mg/dL (11.1 mmol/L).

Fasting plasma glucose ≥126 mg/dL (7.0 mmol/L). Fasting is defined as no caloric intake for at least eight hours. Abnormal fasting blood glucose should be confirmed on another day.

Two-hour plasma glucose ≥200 mg/dL (11.1 mmol/L) during an oral glucose tolerance test (OGTT). The test should be performed using a glucose load containing the equivalent of 75 g anhydrous glucose dissolved in water. Up to one-third of non diabetic kidney transplant recipients develop persistently impaired glucose metabolism by six months post transplantation. Azathioprine and MMF do not have independent diabetogenic effects. A stepwise approach is recommended for treatment of NODAT, starting with nonpharmacologic therapy, including diet, weight reduction, and exercise; followed by oral monotherapy; oral combination therapy; and finally insulin, providing metabolic decompensation has not occurred (which would require earlier insulin initiation). The thiazolinediones may worsen immunosuppression-associated bone loss and are commonly associated with formation of edema, which may necessitate the use of diuretics and may predispose to calcineurin toxicity.

Sharif A, Hecking M, de Vries AP, et al. Proceedings from an international consensus meeting on posttransplantation diabetes mellitus: recommendations and future directions. Am J Transplant. 2014;14:1992.

Q11. Answer FTTFF

Furosemide, bumetanide, torsemide, and ethacrynic acid are loop diuretics.

They act in the medullary and cortical aspects of the thick ascending limb, including the macula densa cells in the early distal tubule. Furosemide, bumetanide, and torsemide, which are sulfonamides, can cause hypersensitivity reactions, usually manifested as a rash or rarely acute interstitial nephritis, similar to those produced by other sulfonamide drugs, however, there is minimal evidence of allergic cross reactivity between sulfonamide antimicrobials and non-antimicrobials.

Brater DC. Mechanism of action of diuretics. Available at: http://www.uptodate.com/contents/mechanism-of-action-of-diuretics?source=search_result&search=loop+diuretics&selectedTitle=2 (Accessd 12 September 2017).

Q12. Answer TTTFT

Q13. Answer TTTTF

Accepted urgent indications for RRT in patients with AKI generally include:
- Refractory fluid overload
- Severe hyperkalemia (plasma potassium concentration >6.5 mEq/L) or rapidly rising potassium levels
- Signs of uremia, such as pericarditis, encephalopathy, or an otherwise unexplained decline in mental status
- Severe metabolic acidosis (pH <7.1)
- Certain alcohol and drug intoxications

Palevsky PM. Renal replacement therapy (dialysis) in acute kidney injury in adults: Indications, timing, and dialysis. Available at: http://www.uptodate.com/contents/renal-replacement-therapy-dialysis-in-acute-kidney-injury-in-adults-indications-timing-and-dialysis-dose?source= search_result&search=indications+for+dialysis&selectedTitle=2%7E150 (Accessed 12 September 2017).

Q14. Answer FFFTT

The thiazide diuretics primarily inhibit sodium transport by action on neutral Na-Cl cotransport in the distal tubule. Distal tubule reabsorb a smaller proportion of the filtered load than the loop of Henle; as a result, the thiazide-type diuretics have a smaller natriuretic effect than loop diuretics and, when given in maximum dose, inhibit the reabsorption of at most 3 to 5% of filtered sodium. Thiazides increase the reabsorption of calcium.

Brater DC. Mechanism of action of diuretics. Available at: http://www.uptodate.com/contents/mechanism-of-action-of-diuretics?source=search_result&search=loop+diuretics&selectedTitle=2 (Accessed 12 September 2017).

Q15. Answer FTFTF

In critically ill patients with renal insufficiency, the initial loading dose (~25 mg/kg) should not be reduced but subsequent dosage adjustments should be made based on renal function and trough serum concentrations.

For patient on vancomycin and intermittent dialysis 5–10 mg/kg should be given after each session in general. For oral Vancomycin no dosage adjustment is required due to low systemic absorption.

Vancomycin initial dosage regimens for patients with impaired renal function (Golightly 2013)

eGFR (mL/minute per 1.73 m^2)	Actual body beight			
	<60 kg	60 to 80 kg	81 to 100 kg	>100 kg
>90	750 mg every 8 hours	1,000 mg every 8 hours	1,250 mg every 8 hours	1,500 mg every 8 hours
50 to 90	750 mg every 12 hours	1,000 mg every 12 hours	1,250 mg every 12 hours	1,000 mg every 8 hours
15 to 49	750 mg every 24 hours	1,000 mg every 24 hours	1,250 mg every 24 hours	1,500 mg every 24 hours
<15[a]	750 mg	1,000 mg	1,250 mg	1,500 mg

[a]Check a random vancomycin level in 24 hours after the dose. If random level is ≤20 mcg/mL, repeat the dose. If random level is >20 mcg/mL, do not re-dose; repeat random level in 12 hours.

Vancomycin: Drug information. Available at: http://www.uptodate.com/contents/vancomycin-drug-information?source=search_result&search=vancomycin&selectedTitle=1%7E150 (Accessed 13 September 2017).

Q16. Answer TFTFF

AKI from aminoglycoside exposure typically manifests after five to seven days of therapy. Hypomagnesemia, hypokalemia, hypocalcemia, and hypophosphatemia are infrequent in AKI due to aminoglycosides.

AKI from aminoglycoside exposure typically is nonoliguric. Aminoglycosides accumulate in the proximal tubule. Pharmacokinetically monitoring aminoglycoside therapy and utilizing a once-daily dosing regimen in selected patients have also demonstrated benefit.

Decker BS, Pharm D, Molitoris BA. Manifestations of and risk factors for aminoglycoside nephrotoxicity. Available at: http://www.uptodate.com/contents/manifestations-of-and-risk-factors-for-aminoglycoside-nephrotoxicity?source=see_link (Acessed 12 September 2017).

Q17. Answer TFFTF

Studies in both humans and animals have shown that saline administration can protect against or ameliorate the amphotericin B-induced decline in GFR.

Amphotericin B nephrotoxicity increases the permeability of the macula densa cells. This may inappropriately activate the tubuloglomerular feedback system and lead to excessive afferent arteriolar vasoconstriction and a fall in GFR. The available lipid-based formulations are amphotericin B lipid complex, amphotericin B cholesteryl sulfate complex and liposomal amphotericin B.

It has been suggested that mixing amphotericin B deoxycholate with fat emulsions may reduce renal dysfunction and infusion-related reactions. However, incomplete and conflicting data exist regarding the safety, efficacy, and stability of these mixtures.

Sterns RH. Amphotericin B nephrotoxicity. Available at: http://www.uptodate.com/contents/amphotericin-b-nephrotoxicity?source=search_result&search=amphotericin+nephrotoxicity&selectedTitle=1%7E150 (Accessed 12 September 2017).

Q18. Answer TTFTT

Kt/V was developed in an era when dialysis utilized small-pore cellulosic dialyzers. Kt/V tends to overestimate delivered dialysis among small-sized or malnourished patients. To achieve the most accurate measure of the Kt/V (referred to as the equilibrated or double-pool Kt/V), it is necessary to use an equilibrated BUN measured from a sample obtained 30 minutes after dialysis has ended

$$Kt/V = -\ln(R - 0.03) + [(4 - 3.5R) \times (UF \div W)]$$

where UF is the ultrafiltration volume in liters, W is the post dialysis weight in kg, and R is the ratio of the post-dialysis to pre-dialysis blood urea nitrogen (BUN).

Qunibi WY, Henrich WL, Prescribing and assessing adequate hemodialysis. Available at: http://www.uptodate.com/contents/prescribing-and-assessing-adequate-hemodialysis?source=search_result&search=kt+v&selectedTitle=1%7E51 (Accessed 12 September 2017).

Q19. Answer FTTFF

QT interval does not increase progressively as hypokalemia worsens. May be caused by proximal RTA due to increased delivery of Na to distal tubule where it is exchanged with K. May be caused by barters syndrome which mimics loop diuretics. For every 1mEq/L that the plasma potassium is below 4.0, there is a total body deficit of 200-400 and not 2000–4000 meq. Trimethoprim may cause hyperkalemia by inducing aldosterone resistance by blocking sodium channel in principal cells.

James NW, Qu Z, Shivkumar K. Electrophysiology of Hypokalemia and Hyperkalemia. Circulation: Arrhythmia and Electrophysiology. 2017; 10:e004667.

Q20. Answer FFFFF

Insulin administration lowers the serum potassium concentration by driving potassium into the cells, primarily by enhancing the activity of the Na-K-ATPase pump in skeletal muscle. Glucose is usually given with insulin to prevent the development of hypoglycemia. However, insulin should be given alone if the serum glucose is ≥250 mg/dL (13.9 mmol/L). Glucose without insulin should not be given since the endogenous insulin secretions cannot be reliable. The effect of insulin begins in 10 to 20 minutes, peaks at 30 to 60 minutes, and lasts for four to six hours. Removal of excess potassium from the body (e.g. with hemodialysis or a gastrointestinal cation exchanger) is sometimes not feasible or may be delayed. Such patients can be treated with either a continuous infusion of insulin or glucose or bolus infusions of insulin with glucose, repeated every two to four hours, with serial monitoring of blood glucose levels.

Mount DB. Treatment and prevention of hyperkalemia in adults. Available at: https://www.uptodate.com/contents/treatment-and-prevention-of-hyperkalemia-in-adults?source=search_result&search=hyperkalemia%20treatment&selectedTitle=1~150 (Accessed 12 September 2017).

CHAPTER 7

Urology, Obstetrics and Gynecology

Mukta Seth

A Type Questions
(One best answer)

1. A 20-year-old primigravida was hospitalized at 37 weeks with regular contractions. She had irregular antenatal visits, which revealed raised blood pressure (BP) between 150/100 and 160/110 mm Hg on admission. Laboratory findings were unremarkable (hemoglobin 12 mg/dL, hematocrit: 37.2%, platelets: 122000/mm^3, glucose: 70 mg/dL, creatinine: 0.58, ALT: 31 U/L, AST: 35 U/L, LDH: 519 U/L), with a trace of proteinuria in the urinalysis. 4 hr after delivery, she developed generalized convulsions.

   One of the following is not a diagnostic feature of eclampsia:
   a. Systolic blood pressure ≥140 mm Hg or diastolic blood pressure ≥90 mm Hg on two occasions at least four hours apart after 20 weeks of gestation
   b. Proteinuria ≥0.3 g in a 24-hour urine specimen
   c. Protein/creatinine ratio ≥0.3
   d. Cerebral edema on Computed Tomography (CT)
   e. Seizures occur anytime before childbirth or during labor in most cases

2. A 30-year-old female, para 3+1, in 36 weeks of pregnancy presented to the Emergency department with a two day history of intermittent fever, night sweats, lower abdominal pain and foul vaginal discharge. Her investigations showed Total Leukocyte Count 16000/cm^2, Procalcitonin 16 mcg/mL and CRP of 80 mg/dL. She was shifted to the ICU in view of falling blood pressure.

   All of the following are acceptable while managing sepsis in pregnancy and puerperal stage *except*:
   a. Inferior Vena Cava (IVC) changes to guide fluid resuscitation can be applied as standard since there are minimal effects of gravid uterus upon it
   b. Surviving Sepsis guideline continues to serve as a cornerstone for the diagnosis and management of maternal sepsis also
   c. Norepinephrine is typically the initial choice of a vasoactive agent
   d. Avoid aortocaval compression after 20 weeks of gestation by maintaining a lateral maternal tilt
   e. Initial volume resuscitation can be applied to restore blood pressure as in nonpregnant state

3. A 28-year-old pregnant woman with a 16-week gestational age fetus was involved in a road car crash resulting in multiple traumas. She was immediately rushed to nearby hospital and required intubation and mechanical ventilation.

   One of the following is FALSE regarding trauma in pregnancy:
   a. Direct trauma to fetus is the most common cause of fetal death
   b. Tranexamic acid, an anti-fibrinolytic agent may be used in pregnancy

c. Focused assessment with sonography for trauma (FAST) is insensitive to detect placental disruption
d. Before 13 weeks of gestation, the uterus is protected by the bony pelvis
e. Kleihauer-Betke test is used to detect Fetal-maternal hemorrhage

4. A 32-year-old nulliparous woman at 40 weeks' of gestation with no known respiratory or heart disease was admitted to the emergency department with complaints of vaginal bleeding and pain. She was accepted in early active labour. ABG analysis showed severe hypoxemia. The chest X-ray showed bilateral perihilar pulmonary edema. ECG revealed only a sinus tachycardia. Endotracheal intubation was immediately performed and was transferred to the ICU. Recorded central venous pressure was 8 mm Hg. Laboratory values revealed mild coagulopathy. Cardiotocography revealed signs of fetal distress and ultrasound showed oligohydramnios of the fetus. Resuscitative measures were undertaken, including fluid resuscitation, inotropic support and volume expansion. Caesarean section was performed immediately but the baby died. Maternal bradycardia and asystole developed and cardiopulmonary resuscitation (CPR) was performed. The patient was declared dead 40 minutes after the onset of resuscitative efforts.

    The most likely diagnosis is:
    a. Acute pulmonary embolism
    b. Amniotic fluid embolism
    c. Acute heart failure
    d. Acute severe asthma
    e. Venous air embolism

5. A 34 years old lady was referred to ICU from a peripheral hospital. She had been admitted there for cough and dyspnea the second week after the delivery of her third child. She also complained of dyspnea and hypertension but declined treatment for hypertension and the dyspnea symptoms were not investigated further. The chest X-ray on admission showed acute pulmonary edema with bilateral pleural effusion and she was commenced on decongestive measures and antibiotics. Echocardiography showed the presence of a severely impaired left ventricular systolic function with EF of 30%, fractional shortening of 11% along with severe mitral regurgitation and moderate tricuspid regurgitation. One of the following is false about Peripartum Cardiomyopathy (PPCM):
    a. Most of the patients recover completely by the end of six months to one year and there is no impact on subsequent pregnancies
    b. Medical therapy is similar to those in patients with acute and chronic systolic HF due to other causes
    c. Generally identified as the development of heart failure during the last month of pregnancy or within 5 months after delivery
    d. PPCM is a diagnosis of exclusion and the time frame and echocardiographic cut-offs are arbitrary
    e. Considered an idiopathic cardiomyopathy without any correlation to coronary artery disease

6. A 33-year-old primiparous woman was admitted to hospital with 33-week pregnancy with swelling, redness and pains in the lower limbs. Homans' sign (pain on passive dorsiflexion of the foot) was positive. Her hemoglobin-9 g%, platelet count-1.5 Lac/cmm, prothrombin time-5.06 (0.8-1.2), partial thromboplastin time ratio-2.21 (0.8-1.2), fibrinogen-866 mg/dL (200-400), ATIII-81 (80-120), D-dimer-.3376 ug/L (0-550).

    Which of the following is most appropriate initially to rule out Deep Vein Thrombosis (DVT) in pregnancy?
    a. D-dimer
    b. Compression duplex ultrasonography
    c. CT pulmonary angiography (CTPA)
    d. V/Q Scan
    e. Echocardiography

7. A 37-year-old pregnant woman at 36 weeks of gestation was admitted to a local hospital with a history of 4 days of fever, sore throat, headache, cough, nausea, vomiting, weakness, and myalgias. On examination, she had tachycardia (128 beats/min), tachypnea (respiratory rate, 42 breaths/min). A diagnosis of ARDS related to suspected severe lower respiratory tract infection was made and she required intubation and mechanical ventilation.

The following is false regarding mechanical ventilation in pregnancy:
a. Maternal PaO$_2$ should be targeted higher (minimum up to 70 mm Hg) than corresponding nonpregnant state
b. Low Tidal Volume ventilation is safe in pregnancy
c. Indication of delivery is signs of fetal hypoxia such as bradycardia, lack of heart rate variability etc.
d. Propofol is the most appropriate sedative during pregnancy since it does not cross the placenta
e. Permissive hypercapnia with PaCO$_2$ of 60 has no adverse effects on fetus but higher levels of CO$_2$ should be avoided

8. A 37 years old woman G1 P0 was diagnosed with a community acquired pneumonia and admitted to the ICU with ARDS. CXR showed bilateral perihilar loss of airspace with air bronchograms and upper lobe diversion. P/F ratio was 60.

   One of the following is false in pregnancy:
   a. Type I respiratory failure are more common in pregnancy as compared to Type II
   b. Pregnancy has worse Mallampati score of airway
   c. Prone position is contraindicated in pregnancy due to already reduced functional residual capacity
   d. Lung protective ventilation and PEEP can be applied similarly as in non pregnant
   e. No mode of ventilation has conclusively been shown to be superior

9. Regarding Venous Thromboembolic (VTE) Disease in Pregnancy, all are true except:
   a. All pregnant women with signs and symptoms suggestive of VTE should have objective testing performed
   b. Treatment with Low Molecular Weight Heparin (LMWH) or Unfractionated Heparin (UFH) is not recommended until the diagnosis is confirmed by objective testing
   c. Magnetic resonance direct thrombus imaging has a high sensitivity and specificity for the diagnosis of iliac-vein thrombosis
   d. Compression ultrasonography is a noninvasive test with high sensitivity and specificity
   e. There is a striking predisposition for DVT to occur in the left leg

10. A 30-year-lady with 36 week of pregnancy develops gradual progressive dyspnea and persistent cough while on treatment for premature uterine contractions. She was not having any significant previous history. On examination she was alert, dyspneic with RR of 32/min, pulse rate of 120/min, blood pressure of 96/60 mm Hg, and basal crepitations on auscultation. 2D Echo revealed LV ejection fraction of 35%, there was no chamber dilation or hypertrophy. Serum BNP was 300 pg/mL. Chest radiograph revealed bilateral symmetrical alveolar opacities. 12 lead ECG shows sinus tachycardia.

    Labs shows Hb 13.0 g/dL, TLC 6.4 × 10 9, Platelet count was 200 × 10/uL

    Which of the following about above condition is true?
    a. ACE inhibitors are recommended for LV dysfunction in pregnancy
    b. The selective sinus node inhibitor Ivabradine reduces the risk of hospital admission and death
    c. Thiazide is generally preferred over loop diuretics and potassium-sparing diuretics
    d. The combination of Hydralazine plus Nitrate (isosorbide dinitrate) is the vasodilator therapy of choice
    e. Beta-adrenergic blocking agents are important components of the treatment regimen

11. A 68-year-old man with end stage renal disease due to diabetic nephropathy underwent a kidney transplant.

    He was previously healthy and in preoperative tests, his hemoglobin level was 12.7 g/dL, packed cell volume was 41%, platelet count was 76,100/mm^3, leukocyte count was 14,400/mm^3, urea level was 57 mg/dL, serum creatinine level was 5.5 mg/dL, and potassium level was 4.8 mmol/L.

    Cyclosporine and Tacrolimus which are commonly used in such patients may cause one of the following electrolyte disorders:
    a. Hypokalemia and Hypermagnesemia
    b. Hyponatremia and Hypokalemia
    c. Hypercalcemia and Hypermagnesemia
    d. Hyperkalemia and Hypomagnesemia
    e. Hypokalemia and Hypermagnesemia

12. A 30-year-old, 56 kg male patient with a history of focal segmental glomerulosclerosis received an ABO-incompatible renal transplantation from his father.

    Oral tacrolimus administration was started 4 days before the operation at an initial dose of 0.15 mg/kg. On postoperative day 5 there was a report of Candida albicans in the ET secretions. The Intensivist thinks Fluconazole to be the best antifungal in this situation.

    One of the following is most appropriate consideration:
    a. Fluconazole can be used as the initial therapy it being C. albicans
    b. Intravenous Posaconazole is more effective against C. albicans than Fluconazole
    c. Liposomal amphotericin B is the safest therapy since nephrotoxicity is minimal on the grafted kidney
    d. Anidulafungin can be given to post transplant patient in view of its minimal interaction with tacrolimus
    e. Candida species being inherently resistant to Voriconazole makes it the worst choice

13. A 23-year-old primigravida, previously healthy with 36 weeks period of gestation was referred from a nursing home with complaints of yellow discoloration of urine and eyes, malaise, anorexia and vomiting since 3–4 days. She had no complaints of pain abdomen, leaking or bleeding per vaginum or decreased fetal movement. On examination she was drowsy, but easily arousable. She was well-hydrated and afebrile. Her blood pressure was 118/70 mm Hg and pulse rate was 74 per min. She had icterus and mild pedal edema. Her cardiovascular and respiratory systems were normal on examination. Investigations revealed hemoglobin of 12.4 g/dL, leucocyte count of 17,700/mm^3 and platelet count 1.7 Lac/cm^2. Her liver function test showed a serum bilirubin of 12.8 mg/dL, alanine aminotransferase 332 IU/L, aspartate aminotransferase 210 IU/L, alkaline phosphatase 150 U/L, total proteins 5.6 g/dL, and albumin 2.4 g/dL. Kidney function tests revealed blood urea 40 mg/dL, serum creatinine 1.7 mg/dL, random blood sugar 67 mg/dL. The coagulation profile showed prothrombin time 52 seconds (12), a partial thromboplastin time >1 min (30) with INR 5.7. Viral markers were negative. Blood gas analysis revealed metabolic acidosis. Ultrasound abdomen showed normal liver and other organs.

    Most likely diagnosis is:
    a. Cholestasis of pregnancy
    b. Viral hepatitis
    c. HELLP syndrome
    d. Acute fatty liver of pregnancy
    e. Severe eclampsia

14. Which of the following drugs commonly used in ICU in pregnant patient does not belong to either category A or B?
    a. Cephalosporins
    b. Macrolides
    c. Acyclovir
    d. Midazolam
    e. Propofol

15. A 56-year ASA I male patient weighing 60 kgs underwent transurethral resection of prostrate (TURP). Patient had no history of any coexisting disease or medications. Preoperative S. Sodium was 142 meq/L, S. Potassium was 3.8 mmol/L, Urea 40 mg%, Creatinine 1.8 mg%. On operating table vitals noted were a Heart Rate of 90 per min, Blood Pressure of 140/90 mm Hg, a normal ECG and SpO$_2$ of 98% with room air. Irrigation fluid used was 1.5% Glycine and resection was done using monopolar instrument. Just as the operation was about to end, patient became increasingly restless, agitated with complaint of nausea vomiting and respiratory distress.

    Pathophysiologically one of the following may be responsible for this condition:
    a. Hyperbilirubinemia
    b. Hyperglycemia
    c. Hypoglycemia
    d. Hyperuricemia
    e. Hyperammonia

16. One of the following is correct about Asthma in pregnancy:
    a. More than 90% of cases improve during pregnancy
    b. Hyperventilation to bring down PaCO$_2$ to less than 28 mm Hg improves uterine flow
    c. MgSO$_4$ can be given during pregnancy
    d. Asthma generally does not affect birth weight

e. Inhaled corticosteroids and short-acting b-agonists are seriously teratogenic

17. **Laboratory criteria for HELLP syndrome include all *except*:**
    a. Haptoglobin concentration (≤25 mg/dL) and schistocytes on blood smear
    b. Total bilirubin ≥1.2 mg/dL (20.52 micromol/L)
    c. Platelet count ≤150,000 cells/microl
    d. Serum AST >2 times upper limit of normal for local laboratory.
    e. All of above

18. **Regarding Management of HELLP syndrome all of following are correct *except*:**
    a. Initial management is to stabilize the mother, assess the fetal condition, and decide whether prompt delivery is indicated.
    b. Severe hypertension is treated with antihypertensive therapy and magnesium sulfate is given to prevent convulsions
    c. For pregnancies ≥23 and <34 weeks of gestation, delivery after a course of corticosteroids should be considered to accelerate fetal pulmonary maturity
    d. Dexamethasone is recommended for treatment of HELLP syndrome
    e. Severe complications of HELLP syndrome are indication for prompt delivery regardless of gestational age

19. **Which of the following sentence regarding physiological adaptation of pregnancy in systemic coagulation is correct?**
    a. Increase in protein C and protein S
    b. Increase in platelet counts
    c. Factors I, II, V, VII, VIII, X, and XII decreases
    d. Activity of the fibrinolytic inhibitors PAI-1 and PAI-2 decreases
    e. There is reduction of Prothrombin Time (PT) and the Activated Partial Thromboplastin Time (APTT)

20. **Which of the following types of Shock can be found on initial presentation of Amniotic Fluid Embolism (AFE)?**
    a. Only cardiogenic shock
    b. Cardiogenic and distributive shock
    c. Cardiogenic and hypovolemic shock
    d. Distributive shock and hypovolemic shock
    e. Cardiogenic, distributive and hypovolemic shock

K Type Questions
[Marked True (T)/False (F)]

1. **A 32-year-old nulliparous woman at 40 weeks' of gestation was admitted to the emergency service with complaints of vaginal bleeding and pain. She had no known respiratory or heart disease. Her condition rapidly deteriorated despite treatment and she died within half an hour of onset of labor. Amniotic fluid embolism (AFE) is strongly suspected as underlying cause.**
    a. There is no one specific test that can confirm the diagnosis of this syndrome.
    b. The finding of squamous cells in the maternal pulmonary circulation on autopsy is neither specific nor sensitive for the diagnosis of AFE.
    c. Hypoxia refractory to oxygen and loss of consciousness requires intubation and mechanical ventilation.
    d. AFE may be prevented by early use of tocolytic agents
    e. Coagulation parameters are mostly preserved

2. **Regarding Venous Thromboembolism (VTE) in Pregnancy**
    a. The incidence of VTE is twice in pregnancy as compare to nonpregnant state
    b. In developed countries pulmonary embolus (PE) is the leading cause of maternal death
    c. Approximately 30% of apparently isolated episodes of PE are associated with silent DVT
    d. Two thirds of cases of DVT occur in the puerperium period
    e. Almost half of pregnancy-related PE occurs in the puerperium

3. **Regarding CT pulmonary Angiogram (CTPA) and Ventilation–perfusion (V/Q) scan in diagnosis of VTE in Pregnancy:**
    a. CTPA delivers significantly higher fetal dose of radiation than V/Q scan
    b. V/Q scan carries a higher risk of childhood cancer
    c. The radiation dose delivered to mothers is higher with V/Q scan than CTPA
    d. V/Q scan carries a higher risk of maternal breast cancer
    e. Perfusion scanning alone may reduce the radiation exposure

4. **Regarding patient receiving prophylactic or therapeutic heparin and neuraxial block (Spinal/Epidural Anesthesia):**
   a. Spinal anesthesia may be performed 12 hours after administration of the last dose of prophylactic LMWH
   b. Intravenous unfractionated heparin (UFH) should be stopped at least 24 hours before placement of a neuraxial blockade, and a normal aPTT should be confirmed
   c. The initiation of prophylactic LMWH should be delayed for at least 12 hours after the removal of an epidural catheter
   d. After neuraxial anesthesia, therapeutic LMWH can be administered after 12 hours postoperatively or post partum.
   e. Treatment with LMWH may be resumed within 12 hours after delivery in the absence of persistent bleeding

5. **A 26-year-lady in first trimester comes to triage with history of one episode of seizures. Her antenatal period until now was uneventful. Her husband says, she was having headache for 1 day prior which was not responding to analgesics. On examination she was comatose, pupils of both sides were equal. HR 100/min, BP 180/110 mm Hg. She was intubated in triage and MRI was performed which revealed symmetrical white matter edema in the posterior cerebral hemispheres, particularly the parieto-occipital regions. Regarding her further management and prognosis:**
   a. Lowering blood pressure should be considered in all patients with above condition
   b. History of cytotoxic drug should be ruled out
   c. Seizure can be controlled with phenytoin
   d. Most patients die of secondary cerebral infarction or hemorrhage
   e. Neurological deficit is common complication

6. **Regarding VTE in Pregnancy:**
   a. The incidence of VTE is twice in pregnancy as compare to nonpregnant state
   b. In developed countries PE is the leading cause of maternal death
   c. Approximately 30% of apparently isolated episodes of PE are associated with silent DVT
   d. Two thirds of cases of deep-vein thrombosis occurred in the puerperium period
   e. Almost half of pregnancy-related PE occur in the puerperium

7. **The following is TRUE about Complicated UTI:**
   a. Organisms are introduced during collection or processing of urine
   b. Common in Immunocompromised host
   c. Multi-drug resistant bacteria is more commonly isolated
   d. Organisms are present in the urine, but are causing no illness or symptoms
   e. Anatomic or functional abnormality of urinary tract is uncommon

8. **Regarding the management of ARDS in pregnancy:**
   a. Low Tidal Volume strategy is a well studied clinical entity and can be applied in the state of pregnancy
   b. Hypercapnia is extremely harmful and all efforts must be taken to bring down $PaCO_2$ to below 30 mm Hg
   c. Higher PEEP should be avoided because it hampers placental circulation
   d. Pregnancy decreases static lung compliance leading to predisposition to Barotrauma
   e. Effect of elevation of diaphragm during pregnancy is nullified by the effect of progesterone on muscles

9. **Regarding anticoagulation therapy during pregnancy and peripartum period:**
   a. Patients with mechanical valve should be continued with oral anticoagulation during labor
   b. The incidence of Heparin Induced Thrombocytopenia (HIT) is low during pregnancy
   c. UFH is preferred during pregnancy since the LMWH has teratogenic effects
   d. Bleeding during labor is not potentiated by prophylactic doses of UFH
   e. Warfarin can be continued during breast feeding

10. **Regarding Amniotic fluid embolism (AFE) syndrome:**
    a. Also called anaphylactoid syndrome of pregnancy
    b. Incidence rate is between 1 and 12 cases per 1000 deliveries
    c. Primiparous is at more risk compared to multiparous
    d. Amniotic fluid is believed to enter the maternal circulation through the endocer-

vical veins, the placental insertion site, or a site of uterine trauma
   e. As many as half of patients develop disseminated intravascular coagulation (DIC)
11. **Regarding trauma in pregnancy:**
   a. If chest tube placement is indicated, consideration should be given to placing the tube one or two interspaces higher than normal
   b. Ultrasound is not useful initial investigations
   c. It is difficult to differentiate between placental abruption and uterine Rupture clinically
   d. Initial laboratory testing should always include Rhesus (Rh) D status of the mother
   e. Anti-D immune globulin should be given to all Rh D negative women of childbearing age following abdominal trauma
12. **A diagnosis of peripartum cardiomyopathy requires the presence of the following criteria:**
   a. Development of cardiac failure in the last month of pregnancy or within 3 months of delivery
   b. Absence of any other identifiable cause for the cardiac failure
   c. Absence of heart disease prior to last month of pregnancy
   d. Echocardiographic evidence of reduced left ventricular function
   e. All of the above
13. **Regarding Peripartum cardiomyopathy:**
   a. ACE inhibitors are contraindicated antepartum but are safe in postpartum and in breastfeeding period
   b. Anticoagulation should be considered in all patients
   c. Immunosuppressives may be beneficial in patients when standard treatment is not effective
   d. Addition of bromocriptine may improve left ventricular function
   e. Peripartum cardiomyopathy is associated with excellent prognosis
14. **Important considerations during resuscitation of obstetric patient are:**
   a. If gestation >26 weeks, use a left lateral tilt to avoid aorto-caval Compression
   b. A definitive airway should be secured as early as possible given the increased risk of aspiration
   c. Summon help immediately; call for an obstetrician, anesthesiologist and Neonatologist
   d. Prepare for perimortem Caesarean section
   e. Defibrillation and cardioversion should be avoided if possible as there is a risk of fetal arrhythmias
15. **Severe pre-eclampsia is characterized by which of the following feature?**
   a. Systolic blood pressure >160 mm Hg or diastolic blood pressure >100 mm Hg on two occasions at least 2 hours apart
   b. Proteinuria: >300 mg in a 24 hr collection
   c. Oliguria: < 100 mL in 24 hr
   d. Visual disturbances
   e. Seizures
16. **Regarding magnesium toxicity and its management:**
   a. At plasma concentration of 3.5 to 5 mmol/L, nausea, flushing, headache, lethargy, drowsiness, and diminished deep tendon reflexes develop
   b. At plasma concentration above 5 mmol/L, the patient is at risk for muscle paralysis, respiratory paralysis, complete heart block, and cardiac arrest
   c. At plasma concentration 2 to 3.5 mmol/L, somnolence, hypocalcemia, absent deep tendon reflexes, hypotension, bradycardia, and ECG changes may occur
   d. In most cases, respiratory failure precedes cardiac collapse.
   e. Specific treatment modalities include: Administration of calcium, Aggressive fluid therapy, loop diuretics and Hemodialysis
17. **Mechanical ventilation considerations when caring for the obstetric patient Include all *except*:**
   a. Aim for a higher PaO_2 or SpO_2 than normal
   b. Maintain reduced $PaCO_2$ levels than normal gestational levels
   c. Avoid high levels of positive end-expiratory pressure in the third trimester
   d. Initiate a trial of spontaneous ventilation as early as possible
   e. Delivery may improve the mechanics of ventilation
18. **Commonly implicated organisms in obstetric sepsis include all *except*:**
   a. *E. coli*

b. Group A, (beta-hemolytic) streptococci
c. Klebsiella species
d. Staphylococcus aureus
e. Bacteroides fragilis

19. 29-year-old primigravida presents in 32 weeks of pregnancy. A diagnosis of HELLP Syndrome was considered. Investigations show, Hemoglobin 7.2 gm%, Total Leukocyte Count 13500/mm³, Platelet Count 48000/mm³, blood urea 41 mg%, serum creatinine 1 mg%, total serum bilirubin 1.8 mg%, and serum alanine aminotransferase 175 units.

Thrombocytopenia may be best managed by:
a. Platelet transfusion when platelet count is less than 20000
b. Dexamethasone is not recommended for maternal benefit
c. Hepatic infarction is common presentation in HELLP syndrome
d. Complicated HELLP syndrome by multi-organ dysfunction should be managed by prompt delivery regardless of gestational age
e. Cesarean section is the preferred mode of delivery

20. A 24-year-old woman, $G_1P_1L_0$ at 34-week gestation was admitted to the hospital with a history of absence of fetal movements, malaise, nausea, vomiting, and yellow colored urine. Ultrasonography revealed death of the 34-week fetus and a fatty liver.

Regarding Acute Fatty Liver of pregnancy (AFLP):
a. It is the most common causes of Jaundice in the first trimester of pregnancy
b. Twin and multiple pregnancy has definitely increased risk of AFLP
c. Up to 50% of the cases show Hyperglycemia requiring insulin infusion
d. Renal failure and coagulopathy are also commonly seen
e. Mild hypoglycemia (up to 60 mg/dL) if any should not be treated since rebound hyperglycemia and dehydration is known clinical entity in AFLP

ANSWER
A Type Answers

Q1. Answer d

In most eclampsia cases CT of the head is normal, but in some it reveals focal lesions, such as cerebral edema, subarachnoid hemorrhage (SAH) or intraparenchymal hemorrhage or occipital symmetric hypodensities. MRI may show reversible low-signal intensities in T1 and high-signal intensities in T2-weighted images.

Cuero MR, Varelas PN. Neurologic Complications in pregnancy. Critical Care Clinics. 2016;32:43-59.

Q2. Answer a

Bedside ultrasound may be useful to guide fluid management, with assessment of IVC size and collapse to various maneuvers, to estimate status of vascular volume and fluid responsiveness. However, use of IVC changes to guide fluid resuscitation in pregnant patients has not been well-studied, and positional effects as well as correlations with vascular volume may differ from the nonpregnant state.

Ryo E, Unno N, Nagasaka T, et al. Changes in the size of maternal inferior vena cava during pregnancy. J Perinat Med. 2004;32(4):327-31.

Q3. Answer a

Before 13 weeks of gestation, the uterus is protected by the bony pelvis. Fetal loss in the first trimester is not secondary to any direct uterine trauma but usually is due to maternal hypotension, with hypoperfusion of the uterus and its contents or the mother's death. Direct fetal injury is extremely rare following blunt trauma, complicating <1% of all significant maternal traumas. Uterine rupture following blunt trauma is also rare, occurring in 0.6% of cases of blunt trauma during pregnancy. Pelvic fractures are specific challenges because hemorrhage from the many dilated venous tributaries can cause significant retroperitoneal blood loss. Pelvic fractures are the most common trauma resulting in fetal death, at a rate as high as 25%.

Mattox KL, Goetzl L. Trauma in pregnancy. Critical Care Medicine. 2005;33(10):S385-S389.

Q4. Answer b

Amniotic fluid embolism (AFE) has dramatic presentation and high rate of mortality. There is no one specific test that can confirm this syndrome. The diagnosis of AFE is based on its clinical presentation and supportive laboratory studies. The diagnosis is therefore made by exclusion of other causes. Any condition that presents as acute cardiorespiratory collapse or massive hemorrhage in the peripartum period must be systematically evaluated. The differential diagnosis includes air or thrombotic pulmonary emboli, septic shock, aspiration pneumonia, acute myocardial infarction, placental abruption, eclampsia, complication of tocolytic therapy with β-sympathomimetics, transfusion reaction and local anesthetic toxicity.

Kahvecd O, Demdrcan A, Keles A, et al. T. Amniotic fluid embolism: A case report. Fırat Tıp Dergisi. 2010;15(1):51-3.

Q5. Answer a

Women with PPCM or history of PPCM should receive counseling regarding the risk of recurrence with subsequent pregnancies. Termination of pregnancy may not prevent relapse. Although limited data are available, patients with PPCM with persistent LV dysfunction (LVEF <50%) or LVEF ≤25% at diagnosis should be advised to avoid a subsequent pregnancy due to the risk of HF progression and death. PPCM should also be advised of the risk of recurrence.

Tsang W, Bales A, Lang R. Peripartum cardiomyopathy: Treatment and prognosis. Available from: https://www.uptodate.com/contents/peripartum-cardiomyopathy-treatment-and-prognosis?source=search_result&search=Peripartum%20Cardiomyopathy&selectedTitle=1~38 [Accessed 7th May, 2017]

Q6. Answer b

Suspected DVT is best assessed by means of compression duplex ultrasonographic examination, including examination of the iliofemoral region.

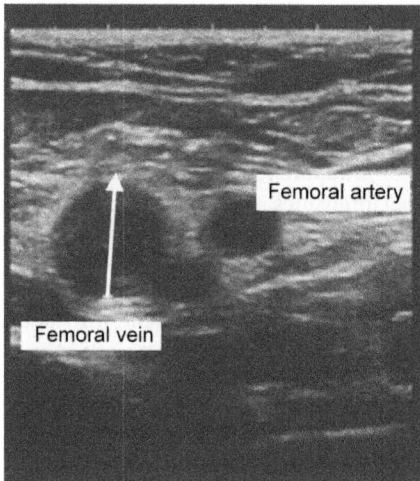

Fig. 1: Ultrasound femoral vessels

This test can safely rule out the diagnosis of deep-vein thrombosis; among women with negative findings on examination.

In a prospective cohort study involving more than 200 pregnant women with suspected DVT, serial compression duplex ultrasonography had a negative predictive value of 99.5% (95% CI, 96.9 to 100). In women with a negative result on ultrasonography in whom clinical suspicion of DVT is high, it may be prudent to repeat the test after 3 to 7 days.

Greer IA. Pregnancy complicated by venous thrombosis. N Engl J Med. 2015;373:540-7.

Q7. Answer d

Several physiologic and anatomic changes in pregnancy promote the incidence of respiratory failure. The fetus needs a maternal PaO_2 greater than 70 mm Hg for sufficient oxygenation. Ventilation should be set regarding the recommendations of the ARDS network. One basic principle is the low-tidal-volume ventilation (4–6 mL/kg predicted body weight). Delivery has small but beneficial effects on the mother. No drug is completely safe for sedation. Propofol, benzodiazepines, opioids etc. cross the placenta. Neonatologist must be aware of the sedation given. Permissive hypercapnia with $PaCO_2$ of 60 mm Hg seems to have no adverse effect on the fetus, but higher levels of CO_2 should be avoided. In delivery, a higher $PaCO_2$ in the mother is associated with a higher APGAR than a lower $PaCO_2$, but a control of maternal pH is essential (goal 7.25–7.35).

Schwaiberger D, Karcz M, Mario M. Respiratory Failure and mechanical ventilation in the pregnant patient. Crit Care Clinics. 2016;(32):85-95.

Q8. Answer c

Physiologic changes of pregnancy predispose to difficulty with mask ventilation and intubation, rapid desaturation during periods and apnea, and high airway pressures during mechanical ventilation. Hypoxic respiratory failure in the parturient can be due to a multitude of causes, both related and unrelated to pregnancy. ARDS is a common final pathway by which many of these etiologies lead to arterial hypoxemia. Treatment of hypoxic respiratory failure should focus on lung-protective ventilation with low tidal volumes and moderate levels of PEEP as well as careful fluid management. For refractory cases, neuromuscular blockade, prone positioning, and extracorporeal membrane oxygenation may be considered. Some have advocated the use of prone positioning (PP) in the most refractory cases of hypoxic respiratory failure in order to improve lung mechanics and gas exchange.

Holly E, Dirk V. Respiratory considerations including airway and ventilation issues in critical care obstetric patients. Obstet Gynecol Clinics. 2016;43:699-708.

Q9. Answer b

All pregnant women with signs and symptoms suggestive of VTE should have objective testing performed expeditiously. Treatment with LMWH or UFH is recommended until the diagnosis is ruled out by objective testing, unless treatment is strongly contraindicated. Compression ultrasonography is a noninvasive test with a sensitivity of 97% and a specificity of 94% for the diagnosis of symptomatic, proximal DVT in the general population. Magnetic resonance direct thrombus imaging, which does not involve radiation exposure and is not harmful to the fetus, has a high sensitivity and specificity for the diagnosis of iliac-vein thrombosis. There is a striking predisposition for DVT to occur in the left leg (approximately 70 to 90% of cases), possibly because of exacerbation of the compressive effects on the left iliac vein due to its being crossed by the right iliac artery.

Paul E, Lauren A. Current Concepts: Venous thromboembolic disease and Pregnancy. N Engl J Med. 2008;359:2025-33. Available from: www.nejm.org/doi/full/10.1056/NEJMra0707993 (Accessed 20th May 2017).

Q10. Answer d

Patients with new or Acute Decompensated Heart Failure (ADHF) most commonly present with progressive dyspnea or perhaps a persistent cough. Gradual onset of symptoms along with findings of 2D Echo, chest radiograph and ECG and BNP levels suggest ADHF failure secondary to use of tocolytic therapy. Important differential diagnoses include preeclampsia/eclampsia, pulmonary embolism, cardiomyopathies, valvular heart diseases, myocardial infarction, pneumonia and amniotic fluid embolism. ACE inhibitors, Angiotensin II receptor blockers (ARBs) which are part of the standard long-term therapeutic regimen in nonpregnant patients with heart failure with reduced ejection fraction, are contraindicated during pregnancy. Beta-adrenergic blocking agents, such as extended release metoprolol, carvedilol and bisoprolol are important components of the treatment regimen for patients with chronic HF due to systolic dysfunction, but should be avoided in acute heart failure. Given lack of evidence of safety ivabradine use in pregnant or nursing women should be avoided. Generally loop diuretics are preferred over thiazide diuretics and potassium-sparing diuretics in pregnancy. The combination of hydralazine plus isosorbide dinitrate is the vasodilator therapy of choice in pregnant women with HF.

Jeanne M, Roberto M, Michael R, et al. Management of heart failure during pregnancy. Uptodate 2016; Topic 3507 Version 14.0, Available from: https://www.uptodate.com/contents/management-of-heart-failure-during-pregnancy (Accessed 26th May 2017).

Q11. Answer d

Calcineurin inhibitors (CNIs) are immunosuppressive drugs, which are used widely to prevent rejection of transplanted organs and treat autoimmune disease. Cyclosporine and tacrolimus decrease potassium excretion and increase magnesium excretion in the urine, with resultant hyperkalemia and hypomagnesemia.

Singapuri MS, Subramanian RM. Renal transplant. Procedures and Complications. Available from: http://www.sccm.org/Communications/Critical-Connections/Archives/Pages/Renal-Transplant---Procedures-and-Complications.aspx (Accessed 17 July, 2017).

Q12. Answer d

Posaconazole is available as only oral formulation. All-cause mortality for invasive fungal infections is reduced by almost 30% by lipid associated formulations when compared with AmB-D. Anidulafungin is free of interactions with other drugs such as prednisone, cyclosporine tacrolimus, mofetil or sirolimus that are metabolized through the liver. Also, dosage adjustments are not required in renally impaired patients and in patients with severe liver disease. Voriconazole shows good in vitro activity against all Candida species, including certain Candida strains that are inherently fluconazole-resistant, and strains of Candida albicans that have acquired resistance to fluconazole and other yeasts, including Cryptococcus neoformans. The interaction of azoles with drugs to prevent graft rejection is significant consideration.

Khana A, El-Charabatyb E, El-Sayeghb S. Fungal infections in renal transplant patients. J Clin Med Res. 2015;7(6):371-8.

Q13. Answer d

Acute fatty liver of pregnancy is characterized by fatty infiltration of hepatocytes. It occurs typically in the third trimester. The association of cases of acute fatty liver of pregnancy with one of the inherited defects in mitochondrial beta-oxidation of fatty acids, long-chain 3-hydroxyacyl CoA dehydrogenase (LCHAD) deficiency. Serum aminotransferase elevations usually ranging from modest values up to 500 int. unit/L. Serum bilirubin levels are also usually elevated. Severely affected patients also have elevations in serum ammonia, prolongation of prothrombin time, and hypoglycemia caused by hepatic insufficiency. The diagnosis of acute fatty liver of pregnancy is usually made clinically based upon the setting, presentation, and compatible laboratory and imaging results. In HELLP syndrome there is hemolysis, elevated liver enzymes, and a low platelet count. Evidence of hepatic insufficiency such as hypoglycemia or encephalopathy and abnormalities in coagulation studies is more consistent with acute fatty liver of pregnancy. Intrahepatic cholestasis of pregnancy (ICP) occurs in the second and third trimester and is characterized by pruritus and an elevation in serum bile acid concentrations. The prothrombin time is usually normal. In viral hepatitis there is predominantly hepatocelluar damage marked by singnificant rise in transaminases. Up to 4-fold rise in alkaline phosphatase (AP) is observed in Cholestasis of pregnancy.

Richard H, Tram T, Keith D, et al. Acute fatty liver of pregnancy. *Update* 2016; Topic 3619 Version 19.0, Available from: https://www.uptodate.com/contents/acute-fatty-liver-of-pregnancy (Accessed 22nd June 2017).

Q14. Answer d

Drugs commonly used in ICU in pregnant patient which belong to category A or B are Dobutamine, Methyldopa, Cephalosporins, Macrolides, Acyclovir, Magnesium Sulfate, Propofol, Paracetamol, NSAIDs (< 28 weeks gestation). Drugs belonging to category C are Norepinephrine/epinephrine, Milrinone, Glyceryl trinitrate/Hydralazine, Digoxin /Adenosine, Fentanyl, Morphine, Haloperidol, Heparins and LMWH, Glucocorticoids, Neuromuscular Blockers. Drugs belonging to category X are ACEI, Diazepam, Midazolam, Lorazepam, NSAIDs >28 weeks Gestation, Fluconazole, Ketoconazole, Warfarin.

Eoin C, Niamh H, Andrew R, et al. Obstetric critical care. 2015. Available from: http://pact.esicm.org/media/Obstetric-critical-care-30-April-2013-final.pdf (Accessed 11th July 2017).

Q15. Answer e

Pathophysiology of TURP Syndrome: 1. Fluid overload: Small amounts of irrigant fluid continuously get absorbed through the open prostatic venous sinuses during TURP. If 1 L of irrigant fluid is absorbed into the circulation within 1 hour, it causes an acute decrease in the serum sodium concentration of 5 to 8 mmol/L. 2. Hyponatremia: Serum sodium concentration of <120 mmol/L is defined as severe TURP syndrome. 3. Hypo-osmolality: The blood-brain barrier is virtually impermeable to sodium but freely permeable to water leading to brain edema. 4. Hyperammonemia: Glycine (used as irrigant during TURP) is metabolized in brain to release ammonia. Hyperammonemic encephalopathy develops as a result of the formation of ammonia. Blood ammonia concentrations >100 mmol/L (normal range 10–35) are associated with neurologic signs and symptoms. 5. Irrigation Fluid: Excess of glycine absorbed into circulation is toxic to heart and retina and may lead to hyperammonemia.

Parua S, Kundu R. Intra operative and ICU management of transurethral resection of prostrate syndrome: A case report. IOSR Journal of Dental and Medical Sciences. 2015;11(I):55-9.

Q16. Answer c

Pregnant females with asthma are at a 46% increased risk of low birth weight. Meta-analysis of two primary studies which examined cleft lip with or without cleft palate indicated that there was a statistically significant risk of this malformation among pregnant females with asthma compared to pregnant females without asthma (RR 1.30, 95% CI 1.01–1.68). Asthma in pregnancy follows rule of 1/3. One third improves, one third deteriorates and one third has no effect on the disease. Hyperventilation can decrease uterine flow and, subsequently, produce fetal acidosis.

Murphy VE, Schatz M. Asthma in pregnancy: a hit for two. Eur Respir Rev. 2014;23:64-8.

Q17. Answer c

Precise Laboratory criteria for HELLP are necessary for research purposes and for predicting maternal complications. We require the presence of all of the following criteria to diagnose HELLP (Tennessee classification):

- Microangiopathic hemolytic anemia with characteristic schistocytes (also called helmet cells) on blood smear. Other signs suggestive of hemolysis include an elevated indirect bilirubin level and a low serum haptoglobin concentration (≤25 mg/dL).
- Platelet count ≤100,000 cells/microL
- Total bilirubin ≥1.2 mg/dL (20.52 micromol/L)
- Serum AST >2 times upper limit of normal for local laboratory (usually >70 international units/L). Some investigators obtain alanine aminotransferase (ALT) levels instead of, or in addition to, AST levels. An advantage of the AST is that it is a single test that reflects both hepatocellular necrosis and red cell hemolysis.

Baha M, Charles J, Keith D, et al. HELLP syndrome. Update 2016; Topic 6778 Version 36.0, Available from: https://www.uptodate.com/contents/hellp-syndrome (Accessed 14th July 2017).

Q18. Answer d

After the diagnosis is confirmed, the initial steps in management are to stabilize the mother, assess the fetal condition, and decide whether prompt delivery is indicated. Severe hypertension is treated with antihypertensive therapy and magnesium sulfate is given to prevent convulsions. HELLP syndrome complicated by multiorgan dysfunction, disseminated intravascular coagulation (DIC), pulmonary edema, liver hemorrhage or infarction, renal failure, abruptio placenta, compromised fetal status, or fetal death is an indication for prompt delivery regardless of gestational age, for pregnancies ≥34 weeks of gestation, delivery is recommended rather than expectant management (Grade 1C). In this population, the potential risks of preterm birth are outweighed by the risks associated with HELLP syndrome. Also delivery is considered in pregnancies <23 weeks of gestation because expectant management is associated with a high-risk of maternal complications without significant improvement in perinatal prognosis. For pregnancies ≥23 and <34 weeks of gestation in which maternal and fetal status are reassuring, delivery is suggested after a course of corticosteroids to accelerate fetal pulmonary maturity rather than expectant management or prompt delivery. Dexamethasone is not recommended for treatment of HELLP syndrome (Grade 1B). Dexamethasone does not accelerate resolution of laboratory abnormalities or reduce the risk of maternal complications.

Baha M, Charles J, Keith D, et al. HELLP syndrome. Update 2016; Topic 6778 Version 36.0, Available from: https://www.uptodate.com/contents/hellp-syndrome (Accessed 14th July 2017).

Q19. Answer e

Pregnancy is associated with changes in several coagulation factors that result in up to 20% reduction of PT and APTT. During pregnancy the concentrations of coagulation factors VII, VIII, IX, X, XII, von Willebrand factor and fibrinogen rise significantly. Plasma fibrinolytic activity is reduced during pregnancy. Tissue plasminogen activator (t-PA) activity decreases during pregnancy. This is due to increase in plasminogen activator inhibitor-1 (PAI-1) and plasminogen activator inhibitor-2 (PAI-2). PAI-1 values increase during pregnancy and normalize at 5 weeks postpartum. Naturally occurring coagulation inhibitors, protein C and protein S significant fall and lead to inhibition of fibrinolysis. Thrombocytopenia, believed to be resulting from hemodilution and other factors is the most common hemostatic abnormality observed in pregnancy. The net effect of these pregnancy-induced changes is to produce a hypercoagulable state, which is a double-edged sword of protection (e.g. hemostasis contributing to reduced blood loss at delivery) and risk (e.g. thromboembolic phenomenon).

Michael R, Charles J, Bernard J, et al. Maternal cardiovascular and hemodynamic adaptations to pregnancy. Update 2015; Topic 443 Version 10.0, Available from: https://www.uptodate.com/contents/maternal-cardiovascular-and-hemodynamic-adaptations-to-pregnancy (14th July 2017).

Q20. Answer b

Initially both cardiogenic and distributive shocks contribute to the presentation of AFE. If the patient survives long enough, hypovolemic shock may contribute as a result of hemorrhage and DIC.

Eoin C, Niamh H, Andrew R, et al. Obstetric critical care. 2015. Available from: http://pact.esicm.org/media/Obstetric-critical-care-30-April-2013-final.pdf (Accessed 11th July 2017).

K Type Answers

Q1. Answer TTTFF

AFE can occur only when there is a breech in the barrier between the amniotic fluid and maternal circulation. If even a small volume of amniotic fluid enters the maternal circulation, the initial hemodynamic response consists of acute pulmonary hypertension and vasospasm complicated by severe hypoxemia and right-sided heart failure, followed by a second phase of more sustained left ventricular failure. The diagnosis is based on exclusion of other causes. Respiratory and cardiovascular supportive therapy is initiated. Laboratory data may be supportive, but they alone can never diagnose or exclude AFE. Laboratory investigations which may be useful include complete blood count, coagulation parameters, arterial blood gases, maternal serum tryptase and plasma zinc coproporphyrin levels, chest X-ray, VQ scan, ECG and echocardiogram. The finding of squamous cells in the maternal pulmonary circulation at autopsy once considered pathognomonic, is neither specific nor sensitive for the diagnosis of AFE. The identification of mucin, however, seems to be a more sensitive indicator of AFE.

Kahvecd O, Demdrcan A, Keles A, et al. Amniotic fluid embolism: A case report. Fırat tıp Dergisi. 2010;15(1):51-3.

Q2. Answer FTTFT

The incidence of VTE increases by a factor of four with pregnancy. The incidence of VTE is estimated at 0.76 to 1.72 per 1000 pregnancies, which is four times as great as the risk in the nonpregnant population. PE is the leading cause of maternal death in the developed world. Current estimates of deaths from PE are 1.1 to 1.5 per 100,000 deliveries in the United States and Europe. Two thirds of cases of DVT occurred in the antepartum period and were distributed relatively equally among all three trimesters. Approximately 30% of apparently isolated episodes of PE are associated with silent DVT. In contrast, 43 to 60% of pregnancy-related episodes of PE appear to occur in the puerperium.

Paul E, and Lauren A. Current concepts: Venous thromboembolic disease and pregnancy. N Engl J Med. 2008;359:2025-33. Available from: www.nejm.org/doi/full/10.1056/NEJMra0707993 (Accessed 20th May 2017)

Q3. Answer FTFFT

V/Q scan delivers a significantly higher fetal dose of radiation than does CTPA (640 to 800 µGy vs. 3 to 131 µGy). Perfusion scanning alone may reduce the radiation exposure. However, the radiation dose delivered to mothers is higher with CTPA than with V/Q scan (2.2 to 6.0 mSv vs. 1.4 mSv). V/Q scan carries a slightly higher risk of childhood cancer while CTPA carries a higher risk of maternal breast cancer (the lifetime risk is up to 13% greater).

Paul E, Lauren A. Current Concepts: Venous Thromboembolic disease and pregnancy. N Engl J Med. 2008;359:2025-33.

Q4. Answer TFTFT

Current guidelines of the American Society of Regional Anesthesia (ASRA) and Pain Medicine suggest that spinal anesthesia may be performed 12 hours after administration of the last dose of prophylactic LMWH and 24 hours after the last dose of therapeutic LMWH (given either once or twice daily). Intravenous UFH should be stopped 6 hours before placement of a neuraxial blockade, and a normal aPTT time should be confirmed. Treatment with LMWH may be resumed within 12 hours after delivery in the absence of persistent bleeding. The initiation of prophylactic LMWH should be delayed for at least 12 hours after the removal of an epidural catheter. After neuraxial anesthesia, therapeutic LMWH should be administered not earlier than 24 hours postoperatively or postpartum and in the presence of adequate hemostasis. Anticoagulation therapy with either LMWH or warfarin is recommended for at least 6 weeks post-partum and for a total of at least 6 months.

Paul E, Lauren A. Current concepts: Venous thromboembolic disease and pregnancy. N Engl J Med. 2008;359:2025-33.

Q5. Answer TTTFF

Reversible Posterior Leukoencephalopathy Syndrome (RPLS) or Posterior Reversible Encephalopathy Syndrome (PRES) is a neurologic syndrome defined by clinical and radiologic features. The typical clinical syndrome includes headache, confusion, visual symptoms, and seizures. Typical MRI findings are consistent with vasogenic edema and are predominantly localized to the posterior cerebral hemispheres. DWI can be helpful in distinguishing RPLS from stroke. Most often it occurs in the setting of hypertensive crisis, preeclampsia, or with cytotoxic immunosuppressive therapy; however, many other clinical settings are described. Blood pressure lowering is recommended in all patients with RPLS. An easily titratable parenteral agent such as nicardipine or labetalol is suggested. Even patients with seemingly normal blood pressure benefit from blood pressure lowering as their baseline blood pressure may be much lower. It is suggested to treat patients who have a seizure with antiepileptic drugs such as phenytoin. Most patients recover within two weeks. In the partum or postpartum setting, it is recommended treating patients with RPLS as though they have preeclampsia or eclampsia. A small number have residual neurologic deficits resulting from secondary cerebral infarction or hemorrhage; some patients die as a result of increased intracranial pressure or as a complication of the underlying condition.

Neill TA. Reversible posterior leukoencephalopathy syndrome. Available from: https://www.uptodate.com/contents/reversible-posterior-leukoencephalopathy-syndrome?source=search_result&search=Reversible%20posterior%20leukoencephalopathy%20syndrome&selectedTitle=1~150 [Accessed 4th July 2017].

Q6. Answer FTTFT

The incidence of VTE increases by a factor of four with pregnancy. The incidence of VTE is estimated at 0.76 to 1.72 per 1000 pregnancies, which is four times as great as the risk in the nonpregnant population. PE is the leading cause of maternal death in the developed world. Current estimates of deaths from pulmonary embolism are 1.1 to 1.5 per 100,000 deliveries in the United States and Europe. Two thirds of cases of deep-vein thrombosis occurred in the antepartum period and were distributed relatively equally among all three trimesters. Approximately 30% of apparently isolated episodes of PE are associated with silent DVT. In contrast, 43 to 60% of pregnancy-related episodes of PE appear to occur in the puerperium.

Paul E, Lauren A. Current Concepts: Venous thromboembolic disease and pregnancy. N Engl J Med. 2008;359:2025-33. Available from: www.nejm.org/doi/full/10.1056/NEJMra0707993 (Accessed 20th May 2017).

Q7. Answer FTTFF

Organisms are introduced during collection or processing of urine is known as contamination.

Complicated UTI is infection associated with factors increasing colonization and decreasing efficacy of therapy such as:
- Anatomic or functional abnormality of urinary tract (enlarged prostate, stone disease, diverticulum, neurogenic bladder, etc.)
- Immunocompromised host
- Multi-drug resistant bacteria

Adult UTI. American Urological Association. Available from: http://www.auanet.org/education/educational-programs/medical-student-education/medical-student-curriculum/adult-uti (Accessed 2nd August, 2017).

Q8. Answer FFFTF

Within the subset of patients with hypoxic respiratory failure who suffer from ARDS, pulmonary consolidations lead to decreased static lung compliance. Because of this decreased compliance, higher inspiratory pressures are required to maintain adequate tidal volumes, subsequently leading to barotrauma and volutrauma. For understanding these mechanisms for lung injury, much research has focused on the effect of limiting tidal volumes during ventilation of patients with ARDS. This requires accepting higher levels of arterial carbon dioxide and the associated effects of respiratory acidosis. Conventional ventilation typically employs tidal volumes of 10 to 15 mL/kg of body weight while low tidal volume ventilation is defined as 5 to 7 mL/kg. Combined with moderate PEEP, this low-volume strategy has been termed lung-protective ventilation and has been shown to decrease overall mortality and increase ventilator-free days in ARDS within the general nonpregnant population. No studies have been performed evaluating the effects of these strategies in parturients.

Ende H, Varelmann D. Respiratory considerations including airway and ventilation issues in critical care obstetric patients. Obstet Gynecol Clin N Am. 43(2016):699-708.

Q9. Answer FTFFT

A subset of pregnant patients requires anticoagulation during pregnancy and/or in the postpartum period. LMW heparin rather than UFH is recommended for all but during the final weeks of the pregnancy since because they are effective and easier to administer than UFH. Warfarin is generally avoided during pregnancy because it crosses the placenta, is a teratogen, and causes fetal anticoagulation throughout the pregnancy. HIT can occur in any patient receiving any amount of heparin; however, the incidence in pregnant women is very low. Anticoagulation during labor should be avoided except in the highest risk settings (e.g. reduced cardiopulmonary reserve and recent pulmonary embolus). The 2012 American College of Chest Physicians (ACCP) guidelines recommends continuation of the following anticoagulants during breastfeeding—1. LMW heparin 2. UFH; 3. Warfarin or other vitamin K antagonists; 4. Danaparoid; 5. Lepirudin.

> Bauer KA. Use of anticoagulants during pregnancy and postpartum. Available from: https://www.uptodate.com/contents/use-of-anticoagulants-during-pregnancy-and-postpartum (Accessed 23rd July, 2017).

Q10. Answer TFFTF

AFE syndrome is also called anaphylactoid syndrome of pregnancy. The incidence rate is between 1 and 12 cases per 100,000 deliveries. Risk factors include precipitous or tumultuous labor, advanced maternal age, cesarean and instrumental delivery, placenta previa and abruption, grand multiparity (≥5 live births or stillbirths), cervical lacerations, fetal distress, eclampsia, and medical induction of labor. Amniotic fluid is believed to enter the maternal circulation through the endocervical veins, the placental insertion site, or a site of uterine trauma. The major clinical findings are the abrupt and fulminant onset of hypotension due to cardiogenic shock, hypoxemia and respiratory failure, disseminated intravascular coagulation, coma or seizures. Disseminated intravascular coagulation (DIC) is a common complication (up to 80%).

Q11. Answer TFTTT

The fetus has low/no chance of survival if the mother is not appropriately managed. If chest tube placement is indicated, consideration should be given to placing the tube one or two interspaces higher than normal because of diaphragmatic displacement in later pregnancy. Ultrasound can rapidly diagnose fetal death, fetal heart rate, fetal movement, multiple pregnancy, fetal extrusion into the abdominal cavity (uterine rupture), and direct fetal injury. It is difficult to differentiate between placental abruption and uterine rupture due to the relatively insensitive and non-specific clinical features that accompany each condition. Initial laboratory testing for the maternal trauma patient should always include Rhesus (Rh) D status of the mother. Anti-D immune globulin should be given to all Rh D negative women of childbearing age following abdominal trauma.

> Eoin C, Niamh H, Andrew R, et al. Obstetric critical care. 2015; 44-45. Available from: http://pact.esicm.org/media/Obstetric-critical-care-30-April-2013-final.pdf (Accessed 11th July 2017).
>
> Moise K, Argoti P. Management and prevention of red cell alloimmunization in pregnancy: a systematic review. Obstet Gynecol. 2012;120(5):1132-9. PMID 23090532.

Q12. Answer FTTTF

Peripartum cardiomyopathy is a diagnosis of exclusion. A diagnosis of peripartum cardiomyopathy requires the presence of the following FOUR criteria:
1. Development of cardiac failure in the last month of pregnancy or within 5 months of delivery (~78% of cases)
2. Absence of any other identifiable cause for the cardiac failure
3. Absence of heart disease prior to last month of pregnancy
4. Echocardiographic evidence of reduced left ventricular function (Ejection fraction <45% and/or Fractional shortening <30%, End-diastolic dimension >2.7 cm/m^2).

> Eoin C, Niamh H, Andrew R, et al. Obstetric critical Care. 2015. Available from: http://pact.esicm.org/media/Obstetric-critical-care-30-April-2013-final.pdf (Accessed 11th July 2017).

Q13. Answer TTTTF

ACE inhibitors are contraindicated antepartum due to potential teratogenic effects but are safe in postpartum and in breastfeeding mothers. Anticoagulation should be considered in all patients with peripartum cardiomyopathy because of increased risk of VTE. Immunosuppressive (if myocarditis proven on biopsy) or immunomodulatory therapy may be beneficial in patients when standard treatment has not yielded an adequate response. In a recent pilot study, the addition of bromocriptine to standard therapy has shown improvement in left ventricular function in patients with peripartum cardiomyopathy. These results need to be confirmed by randomized controlled trials. Peripartum cardiomyopathy is associated with a relatively poor prognosis with mortality ranging from 15 to 50%.

<small>Eoin C, Niamh H, Andrew R, et al. Obstetric critical Care. 2015; 29. Available from: http://pact.esicm.org/media/Obstetric-critical-care-30-April-2013-final.pdf (Accessed 11th July 2017).</small>

Q14. Answer FTTTF

The principles of resuscitation are the same as for the non-obstetric patient but incorporate additional issues outlined below.
- Summon help immediately; call for an obstetrician, anesthesiologist and neonatologist
- Commence cardiopulmonary resuscitation according to advanced life support algorithms
- If gestation >20 weeks, use a left lateral tilt to avoid aortocaval compression
- A definitive airway should be secured as early as possible given the increased risk of aspiration
- Establish large bore IV access; initiate aggressive volume resuscitation unless suspicious of pre-eclampsia/eclampsia
- Defibrillation and resuscitation drugs should be administered according to established algorithms
- Prepare for Caesarean section

Although there is a small risk of inducing fetal arrhythmias, cardioversion and defibrillation are considered safe at all stages of pregnancy. If there has not been a return of spontaneous circulation (ROSC) as the resuscitation effort approaches 4 minutes and the gestational age is >20 weeks, emergency caesarean section should be performed if resources and expertise are available.

<small>Eoin C, Niamh H, Andrew R, et al. Obstetric critical care. 2015; 35. Available from: http://pact.esicm.org/media/Obstetric-critical-care-30-April-2013-final.pdf (Accessed 11th July 2017).</small>

<small>Soar J, Perkins G, Abbas G, et al. European Resuscitation Council Guidelines for Resuscitation 2010 Section 8. Cardiac arrest in special circumstances: Electrolyte abnormalities, poisoning, drowning, accidental hypothermia, hyperthermia, asthma, anaphylaxis, cardiac surgery, trauma, pregnancy, electrocution. Resuscitation. 2010;81(10):1400-33. PMID 20956045.</small>

<small>Royal College of Obstetricians and Gynaecologists. Maternal collapse in pregnancy and the puerperium: Green-top guideline No. 56. Available from http://www.rcog.org.uk/files/rcog-corp/GTG56.pdf (Accessed 10 July 2017).</small>

Q15. Answer FFFTT

Severe preeclampsia is more likely to require critical care and is diagnosed by the presence of more severe blood pressure elevation and significant organ dysfunction as noted below.
- Systolic blood pressure : >160 mm Hg or diastolic blood pressure >110 mm Hg on two occasions at least 2 hours apart
- Proteinuria: >5 g in a 24 hr collection
- Oliguria: < 500 mL in 24 hrs
- Elevated serum creatinine
- Pulmonary edema or cyanosis
- Persistent headaches
- Visual disturbances
- Seizures
- Epigastric or right upper quadrant pain and/or elevated liver function tests
- Thrombocytopenia and/or deranged coagulation tests
- Oligohydramnios, decreased fetal growth or placental abruption

<small>Eoin C, Niamh H, Andrew R, et al. Obstetric critical care. 2015:18-19. Available from: http://pact.esicm.org/media/Obstetric-critical-care-30-April-2013-final.pdf (Accessed 11th July 2017).</small>

Q16. Answer FTFTT

At plasma magnesium concentration of 2 to 3.5 mmol/L (4.8–8.4 mg/dL), nausea, flushing, headache, lethargy, drowsiness, and diminished deep tendon reflexes develop. When plasma magnesium concentration reaches 3.5 to 5 mmol/L (8.4–12 mg/dL), somnolence, hypocalcaemia, absent deep tendon reflexes, hypotension, bradycardia, and ECG changes may occur. At plasma magnesium concentration above 5 mmol/L (12 mg/dL), the patient is at risk for muscle paralysis, respiratory paralysis, complete heart block, and cardiac arrest. In most cases, respiratory failure precedes cardiac collapse. Specific treatment modalities for hypermagnesemia include administration of calcium, e.g. 10 mL of 10% calcium gluconate in the patient with cardiorespiratory compromise, aggressive fluid therapy, loop diuretics and hemodialysis.

Eoin C, Niamh H, Andrew R, et al. Obstetric critical care. 2015; 24. Available from: http://pact.esicm.org/media/Obstetric-critical-care-30-April-2013-final.pdf (Accessed 11th July 2017).

Q17. Answer FTFFF

In obstetric patient there should be aim for a higher PaO_2 or SpO_2 than normal to reduce the risk of fetal hypoxia in a potentially compromised fetoplacental circulation. Gestational $PaCO_2$ should be maintained at normal levels because maintenance of the fetomaternal CO_2 gradient is important for fetal CO_2 excretion. Also hypocapnia produces placental vasoconstriction and reduced uteroplacental perfusion. High levels of positive end-expiratory pressure should be avoided in the parturient greater than 20 weeks gestation as it may further impair venous return and cardiac output. Spontaneous ventilation trial should be given as early as possible to avoid positive intra-thoracic pressure. Delivery may improve the mechanics of ventilation. Each case should be considered individually along with maternal and fetal concerns in the decision-making process.

Eoin C, Niamh H, Andrew R, et al. Obstetric critical care. 2015; 53. Available from: http://pact.esicm.org/media/Obstetric-critical-care-30-April-2013-final.pdf (Accessed 11th July 2017).

Lapinsky S, Posadas C, McCullagh I. Clinical review: Ventilatory strategies for obstetric, brain-injured and obese patients. Crit Care. 2009;13(2):206. PMID 19291279.

Cole D, Taylor T, McCullough D, et al. Acute respiratory distress syndrome in pregnancy. Crit Care Med. 2005; 33(10 Suppl): S269-78. PMID 16215347.

Q18. Answer TTTTF

Commonly implicated organisms in obstetric sepsis include *E. coli*, Group A, (beta-hemolytic) streptococci, Klebsiella species, Staphylococcus aureus. As a result of the increasing prevalence of sepsis related maternal mortality, Centre for maternal and child enquiries (CMACE) have now issued guidelines on appropriate antibiotic strategies for the septic obstetric patient.

Cantwell R, Clutton-Brock T, Cooper G, et al. Saving mothers' lives: Reviewing maternal deaths to make motherhood safer: 2006-2008. The Eighth Report of the Confidential Enquiries into Maternal Deaths in the United Kingdom. BJOG 2011; 118 Suppl 1: 1-203. Available from: http://www.hqip.org.uk/cmace-reports (Accessed 12th July 2017).

Eoin C, Niamh H, Andrew R, et al. Obstetric critical care. pact.esicm.org 2015; Page 58. Available from: http://pact.esicm.org/media/Obstetric-critical-care-30-April-2013-final.pdf (Accessed 11th July 2017).

Q19. Answer TTFTF

Actively bleeding patients with thrombocytopenia should be transfused with platelets. Platelet transfusion may be indicated to prevent excessive bleeding during delivery if the platelet count is less than 20,000 cells/microL, but the threshold for prophylactic platelet transfusion in this setting is controversial. The decision depends on patient specific factors; consultation with the hematology service may be helpful. If cesarean delivery is planned, platelet transfusion may be required. Some experts recommend platelet transfusion to achieve a preoperative platelet count greater than 40,000 to 50,000 cells/microL, but the minimum count before a neuraxial procedure is controversial and depends on factors in addition to platelet concentration.

Sibai BM. HELLP syndrome. Available from: https://www.uptodate.com/contents/hellp-syndrome?source=search_result&search=hellp%20syndrome%20management&selectedTitle=1~87 [Accessed 14th April 2017].

Q20. Answer FTFTF

AFLP occurs in 1 of 7,000 to 16,000 pregnancies, primarily in the third trimester. The incidence is higher in primigravid a women, multiple gestations, and pregnancies with a male fetus. The exact pathophysiology is unknown. It is thought that AFLP is caused by microvesicular fatty infiltration of the hepatocytes. This accumulation results in hepatotoxicity and eventually leads to liver failure. Though rare, the maternal and neonatal mortality rates are high, up to 18% and 55%, respectively. Hypoglycemia is a common occurrence and should be promptly treated.

Vora KS, Shah VR, Parikh GP. Acute fatty liver of pregnancy: A case report of an uncommon disease. Indian J Crit Care Med. 2009;13(1):34-6.

CHAPTER

Endocrinology and Metabolism

Mohit Mathur, Amit Singh, Yash Javeri

A Type Questions
(One best answer)

1. A 24-year-old wrestler with no prior comorbidity presented to ER with c/o brief period of unconsciousness when he was going to toilet from bed at 2 am. He was feeling lethargic and giving history of similar episodes in past. There was no history of fever, vomiting but having mild abdominal pain. His vital parameters revealed heart rate of 120/min and blood pressure of 70/40 mm Hg. Fluid resuscitation was done with 2 L of normal saline but blood pressure did not improve. Vasopressor support was started under invasive hemodynamic monitoring. All relevant investigations including cultures were sent and broad spectrum IV antibiotics were started. Lab investigations revealed normal blood counts, normal LFT, urea-30, creatinine of 1.4, sodium-125, k-6.4. ECG showed peaked T waves. What is the most probable diagnosis?
   a. Septic shock
   b. Adrenal insufficiency
   c. Myxedema coma
   d. Pancreatitis
   e. Acute myocardial infarction

2. Considering above case, which statement is correct?
   a. Give IV dexamethasone, send baseline plasma cortisol and ACTH level, if cortisol comes low then do ACTH stimulation test
   b. Send baseline plasma cortisol and ACTH level, give IV hydrocortisone; if cortisol comes low then do ACTH stimulation test but after switching to dexamethasone for 24–36 hrs
   c. Do not give any steroid; send serum cortisol level
   d. Empirically supplement steroids. There is no benefit of measuring levels of cortisol and ACTH
   e. Give thyroxine

3. Which of the following statement is true about Waterhouse-Friderichsen syndrome?
   a. It is almost always associated with meningococcal infection
   b. Having 100% mortality
   c. It is associated with hemorrhage in pituitary gland
   d. Treatment is parenteral administration of steroids
   e. If treatment started early, most of the patients recover

4. A 29-year-old woman presented to emergency with complaints of altered mental status, polyuria and polydipsia. She is not having any past medical history except that she had postpartum hemorrhage (PPH) 2 years back. At that time total abdominal hysterectomy was done. Initial workup showed pancytopenia and sodium of 160 mEq/L. Blood sugar-170 mg/dL. Serum osmolality is 350 mOsm/kg and urine osmolality 150 mOsm/kg. DDAVP Results

of water deprivation test and desmopressin challenge test are following:

	Water deprivation	DDAVP challenge
Urine osmolality (mOsm/kg)	150	800

What is the diagnosis?
   a. Nephrogenic diabetes insipidus (DI)
   b. Sheehan's syndrome
   c. SIADH
   d. Psychogenic polydipsia
   e. Diabetes mellitus

5. A 45-year-old male was admitted in ICU after head injury in a road traffic accident. His CT head showed contusion in temporal-parietal region and craniotomy was done for the same. On 5th post-operative day he developed hyponatremia with worsening GCS. ICU resident planned to administer 3% saline. Urine sodium came out as 40 mEq/L. A provisional diagnosis of Syndrome of Inappropriate Antidiuretic Hormone Secretion (SIADH)/cerebral salt wasting (CSW) syndrome was made. Which laboratory test or clinical finding will help best in differentiating between the two?
   a. Fraction excretion of urea pre and post-correction of sodium with 3% saline
   b. Fraction excretion of uric acid pre and post-correction of sodium with 3% saline
   c. Fractional excretion of sodium pre and post-correction of sodium with 3% saline
   d. Assessing volume status
   e. Urine output

6. Which of the following statement is not correct regarding sodium bicarbonate administration in diabetic ketoacidosis (DKA)?
   a. Can cause hypokalemia and arrhythmias
   b. Correct intracellular acidosis within 5 minutes of administration
   c. Reduction in intravenous chloride load
   d. It reduces the cardiac irritability
   e. Should be usually avoided in DKA in mild to moderate acidosis

7. A 48-year-old male was shifted to ICU from operating room after excision of adrenal glands for pheochromocytoma. He was on phenoxybenzamine 20 mg BD in preoperative period. Which of the following statement is FALSE regarding his management in post-operative period?
   a. Hypotension can be severe requiring large amount of fluid administration
   b. Vasopressin will be choice of vasopressor in this patient
   c. Rebound hyperglycemia is common and requires intensive sugar monitoring and insulin supplementation
   d. Steroid supplementation can be considered
   e. Phenoxybenzamine is irreversible non-selective alpha blocker

8. Which of the following is not a feature of refeeding syndrome?
   a. Hypokalemia
   b. Hypomagnesemia
   c. Hypophosphatemia
   d. Hypoglycemia
   e. Hyponatremia

9. Which of the following is not a causative factor for hypophosphatemia?
   a. Hungry bone syndrome
   b. Volume expansion
   c. Recovery from malnutrition
   d. Hypoventilation
   e. Kidney transplantation

10. A 27-year-old female was shifted to ICU from ward with complaints of nausea, vomiting, abdominal distension and decreased urine output. Her blood pressure and heart were 80/40 mm Hg and 120/min respectively. She was on treatment for infertility for 1 year and 2 days back she was taken for ovum pick up. USG abdomen was done showing massive ascites and bilateral mild pleural effusion. What is the most probable diagnosis?
    a. Septic shock
    b. Hemorrhagic shock
    c. Acute liver failure
    d. Anti-phospholipid antibody syndrome
    e. Ovarian hyperstimulation syndrome

11. Which of the following is not correct about tumor lysis syndrome?
    a. Usually occurs in patient with acute leukemia and non- Hodgkin's lymphoma
    b. Can lead to renal failure
    c. Large cell mass of tumor is one of the risk factor
    d. Causes hyperuricemia, hyperphosphatemia, hypercalcemia and hyperkalemia

e. Adequate hydration, allopurinol and rasburicase are treatment choices

12. A 35-year-old lady on treatment for UTI with levofloxacin presented to hospital with complaints of fever, vomiting, confusion and agitation. She was apparently alright 3 months back but started to have palpitations on and off since then. On examination she is agitated, her pulse rate is 140/min irregularly irregular, BP of 180/70 mm Hg and having temp of 104.5°F. Her ECG is showing atrial fibrillation. There is no focal neurological deficit and no neck rigidity. Which of the following statement is NOT CORRECT about her management?
    a. Beta blockers should be started
    b. Levofloxacin should be stopped
    c. Aggressive management for temperature control should be initiated
    d. IV hydrocortisone can be given
    e. Lithium therapy is option in this patient

13. A 37-year-old patient known hypothyroid presented to hospital with c/o polyuria, polydipsia. She was having high prolactin. DDAVP challenge test was done and patient was diagnosed as central diabetes insipidus. MRI brain done showing following finding:

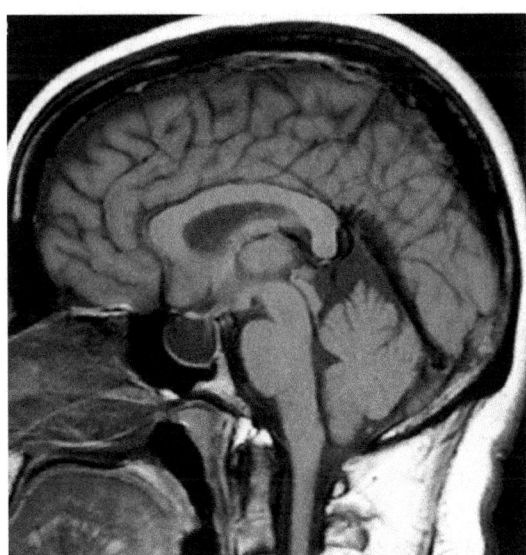

What is the diagnosis?
    a. Pituitary adenoma
    b. Pituitary necrosis
    c. Empty sella syndrome
    d. Sheehan syndrome
    e. Intra-cranial space occupying lesion

14. Which of the following drug is not associated with magnesium deficiency?
    a. Proton pump inhibitors
    b. Aminoglycosides
    c. Epinephrine
    d. Amphotericin B
    e. Acetylsalicylic acid

15. A 55-year-old patient with past history of coronary artery disease was shifted to ICU post-exploratory laparotomy after intestinal obstruction. Intra-operatively he received IV furosemide 20 mg for low urine output. ABG done in ICU were showing following results: pH-7.54, PO_2-90 on 2 Ltr O_2 by nasal prongs, HCO_3-40, lactate-2.5, K^+-4.0 mEq/L, Urine Cl^- - 13 mEq/L

What should be best management to correct his alkalosis?
    a. Aldosterone antagonist
    b. Hydrochloric acid infusion
    c. Normal saline
    d. Potassium supplementation
    e. Acetazolamide

16. Which of the following is not associated with hyperlactatemia?
    a. Thiamine deficiency
    b. Epinephrine
    c. Severe alkalosis
    d. Antiretroviral agents
    e. Diuretics

17. Which of the statement is correct about kayexalate (polystyrene sulphonate)?
    a. It is anion exchange resin
    b. It should be taken with glycerol to prevent loose motions
    c. 1 gm of resin binds with 0.25 mEq of potassium
    d. Can only be given orally
    e. It may cause necrotic lesion in the bowel

18. Which of the following statement is incorrect about use of hydrocortisone?
    a. Hydrocortisone should be used in doses of 200 mg over 24 hrs in infusion
    b. Hydrocortisone infusion can reduce mortality by upto 6-9% in septic shock cases
    c. Hydrocortisone hastens the reversal of shock
    d. Hydrocortisone does not reduce the development of septic shock in patient with severe sepsis (now sepsis)

e. Hydrocortisone hasten the recovery of shock in those patients in whom shock ultimately reversed

19. A 60-year-old male, known case of carcinoma prostate with bone metastasis presented to emergency with complaints of multiple episodes of vomiting followed by an episode of seizure. He is having no other comorbidity. Arterial Blood gas was done showing following findings: pH-7.37, PO_2-90 on room air, PCO_2- 32, HCO_3- 23, Na^+ -136 mEq/L, K^+ -3.6 mEq/L, Chloride - 90 mEq/L RBS - 300 mg%.
    Urine ketones - negative
    Osmolal gap - normal
    Poisoning is suspected.

    What is the most appropriate treatment?
    a. Normal saline bolus and insulin infusion
    b. IV fomepizole
    c. Urine alkalinization
    d. Flumazenil
    e. Antibiotics

20. A 50-year-old female (Wt 70 kg) with past history of diabetes and chronic alcoholism is admitted in ICU with c/o severe generalized weakness and body ache. Her vital parameters are HR-110/min, BP-120/84 mm Hg, and SPO_2- 98% on room air. She is conscious and fully oriented. After initial fluid resuscitation her urine output is around 25 mL per hour and tea colored. Her lab parameters are following: Complete blood count – normal, BUN - 190 mg%, Creatinine - 3.1 mg %, Na^+ - 134 mEq/L, K^+ - 6.7 mEq/L, HCO_3 - 24 mEq/L, Chloride – 110 mEq/L, PH - 7.38, Blood sugar- 170 mg %, Uric acid - 10.1 mg/dL, Serum osmolality - 360 mg%

    What is the most probable diagnosis?
    a. Severe dehydration
    b. Tumor lysis syndrome
    c. Methanol poisoning
    d. Rhabdomyolysis
    e. Diabetic ketoacidosis

21. In the above scenario all of the following drugs may be responsible for rhabdomyolysis, *except*:
    a. Simvastatin
    b. Cocaine
    c. Aspirin
    d. Carbon monoxide
    e. Tramadol

22. A 26-year-old male was found unconscious in car parked in garage on Sunday morning. He was immediately taken to hospital by neighbors. Saturation gap measured is more than 10%. Carbon monoxide poisoning is suspected.

    Which of the following statement is correct?
    a. Half-life of carboxyhemoglobin is approximately 100 minutes
    b. Half-life of carboxyhemoglobin is decreased to 50 minutes when treated with 100% O_2
    c. Delayed neurological complications are uncommon in follow up cases
    d. Half-life of carboxyhemoglobin is decreased to 23 minutes when treated with hyperbaric O_2 therapy with 3 ATA (absolute atmosphere)
    e. Hyperbaric O_2 therapy should not be given to pregnant patient

23. Which of the following statement is correct regarding studies for glucose control in ICU?
    a. Van den Berghe et al. (2001) took medical patients and showed significant mortality benefit with intensive glycemic control
    b. Van den Berghe et al. (2006) took surgical patients and showed significant mortality benefit with intensive glycemic control
    c. Van den Berghe et al. (2006) took medical patients and showed no mortality benefit but morbidity benefit with intensive glycemic control
    d. In NICE-SUGAR study (2009) there was no difference in mortality between intensive versus conventional therapy
    e. Glucose level in ICU should be kept between 90 and 150 mg/dL

24. All of the following drugs cause hypoglycemia except:
    a. Levofloxacin
    b. Salicylates
    c. Quinine
    d. Salbutamol
    e. Alcohol

25. A 50-year-old woman presented to emergency department with complaints of decreased level of consciousness since last 4–5 days. There is no history of fever. She is having past history of diabetes mellitus, mitral stenosis and atrial fibrillation. Her current medications are metformin 500 mg twice a day, warfarin 2 mg

once a day, amiodarone 200 mg once a day. Her general examination revealed heart rate of 52/min, Blood pressure of 120/76 mm Hg, temperature of 35 degree Celsius and she is maintaining saturation on room air. Her GCS is 10/15 and there is no focal neurological deficit. She is having dry skin and cold extremities. No neck rigidity is found. On laboratory investigations her complete blood count, and electrolytes, are unremarkable. Renal parameters showed creatinine of 1.6 and urea of 46. NCCT head showed no abnormality. What will be next best course of action?

a. CSF examination, blood culture, empirical antibiotics
b. MRI brain to rule out ischemic stroke
c. T3, T4, TSH and cortisol
d. Stop Amiodarone
e. EEG

K Type Questions
[Marked True (T)/False (F)]

1. In hyperthyroidism:
   a. Normal TSH level almost always excludes hyperthyroidism
   b. Propranolol is drug of choice for thyroid storm; it relieves not only tachycardia, agitation but also blocks of conversion of T4 to T3
   c. Volume resuscitation should not be done in thyroid storm as there is risk of heart failure
   d. Steroids are having no role in thyroid storm
   e. Hyperthermia is usual finding in thyroid storm

2. Regarding hypokalemia:
   a. If serum potassium decreases by 0.3 mEq/L total body potassium deficit more than 100 mEq
   b. Urinary potassium does not help in establishing the cause of hypokalemia
   c. 6 mEq IV Potassium chloride can be given over 1 minute in case of cardiac arrest through central line
   d. Transtubular potassium gradient is calculated to differentiate between renal and extra-renal cause
   e. Chronic mild hypokalemia increases the progression of kidney dysfunction and should be treated

3. Following are the causes of normal anion gap metabolic acidosis:
   a. Diarrhea
   b. Parenteral alimentation
   c. Vomiting
   d. Salicylate poisoning
   e. Bartter syndrome

4. Management of diabetic ketoacidosis includes:
   a. Insulin should be started immediately followed by 15–20 mL/kg bolus of isotonic fluid in 1st hour
   b. Insulin infusion should be continued until ketonuria persist
   c. Insulin infusion should be continued until anion gap closes
   d. Insulin should be stopped once blood sugar normalizes
   e. Normal saline should be continued till corrected sodium normalizes then start 0.45% saline to prevent normal anion gap acidosis

5. Regarding magnesium retention test:
   a. If less than 80% of infused magnesium is recovered in urine, hypomagnesaemia may be present
   b. If more than 80% magnesium is recovered in urine hypomagnesemia is unlikely
   c. Urine spot magnesium is measured
   d. 6 g $MgSO_4$ is infused over 1 hour
   e. This test is reliable even in renal failure

6. Management of hypercalcemia includes:
   a. Fluid replacement followed by diuretics
   b. Zoledronate and gallium nitrate can lead to renal failure
   c. Calcitonin is having rapid response
   d. Tachyphylaxis is common with calcitonin and can be reduced by glucocorticoids
   e. Glucocorticoid is not effective in hypercalcemia associated with malignancies

7. A 55-year-old male was admitted to ICU with right sided pneumonia and septic shock. He was mechanically ventilated as he was hemodynamically unstable and severely tachypneic. Initial ABG was showing severe metabolic acidosis. Urine legionella antigen came as positive. Gradually pneumonia recovered after antibiotic course (azithromycin) and vasopressors were tapered off after 4 days. Oxygenation and ventilation parameters became stable

for weaning. Weaning was tried but failed for 2 consecutive days. Serum electrolytes sent showed: Mg^{+2} - 1.7 mEq/L, Na^+ -136 mEq per L, K^+ - 4.1 mEq per L, Phosphate - 0.7 mg per dL, Ionized Ca^{+2} -4.8 mg/dL
Regarding phosphate:
   a. Low phosphorus may be responsible for failed weaning
   b. IV Phosphate supplementation should be done in all patients with serum PO_4^{-3} less than 1.5 mg /dL
   c. Normal value of serum phosphate is 2.5-5.0 mg/dL
   d. Legionella infection is a risk factor for hypophosphatemia
   e. Azithromycin and metabolic acidosis are risk factors

8. Causes of metabolic alkalosis include:
   a. Liddle syndrome and Bartter syndrome
   b. Acetazolamide
   c. Ampicillin
   d. Licorice ingestion
   e. Linezolid

9. A 42-year-old lady is admitted to ICU with community acquired pneumonia with septic shock. She is having past medical history of diabetes and is on metformin 1000 mg daily. Her thyroid profile is having following findings: Low TSH (0.1 mU/mL, normal free T4 1.0 ng/dL, low T3 (40 ng/dL).
Which of the following statement is correct regarding the management of this patient?
   a. Supplement IV T3
   b. Supplement oral levothyroxine
   c. This profile of thyroid hormones can be due to sepsis
   d. No treatment is required
   e. Dopamine infusion is one of the causes

10. Regarding DKA:
    a. Occurs only in type 1 diabetes mellitus
    b. Potassium supplementation should be started if potassium level is below 5.5 mEq/L
    c. Detection of ketone in urine is necessary for the diagnosis
    d. Insulin infusion should always be preceded by bolus
    e. Cerebral edema is more common in adults

11. A 37-year-old male presented to emergency in state of shock. He is complaining of severe headache and double vision. Family is giving past history of pituitary adenoma and he is recently started on bromocriptine? Pituitary apoplexy is suspected.
    a. This condition is precipitated by bromocriptine
    b. MRI brain should be done in acute setting
    c. Treatment is neurosurgical intervention and steroids
    d. Meningeal signs are absent
    e. Long-term hormone replacement is usually not required

12. Anion gap is increased in:
    a. Severe hypophosphatemia
    b. Methanol poisoning
    c. Propylene glycol poisoning
    d. Diabetic ketoacidosis
    e. Respiratory and metabolic alkalosis

13. Antidiuretic hormone (ADH):
    a. Arginine vasopressin
    b. Produced in posterior pituitary
    c. Acts at proximal convoluted tubule and increases water reabsorption
    d. Acts at collecting duct decreases water absorption
    e. Acts at proximal convoluted tubule and increases water reabsorption

14. Pheochromocytomas:
    a. Arise from adrenals only
    b. Secrete mainly noradrenaline
    c. Are associated with MEN type 2
    d. In symptom control beta blockade should start before alpha blockade
    e. Onset of postural hypotension is a marker of optimum preoperative control

15. In Hyperosmolar Hyperglycemic State (HHS):
    a. Hyperglycemia is less marked than in DKA
    b. Thrombotic complications are rare
    c. Onset may be over several days
    d. Sr. osmolarity is usually > 320 mOsm/kg
    e. There is never any ketosis

16. Laboratory abnormalities seen in rhabdomyolysis include:
    a. Hypokalemia
    b. Hypophosphatemia
    c. Hyperkalemia
    d. Hypocalcemia
    e. Fraction excretion of sodium < 1%

17. Serotonin syndrome is characterized with:
    a. Autonomic hypoactivity
    b. Hyperreflexia
    c. Altered mental status

d. Can occur with linezolid therapy in ICU
e. Bromocriptine is drug of choice

18. **Contrast induced nephropathy (CIN):**
    a. Hypotension is a risk factor
    b. Low osmolarity contrast agents are safe then high osmolarity contrast agents
    c. FENa > 1%
    d. It is a common cause of pre renal failure
    e. Manifest in first 24 hrs

19. **Features of hepatorenal syndrome (HRS) include:**
    a. Pre-renal AKI
    b. Urine sodium> 10 mEq/L
    c. Urine osmolality < Plasma osmolality
    d. Proteinuria < 500 mg/dL
    e. Serum creatinine > 2.0 mg/dL

20. **Hartmaan's solution:**
    a. Sodium content is 142 mEq/L
    b. Chloride content is 130 mmol/L
    c. It contains 5 mEq/L potassium
    d. It does not have any calcium
    e. Osmolarity is 291 mOsmol/L

21. **A-a gradient in increased in:**
    a. Thromboembolism
    b. Low inspired oxygen
    c. Ventricular septal defect
    d. COPD
    e. TRALI

22. **Type 4 Renal tubular acidosis is characterized by:**
    a. Aldosterone excess
    b. Plasma bicarbonate level > 15 mEq/L
    c. Urine pH > 5.3
    d. Hypokalemia
    e. Urinary anion gap - positive

23. **Hypocalcemia in septic shock:**
    a. More common in gram-negative in comparison to gram- positive septicemia
    b. Is mediated by effect of procalcitonin
    c. Correction leads to improvement in hemodynamics
    d. Correction leads to better outcome
    e. Indication for IV replacement is symptomatic patient or ECG changes

24. **Clinically significant hypophosphatemia is relevant in following condition:**
    a. Continuous renal replacement therapy
    b. Total parenteral nutrition
    c. Chronic alcoholism
    d. Volume expansion
    e. Respiratory acidosis

ANSWER

A Type Answers

Q1. Answer b

This case may be secondary adrenal insufficiency. It may be because of two reasons: (1) Patient is an athlete and may be taking steroids. Sudden withdrawal of steroids can lead to adrenal insufficiency which is a life threatening emergency. Syncope attacks in past, hyponatremia and hyperkalemia also raise further suspicion. (2) Overtraining Syndrome (OS) - Running, or any aerobic training in moderation, has a positive effect on health. There is a point of diminishing returns, where chronic stress from overtraining, which is common in runners, may be linked to problems in the adrenal gland. OS has been linked with adrenal insufficiency. There is a direct link between stress and the adrenal glands, and the physical stress of overtraining may cause the hormones>produced in these glands to become depleted. OS has been described as chronic fatigue, burnout and staleness, where an imbalance between training/competition, versus recovery occurs. Training alone is seldom the primary cause. In most cases, the total amount of stress on the athlete exceeds their capacity to cope. A triggering stressful event, along with the chronic overtraining, pushes the athlete to start developing symptoms of overtraining syndrome, which is far worse than classic overtraining. Overtraining can be a part of healthy training, if only done for a short period of time. Chronic overtraining is what leads to serious health problems, including adrenal insufficiency. Severe overtraining over an extended period can result in adrenal depletion. An Addison-Type OS, where the adrenal glands are no longer able to maintain proper hormone levels and athletic performance is severely compromised has been described by researchers.

Brooks K, Carter J. Overtraining, Exercise, and Adrenal Insufficiency. J Nov Physiother. 2013;16(3):125.

Q2. Answer b

Base line sample of cortisol and ACTH should be taken and steroids should be started immediately. Hydrocortisone should be given initially because it is also having mineralocorticoid activity which may be needed in adrenal insufficiency. It should be switched to dexamethasone as it interferes with ACTH stimulation test (Should be done once patient becomes hemodynamically stable). However some physicians prefer to give dexamethasone initially and do ACTH stimulation test first. Empirical supplementation can be done in septic shock.

Savage MW, Mah PM, Weetman AP, Newell-Price J. Endocrine emergencies. Postgraduate Medfical Journal. 2003;80(947).

Q3. Answer d

Waterhouse-Friderichsen syndrome is most commonly occurs with meningococcal infection but can occur with other infections also e.g. *Streptococcus pneumoniae,* Staphylococcus *aureus, Hemophilus influenza,* β-hemolytic *streptococcus* group A. It is a highly fatal disease but does not carry 100% mortality. Disseminated intravascular coagulation is the phenomenon which leads to adrenal hemorrhage. It is treated with steroids along with treatment of underlying disease. Even if treatment is started early, mortality is very high.

Sonavane A, Baradkar V, Salunkhe P, et al. Waterhouse-Friderichsen syndrome in an adult patient with meningococcal meningitis. Indian J Dermatol; 2011;56(3):326-8.

Q4. Answer b

Above findings correlate with central diabetes insipidus. After desmopressin challenge, urine osmolality increased so cause of DI is central. Sheehan syndrome causes pituitary necrosis and is a consequence of PPH. Pancytopenia is common.

Shivaprasad C. Sheehan's syndrome: Newer advances. Indian J Endocrinol Metab. 2011;15(Suppl3): S203-S7.

Q5. Answer b

Clinician usually encounter problem when treating hyponatremia. Whether to restrict fluid or to supplement salt and water is most of the time a difficult decision. Both conditions are associated with intracranial pathology, urine Na>20 mEq/L, low serum uric acid and high fractional excretion of uric acid (>11%). Only difference is volume status. SIADH is a euvolumic state and CSW is hypovolemic. Assessment of volume status is most of the time difficult in ICU. Fractional excretion of urate after correction of sodium by 3% saline reduces FE(urate) to less than 11% in SIADH and remains same in case of CSW.

<small>Maesaka JK, Imbriano L, Mattana J, et al. Differentiating SIADH from Cerebral/Renal Salt Wasting: Failure of the Volume Approach and Need for a New Approach to Hyponatremia. J Clin Med. 2014;3(4):1373-85.</small>

Q6. Answer b

Sodium bicarbonate administration increases intracellular acidosis as CO_2 crosses cell membrane and bicarbonate cannot.

<small>Savage MW, Mah PM, Weetman AP, et al. Endocrine emergencies. Postgrad Med J. 2004;80:506-5.</small>

Q7. Answer c

Vasodilatation occurs in post-operative period which can lead to severe hypotension. 4-6 L saline administration may be required. Hypoglycemia occurs due to rebound hyperinsulinemia. Patients may land into adrenal insufficiency so steroid supplementation may be needed.

<small>Därr R, Lenders JW, Hofbauer LC, et al. Pheochromocytoma - update on disease management. Ther Adv Endocrinol Metab. 2012;3(1):11-26.</small>

Q8. Answer d

Refeeding syndrome occurs in severely malnourished patients after starting nutritional support. When carbohydrate introduced in these patients there is intracellular shift of phosphate, potassium and magnesium in cells leading to drop in serum level of these electrolytes. This syndrome is associated with hyperglycemia.

<small>Mehanna HM, Moledina J, Travis J. Refeeding syndrome: what it is, and how to prevent and treat it. BMJ. 2008;336(7659):1495-8.</small>

Q9. Answer d

Respiratory alkalosis (hyperventilation) causes hypophosphatemia due to intracellular shift. Volume expansion increases urinary excretion of phosphate.

<small>Weisinger J, Bellorín-Font E. Magnesium and phosphorus. The Lancet. 1998;352(9125):391-6.</small>

Q10. Answer e

Although septic shock and hemorrhagic shock cannot be ruled out but most probable diagnosis is ovarian hyperstimulation syndrome. Beta Human chorionic gonadotropin (hCG) and its analogue given in treatment of infertility are responsible for development of this syndrome.

<small>Kumar P, Sait SF, Sharma A, et al. Ovarian hyperstimulation syndrome. J Hum Reprod Sci. 2011;4(2):70-5.</small>

Q11. Answer d

Tumour lysis syndrome occurs usually after treatment of lymphomas and leukemias. It occurs due to lysis of tumor cells. Hypocalcemia occurs rather than hypercalcemia.

<small>Howard SC, Jones DP, Pui CH. The tumor lysis syndrome. N Engl J Med. 2011;364(19):1844-54.</small>

Q12. Answer b

The patient may be in thyroid storm. History of palpitations, widened pulse pressure and atrial fibrillation favors the diagnosis. Urinary tract infection is a precipitating event. Waiting for investigation can be fatal so treatment should be started on clinical grounds. Treatment options are Beta blockers, hydration, propylthiouracil, lugol's iodine and lithium with aggressive temperature control.

<small>Carroll R, Matfin G. Endocrine and metabolic emergencies: thyroid storm. Ther Adv Endocrinol Metab. 2010;1(3):139-45.</small>

Q13. Answer c

The pituitary gland sits in sella turcica, which is a saddle like compartment present at the base of the skull. When the pituitary gland shrinks or becomes flattened it cannot be seen on the MRI scan making it look like an empty sella. This is called as empty sella syndrome. It is a damaged pituitary gland, & look like as empty sella on scan.

<small>Aruna P, Sowjanya B. Partial Empty Sella Syndrome: A Case Report and Review. Indian J Clin Biochem. 2014;29(2):253-6.</small>

Q14. Answer e
Following drugs causes hypomagnesemia: (1) Proton pump inhibitors, (2) Amphotericin B, (3) Aminoglycosides, (4) Epinephrine, (5) Cyclosporine, (6) Cisplatin, (7) Pentamidine, (8) Loop and thiazide diuretics etc.

Panahi Y, Mojtahedzadeh M, Najafi A, et al. The role of magnesium sulfate in the intensive care unit. EXCLI J. 2017;16:464-82.

Q15. Answer c
Urinary chloride differentiates between chloride responsive and chloride resistant alkalosis. If urinary chloride is less than 15 mEq/L than it is chloride responsive and if >25 mEq/L than it is resistant. In this case chloride supplementation is required with normal saline. Acetazolamide is used in chloride resistant alkalosis. Hydrochloric acid infusion is used in case of emergency or if normal saline is contraindicated due to fluid overload.

Hennessey I, Japp A. Arterial Blood Gases Made Easy. Churchill Livingstone 1 edition (18 Sep 2007).

Q16. Answer e
Severe alkalosis can increase lactate in blood as activity of pH dependent enzymes in glycolytic pathway is increased. Diuretics do not cause rise in lactates.

Galla JH. Metabolic Alkalosis. J Am Soc Nephrol. 2000;11:369-75.

Q17. Answer e
It is a cation-exchange resin. It should be taken with glycerol and can be given orally as well as retention enema. It binds 0.65 mEq of potassium per gm of resin. It rarely can cause necrotic lesion in intestine.

Potassium. In: Marino's The ICU Book 4th edition, New Delhi, India; 2014.p.684

Q18. Answer e
Infusion of stress doses of hydrocortisone reduced the time to cessation of vasopressor therapy in human septic shock. This was associated with a trend to earlier resolution of sepsis-induced organ dysfunctions. Overall shock reversal and mortality were not significantly different between the groups in this low-sized single-center study. No mortality benefit.

Keh D, Trips E, Marx G et al. Effect of Hydrocortisone on Development of Shock Among Patients With Severe Sepsis. The HYPRESS Randomized Clinical Trial. JAMA. 2016;316(17):1775-85.

Q19. Answer c
Following are the findings in this patient: (1) High anion gap (23) so there is hidden acidosis despite normal HCO_3, (2) Respiratory alkalosis, (3) Normal osmolal gap. Normal osmolal gap rules out alcohol poisoning. Diabetic ketoacidosis is associated with only high anion gap metabolic acidosis. This case is having respiratory alkalosis with metabolic acidosis which is hallmark of salicylate poisoning. Patient may have overused analgesic. Fluid resuscitation and urine alkalinization is first line treatment. In severe poisoning dialysis may be required.

Dargan P, Wallace C, Jones A. An evidence based flowchart to guide the management of acute salicylate (aspirin) overdose. Emerg Med J. 2002;19(3):206-9.

Q20. Answer d
Although severe dehydration can lead to this clinical picture but tea colored urine should raise suspicion of rhabdomyolysis. Methanol poisoning is ruled out as there is normal osmolal gap (Calculated serum osmolality is 360). There is no history of tumor or chemotherapy so tumor lysis syndrome is ruled out although it can have similar presentation. Alcohol intake is one of the most common cause of rhabdomyolysis. Diabetic ketoacidosis is unlikely as there is normal anion gap and normal blood sugar.

Hunter JD, Gregg K, Damani Z. Rhabdomyolysis. Continuing Education in Anaesthesia Critical Care & Pain. 2006;6(4):141-3.

Q21. Answer e
Both prescribed medications and drugs of abuse have been implicated in rhabdomyolysis. Alcohol, heroin, cocaine, amphetamines, methadone, and D-lysergic acid diethylamide (LSD) have been implicated. Coma induced by alcohol, opioid overdose, or other central nervous system (CNS) depressants leads to immobilization

and ischemic compression of muscle. Some drugs, including statins and colchicine, are direct myotoxins. Statins can increase the risk of rhabdomyolysis in patients with other predisposing conditions, such as hypothyroidism or an inflammatory myopathy. Drug-induced agitation states, drug-induced seizures, dystonic reactions, and cocaine-induced hyperthermia are associated with excess muscle energy demands. Drug-drug interactions may be responsible for rhabdomyolysis in some individuals. The nature of the interactions varies. As an example, some drugs interfere with the clearance of statins and lead to elevated plasma levels; offending agents include macrolide antibiotics (e.g. erythromycin and clarithromycin), cyclosporine, gemfibrozil, and some protease inhibitors used in the treatment of HIV infection. In some individuals exposed to drugs, multiple mechanisms may contribute to muscle damage; as an example, rhabdomyolysis with alcoholic binges may result from a combination of hypokalemia, hypophosphatemia, coma, agitation, and direct muscle toxicity. Dietary supplements used for weight loss or enhanced physical performance, which typically contain multiple ingredients, may lead to rhabdomyolysis, possibly as a result of metabolic stress. Metabolic poisons, such as carbon monoxide, which lead to insufficient muscle energy production and snake venoms are also implicated. Mushroom poisoning and an unidentified toxin found in certain types of fish may cause rhabdomyolysis within 24 hours of ingestion.

Torres PA, Helmstetter JA, Kaye AM, et al. Rhabdomyolysis: Pathogenesis, Diagnosis, and Treatment. Ochsner J. 2015;15(1):58-69.

Q22. Answer d

Half-life of carboxyhemoglobin is 320 minutes on room air which reduces to 72 minutes after 100% oxygen therapy and to 23 minutes after hyperbaric oxygen therapy with 3 ATA (atmosphere).

Blumenthal I. Carbon monoxide poisoning. J R Soc Med. 2001;94(6):270-2.

Q23. Answer c

Van den berghe et al. in 2001 compared patients under intensive glycemic control and conventional therapy in surgical patients in ICU and showed mortality benefit in intensive group. In 2006, he took non-surgical patients and used same protocol and showed that patient on intensive sugar control did not show any overall mortality benefit even increased mortality in patients who stayed less than 3 days in ICU. NICE-SUGAR STUDY showed increased mortality in intensive group but trauma patients and patient on steroids showed mortality benefit in intensive group. Recommended target for blood sugar in ICU is less than 180 mg%.

N Engl J Med. 2001;345:1359-1367DOI: 10.1056/NEJMoa011

N Engl J Med. 2006;354:449-461DOI: 10.1056/NEJMoa052521

N Engl J Med. 2009;360:1283-1297DOI: 10.1056/NEJMoa0810625

Q24. Answer d

All above mentioned drugs causes hypoglycemia except salbutamol. Beta 2 agonist causes hyperglycemia.

Mukherjee E, Carroll R, Matfin G. Endocrine and metabolic emergencies: hypoglycaemia. Ther Adv Endocrinol Metab. 2011; 2(2):81-93.

Q25. Answer c

This patient is most likely having features of myxedema coma. Ischemic stroke is unlikely although it is common complication of atrial fibrillation as patient is having no focal neurological deficit and CT should pick up stroke after 4 days. There is no history of fever and signs of meningitis. Decreased level of consciousness, bradycardia, hypothermia and history of taking amiodarone all suggest hypothyroidism. Adrenal insufficiency is common with thyroid dysfunction so sending cortisol level is a wise decision.

Adrenal and Thyroid Dysfunction. In: Marino's The ICU Book 4th edition, New Delhi, India;2014. p. 895.

K Type Answers

Q1. Answer TTFFT

Although thyroid storm can precipitate high output heart failure but volume resuscitation is required to replace fluid losses. It is associated with relative adrenal insufficiency so replacement with hydrocortisone is recommended.

Adrenal and Thyroid Dysfunction. In: Marino's The ICU Book 4th edition, New Delhi, India; 2014. p.893-895.

Q2. Answer TFTTT

Decrease in 100 mEq total body potassium correlates with 0.3 mEq fall in serum potassium. Urine potassium >20 mEq/L suggest renal cause.

Asmar A, Mohandas R, Wingo CS. A physiologic-based approach to the treatment of a patient with hypokalemia. Am J Kidney Dis. 2012;60(3):492-7.

Q3. Answer TTFFF

Diarrhea and parenteral fluid therapy causes normal anion gap acidosis. Vomiting and Bartter syndrome causes metabolic alkalosis. Salicylate poisoning is associated with high anion gap metabolic acidosis.

Metabolic acidosis and alkalosis. In: Irwin & Rippe's Manual of intensive Care Medicine. 6th edition 2014. p.411-416.

Q4. Answer FFTFT

In diabetic ketoacidosis always resuscitate first before starting insulin. If insulin is started early then it leads to further dehydration. Disappearance of ketones and euglycemia is not the criteria to stop insulin infusion. Insulin should be stopped once anion gap closes. Normal saline should be replaced by 0.45% saline once sodium is normalized or hyperchloremia is developing.

Gosmanov AR, Gosmanova EO, Dillard-Cannon E. Management of adult diabetic ketoacidosis. Diabetes Metab Syndr Obes. 2014;7:255-64.

Q5. Answer FTFTF

If less than 50% of infused magnesium is recovered in urine than there is possibility of magnesium deficiency and if more than 80% magnesium is found in urine than it is unlikely. 24 hr urinary magnesium is measured. 6 gm of magnesium is infused over 1 hr. This test is not valid in renal failure patients.

Magnesium. In: Marino's The ICU Book 4th edition, New Delhi, India; 2014. p.693.

Q6. Answer FTTTF

Hypercalcemia is volume contracted state because of diuresis induced by it. Diuretics are now a days not recommended in treatment of hypercalcemia until and unless there is fluid overload. Calcitonin has rapid onset of action but tachyphylaxis is an issue. Glucocorticoids reduce this effect. Gallium nitrate and zolidronic acid both are nephrotoxic.

Richard Carroll and Glenn Matfin. Endocrine and metabolic emergencies: hypercalcaemia. Ther Adv Endocrinol Metab. 2010;1(5):225(234).

Q7. Answer TFTTF

Hypophosphatemia causes respiratory muscle weakness due to low energy phosphate availability. It should be supplemented by IV route when phosphate level is below 1.0 mg/dL. Normal value is 2.5–5.0 mg/dL. Legionella infection, aminoglycosides, diuretics, metabolic acidosis, respiratory alkalosis, antiretroviral drug, insulin are risk factors not azithromycin.

Pesta DH, Tsirigotis DN, Douglas E, et al. Hypophosphatemia promotes lower rates of muscle ATP synthesis. FASEB J. 2016;30(10):3378-87.

Q8. Answer TFTTF

Liddle syndrome, Bartter syndrome, ampicillin and licorice ingestion cause metabolic alkalosis. Acetazolamide is used in treatment of metabolic alkalosis. Linezolid is associated with lactic acidosis.

Galla JH. Metabolic Alkalosis. J Am Soc Nephrol. 2000;369-75.

Q9. Answer FFTTT

Above patient is having non thyroidal illness syndrome (NTIS). Sepsis, dopamine and corticosteroids suppresses TSH secretion. No treatment is usually required and thyroid profile becomes normal after recovery from critical illness.

Goldberg PA, Inzucchi SE. Critical issues in endocrinology. Clin Chest Med. 2003;24(4):583-606.

Q10. Answer FTFFF

DKA is more common with type 1 diabetes mellitus but can occur in type 2 also. Potassium supplementation should be done whenever K level goes below 5.5 mEq/L. Initial urinary ketone may be 3-hydroxybutyric acid which is not detected by ketostix. Insulin bolus is not necessary. Cerebral edema is more common in children.

Savage MW, Mah PM, Weetman AP, et al. Endocrine emergencies. Postgraduate Medfical Journal. 2003;80(947).

Q11. Answer TFTFF

Pituitary apoplexy is precipitated by head injury, bromocriptine, diabetes, dialysis and radiation therapy. CT head should be done in acute settings. Clinical features include headache, meningeal signs and ocular palsies. It is associated with cortisol and thyroid hormone deficiency so hormone replacement and immediate surgical decompression is the treatment.

Goldberg PA, Inzucchi SE. Critical issues in endocrinology. Clin Chest Med. 2003;24(4):583-606.

Q12. Answer FTFTT

High anion gap can be present in methanol poisoning, hyperphosphatemia, diabetic ketoacidosis. It can also be present with respiratory and metabolic alkalosis. Propylene glycol poisoning is associated with normal anion gap. Osmolal gap will be increased in this poisoning.

Lee S, Kang KP, Kang SK. Clinical usefulness of the serum anion gap. Electrolyte Blood Press. 2006;4(1):44-6.

Q13. Answer TFFFT

ADH is arginine vasopressin. It is produced in hypothalamus and stored and secreted from posterior pituitary. Its primary action is on collecting duct and leads to water reabsorption. It also increases water reabsorption from distal convoluted tubule.

Sawyer WH. Evolution of antidiuretic hormones and their functions. 1967;42(5):678-86.

Q14. Answer FTTFT

Pheochromocytomas are rare endocrine tumors that can present insidiously and remain undiagnosed until death or onset of clear manifestations of catecholamine excess. They are often referred to as one of the 'great mimics' in medicine. These tumors are heterogeneous group of chromaffin cell neoplasms with different ages of onset, secretory profiles, locations, and potential for malignancy according to underlying genetic mutations. These aspects all have to be considered when the tumor is encountered, thereby enabling optimal management for the patient. This is not only important for surgical management of patients, but also for post-surgical follow-up and screening of disease in patients with a hereditary predisposition to the tumor. While preoperative management has changed little over the last 20 years, surgical procedures have evolved so that laparoscopic resection is the standard of care and partial adrenalectomy should be considered in all patients with a hereditary condition. Follow-up testing is essential and should be recommended and ensured on a yearly basis. Patients and family members with identified mutations then require an individualized approach to management. This includes consideration of distinct patterns of biochemical test results during screening and the appropriate choice of imaging studies for tumor localization according to the mutation and associated differences in predisposition to adrenal, extra-adrenal and metastatic disease.

Därr R, Lenders JW, Hofbauer LC, et al. Pheochromocytoma - update on disease management. Ther Adv Endocrinol Metab. 2012;3(1):11-26.

Q15. Answer FFTTF

HHS is a complication of diabetes mellitus in which high blood sugar results in high osmolarity without significant ketoacidosis. Symptoms include signs of dehydration, weakness, legs cramps, trouble seeing, and an altered level of consciousness. Onset is typically over days to weeks. Diagnosis is based on blood tests finding a blood sugar greater than 30 mmol/L (600 mg/dL), osmolarity greater than 320 mOsm/kg, and a pH above 7.3. Hyperglycemia is more marked than DKA. Arterial thromboembolic events, such as myocardial infarction, cerebrovascular accidents and peripheral and mesenteric arterial thrombosis, occur frequently in HHS. The higher circulating ratio of insulin/glucagon in patients with HHS prevents ketogenesis and the development of ketoacidosis. The term hyperglycemic hyperosmolar nonketotic coma (HHNK) was replaced with "hyperglycemic hyperosmolar state" to reflect the fact that many patients present without significant decline in the level of consciousness (less than one-third of patients present with coma) and because many patients can present with mild to moderate degrees of ketosis. In some studies, up to 20% of patients with severe hyperglycemia and hyperosmolarity were reported to have combined features of HHS and DKA.

Savage MW, Mah PM, Weetman AP, et al. Endocrine emergencies. Postgraduate Medfical Journal. 2003;80:947.

Q16. Answer 16. FFTTT

Rhabdomyolysis causes Hyperkalemia, Hyperphosphatemia, Hypocalcemia, Hyperuricemia, FENa < 1%.

Keltz E, Khan FY, Mann G. Rhabdomyolysis. The role of diagnostic and prognostic factors. Muscles Ligaments Tendons J. 2013;3(4):303-12.

Q17. Answer FTTTF

Serotonin syndrome is characterized by- altered mental status, autonomic hyperactivity and neuromuscular abnormalities. It is precipitated by factors that interferers with serotonergic pathways like SSRIs, MAO inhibitors, linezolid and meperidine. Treatment of the condition is benzodiazepine, short acting beta blockers and cyproheptadine. Bromocriptine is drug of choice for neuroleptic malignant syndrome.

Volpi-Abadie J, Kaye AM, Kaye AD. Serotonin syndrome. Ochsner J. 2013;13(4):533-40.

Q18. Answer TTFFF

IV contrast causes acute tubular necrosis (Renal AKI) not pre renal AKI. Low osmolarity contrast are more safe. Usually in renal AKI, FENa is > 1% but in CIN FENa is less than 1%. It manifests 3–5 days after exposure of radio-contrast agents.

Kollen M, Isakow W, Acute Kidney Injury, The Washington Manual of Critical Care, second edition,china. 2012. p 358-59.

Q19. Answer TFFTF

Diagnostic criteria of HRS:

Major Criteria:
  i. Advanced hepatic failure and portal hypertension.
  ii. Serum creatinine > 1.5 mg/dL or 24 hr creatinine clearance < 40 mL/min.
  iii. Absence of shock, bacterial infection and current or recent use of nephrotoxic drugs
  iv. No sustained improvement in renal function following diuretic withdrawal and expansion of plasma volume with 1.5 L of isotonic saline.
  v. Proteinuria < 500 mg/dL

Additional Criteria:
  i. Urine volume < 500 mL/day.
  ii. Urinary sodium < 10 mEq/L.
  iii. Urinary osmolality greater than plasma osmolality.
  iv. Urine red blood cells < 50 per hpf.
  v. Serum sodium < 130 mEq/L.

Low G, Alexander GJM, Lomas DJ. Hepatorenal Syndrome: Aetiology, Diagnosis, and Treatment. Gastroenterology Research and Practice. 2015; Article ID 207012.

Q20. Answer FFFFF

Hartmann solution contains:
Na^+ - 130 mEq/L
Chloride - 109 mEq /L
K^+ - 4 mEq /L
Magnesium - 0
Calcium – 2.17 mEq/L
Buffer-28 mmol/L

Osmolarity-273 mOsmol/L

Osmolality-254 mOsmol/Kg

Severs D. Hoorn EJ. Rookmaaker MB. A critical appraisal of intravenous fluids: from the physiological basis to clinical evidence. Nephrology Dialysis Transplantation. 2015;30(2):178-87.

Q21. Answer TFTTT

A-a gradient is increased in all of the above options except low inspired oxygen. A-a gradient remains normal at high altitude and low FiO_2.

Sarkar M, Niranjan N, Banyal PK. Mechanisms of hypoxemia. 2017;34(1):47-60.

Q22. Answer FTFFT

Type 4 renal tubular acidosis (RTA) occurs due to aldosterone excess. Plasma bicarbonate is more than 15 mEq/L. Potassium level is < 5.3 mEq/L and plasma potassium always high. Urinary anion gap is positive in type 1 and type 4 RTA.

Rodríguez-Soriano J, Vallo A. Renal tubular acidosis. Pediatr Nephrol. 1990;4(3):268-75.

Q23. Answer TTTFT

Hypocalcemia in septic shock is more common in gram-negative in comparison to gram- positive septicemia. Hypocalcemia during sepsis occurred in previously normocalcemic patients and was multifactorial in origin, resulting from acquired parathyroid gland insufficiency, renal 1 alpha-hydroxylase insufficiency, vitamin D deficiency, and acquired calcitriol resistance. It is mediated is also mediated by the effect of procalcitonin. Correction leads to improvement in hemodynamics. Indication for IV replacement is symptomatic patient or ECG changes but its correction does not lead to better outcome.

Baruscotti M, Bucchi A, Difrancesco D. Physiology and pharmacology of the cardiac pacemaker ("funny") current. Pharmacol Ther. 2005;107(1):59-79.

Q24. Answer TTTTF

Hypophosphatemia is commonly missed due to nonspecific signs and symptoms, but it causes considerable morbidity and in some cases contributes to mortality. Three primary mechanisms of hypophosphatemia exist: increased renal excretion, decreased intestinal absorption, and shifts from the extracellular to intracellular compartments. Renal hypophosphatemia can be further divided into fibroblast growth factor 23-mediated or non-fibroblast growth factor 23-mediated causes. Proper diagnosis requires a thorough medication history, family history, physical examination, and assessment of renal tubular phosphate handling to identify the cause. During the past decade, our understanding of phosphate metabolism has grown greatly through the study of rare disorders of phosphate homeostasis. Treatment of hypophosphatemia depends on the underlying disorder and requires close biochemical monitoring.

Imel EA, Econs MJ. Approach to the hypophosphatemic patient. J Clin Endocrinol Metab. 2012;97(3):696-706.

CHAPTER 9

Oncology

Vijaya Patil, Amol Kothekar, Jacob George

A Type Questions
(One best answer)

1. **Drugs used in management of hypercalcemia include all of the following *except*:**
   a. Steroids
   b. Diuretics like thiazides and amiloride
   c. Calcitonin
   d. Zoledronic acid
   e. Loop diuretics

2. **Diagnostic criteria of syndrome of inappropriate antidiuretic hormone secretion (SIADH) include all of the following *except*:**
   a. Decreased serum osmolality of less than 275 mOsm/kg
   b. Increased urinary osmolality of more than 100 mOsm/kg of water
   c. Fe Na > 40%
   d. Serum uric acid less than 4 mg/dL
   e. Correction of hyponatremia by fluid restriction

3. **A 68-year-old female, known case of carcinoma of breast, is receiving cyclophosphamide based chemotherapy. After the first cycle of chemotherapy, she is brought to the casualty with complaints of loose motions, increased somnolence, and lethargy since midnight. In casualty on examination, her heart rate is 88/min, BP 110/76 mm Hg, and respiratory rate is 14/min. GCS is E2M5V2. Pupils are bilaterally equal in size and reacting to light. In casualty, she suddenly developed a seizure that lasted for 2 minutes. Lab reports showed glucose of 110, serum sodium of 118, and urea of 33.** Which of the following steps represent further adequate management?
   a. Immediate correction of serum sodium to 135 mEq/dL
   b. Mannitol 20% 100–150 mL to reduce cerebral oedema immediately
   c. 2 mL/kg of 3% saline over 20 minutes immediately
   d. Immediate intubation under rapid sequence induction (RSI) followed by emergency CT scan of brain
   e. Normal Saline 100 mL/ hour for 6 hours

4. **According to Bishop Cairo classification, all are features of clinical Tumor Lysis Syndrome (TLS) *except*:**
   a. Renal insufficiency
   b. Cardiac arrhythmia
   c. Elevated Potassium ≥ 7.0 mEq/L or 50% increase from baseline
   d. Seizure
   e. Sudden death

5. **A 50-year-old male presented with testicular mass and abdominal nodes. He underwent an orchidectomy with retro peritoneal lymph node dissection. Post-op the resident noted that the drains placed began to drain at 70 mL/hr resulting in over 1.5 liter of output in 24 hours. Which of the following describes the correct management in this patient?**
   a. Octreotide 100 μg thrice daily
   b. Do a thromboelastogram and replace FFP and cryoprecipitate accordingly
   c. Keep the patient NPO and initiate discussion for total parenteral nutrition (TPN)

d. Resuscitate the patient with blood, plasma and platelets in ratio of 1:1:1 for the fluid lost

6. A 46-year-old female, a known case of periampullary carcinoma underwent Whipple's surgery. Pre-operatively she had poor oral intake for almost 3 months duration and gives history of weight loss of 18 kg. Post-surgery she was initiated on full nasojejunal feeds by POD3. After 2 days, she is found to be hypothermic, disoriented and drowsy. Her lab reports are positive for hypokalemia, hypomagnesemia and hypophosphatemia. Her blood sugars are also elevated (300 mg/dL) though she was non diabetic. Which of the following statements are true?
    a. The patient is probably septic and requires fluid resuscitation @ 30 mL/kg
    b. Insulin infusion needs to be started immediately as symptoms may be due to elevated sugars
    c. Haloperidol can be used to treat the disorientation
    d. Urgent administration of vitamin B1
    e. Start parenteral nutrition @40 mL/hr

7. A 65-year-old male, diagnosed as metastatic small cell carcinoma of the lung on palliative chemotherapy - presents with acute onset fever [temperature 103°F (39.4°C)], nonproductive cough and dyspnea. There is no history of vomiting or diarrhea. Chest X-ray shows a left lower zone consolidation. Lab reports are positive for absolute neutrophil count (ANC) of 450. Which of the following best describes appropriate management in this case?
    a. Meropenem and amikacin - for double GNB coverage
    b. Empiric Amphotericin B alone
    c. Meropenem as single agent after blood cultures
    d. Urgent removal of all invasive lines
    e. Meropenem and caspofungin

8. A 40-year-old male, known case of hepatoblastoma undergoing excision suffered an injury to inferior vena cava (IVC) intra-operatively. He started to bleed profusely and required 14 packed cells, and 16 FFP along with 8 Cryoprecipitate intra-operatively along with crystalloids and colloids. The raw area from liver continued to ooze and hence the abdomen was packed, and he was shifted to ICU for further management.

In the ICU, he was having a temperature of 33-degree, heart rate of 156, MAP of 65 on 0.3 µg/kg/min of noradrenaline. Urine output was 15 mL/hr. Drainage continued to be high and it was decided to administer factor 7. Which of the following is most appropriate?
    a. Hypothermia should be corrected prior administering factor 7
    b. The resuscitation should be ongoing, replacing PC FFP and Plc in ratio of 1:1:5
    c. Factor 7 has proven role in arresting post-operative bleeding in liver surgery
    d. Factor 7 should be repeated in multiple doses every 30 minutes till the bleeding is stopped.
    a. Recombinant factor VIIa should be avoided in blunt trauma

9. A 58-year-old female, with no other comorbid illness is posted for pylorus preserving pancreato-duodenectomy. Intra-operatively the mass was adherent to the spleen necessitating splenectomy.

Suggestion for vaccination with pneumococcal vaccine - the best option is:
    a. Administering vaccine intra-op immediately
    b. Administering vaccine in immediate post-op period
    c. Administering vaccines after 2-3 weeks of surgery
    d. No need of vaccination as she is immunocompetent with no comorbidities
    e. Administering vaccines after 3-6 months of surgery

10. A 65-year-old female, post-operative case of subtotal thyroidectomy is shifted to the recovery with complaints of agitation and hypertension on emergence. The ICU registrar after complete examination arrived at a diagnosis of emergence delirium, and administered 5 mg of haloperidol. Overnight she was stable though she required one more dose of haloperidol for delirium. She was shifted to the ward the next day as was relatively better. 3 days later, a reference was sent to the ICU to assess the patient with fever. On examination patient is drowsy, responding to pain. Pupils equal and reacting to light. No

focal neurological deficit. She is shivering, febrile (T-105°F) hypertensive (MAP 110 mm Hg) and having a HR 140/min and muscular rigidity. The ward registrar recorded history of mild fever for the past 2 days that did not respond to acetaminophen. She was on amox–clav injection and her blood and urine cultures of last 2 days have been sterile. A procalcitonin sent over past 3 days have been consistently less than 0.15. The surgical site seemed satisfactory with no erythema. The best management in this case will be:
   a. Administer 5 mg haloperidol IV as she had responded prior to it
   b. Hike up the antibiotics empirically to Meropenem and Vancomycin
   c. Dantrolene 2.5 mg/kg IV immediately, intubate and shift to ICU
   d. Urgent iv Midazolam followed by enteral Bromocriptine, shift to ICU for observation
   e. Continue same treatment under monitoring in the ICU

11. An 8-year-old child – known case of acute lymphoblastic leukemia (ALL) on chemotherapy presented with fever, altered sensorium and hypotension. He is neutropenic (ANC 50) and is already on meropenem and Vancomycin for 3 days. Blood culture taken immediately after ICU admission was positive for Candida albicans. CSF analysis shows no cells with low sugars and elevated proteins. Regarding further management which of the following is correct?
   a. Candida meningitis is unlikely in view of absence of any cells on CSF
   b. Echinocandins are the preferred agent in view of suspected meningitis and hypotension
   c. Fluconazole crosses blood brain barrier poorly and hence intrathecal fluconazole might be needed for disease eradication
   d. Amphotericin B + Flucytosine is the recommended treatment for this child

12. Which of the following is not a feature of acute graft versus host disease (GVHD)?
   a. Painful rash
   b. Bloody diarrhea
   c. Upper GI bleed
   d. Hemorrhagic conjunctivitis
   e. Keratoconjunctivitis sicca

13. Regarding radiation recall all are true *except*:
   a. It is also known as radiosensitization
   b. Is an acute inflammatory reaction confined to previously irradiated areas that can be triggered when chemotherapy agents are administered after radiotherapy
   c. Most commonly reported with doxorubicin, taxanes, and the antimetabolites like gemcitabine and capecitabine
   d. Drugs like, antituberculosis drugs, and simvastatin can also cause radiation recall
   e. It can occur months or even many years after irradiation

14. A 62-year-old male operated for total esophagectomy was shifted to the ICU on 4th post-operative day with complaints of tachypnea and tachycardia. His BP was 160/70 mm Hg, ECG showed atrial fibrillation (AF) with fast ventricular rate and had bilateral rhonchi. Which of the following statements is correct?
   a. Start patient on inhaled steroids as B2 agonists may cause further tachycardia
   b. Start IV Amiodarone and give trial of NIV for respiratory failure
   c. Intubate the patient and get urgent bedside endoscopy and contrast CT chest done as patient is most likely to have mediastinitis following anastomotic leak
   d. Get urgent cardiology reference as this might be acute coronary syndrome
   e. One can use bedside contrast X-ray to look for anastomotic leak instead of CT scan

15. A 42-year-old male was readmitted to ICU on 3rd postop day after retroperitoneal lymph node dissection surgery with hypotension and tachycardia. His abdominal drain output was 400 mL and 270 mL on first 2 postop days and had increased to 1200 mL on third day when the patient was allowed oral diet. All the following statements are true *except*:
   a. Patient is likely to have chylous ascites
   b. The presence of chylomicrons and a triglyceride level > 110 mg% confirm the diagnosis of a chylous leak
   c. Chyle generally has pH <7.3
   d. High-volume leakage (>1000 mL/day) should be aggressively treated either surgically or with interventional radiology
   e. One can use octreotide as an adjunct to reduce chyle production

16. A 22-year-old male who presented with right inguinal lymphadenopathy was diagnosed to have Hodgkin's lymphoma. He was started on ABVD regimen (Adriamycin, Bleomycin, Vincristine, Dacarbazine). Two weeks after 4th cycle of chemotherapy patient presented with complaints of progressive exertional dyspnea and dry cough. Which of the following statements is not true as regards to bleomycin induced pulmonary toxicity?
    a. Repeated systemic administration of bleomycin and total cumulative dose more than 450 units are risk factors associated with bleomycin induced lung fibrosis
    b. Decrease in DLCO is one of the earliest manifestations of bleomycin lung toxicity
    c. Lung specimens from subjects with bleomycin-induced lung injury typically demonstrate subpleural lung injury and fibrosis
    d. Thoracic irradiation increases the risk of bleomycin-induced lung toxicity
    e. Younger patients are more prone for bleomycin induced toxicity

17. A 56-year-old lady known operated case of papillary Ca Thyroid presented to hospital with 4 weeks history of backache unresponsive to paracetamol and Diclofenac. On examination there was localised tenderness in L1, L2 region but otherwise back appeared normal. She was advised to get MRI spine done. 1 week later patient presented with weakness of both lower limbs and inability to stand. Which is correct statement?
    a. Thyroid carcinoma is most common cause for malignant spinal cord compression (MSCC)
    b. Sensory loss is commonest presentation of MSCC
    c. Radiotherapy is always better option for these patients than surgery
    d. Mechanism of MSCC is same in adults and children
    e. MSCC may be an initial manifestation of cancer

18. A 32-year-old girl weighing 60 kgs, diagnosed case of pituitary adenoma underwent hypophysectomy. She had significant blood loss and hemodynamic instability. She received 4.5 L of crystalloid, 3 units of blood and 1 L of colloid during intraoperative period. 4 hours postoperatively her urine output increased to 200–250 mL/hr which persisted for more than 4 hours. Patient remained hemodynamically stable. Correct management options would be:
    a. Give IV/intranasal desmopressin
    b. Monitoring S. electrolytes and treating only if S Na is >145 mEq/L
    c. Replacing each hours loss in next hour with use of 0.33% saline
    d. Use Desmopressin if urine osmolality is < 300 mOsm/kg

19. A 54-year-old averagely built male presented to casualty with complaints of loose motions and vomiting of 3 days duration and breathlessness of 1 day. In casualty patient was found to be drowsy, pulse rate of 86/min, regular and BP of 70/40 mm Hg. He was shifted to ICU with diagnosis of hypovolemic shock/GI sepsis. His past history revealed he was case of Ca larynx and had undergone concurrent chemo radiation 4 years prior. His disease responded well and was disease free. In ICU patient was intubated in view of GCS of 10, was fluid resuscitated with 3 lit of 0.9% NS and was started on noradrenaline to get MAP above 65 mm Hg. Patients hemodynamics stabilized with next 8 hours and was off noradrenaline. He was maintaining good oxygenation on minimum ventilatory support. However patient continued to be drowsy responding only to deep painful stimuli. His S. electrolytes were normal except low S Na (118 mEq/L). What amongst following is most relevant investigation?
    a. CT/MRI brain
    b. S. Cortisol levels
    c. S. Ammonia level
    d. Thyroid function tests
    e. CSF studies

20. A 42-year-old female was admitted to ICU with c/o perioral twitching and carpopedal spasm 36 hours after undergoing total thyroidectomy for papillary Carcinoma Thyroid. Regarding hypocalcemia management the correct strategy is:
    a. Calcium gluconate is preferred over calcium chloride because it causes less tissue necrosis if extravasated
    b. All post-thyroid surgery hypocalcemic patients should be treated with IV calcium

c. Acute symptomatic hypocalcemia should receive 50 mg elemental calcium every 6 hours
d. Presence of preoperative Vitamin D deficiency increases risk of postop hypocalcemia

21. A 45-year-old lady with breast cancer presented to Emergency Department with complaints of fever for one week after receiving chemotherapy. On examination, she was hemodynamically stable and her temperature was 39.5°C. There was no evidence of mucositis. Central line insertion site looked clean. Which of the following is most appropriate choice of initial antibiotics?
    a. Cefepime
    b. Meropenem plus Vancomycin
    c. Cefepime plus Aminoglycoside
    d. Cefepime plus Vancomycin
    e. Meropenem plus Caspofungin

22. A 45-year-old lady with breast cancer was admitted to ICU with febrile neutropenia and hypotension not responding to fluid boluses. On admission to ICU she had received meropenem and vancomycin. She required noradrenaline only for short duration of 6 hours. On third day of ICU admission when she was ready to be discharged to the ward, she was afebrile but continued to be neutropenic. What should be next course of management regarding her empiric antibiotic therapy?
    a. Discontinue after negative blood culture
    b. Discontinue after 48 to 72 hours after the last fever
    c. Continue for a total of 7 days
    d. De-escalate, and continue antibiotic therapy till resolution of neutropenia

23. A patient with AML and prolonged neutropenia, with fever and cough, was started on piperacillin+tazobectum, teicoplanin and fluconazole. Patient is hemodynamically stable but with PF ratio of 170. His CT chest after 48 hours showed bilateral lung consolidation and has positive serum galactomannan. Which one is most appropriate step?
    a. Change to voriconazole
    b. Do not act on S Galactomannan as it may be falsely positive
    c. Escalate to caspofungin
    d. Send for BAL fungal culture and cytology and based on results add voriconazole
    e. Start patient on Amphotericin-B

24. Which of the following patient require Prophylaxis against invasive Aspergillus infections?
    a. Acute myeloid leukaemia (AML)
    b. Non-Hodgkin's lymphoma
    c. Carcinoma breast
    d. Acute LL

25. A 29-year-old female with AML on induction chemotherapy presents with febrile neutropenia and hypotension to ICU. She has a PICC line in situ and Central Line Associated Blood Stream Infection (CLABSI) is suspected. She receives broad spectrum antibiotics after paired blood culture. Removal of catheter is recommended in which of the following organism:
    a. Staphylococcus aureus
    b. Pseudomonas aeruginosa
    c. Fungi
    d. All of the above
    e. None of the above

26. A 45-year-old male is admitted to ICU with cough, dyspnea and facial swelling and cervical lymphadenopathy. X-ray chest shows widening of superior mediastinum and no pleural effusion. There is no prior history of insertion of central line. Patient is intubated and ventilated. Most appropriate step in disease management would be:
    a. Supraclavicular lymph node biopsy
    b. Thoracotomy and excision of mediastinal mass
    c. Temporizing emergency mediastinal irradiation
    d. Cyclophosphamide and steroids

27. In above patient, which of the following diagnosis is MOST UNLIKELY?
    a. Small cell lung cancer (SCLC)
    b. Diffuse large cell lymphoma
    c. Lymphoblastic lymphoma
    d. Hodgkin's lymphoma
    e. None of the above

28. Which of the following is true regarding pleural effusion in cancer patients?
    a. Malignant pleural effusion (MPE) in a solid tumor indicates advanced disease

b. Pleural fluid cytology is highly accurate in diagnosis
c. Re-expansion pulmonary (RPE) edema is very common and fluid more than 500 ml should not be drained
d. All of the above

29. Coronary vasospasm is seen with which of the following drug?
    a. Epirubicin
    b. Bleomycin
    c. Cyclophosphamide
    d. Capecitabine

30. A 45-year-old male with no past history of cancer presents to the Emergency Department with acute onset of loss of power of both lower limbs with bladder and bowel involvement. MRI shows evidence of Metastatic Spinal Cord Compression (MSCC). Which of the following is MOST UNLIKELY cause?
    a. Small-cell carcinoma of Lung
    b. Non-Hodgkin's lymphoma
    c. Myeloma
    d. Colon cancer

31. A 20-year-old male, with acute promyelocytic leukemia (APL), presents to ICU with fever, hypotension, dyspnea, and pulmonary infiltrates in chest radiograph. Regarding APML, which of the following is true?
    a. Differentiation syndrome is quiet common and can affect up to 25% of patients with APL
    b. Steroids are not effective for treatment of Differentiation syndrome
    c. Patients with presentation WBC more than 10,000/mcL have better prognosis
    d. None of the above

32. In which of the cancer, vasculitis is generally NOT observed?
    a. Small cell carcinoma of lung
    b. Squamous cell carcinoma of esophagus
    c. Prostate cancer
    d. Hairy cell leukemia

33. Which of the malignance is not associated with thromboembolic events?
    a. Ovary
    b. Pancreas
    c. Liver
    d. Acute promyelocytic leukemia (APML)

34. A 23-year-old lady with Gestational trophoblastic neoplasms (GTNs) with pulmonary metastasis is admitted to ICU with respiratory failure. Which of the following statements are true?
    a. GTNs with pulmonary metastasis has poor prognosis due to low cure rates
    b. Liver and spleen are most common sites of metastasis
    c. Patients with liver, brain, kidney, gastrointestinal tract, and spleen metastasis have highest risk of death
    d. All of the above

35. Which of the following drug is not commonly associated with veno-occlusive disease (VOD) of the liver?
    a. Gemtuzumab ozogamicin
    b. Dactinomycin
    c. Oral busulfan
    d. Defibrotide

36. A 14-year-old boy with acute lymphocytic leukemia (ALL) with febrile neutropenia and pneumonia is admitted to ICU. He has received L-asparaginase. Which of the following is not a common toxicity of L-asparaginase?
    a. Bleeding
    b. Thromboembolic events
    c. Acute pancreatitis
    d. Myelosuppression

37. Which of the following is correct statement regarding Multinational Association for Supportive Care in Cancer Risk-Index Score (MASCC)?
    a. Higher the score, greater is risk of complications
    b. Outpatient status denote lower risk
    c. Age > 60 years denote lower risk
    d. Presence of diabetes mellitus indicate greater risk
    e. All statements are correct

38. A 62-year-old known case of carcinoma breast, treated with neo adjuvant chemotherapy underwent surgery. Her tumor was positive for estrogen and progesterone receptors and negative for Herceptin2 receptors. She came back with recurrence after 2 years for which she was receiving gemcitabine and docetaxel. At the end of 3rd cycle patient presented to emergency department with fever, diarrhea

and breathlessness. On examination patient was drowsy responding to painful stimuli, hypotensive with systolic BP of 65 mm Hg, pulse rate of 132/min, regular, tachypnic with respiratory rate of 42/min, and febrile (T 103°F). On examination patient had grade 3 mucositis. Her WBC count showed severe neutropenia (ANC- 0.12/cm^2). You have been called to decide for further plan and transfer to ICU. Which is the best strategy?
   a. This patient should not be admitted to ICU as she is metastatic and in neutropenic septic and triaged to palliative care ward
   b. Admitted to ICU but should not be for aggressive management
   c. Should be treated aggressively for first 24 hours and if does not respond initiate end of life discussion with family
   d. Should be admitted to ICU for ICU trial with aggressive management for 3–5 days
   e. Relatives should be counselled to take her home

39. A 4-year-old child diagnosed case of ALL undergoing induction chemotherapy with L Asperginase, vincristine and dexamethasone presented to ICU with generalised tonic clonic seizures for which he received IV midazolam and levetiracetam in the ward. He is neutropenic with ANC count of 0.03/cm^2, and platelets 92,000/cm^2. On admission to ICU child was drowsy (E1V1M5), pupils bilaterally equal responding to light, moving all 4 limbs, had HR of 124/min, regular, and BP 140/96 mm Hg. He has unobstructed breathing at the rate of 20/min. Mother gave history that child was continuously crying and complaining of intermittent severe headache for last 8 hours. Oncologist got his CT head done 4 hours prior to rule out intracranial bleed which was negative. What would be your priority at this point?
   a. Immediate intubation and mechanical ventilation
   b. CSF studies to look for meningitis
   c. Continuous EEG monitoring
   d. Control of blood pressure followed by MRI
   e. Repeat CT head

40. Multinational Association of Supportive Care in Cancer (MASCC) is used for:
   a. To decide on end of life care
   b. To decide on fitness for chemotherapy or surgery
   c. To identify those suitable febrile neutropenic patients for outpatient antibiotic therapy
   d. None of these

41. A 38-year-old female a case of AML–M2 on induction chemotherapy presented with fever and abdominal pain of 5 days duration. She was initially managed at local hospital with Meropenem and Amikacin. However, as fever persisted, she was referred to main centre. On examination, she is toxic, HR 156/min, MAP 64 mm Hg and RR of 30. Clinical examination is positive for mucositis, oral lesions suggestive of candidiasis and hepatosplenomegaly. Lab reports were suggestive of neutropenia and elevated alkaline phosphatase. Blood cultures are negative. CT abdomen demonstrated multiple focal lesions in liver and spleen, occasionally with peripheral enhancement. Most likely diagnosis would be:
   a. Hydatid disease
   b. Hepatosplenic candidiasis
   c. Malaria
   d. Disease progression

42. A 50-year-old male, recipient of HSCT 4 days prior was shifted to ICU with temperature of 38.3°C, erythrodermic rash involving face, trunk and upper limb and progressive dyspnoea of 2 days duration. He was drowsy but arousable, tachypnoeic with RR of 30/min, maintaining saturation on room air of 98%. His WBC count is 9,000/cm^2, Chest X-ray showed diffuse bilateral pulmonary infiltrates. Lab showed mild transaminitis. Which of the following would fit the description of the current condition?
   a. GVHD
   b. Cardiogenic pulmonary edema
   c. Engraftment syndrome
   d. Ventilator associated pneumonia

43. A 58-year-old female, known case of mucinous carcinoma of ovary, presented to the casualty with breathing difficulty of 3 hours duration. On examination, she has a heart rate of 140/min, regular and low volume, BP 106/50 mm Hg, respiratory rate 30/min and the entire right lower limb is swollen and tender. Chest is clear to auscultation with no evidence of

pleural effusion, rhonchi or consolidation. Which of the following investigations aid in diagnosis of pulmonary embolism in the emergency department?
   a. Compression ultrasound of lower limb
   b. High sensitivity D dimer assay
   c. CT pulmonary angiography
   d. Bedside ECHO

44. A 76-year-old female, known case of esophageal adenocarcinoma, presented to the casualty with acute onset of breathing difficulty of 1 hour duration. On examination, she has a heart rate of 156/min, regular and low volume, BP 76/50, respiratory rate 35/min. Chest is clear to auscultation. Which of the following scoring systems accurately predict the risk of pulmonary embolism (PE) in malignancy patients?
   a. Modified Geneva score
   b. Modified Wells score
   c. Ramsay score
   d. Khorana score

45. A 72-year-old male, known case of sacral chordoma, underwent excision surgery with VY plasty. Postop he was started on UFH 5000 units twice daily as DVT prophylaxis. On postop day 4, despite being on heparin prophylaxis, he developed DVT of the left lower limb. Routine investigations were normal, except for a mild thrombocytopenia (Platelets 100,000/cmm, pre op being 300,000/cm^2). Which of the following statements are true regarding further management of the DVT?
   a. Increase the dosage of heparin to thrice daily/ infusion of Heparin to maintain aPTT in range of 45–70 sec
   b. Add on warfarin immediately as he is already on heparin
   c. Change to Argatroban immediately and continue Argatroban
   d. Add on DVT stockings, and change to LMWH twice a day

46. All the following are indications for empiric antibiotics against gram-positive organisms in patients with febrile neutropenia *except*:
   a. Hemodynamic instability
   b. Radiologic evidence of pneumonia
   c. Skin and soft tissue infection
   d. Patients on Voriconazole prophylaxis now presenting with oral mucositis

47. The drug used to prevent anthracycline associated cardiotoxicity is:
   a. Dextromethorphan
   b. Dexmedetomidine
   c. Dexrazoxane
   d. Desferrioxamine

48. All are true about Tumor Lysis Syndrome (TLS) *except*:
   a. Hypocalcemia needs to be treated even in absence of symptoms
   b. Sevelamer should be given for hyperphosphatemia
   c. Urinary alkalinization increases uric acid solubility but decreases calcium phosphate solubility
   d. Hematolymphoid malignancies have high chance of developing TLS as compared to solid organ malignancies

49. Regarding Pneumocystis pneumonia (PCP) in malignancy, false statement is:
   a. Prophylaxis is needed in patients with malignancy in whom CD4 count < 200/mcl
   b. Prophylaxis is needed in patients receiving glucocorticoids for one month or more
   c. Belongs to fungal group
   d. Dapsone + Atovaquone is the treatment of choice for patients with history of Sulfa allergy

50. A 22-year-old male, under diagnostic evaluation for hematologic malignancy is referred to ICU in view of worsening tachypnea. His labs are positive for a WBC count of 60000/cm^2, and PLC 638000/cm^2. CXR revealed bilateral diffuse interstitial infiltrates. Bedsides this ECHO revealed normal cardiac function with no pericardial effusion. He is maintaining 100% saturation on 4 litres by simple face mask. However, a simultaneous ABG showed PaO$_2$ of 50 mm Hg. The current scenario is best explained by:
   a. ARDS
   b. Methemoglobinemia
   c. Leucocyte larceny
   d. Acute left ventricular failure

51. Fever in neutropenic patients is defined as:
   a. A single oral temperature of ≥38.3°C (101°F)
   b. A temperature of ≥38.0°C (100.4°F) sustained over 30 minutes period
   c. A single oral temperature ≥38.0°C (100.4°F)
   d. Persistent oral temperature of ≥38.3°C (101°F) for more than half an hour period

52. An 8-year-old male child, known case of Burkitt's lymphoma on chemotherapy presents to the emergency room with complains of abdominal distension, loose stools, bloody diarrhea, and fever of 3 days duration. On examination, his heart rate is 160/minute, MAP 46 mm Hg, and has distended and tender abdomen, there is no hepatosplenomegaly and no bowel sounds appreciated. Further information regarding diagnosis can be attained by
    a. Barium enema
    b. Erect X-ray abdomen
    c. Colonoscopy
    d. Contrast CT abdomen

53. A 6-year-old female child, with leukemia, on chemotherapy, presented with fever, hypotension and respiratory distress 2 weeks after induction chemotherapy. She was intubated and initiated on vasopressors and broad spectrum antibiotics. However, she continued to deteriorate clinically. All cultures including blood culture sent twice were negative. Rectal swab showed E. coli – MDR, sensitive to Fosfomycin and Colistin. She had a hemoglobin of 5.7, platelet count of 90000/cm^2, bilirubin 4.5 mg%, AST, ALT both more than 500 U/lit, and progressive increase in vasopressor requirements. A serum ferritin sent on day 3 was 56,000 ng/mL, LDH was 1200 U/lit, Serum triglycerides were 1200 mg%. Serum procalcitonin < 0.5. Which of the following steps would be appropriate in further management of the condition?
    a. Liver biopsy and transplant work up
    b. Bone marrow biopsy to look for hemophagocytosis
    c. Anti-fungal therapy as empirical treatment, in view of worsening shock and low procalcitonin
    d. Escalate antibiotics to cover for MDR E. coli

54. A 34-year-old female, diagnosed case of APML, initiated on chemotherapy with Retinoic acid presented with high grade fever, hypotension, dyspnea, weight gain of more than 5 kg over the past 3 days. A chest X-ray taken on bed side revealed interstitial thickening and peri bronchial cuffing, right sided upper lobe consolidation along with nodular opacities in all zones of lung and bilateral mild pleural effusion. All the following are appropriate actions for this patient *except*:
    a. Broad spectrum antibiotics
    b. High dose steroids
    c. Heparin
    d. Voriconazole

55. A 45-year-old male, case of ALL on treatment, presents with respiratory distress and features of septic shock. He is initiated on broad spectrum antibiotics and caspofungin (as he was already on daily voriconazole and weekly Trimethoprim+Sulfamethoxazole). Serum galactomannan has been sent and results are awaited. The following statement is true regarding anti-fungal therapy:
    a. Voriconazole is prophylactic and caspofungin is pre-emptive
    b. Voriconazole is empiric and caspofungin is targeted
    c. Both Voriconazole and caspofungin are pre-emptive
    d. Voriconazole is prophylactic and caspofungin is empiric

56. Rasburicase is contraindicated in which of the following condition:
    a. Porphyria
    b. G6PD deficiency
    c. Malaria
    d. Uncontrolled bronchial asthma

57. A 56-year-old male, known case of carcinoma buccal mucosa, underwent segmental mandibulectomy with flap reconstruction 3 month back. He was undergoing postoperative concurrent chemotherapy and radiotherapy from local hospital. He presented to casualty with complaints of breathing difficulty, fever with cough of 3 days duration. On examination, he is found to be tachypneic (33/min), tachycardic (130/min) and hypotensive (MAP 60 mm Hg). He was saturating 60% on room air that improved to 85% with 10 litre oxygen on a non-rebreathing mask (NRBM). All of the following are appropriate in management *except*:
    a. Application of high-flow nasal cannula (HFNC) instead of NRBM, at 60 L/min flow and 100% FIO$_2$

b. Immediate intubation
c. Crystalloid bolus @ 20 mL/kg
d. Collection of blood culture and immediate administration of antibiotics

58. A 46-year-old male, known case of non-Hodgkin's lymphoma on treatment, presented to emergency room with complaints of fever and respiratory distress of 2 days duration. On examination, he was drowsy, heart rate of 134/min, respiratory rate of 30/minute, and blood pressure of 96/40 mm Hg. CNS examination revealed an obtunded sensorium, non-comprehensive sounds, and localizing pain. No focal neurological deficits were elicited. Crepitation was present bilaterally, more towards bases. Lab investigations showed Hb of 6.8 gm%, total WBC count 300/cm^2, platelet 20000/cm^2, urea 96 mg%, S creatinine 3.1 mg%, INR 3.6, bilirubin of 4.5 mg%, transaminase 660/450 U/lit, LDH 2500 U/lit. All the following interventions would be appropriate, *except*:
    a. Urgent broad spectrum antibiotics
    b. Correction of platelets by transfusion
    c. Correction of INR by FFP transfusion
    d. Plasma exchange

K Type Questions
[Marked True (T)/False (F)]

1. A 56-year-old male, diagnosed case of Hodgkin's lymphoma on chemotherapy with RCHOP regime, presented with chest tightness, half an hour after starting chemotherapy. ECG showed ST elevation in leads V2-V4. Echocardiography showed reduced motion of anterior wall and a decreased left ventricular ejection fraction. A Coronary angiography documented the absence of significant coronary artery disease. Which of the following drugs are associated with myocardial infarction?
    a. Vincristine
    b. Rituximab
    c. Gemcitabine
    d. 5 FU
    e. Cyclophosphamide

2. Symptoms of hypercalcemia are:
    a. Diarrhea
    b. Lethargy
    c. Abdominal pain
    d. QT prolongation

3. Regarding malignant spinal cord compression (MSCC):
    a. Steroids are the treatment of choice
    b. Radiation therapy is a main stay in treatment
    c. Role of surgery is limited to patients who are paraplegic for more than 48 hours
    d. Surgery is useful only for tumours arising from spinal cord/CNS

4. In patients with raised ICP, the triad of Cushing response include:
    a. Hypertension with narrow pulse pressure
    b. Bradycardia
    c. Irregular respiratory rate
    d. Pupillary asymmetry

5. A 72-year-old male, is being evaluated for recurrent epistaxis, and headache for 1-month duration. He is also suffering from blurring of vision and excessive fatigability and melena for the past 3 months. His clinical examination is otherwise normal. He has mild anemia, elevated ESR and Serum protein electrophoresis showed a strong positive band for monoclonal IgM. Urine analysis also revealed Bence Jones proteins. A clinical diagnosis of hyperviscosity syndrome secondary to multiple myeloma was made. Which of the following conditions are associated with hyperviscosity syndrome?
    a. Hyponatremia
    b. Hypercalcemia
    c. Retinal hemorrhage
    d. Platelet dysfunction

6. A diagnosis of idiopathic pulmonary syndrome (IPS) can be made by:
    a. Multilobar infiltrates on thoracic imaging
    b. Excellent response to steroids
    c. Respiratory distress that occurs within 2 weeks of engraftment
    d. Lung biopsy revealing interstitial pneumonia pattern

7. A 72-year-old male a case of carcinoma of upper esophagus underwent chemoradiation for the same. 3 months later, he presents with cough of 2 weeks duration and left lower pneumonia. Bronchoscopy reveals a tracheoesophageal fistula, just above the carina. Which of the following are appropriate for further management of the patient condition?

a. Surgical intervention and closure of fistula
   b. Endoscopic stent placement
   c. Nasojejunal tube insertion for feeding
   d. Refer for concurrent CTRT

8. **The mechanism for hypercalcemia in malignancy is:**
   a. Secretion of parathormone like peptide
   b. Ectopic PTH production
   c. Local osteolysis from bone metastasis
   d. Increased Vitamin D secretion

9. **A 14-year-old male, newly diagnosed case of AML is referred to ICU in view of SVC syndrome and respiratory distress with stridor. HR is 160/min, BP 76/45 mm Hg and afebrile. All the following are immediate measures in managing this case *except*:**
   a. Prepare for difficult intubation in view of upper airway edema
   b. Hydrocortisone 100 mg IV stat (debatable)
   c. Continuous nebulized adrenalin to reduce airway edema
   d. IV access preferably on left upper limb

10. **A 12-year-old male, AML on induction chemotherapy with Trimethoprim+Sulfamethoxazole and Voriconazole prophylaxis, presented to the casualty with fever, left sided facial pain, left sided periorbital cellulitis, with a black necrotic discharge from the nose of 2 days duration. Regarding this case, the following are true:**
    a. Biopsy of the necrotic material will show non-septate hyphae with right angles and ribbon-like appearance
    b. Blood cultures are diagnostic in most of the cases
    c. Voriconazole is an effective drug in both aspergillosis and mucormycosis
    d. Galactomannan and 1- 3 beta d glucan cannot be used to screen patients with mucormycosis

11. **Regarding Radiation pneumonitis:**
    a. Generally presents 6-8 months after completion of radiotherapy
    b. Hilar adenopathy and cavitations are common occurrences
    c. Chronic obstructive pulmonary disease (COPD) is one of the important risk factor
    d. Lung infiltrates are confined to the original radiation exposure fields
    e. It is rare with fractionated total doses of less than 20 Gy

12. **Regarding Neutropenic Enterocolitis:**
    a. Observed only in hematolymphoid malignancies and not seen with solid tumors
    b. Clostridial species are the most common anerobic pathogens
    c. Prompt surgical treatment is indicated
    d. Never extends to colon
    e. CT scan findings are common

13. **A 21-year-old lady with non-Hodgkin's lymphoma has presented to casualty with febrile neutropenia. Which of the following statement is truer regarding role of Hematopoietic Growth Factors (G-CSF or GM-CSF) in Management?**
    a. Prophylactic use of myeloid CSFs has not been shown to reduce the incidence of neutropenic fever or all-cause mortality
    b. Prophylactic use of myeloid colony-stimulating factors should be considered for patients with anticipated risk of fever and neutropenia is >20%
    c. Prophylactic Hematopoietic Growth Factors are contraindicated in older patients
    d. Therapeutic Hematopoietic Growth Factors are not generally recommended for treatment of established fever and neutropenia
    e. Therapeutic Hematopoietic Growth Factors offer survival benefit

14. **Regarding Hyperviscosity syndrome:**
    a. Level of increased viscosity fairly correlates with severity of symptoms
    b. It is more common in patients with IgG myeloma than Waldenstrom Macroglobulinemia with IgM
    c. Plasmapheresis can reduce symptoms and prevent organ damage
    d. Mental status changes and respiratory pulmonary distress are important symptoms to watch for

15. **A 10-year-old male child is getting evaluated for history on and off fever since 2 months, has baseline Total WBC count of 60,000 with 37% blasts. Admitted to hospital with diagnosed of acute leukemia, presents to ICU with respiratory distress. On examination, dirty sloughed lesion over the hard palate on left side is seen. CT reveals sinusitis of the left maxillary and anterior ethmoid sinus.**

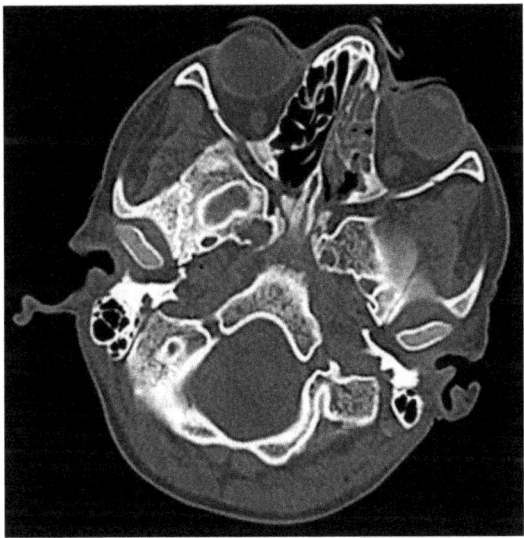

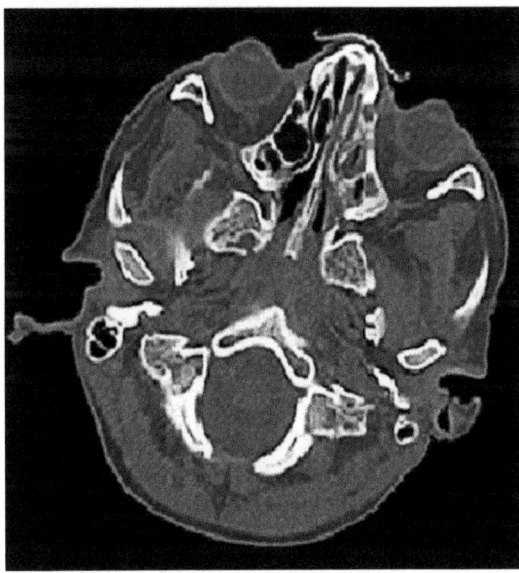

Patient is started on antifungals suspecting possible Mucormycosis. Regarding Mucormycosis:

a. Typically involvement is sinus or pulmonary
b. Amphotericin B and early surgical debridement is the treatment of choice
c. Posaconazole can be used for salvage therapy
d. Voriconazole is equally effective
e. Echinocandins are fairly active and can be used

16. Which of the following is true?
    a. Dexamethasone should be avoided before a tissue diagnosis if CNS lymphoma is suspected
    b. Freshly frozen plasma may be required with anticoagulation in L-asparaginase induced dural sinus thrombosis
    c. Choriocarcinoma can have brain metastasis with hemorrhagic transformation
    d. Whole brain irradiation is not useful in leukostasis

17. A 30-year male patient with AML on Day 10 of induction chemotherapy presented with febrile neutropenia in OPD. Peripheral blood and PICC blood cultures were sent; started on first line antibiotics with cefoperazone + sulbactum, amikacin and admitted to the ICU. Fever persisted, and antibiotics hiked up to Meropenem on day 2. Patient continued to be neutropenic and febrile though hemodynamically stable. A call from microbiology resident informed that patient has growth of candida from both (peripheral and catheter) blood samples. Identify the true statements:
    a. Start patient on injection fluconazole as patient is hemodynamically stable
    b. Start any Echinocandin
    c. Daily or alternate day blood culture to decide duration of therapy
    d. Do an urgent dilated retinal examination to see for metastatic complication

18. A 36-year-old female, known case of Ca breast, presented to the emergency with 3 episodes of vomiting, and acute onset of drowsiness for 4 hours. She had received her chemotherapy on the previous day. Her previous lab investigations were normal; however the current lab investigation show sodium-106 mmol/L. Which of the following drugs are responsible for hyponatremia in cancer patients?
    a. Cisplatin
    b. Mithramycin
    c. Cylophosphamide
    d. Adriamycin

ANSWER

A Type Answers

Q1. Answer b

Patients with severe hypercalcaemia require hospital admission and aggressive hydration with 200-250 mL saline hourly unless contraindicated due to cardiac disease or renal dysfunction. Aggressive rehydration acts by 2 mechanisms: (1) it dilutes S. Calcium due to increase in volume and (2) induces calciuria by increasing GFR. Thiazide diuretics decrease renal excretion by 50-150 mg/day and hence are contraindicated. However loop diuretics increase calcium excretion by kidneys and hence may be used. Bisphosphonates inhibit the osteoclast's' activity and are highly efficacious agents in reducing calcium levels, although they have a delayed onset of action. The safety of bisphosphonates in kidney injury is not clear. Calcitonin acts within 2 hours by inhibiting bone resorption and reducing renal reabsorption of calcium. However, it is short acting, and tolerance to its action develops rapidly. Denosumab is a RANKL monoclonal antibody that inhibits the activation, maturation, and osteoclast function and can be administered even to those with a creatinine clearance of less than 30 ml/min. Hemodialysis may be done in cases where intractable hypercalcemia is life threatening. Severe hypercalcemic crisis associated with parathyroid adenoma is rare in oncologic practice and might require surgical excision of parathyroid gland. Hypercalcemia from causes like granulomatous disorders or lymphoma respond well to corticosteroids.

Minisola S. The diagnosis and management of hypercalcaemia. BMJ (British Med Journal). 2015;(350):h2723.

Q2. Answer c

SIADH is a common cause of hyponatremia occurring in patients with malignancy. In persons with SIADH, the non-physiological secretion of arginine vasopressin (AVP) results in enhanced water reabsorption, leading to dilutional hyponatremia. In the absence of hypovolemia, thyroid or adrenal dysfunction and in the setting of low plasma osmolality, a urinary osmolality of 100 mOsm per kilogram of water is usually diagnostic of SIADH. Hypouricemia, low blood urea, and a urinary sodium level greater than 40 mmol per litre are being used as measures of assessing euvolemic status. A FeNa> 1 (not 40) and a FeUrea> 55% is also suggestive of SIADH, if the patient has not received 3% hypertonic saline or diuretics before sampling. SIADH patients fail to correct hyponatremia after 0.9% saline infusion and rather may have worsening of hyponatremia. Correction of hyponatremia is usually achieved through fluid restriction and in case of medical emergencies through hypertonic saline.

Ellison DH, Berl T. The Syndrome of Inappropriate Antidiuresis. N Engl J Med. 2007;356(20):2064-72.

Q3. Answer c

This patient has presented with a seizure after undergoing chemotherapy with Cyclophosphamide a drug known to cause acute hyponatremia. Lab reports are suggestive of profound and severely symptomatic hyponatremia. Severely symptomatic hyponatremia is an acute emergency, if left untreated may lead to permanent brain damage or death. Available data suggest that this can be reversed by rapidly increasing the serum sodium concentration immediately. Management will be administering 2 mL/kg of 3% saline immediately over 20 minutes. Sensorium is expected to improve after rapid administration of 3% saline. However, in case the sensorium does not improve even after a rise in serum sodium by 5 mmol/L or worsens, further investigation from history, and imaging may be warranted after securing airway. These patients are borderline patients and require intense monitoring of sensorium to decide on airway protection. In the event of on-going worsening or even not improvement, then airway needs to be protected. A rapid correction of sodium more than 10 mmol/L/day is not advocated in view of possibility for osmotic demyelination. Cerebral edema is due to hyponatremia and in these patients 3% Saline is preferred over mannitol.

Spasovski G, Vanholder R, Allolio B, et al. Clinical practice guideline on diagnosis and treatment of hyponatremia. Nephrol Dial Transplant. 2014;29(SUPPL. 2):1-39.

Q4. Answer c

According to Bishop Cairo classification TLS is classified as Lab TLS and Clinical TLS. Criteria for Lab TLS are – uric acid level ≥ 8 mg% or 25% increase from baseline, K level ≥ 6.0 mEq/L or 25% increase from baseline, phosphorous ≥6 mg% in children, phosphorous concentration ≥4.5 mg% or 25% increase from baseline in adults and calcium level ≤7 mg% or 25% decrease from baseline. Two or more of these criteria within 3 days prior to or 7 days after initiation of chemotherapy confirm diagnosis of Lab TLS. However, many cancers with high tumor load (such as hematolymphoid malignancy) can undergo spontaneous tumor lysis prior to initiation of chemotherapy.

A patient has lab TLS with 1 or more of these signs who show any cardiac arrhythmia, seizure or sudden death is classified as clinical TLS.

Cairo MS, Bishop M. Tumour lysis syndrome: new therapeutic strategies and classification. Br J Haematol. 2004;127(1):3-11.

Q5. Answer c

Patients undergoing surgeries for retroperitoneal dissection, Whipple's procedure, neck dissection and esophageal surgeries are at high risk for post-operative chyle leak. High drain output in the immediate post-operative period with characteristic color is diagnostic. It can be confirmed by testing the drain fluid for triglycerides. Decreasing oral fat or changing the feed to medium chain triglycerides or TPN reduces chyle flow, and might help in spontaneous closure of small leaks. If symptomatic, patients might require paracentesis although it may cause immunosuppression and electrolyte imbalance. Somatostatin analoges like octreotide are effective in reducing cholorrhea and may be attempted prior to any surgical approach. Percutaneous image guided embolization of thoracic duct is of increasingly popular upcoming centres of interventional radiology. Surgical approaches like peritoneovenous shunt or re exploration and ligation of thoracic duct are the other options that may also be attempted, despite their associated high morbidity.

Kaas R, Rustman LD, Zoetmulder FA. Chylous ascites after oncological abdominal surgery: incidence and treatment. Eur J Surg Oncol. 2001;27(2):187-9.

Q6. Answer d

This patient has developed refeeding syndrome that may occurs once feeding is initiated in malnourished patients. Refeeding causes an insulin surge, resulting potentially fatal electrolyte and fluid imbalance. The clinical picture is characterised by abnormal glucose intolerance, hypokalaemia, hypophosphatemia and hypomagnesemia. Concomitant thiamine deficiency is also present as thiamine stores are rapidly exhausted. Patients with chronic alcoholism, postoperative patients, patients with chronic malnutrition like prolonged fasting or malabsorption, cancer patients etc. are at high risk for refeeding syndrome. It can be avoided by providing no more than 50% of energy requirements in high risk patients with concomitant vitamin supplementation. The feeding can then be gradually increased with close clinical and biochemical monitoring. Although post-operative sepsis and septic shock can be a differential diagnosis in the clinical scenario, the laboratory parameters are more favourable for refeeding syndrome. Although this patient has hyperglycemia, in the setting of hypokalemia, upfront initiation of insulin causes precipitous fall of potassium. Hence, dyselectrolytemia needs to be corrected before initiating insulin in this patient.

Mehanna HM, Moledina J, Travis J. Refeeding syndrome: what it is, and how to prevent and treat it. Bmj. 2008;336(7659):1495-8.

Q7. Answer c

This patient is suffering from pneumonia and with no other focus of infection. Double coverage for pneumonia is not shown to offer added advantage and currently is not recommended. Empirical antifungals are indicated only if the patient is not improving even after 3 days of adequate antimicrobial therapy. When a source of infection is evident, urgent removal of lines are also not required. A broad spectrum antibiotic like cefepime, piperacillin tazobactam or meropenem as a single agent that is later deescalated according to culture and sensitivity results will be the appropriate management in this case.

Freifeld AG, Bow EJ, Sepkowitz KA, et al. Clinical practice guideline for the use of antimicrobial agents in neutropenic patients with cancer: 2010 Update by the Infectious Diseases Society of America. Clin Infect Dis. 2011;52(4).

Q8. Answer a

Recombinant Factor VIIa may be used as an adjunctive to treat massive bleeding in conditions where surgical intervention and conventional therapies have failed to control bleeding. Any factor that may affect coagulation including hypothermia, acidosis, coagulopathy should be corrected whenever possible. Hypothermia impairs platelet function, and clotting factors especially at temperatures below 34 degrees. For optimal effects, the platelets should be maintained at a level more than $50,000 \times 10^9/l$; fibrinogen more than 500 mg%, and acidosis should be avoided, preferably maintaining pH ≥ 7.20. In cases of massive transfusions, blood products should be transfused preferably in a ratio of 1:1:1. There is no evidence of benefit for rFactor 7 in routine surgeries, or liver diseases. Usually administered dose is 200 μg/kg, followed by two doses of 100 μg/kg, administered at 1 and 3 hours after the first dose, while monitoring for thromboembolic complications. Current evidence suggests recombinant factor VIIa is more useful in blunt trauma rather than penetrating trauma.

Vincent JL, Rossaint R, Riou B, et al. Recommendations on the use of recombinant activated factor VII as an adjunctive treatment for massive bleeding—a European perspective. Crit Care. 2006;10(4):R120.

Q9. Answer c

After splenectomy, all persons should receive pneumococcal and meningococcal vaccine, ideally two weeks before elective splenectomy, or two weeks after emergency splenectomy.

Howdieshell TR, Heffernan D, Dipiro JT. Surgical Infection Society Guidelines for Vaccination after Traumatic Injury. Surg Infect (Larchmt). 2006;7(3):275-303.

Q10. Answer d

This patient is suffering from neuroleptic malignant syndrome (NMS), manifested by altered mental status, muscular rigidity, hyperthermia, and dysautonomia. It has an incidence of 0.02%–3% and a mortality of 10%–20%. The common agents like haloperidol used for managing ICU delirium can trigger NMS even after withdrawal of the drug. Management will be benzodiazepines to ameliorate the catatonia, and urgent dopaminergic agonists like Bromocriptine, and avoiding further incriminating drugs. The differential diagnosis is usually serotonin syndrome and it might be difficult to differentiate the two at times. There is no evidence of infection as visualised form surgical site, clinical examination and a consistently low procalcitonin with negative blood cultures. Hence option (b) is not correct. Malignant hyperthermia (MH) is unlikely in the absence of a precipitating event hence option (c) is wrong

Sevransky JE, Bienvenu OJ, Neufeld KJ. Treatment of four psychiatric emergencies in the intensive care unit. Crit Care Med. 2012;40(9):2662-70.

Q11. Answer d

Q12. Answer e

GVHD is immune mediated phenomenon between donor and recipient. Acute GVHD involves skin (dermatitis), liver (hepatitis) and gastrointestinal tract (enteritis) and develops within 100 days after allogeneic hematopoietic-cell transplantation (HCT). Chronic GVHD develops after 100 days and can involve eyes, gut, lungs, neuromuscular system and joints. In addition to allogeneic HCT, GVHD is also seen in solid organs transplant and transfusion of non-irradiated blood products. Dry eye disease, also known as dry eye syndrome (DES), Kerato conjunctivitis sicca, and keratitis sicca, is a multifactorial disease of the tears and the ocular surface that results in discomfort, visual disturbance, and tear film instability with potential damage to the ocular surface.

Socié G, Blazar BR. Acute graft-versus-host disease: from the bench to the bedside. Blood. 2009;114(20):4327-36.

Q13. Answer a

Radio sensitization is the use of a drug that makes tumor cells more sensitive to radiation therapy and these drugs are also known as radio enhancers whereas radiation recall is an acute inflammatory reaction confined to previously irradiated areas that can be triggered when chemotherapy agents are administered after radiotherapy. Thus one is intended phenomenon whereas other is unintended side effect. One of the important features of radiation recall is that the reaction affects skin or other organs that was previously quiescent and apparently normal. The area affected clearly corresponds to an area previously irradiated. The time interval between end of radiation therapy and administration of the precipitating chemotherapy varies widely in cases of radiation recall. The onset of the symptoms usually occurs within days to a few weeks after exposure to the precipitating chemotherapy drug, frequently after the first dose and sometimes during or immediately after intravenous administration. Radiation recall dermatitis is classified in 5 stages, stage 1 being mild dermatitis to stage 5 being death.

Burris HA, Hurtig J. Radiation recall with anticancer agents. Oncologist. 2010;15(11):1227-37.

Q14. Answer c

Changes in heart rate, often in the form of AF, can be the first and only indicator of anastomotic insufficiency. This is especially important in cases without prior heart conditions where AF occurred for the first time after surgery and requires further immediate investigation. Early symptoms of incipient sepsis can be as subtle as changes in the patient's subjective general condition (e.g. persisting pain) and minor changes in neurological status, such as reduced compliance. Contrast CT and endoscopy are widely regarded as the gold standard diagnostics. While a single method may miss some leaks and be unable to provide certain information (e.g. CT cannot determine vascularization and endoscopy cannot supply topical information), their combination delivers a powerful picture of the patient's status. X-ray based contrast radiology is quickly performed, but suffers from reduced sensitivity and can miss up to 50% of anastomotic leakages.

Griffin SM, Lamb PJ, Dresner SM, et al. Diagnosis and management of a mediastinal leak following radical esophagectomy. Br J Surg. 2001;88:1346-51.

Q15. Answer c

Chyle has a fat content of 0.4-4.0 g/dL, a protein content of approximately 3 g/dL, a pH of greater than 7.5, and a specific gravity of greater than 1.010 g/dL. Nutritional status can be optimized with the administration of a low-fat, high-protein and medium-chain triglyceride diet. In severe cases, complete bowel rest and TPN may be required.

Q16. Answer e

The risk of bleomycin-induced lung toxicity is higher in older patients. Age over 40 years was associated with a 2.3-fold higher risk of pulmonary complications.

O'Sullivan J M, Huddart R A, Norman A R, et al., Predicting the risk of bleomycin lung toxicity in patients with germ-cell tumors. Annals of Oncology. 2003;14(1):91-6.

Q17. Answer a

Usually Severe local back pain is first symptom (80–90% of the time) that is aggravated by lying down due to distension of venous plexus. Motor weakness is second most common symptom occurring in 60-80% patients. Prostate cancer, breast cancer, and lung cancer each account for 15-20% of adult patients with MSCC. In children the cause and mechanisms of MSCC are different than in adults. Neuroblastoma, Ewing's sarcoma, Wilms' tumor, lymphoma, soft-tissue sarcoma, and bone sarcoma are the most common tumor types that lead to compression in children. Also in children compression is more likely to be caused by paravertebral masses that impinge on the spinal cord directly, rather than by involvement of bony elements in the spine. Although most MSCC develops in patients known to have cancer, 8-34% arises as an initial manifestation of Cancer. MSCC is a common presentation of cancer of unknown primary origin, non-Hodgkin lymphoma, myeloma, and lung cancer. Results of a multicentre comparison of surgical decompression and radiation with radiotherapy alone concluded that patients with spinal-cord compression who were treated with radical, direct decompressive surgery and postoperative radiotherapy regained the ability to walk more often and maintained it longer than did patients treated with radiation alone. Surgery permits most patients to remain ambulatory and continent for the remainder of their lives whereas patients given radiation alone spend about two-thirds of their remaining time unable to walk and incontinent.

Bach F, Larsen BH, Rohde K. Metastatic spinal cord compression. Occurrence, symptoms, clinical presentations and prognosis in 398 patients with spinal cord compression. Acta Neurochir. 1990;107:37.

Q18. Answer b

The diagnosis of Central Diabetes Incipidus (CDI) should be made with caution in postoperative patients as intra-operative fluid overload may present with hypo-osmolar polyuria in postoperative period. It is also important to rule out glycosuria and hyperglycemia, especially if the patient is known diabetic or on dexamethasone. Diagnosis of CDI is made on the basis of clinical and biochemical findings and should not be based on only clinical findings. The CDI patient may develop a sudden onset of polyuria (urine output >2.5 mL/kg/h) and polydipsia, usually within the first 24–48 h after neurosurgery. Plasma osmolality is increased (>300 mOsm/L), and urine osmolality is decreased with a urine/plasma osmolality ratio <1. As long as fluids are replaced, CDI is not life-threatening. Desmopressin (DP) can be started to reduce the total daily fluid intake/output. It can be given at an initial dose of 50–100 µg (tablets) orally, 5–10 µg intranasally or 30–60 µg sublingually. Each subsequent dose of DP should be given after the demonstration of dilute urine with an osmolality <200 mosm/L or a specific gravity <1.005, and a urine output of >2.5 mL/kg/h for >2 h. Treatment results in the reduction of urine output, with the effect lasting for 6–18 h, and doses should be titrated according to the daily total urine output. Regular Desmopressin should only be prescribed when CDI is stable and permanent.

Q19. Answer d

Hypothyroidism may occur in up to 48% of patients treated for head and neck malignancies. It has been observed after radiation, surgery, and combined-modality therapies. The onset of hypothyroidism may be as early as 4 weeks and as late as 5 or 10 years after completion of therapy. Hypothyroidism is a frequent late effect after definitive radiotherapy. The size of the thyroid gland and the radiation dose to the gland are key factors in the development of radiation induced hypothyroidism.

> Matthew CM, Agrawal A. Hypothyroidism in post radiation head and neck cancer patients: incidence, complications, and management. Current Opinion in Otolaryngology & Head & Neck Surgery. 2009;17(2):111-5.

Q20. Answer a

Incidence of postop hypocalcemia after thyroid surgery is around 28%. Majority of these patients have transient hypocalcemia. Incidence of permanent hypocalcemia is much lower, around 0.9%. Main risk factors for postoperative hypocalcemia are thyroid cancer, nodal dissection, and female gender. Only symptomatic hypocalcemic patients and asymptomatic patients with an acute decrease in serum corrected calcium to ≤7.5 mg/dL should receive corrections with IV calcium. Either 10% calcium gluconate (90 mg of elemental Ca/10 mL) or 10% calcium chloride (270 mg of elemental Ca/10 mL) diluted in 50 ml of 5% dextrose should be infused over 10–20 minutes. This should be followed by continuous infusion of 0.5 to 1.5 mg/kg of elemental calcium per hour. Continuous infusion can be prepared by adding 11 g of calcium gluconate (equivalent to 990 mg elemental Ca) to 1 litre of 0.9% NS or 5% D and administered at rate of 50 mL/hour (equivalent to 50 mg/hour). The dose can be adjusted to maintain the serum calcium concentration at the lower end of the normal range.

> Puzziello A, Rosato L, Innaro N, et al. Hypocalcemia following thyroid surgery: incidence and risk factors. A longitudinal multicenter study comprising 2,631 patients. Endocrine. 2014;47(2):537-42.

Q21. Answer a

High-risk patients require hospitalization for IV empirical antibiotic therapy; monotherapy with an antipseudomonal β-lactam agent, such as cefepime, a carbapenem (meropenem or imipenem-cilastatin), or piperacillin-tazobactam, is recommended.

Other antimicrobials (aminoglycosides, fluoroquinolones, and/or vancomycin) may be added to the initial regimen for management of complications (e.g. hypotension and pneumonia) or if antimicrobial resistance is suspected or proven.

Vancomycin (or other agents active against aerobic gram-positive cocci) is not recommended as a standard part of the initial antibiotic regimen for fever and neutropenia. These agents should be considered for specific clinical indications, including suspected catheter-related infection, skin or soft-tissue infection, pneumonia, or hemodynamic instability.

> Alison GF, Eric JB, Kent A et al. Clinical Practice Guideline for the Use of Antimicrobial Agents in Neutropenic Patients with Cancer: 2010 Update by the Infectious Diseases Society of America. IDSA GUIDELINES. Clinical Infectious Diseases. 2011;52(4):e56-e93.

Q22. Answer d

In patients with clinically or microbiologically documented infections, the duration of therapy is dictated by the particular organism and site. Appropriate antibiotics should continue for at least the duration of neutropenia (until ANC is> 500 cells/mm³) or longer if clinically necessary. In patients with unexplained fever, it is recommended that the initial regimen be continued until there are clear signs of marrow recovery; the traditional endpoint is an increasing ANC that exceeds 500 cells/mm³. Alternatively, if an appropriate treatment course has been completed and all signs and symptoms of a documented infection have resolved, patients who remain neutropenic may resume oral fluoroquinolone prophylaxis until marrow recovery.

> Alison GF, Eric JB, Kent A et al. Clinical Practice Guideline for the Use of Antimicrobial Agents in Neutropenic Patients with Cancer: 2010 Update by the Infectious Diseases Society of America. IDSA GUIDELINES. Clinical Infectious Diseases. 2011;52(4):e56-e93.

Q23. Answer a

Even though false positive galactomannan is known with antibiotics like piperacillin+tazobectum, carbapenems, ceftriaxone, amox-clav and cefepime, this patient is high risk for Aspergillus infection due to underlying hematolymphoid malignancy and prolonged neutropenia. Waiting for BAL fungal culture and cytology before starting voriconazole may lead to worsening of patient. In patients with invasive aspergillosis, initial therapy with voriconazole leads to better responses and improved survival with fewer severe side effects than initial therapy with amphotericin B.

> Herbrecht R, Denning DW, Patterson TF et al. Voriconazole versus Amphotericin B for Primary Therapy of Invasive Aspergillosis. N Engl J Med. 2002;347:408-15.

Q24. Answer a

Prophylaxis against invasive Aspergillus infections with posaconazole should be considered for selected patients >13 years of age who are undergoing intensive chemotherapy for AML or myelodysplastic syndrome (MDS) in whom the risk of invasive aspergillosis without prophylaxis is substantial.

> Alison GF, Eric JB, Kent A et al. Clinical Practice Guideline for the Use of Antimicrobial Agents in Neutropenic Patients with Cancer: 2010 Update by the Infectious Diseases Society of America. IDSA GUIDELINES. Clinical Infectious Diseases. 2011;52(4):e56-e93.

Q25. Answer d

When CLABSIs occur in the ICU, physicians must be prepared to recognize and treat them. Prevention of these infections requires careful attention to optimal catheter selection, insertion and maintenance and to remove when they are no longer needed or are infected.

> Alison GF, Eric JB, Kent A et al. Clinical Practice Guideline for the Use of Antimicrobial Agents in Neutropenic Patients with Cancer: 2010 Update by the Infectious Diseases Society of America. IDSA GUIDELINES. Clinical Infectious Diseases. 2011;52(4):e56-e93.

Q26. Answer a

Biopsy of a palpable supraclavicular node was rewarding in two-thirds of the reported attempts. Small Cell Lung Carcinoma (SCLC) and non-Hodgkin's lymphoma (NHL) often involve the bone marrow. Temporizing emergency mediastinal irradiation before biopsy is rarely used because it may preclude proper interpretation of the specimen in almost half of the patients with malignancy-induced superior vena cava syndrome (SVCS), surgical intervention should be considered only after other therapeutic maneuvers with irradiation, chemotherapy, and stenting have been exhausted. Choice of treatment is based on histologic diagnosis. Treatment like Cyclophosphamide is generally not started before tissue diagnosis.

> Hellman D, Rosenberg's Cancer: Principles & Practice of Oncology. 10th edition. 2014. Chapter 143: Superior Vena Cava Syndrome 2123.

Q27. Answer d

Hodgkin's lymphoma commonly involves the mediastinum, but it rarely causes SVCS.

> DeVita, Hellman, and Rosenberg's Cancer: Principles & Practice of Oncology. 10th edition. 2014. Chapter 143: Superior Vena Cava Syndrome 2123.

Q28. Answer a

Unilateral pleural effusions in patients with a history of malignancy raise the possibility of MPE. Its presence frequently indicates advanced disease, and the overall prognosis of patients with MPE depends largely on the underlying type of malignancy and the extent of primary disease. Initial cytology from the pleural fluid is positive in approximately 66% of patients with MPE. However, the overall incidence of clinically significant RPE is low. The overall incidence of clinically significant RPE is low and thoracic surgeons routinely remove >1.5 L of pleural effusion without serious sequelae during thoracoscopic procedures to treat various conditions.

DeVita, Hellman, and Rosenberg's Cancer: Principles & Practice of Oncology. 10th edition. 2014. 127. Malignant Pleural and Pericardial Effusions.

Q29. Answer d

Capecitabine, an oral prodrug of 5-fluorouracil (5-FU), is approved for early-stage and advanced colorectal cancer and metastatic breast cancer. Cardiotoxicity of 5-FU and capecitabine is well described in the literature. Electrocardiogram test may show no acute ischemic changes.

DeVita, Hellman, and Rosenberg's Cancer: Principles & Practice of Oncology. 10th edition. 2014. Chapter 36: Antimetabolites 395.

Q30. Answer d

MSCC as the primary manifestation of a malignancy is more common in non-Hodgkin lymphoma, myeloma, and lung cancer, especially the small-cell variant. Colon and prostate cancers seem to have a predilection for the lumbosacral spine.

DeVita, Hellman, and Rosenberg's Cancer: Principles & Practice of Oncology. 10th edition. 2014. 121 Spinal Cord Compression.

Q31. Answer a

Differentiation syndrome can be a life-threatening complication of APL and ATRA treatment. As the granule-laden promyelocytes differentiate, the granular products induce pulmonary edema and fluid retention. Fever and weight gain are common symptoms of differentiation syndrome. Treatment includes steroids and management of coagulopathy. Differentiation syndrome may affect as many as 10% to 25% of patients with APL 10% to 25 % of patients will develop the APL differentiation syndrome (APLDS) characterized by fever, weight gain/edema, pleural effusions, and pulmonary infiltrates; the TLC is often elevated. Steroids (e.g., methylprednisolone 45 mg intravenous daily with subsequent tapering) are effective for treatment of APLDS. The principal prognostic factor in untreated APL is initial WBC. Patients with TLC less than 10,000/mcL will have complete response (CR) rates greater than 90% with idarubicin plus ATRA, while patients with higher WBC counts will have CR rates of 70% to 85%.

DeVita, Hellman, and Rosenberg's Cancer: Principles & Practice of Oncology. 10th edition. 2014. Chapter 131: Management of Acute Leukemias1935.

Q32. Answer a

Vasculitis is observed in 4.5% to 8% of malignancies; it is found in solid tumors (most commonly lung non-small cell), squamous cell carcinoma of oesophagus, and prostate, as well as in hematologic malignancies (hairy cell leukemia, lymphomas and rarely multiple myeloma).

DeVita, Hellman, and Rosenberg's Cancer: Principles & Practice of Oncology. 10th edition. 2014. Chapter 153: Paraneoplastic Syndromes 2227.

Q33. Answer d

The majority of cancers associated with thromboembolic events are clinically evident and have been previously diagnosed at the time of the event. However, thromboembolism can precede the diagnosis of malignancy. The risk is highest for cancers of the ovary, pancreas, and liver. Patients with APML generally present with bleeding and coagulopathy.

DeVita, Hellman, and Rosenberg's Cancer: Principles & Practice of Oncology. 10th edition. 2014. Chapter 153: Paraneoplastic Syndromes 2223.

Q34. Answer c

DeVita, Hellman, and Rosenberg's Cancer: Principles & Practice of Oncology. 10th edition. 2014. Chapter 103: Gestational Trophoblastic Neoplasms1365.

Oncology

Q35. Answer d

Hepatic VOD is a major manifestation of liver toxicity associated with conventional and high-dose chemotherapy in children affected by hematologic malignancies and certain solid tumors. Clinically, patients present with jaundice, painful hepatomegaly, and fluid retention, which may evolve into multi-organ failure, a hallmark of severe disease. Gold standard investigations being hepatic-venous pressure gradient and biopsy. Out of all treatment options, Defibrotide, a novel oligonucleotide with antithrombotic and antiplatelet aggregating properties, and endothelial-stabilizing effects is found to be most effective.

> DeVita, Hellman, and Rosenberg's Cancer: Principles & Practice of Oncology. 9th edition. 2011. Chapter 155: Allogeneic Stem Cell Transplantation. 2247.

Q36. Answer d

> DeVita, Hellman, and Rosenberg's Cancer: Principles & Practice of Oncology. 10th edition. 2014. Chapter 43: Miscellaneous Chemotherapeutic Agents 457.

Q37. Answer b

Characteristic	Weight
Burden of febrile neutropenia with nor or mild symptoms	5
No hypotension (systolic BP > 90 mm Hg)	5
No chronic obstructive pulmonary disease	4
Solid tumor or hematological malignancy with no previous funga infection	4
No dehydration requiring parenteral fluids	3
Burden of febrile neutropenia with moderate symptoms	3
Outpatient status	3
Age <60 years	2

The points attributed to the variable "burden of febrile neutropenia" are not cumulative. The maximum theoretical score is therefore 26. A score of ≥ 21 is considered low risk and a score of < 21 as high risk (positive predictive value of 91%, specificity of 68%, and sensitivity of 71%).

> IDSA febrile neutropenia 2010: Clinical Practice Guideline for the Use of Antimicrobial Agents in Neutropenic Patients with Cancer: 2010 Update by the Infectious Diseases Society of America. Clinical Infectious Diseases 2011;52(4):e56-e93.

Q38. Answer d

Till early 90's cancer patients requiring ICU admission and mechanical ventilation had very low survival rate worldwide, which discouraged ICU admission for these patients. However, over last 2 decades this picture has changed dramatically. With development of newer anticancer agents many cancers can be controlled, though not cured with good quality of life. Especially for patients with good performance status and potentially controllable cancers if treated aggressively in time outcome may be changed positively including those who need mechanical ventilation or vasopressors. Treatment-limitation decisions should be considered only after at least 6 days of fully aggressive ICU management. Cancer patients who required intubation, vasopressors, or dialysis after day 3 have very grim prognosis. This patient has metastatic breast cancer, but is hormone positive and thus may have good prognosis. Her present condition is probably due to GI sepsis secondary to her mucositis and there is good chance that she will survive with timely proper antibiotics and supportive treatment.

> Elie A, Corinne A, Caroline B et al. Improved survival in cancer patients requiring mechanical ventilatory support: Impact of noninvasive mechanical ventilatory support. Critical Care Medicine. 2001;29(3):519-25.

Q39. Answer d

Most probably this child is in postictal state and since has unobstructed breathing does not need immediate intubation. Child can be nursed in lateral position with close monitoring. His pupils are bilateral equal and normally reacting to light, there is no lateralising sign and also his platelet counts are near normal. Plain CT scan 4 hours prior is normal. Probability of him having intracranial bleed is less likely. Most likely this child is suffering from Posterior reversible encephalopathy syndrome (PRES). PRES usually presents with headache, seizures, status epilepticus, altered consciousness, and visual disturbance of short duration. Hypertension is a common finding and is seen in around 70% of patients. MRI is diagnostic and typical findings are of bilateral white matter abnormalities (mainly suggestive of vasogenic edema) in vascular watershed areas in the posterior regions of both cerebral hemispheres, affecting mostly the occipital and parietal lobes. Less frequently similar changes may be seen in other parts of brain like frontal lobe, temporal lobe or cerebellar hemispheres. Even basal ganglion and brain stem can get involved. Commonly seen in patients with eclampsia, CRF or severe hypertension, it is also seen in patients on immunosuppressive agents. The exact cause of PRES is not known, but the most popular theory is that severe hypertension causes interruption to brain autoregulation resulting in interstitial extravasation of proteins and fluids, causing vasogenic edema.

Treatment mainly consists of treatment of underlying cause antiepileptic medications and control of high blood pressure. If properly managed clinical syndrome resolves within a week though MRI changes may take days to weeks to disappear.

Hobson EV, Craven I, Blank C. Posterior Reversible Encephalopathy Syndrome: Truly Treatable Neurologic Illness. Perit Dial Int. 2012;32(6):590-4.

Q40. Answer c

MASCC prognostic index is developed to identify malignancy patients with infections yet suitable for outpatient antibiotic therapy. A greater than or equal to identified negligible risk patients while a lesser score identified patients at high risk of developing bacteraemia and death.

Thirumala R, Ramaswamy M, Chawla S. Diagnosis and Management of Infectious Complications in Critically Ill Patients with Cancer.Crit Care Clin. 2010;26(1):59-91.

Klastersky J, de Naurois J, Rolston K, et al. Management of febrile neutropaenia: ESMO clinical practice guidelines. Ann Oncol. 2016; 27(Supplement 5):v111-8.

Q41. Answer b

This patient is at high risk for invasive fungal infection. Hepatosplenic candidiasis occurs in leukemia patients with febrile neutropenia after chemotherapy. Clinical features include fever, right upper quadrant pain and repeatedly negative blood cultures and negative workup for malaria. Laboratory report shows elevated alkaline phosphatase. These patients have hepatosplenomegaly and imaging demonstrates multiple focal lesions, with peripheral enhancement on USG or CT. A targeted biopsy is generally required for diagnosis. Treatment includes amphotericin B or its liposomal preparation administered for 10 to 14 days and continued with fluconazole for 3- 6 months until radiologic resolution of illness. The differential diagnosis usually involves disseminated tuberculosis, malaria or disseminated malignancies. However, a biopsy will usually prove or disprove the same.

Thirumala R, Ramaswamy M, Chawla S. Diagnosis and Management of Infectious Complications in Critically Ill Patients with Cancer. Crit Care Clin. 2010;26(1):59-91.

Pappas PG, Kauffman CA, Andes DR, et al. Clinical Practice Guideline for the Management of Candidiasis: 2016 Update by the Infectious Diseases Society of America. Clin Infect Dis. 2015;62(4):e1-50.

Q42. Answer c

Engraftment syndrome is a clinical syndrome that presents with low grade fever, erythrodermatitis, and noncardiogenic pulmonary oedema. The exact aetiology is unclear. The presentation usually occurs within 72-96 hours of engraftment and coincides with neutrophil recovery. This has to be differentiated from acute GVHD, CHF, and also infectious complications that may occur at the similar time frame. Criteria for the diagnosis of engraftment syndrome include major criteria: temperature ≥38.3°C without an infectious aetiology, rash involving more than 25% of body surface area, and diffuse pulmonary infiltrates causing hypoxia. Minor criteria include organ dysfunction including hepatic dysfunction, renal insufficiency, weight gain ≥2.5% of baseline body weight, and transient encephalopathy. Diagnosis is made by the presence of three major or two major and one minor criterion. Management includes cessation of granulocyte-colony stimulating factor (GCSF), and supportive. Prognosis is usually good.

>   Soubani AO, Pandya CM. The spectrum of noninfectious pulmonary complications following hematopoietic stem cell transplantation. Hematol Oncol Stem Cell Ther. 2010;3(3):143-57.

Q43. Answer a

This patient is a known case of pelvic malignancy and at elevated risk for pulmonary embolism (PE). According to the ESC guidelines of 2014 for PE, high sensitivity D dimer assay can be used to rule out PE in cases with low or intermediate risk. It cannot be used to diagnose PE. Bedside echocardiography may help to rule out other causes of hemodynamic instability. It may also be useful if signs like right ventricle (RV) dilation with an increased RV-LV ratio, hypokinesia of the free wall of RV (McConnell's sign), and decreased tricuspid annulus plane systolic excursion can be elicited. These signs of RV overload or RV dysfunction are not specific only to PE. The negative predictive value for echocardiography in PE is 40 – 50% and although transthoracic echocardiography (TTE) has a high specificity of 83%, the sensitivity in diagnosing PE is only 53%, especially in hemodynamically stable patient. A negative compression ultrasound cannot rule out PE in high risk patients. However, as she is having symptoms of deep vein thrombosis (DVT), a compression ultrasound showing proximal DVT may diagnose PE. If compression ultrasound is negative, then CT angiography must be done.

>   Konstantinides SV, Torbicki A, Agnelli G, et al. 2014 ESC Guidelines on the diagnosis and management of acute pulmonary embolism. Eur Heart J. 2014;35(43):3033-80.

Q44. Answer d

Scoring systems for prediction of DVT and PE have been well established and validated in general population (e.g. well's score, Geneva score, modified Wells score and Modified Geneva score) however they are not validated for cancer patients, and rather have points included for malignancy. Scores that have been developed and validated in cancer patients include Khorana score, Vienna CATS score, PROTECHT and CONKO. All of them have been validated in cancer patients. Khorana score is an easy score that can be used bedside without the requirement of any lab investigations and comprises of baseline characteristics of the tumor type BMI and pre-chemotherapeutic hemogram (Hb, WBC count and platelet count). Vienna CATS score requires laboratory value of D – dimer and soluble P selectin, apart from all the variables included in Khorana score. PROTECHT takes into consideration the baseline characteristics as in Khorana scoring system and chemotherapeutic regime while CONKO score takes into consideration the baseline characteristics and WHO performance status.

>   Van Es N, Di Nisio M, Cesarman G, et al. Comparison of risk prediction scores for venous thromboembolism in cancer patients: a prospective cohort study. Haematologica. 2017;102(9):haematol. 2017.169060.

Q45. Answer c

This patient most probably is suffering from heparin induced thrombocytopenia (HIT). HIT is clinically diagnosed based on the timing of thrombocytopenia and heparin exposure, the severity of platelet drops, development of systemic thrombosis, in the absence of other factors causing thrombocytopenia (4 T score). A HIT Expert Probability score has also been developed, based on literature review and retrospective data identifying eight clinical features of HIT. A cut off value of 2 for the HIT Expert Probability score, had 100% sensitivity and 60% specificity for the diagnosis of HIT (compared to 44% specificity of 4T score). However, in patients with malignancy, the disease per se or the chemotherapy agents may cause a thrombocytopenia, leading to under diagnosis of HIT in this sub group and both the scores have not been validated in this setting. Considering HIT as a prothrombotic state, an increase in heparin dosage will worsen the thrombocytopenia and systemic thrombosis. Addition of warfarin without bridging can initially worsen the pro-thrombotic state and thrombosis. Although the incidence of HIT is less with LMWH, once HIT is established, they are not preferred. Direct acting thrombin inhibitors like lepirudin and Argatroban are the preferred agents in such cases.

>   Miriovsky BJ, Ortel TL. Heparin-induced thrombocytopenia in cancer. JNCCN J Natl Compr Cancer Netw. 2011;9(7):781-7.

Q46. Answer d

IDSA guidelines identify certain high-risk groups who may benefit from empirical coverage for gram-positive organism. They include evidence of sepsis or septic shock (Hemodynamic instability), pneumonia on imaging, an initial positive blood culture report for gram-positive bacteria, before final identification and susceptibility testing is available, suspected CRBSI, Skin or soft-tissue infection at any site, colonization with methicillin-resistant Staphylococcus aureus MRSA), vancomycin-resistant enterococcus (VRE), or penicillin-resistant Streptococcus pneumoniae and patients with severe mucositis, on fluoroquinolone prophylaxis with ceftazidime as empirical therapy.

Freifeld AG, Bow EJ, Sepkowitz KA, et al. Clinical practice guideline for the use of antimicrobial agents in neutropenic patients with cancer: 2010 Update by the Infectious Diseases Society of America. Clin Infect Dis. 2011;52(4).

Q47. Answer c

Dexrazoxane is a FDA approved drug that significantly reduces the incidence of anthracycline-induced congestive heart failure (CHF) irrespective of pre-existing cardiac risk factors or whether the drug is given before the first dose of anthracycline or until cumulative doxorubicin dose is ≥ 300 mg/m^2.

Cvetkovi RS, Scott LJ. Dexrazoxane. Drugs. 2005;65(7):1005-24.

Q48. Answer a

TLS is an oncologic emergency due to lysis of tumor cells releasing large amount of intra cellular metabolic components causing end organ damage and even death. Hyperkalemia, hyperuricemia, hyperphosphatemia and hypocalcemia are the common metabolic abnormalities seen with TLS. Hypocalcemia is usually secondary to hyperphosphatemia and calcium phosphate crystallisation. Supplementing calcium in patients with TLS and hypocalcemia might increase the risk of calcium phosphate crystallization and further worsening of kidney injury. Calcium should be administered only in the case life threatening arrhythmia, cardiac arrest, or seizures.

Mirrakhimov AE. Tumor lysis syndrome: A clinical review. World J Crit Care Med. 2015;4(2):130.

Q49. Answer d

Pneumocystis jirovecii pneumonia was initially classified as a protozoan due to the occurrence of trophic and cyst forms. Based on RNA analysis, it has been reclassified as an ascomycetous fungus. It affects severely immunocompromised patients such as those undergoing treatment for cancer or those with HIV infection. Corticosteroid use of more than 1 month is also a predisposing factor for PCP pneumonia. A specific dose or duration of steroids that increases the risk significantly has not been identified although there are recommendations for starting prophylaxis in patients receiving ≥ 20 mg prednisolone equivalent/day for ≥ 1 month. Early recognition is crucial for management as it has a high mortality in patients with hematological malignancies and transplant recipients. Although lymphocytopenia and low CD4 counts have been documented as elevated risk for PCP pneumonia, no cut off for CD4 has been identified as a threshold to initiate prophylaxis as compared with HIV and AIDS. Those patients who develop allergies to cotrimoxazole will also cross react to dapsone. Hence dapsone should be avoided in patients with sulpha allergy. Primaquine and Clindamycin or aerosolized pentamidine may be tried in those with documented sulpha allergies.

Cordonnier C, Cesaro S, Maschmeyer G, et al. Pneumocystis jirovecii pneumonia: Still a concern in patients with haematological malignancies and stem cell transplant recipients. J Antimicrob Chemother. 2016;71(9):2379-85.

Maertens J, Cesaro S, Maschmeyer G, et al. ECIL guidelines for preventing Pneumocystis jirovecii pneumonia in patients with haematological malignancies and stem cell transplant recipients. J Antimicrob Chemother. 2016;71(9):1-8.

Q50. Answer c

Spurious hypoxemia in leukemia is due to oxygen consumption by leukemic cells before analysis. The diagnosis is made by a patient having normal saturation but very low PaO$_2$ on ABG. The clinical laboratory dissociation is diagnostic of leucocytosis larceny. All the given choices other than (c) cannot explain the difference between oxygen saturation and PaO$_2$.

Sacchetti A, Grynn J, Pope A, et al. Leukocyte larceny: spurious hypoxemia confirmed with pulse oximetry. J Emerg Med. 1990;8(5):567-9.

Oncology

Q51. Answer a

IDSA defines febrile neutropenia as "as a single oral temperature measurement of >38.3°C (101°F) or a temperature of >38.0°C (100.4°F) sustained over a 1-h period."

<small>Freifeld AG, Bow EJ, Sepkowitz KA, et al. Clinical practice guideline for the use of antimicrobial agents in neutropenic patients with cancer: 2010 Update by the Infectious Diseases Society of America. Clin Infect Dis. 2011;52(4).</small>

Q52. Answer d

This child is probably suffering from neutropenic enterocolitis or typhilitis which occurs after intensive chemotherapy for acute leukemia, neutropenia from other causes, and in those receiving immunosuppressive therapy for HSCT or solid tumours. Mucosal edema, ulceration, necrosis, and focal hemorrhage in the terminal ileum, cecum, and right colon lead to bacterial translocation and bacteraemia or candidemia. Patients present with fever, abdominal distension and tenderness, diarrhea etc. Initial management includes nasogastric decompression, intravenous fluids, and broad-spectrum antibiotics. Barium enema is usually contraindicated, as they are at high risk of potential perforation. Water-soluble contrast may demonstrate rigidity and thickening of the cecum. Plain abdominal X-ray findings usually are nonspecific and may even be normal. Colonoscopy or sigmoidoscopy are relatively contraindicated due to risk of perforation and associated thrombocytopenia. Abdominal CT is one of the most important diagnostic studies and has relatively low false negative rate (around 15%). The main finding is caecal thickening, fluid filled caecum, peri-caecal inflammation and presence of gas in portal venous circulation. It can also detect free air in abdomen in case of perforation. Apart from perforation surgical intervention will also be needed in case of persistent bleeding or clinical deterioration. However, surgical intervention is preferably deferred till the recovery of neutropenia.

<small>Thirumala R, Ramaswamy M, Chawla S. Diagnosis and Management of Infectious Complications in Critically Ill Patients with Cancer. Crit Care Clin. 2010;26(1):59-91.</small>

Q53. Answer b

This child is probably suffering from hemolymph phagocytosis (HLH). HLH is a clinical diagnosis based on clinical features and laboratory parameters in patients at high risk for developing this condition. T cell malignancies, DLBCL, NHL and aggressive chemotherapies for leukemia or lymphoma are high risk conditions for developing HLH. There is dysregulated activation of immune system with activated macrophages and lymphocytes and inflammatory cytokines resulting in tissue infiltration, hemophagocytosis, and organ damage. This condition is common in pediatric age group, although adults also may be affected. The criteria for diagnosing HLH are fever, bicytopenia (at least) in the peripheral blood smear, hypertriglyceridemia and/or hypofibrinogenemia, hyperferritinemia, splenomegaly, hemophagocytosis in bone marrow, spleen, or lymph nodes, low or absent NK-cell activity, and high levels of soluble interleukin-2 (CD25). Five of eight criteria must be fulfilled to make a diagnosis of HLH. All these conditions may occur otherwise in malignancy, masking the diagnosis (e.g. bone marrow suppression causing bicytopenia, sepsis causing fever and hemophagocytosis, blood transfusions causing hyperferritinemia). Organ damage is evident, and will require supportive treatment. Management includes immunosuppression by cyclosporine, etoposide, dexamethasone and intrathecal methotrexate. In this case, no focus of infection could be identified despite aggressive investigations. Repeatedly negative blood cultures, with low procalcitonin and elevated parameters like high ferritin and triglycerides probably suggests HLH as a non-infectious cause of deterioration of this child.

<small>Tang Y, Xu X. Advances in hemophagocytic lymphohistiocytosis: pathogenesis, early diagnosis/differential diagnosis, and treatment. Scientific World Journal. 2011; 22(11):697-708.</small>

<small>Gupta AA, Tyrrell P, Valani R, et al. Experience with hemophagocytic lymphohistiocytosis /macrophage activation syndrome at a single institution. J Pediatr Hematol Oncol. 2009;31(2):81-4.</small>

Q54. Answer c

This female is probably suffering from differentiation syndrome or the Retinoic acid syndrome (ATRA syndrome). It manifests as breathlessness with infiltrates on chest X-ray, unexplained fever that can be high grade also, weight gain of more than 5 kg, pleural effusion, and renal failure occurring in the initial weeks of therapy with trans retinoic acid. The clinical features overlap with those of underlying infection and differentiating the two might be difficult. These patients are at high risk for spontaneous intra-cranial bleed. Hence, they need to be closely monitored for coagulation abnormalities, DIC and thrombocytopenia. Supportive care in view of ventilatory support, dialysis, and empirical antibiotics and antifungals are usually initiated. The management is high dose steroids that reverse the symptoms of ATRA. Heparin or other anti-coagulation agents are preferably avoided in view of their bleeding tendency.

Montesinos P, Sanz MA. The differentiation syndrome in patients with acute promyelocytic leukemia: Experience of the pethema group and review of the literature. Mediterr J Hematol Infect Dis. 2011;3(1).

Q55. Answer d

- Prophylactic antifungal treatment refers to the administration of an antifungal agent to patients at risk of invasive fungal infection even without attributable signs and symptoms. Prophylactic Anti-fungal agents are given to patients undergoing chemotherapy, in the absence of any signs or symptoms of disease.
- Empiric anti-fungal treatment is defined as the initiation of antifungal agents in patients at high risk of invasive fungal infections with established clinical signs and symptoms before microbiological documentation (e.g. Anti-fungal given to patients presenting with septic shock, along with broad spectrum antibiotics).
- Pre-emptive therapy is administration of antifungal agents in patients with sign and symptoms of invasive fungal infection and also has a diagnostic test positive for the same, suggesting fungal infection. Antifungal agents initiated after a positive beta glucan or galactomannan test.
- Targeted therapy is initiation of antifungal based on identification of species after a culture sensitivity report.

Zaragoza R, Pemán J, Salavert M, et al. Multidisciplinary approach to the treatment of invasive fungal infections in adult patients. Prophylaxis, empirical, preemptive or targeted therapy, which is the best in the different hosts? Ther Clin Risk Manag. 2008;4(6):1261-80.

Q56. Answer b

In tumor lysis syndrome (TLS), excessive uric acid is produced from break down of intracellular nucleic acid of tumor cells. Human beings lack the enzyme urate oxidase that converts uric acid into water soluble allantoin. This results in accumulation of uric acid crystals and urate nephropathy, and is one of the crucial factor in development of TLS. Allopurinol inhibits xanthine oxidase; the enzyme which converts xanthine into uric acid, thus decreasing uric production. However, this can still lead to xanthinuria and also cause acute interstitial nephritis. Patients presenting with pre-existing kidney disease requires dose modification of allopurinol. FDA has approved the use of rasburicase a recombinant urateoxidase that converts uric acid into water soluble allantoin. In patients at medium to substantial risk of developing TLS or those who present with substantially raised uric acid levels at base line, the dosage recommended is 0.1mg/kg – 0.2 mg/kg. It is relatively a safe but costly drug and needs parenteral administration. The safety in pregnant or lactating patients is not established. It is also contraindicated in patients with G6PD deficiency as these patients are at elevated risk for haemolysis and methemoglobinemia.

Jacobsen NEB, Beck SDW, Foster RS. Oncologic emergencies. Emergencies Urol. 2007;26:142-71.

Mirrakhimov AE. Tumor lysis syndrome: A clinical review. World J Crit Care Med. 2015;4(2):130.

Q57. Answer b

This patient has presented with respiratory distress and shock. Airway protection and mechanical ventilation will be of utmost importance in such patients. However, this patient will have an anticipated difficult (anatomical and physiological) airway in view of recent surgery with flap reconstruction. Hence getting an airway expert help and preparations for an emergency tracheostomy standby should be initiated while continuing other management for septic shock as per guidelines. Of the choices given, immediate intubation under RSI might convert the situation to a cannot intubate or cannot ventilate one. Hence that is the not appropriate choice.

Myatra SN, Ahmed SM, Kundra P, et al. The all India difficult airway association 2016 guidelines for tracheal intubation in the intensive care unit. Indian J Anaesth. 2016;60(12):922-30.

Q58. Answer c

This is a neutropenic patient presenting with fever, altered mentation, hypotension and tachypnea. He is also having deranged liver and renal function also. Neutropenia places him at elevated risk for infections, and he requires urgent blood cultures followed by initiation of empirical antibiotics. The constellation of altered mental status, elevated RFT and LFT along with neutropenia and thrombocytopenia can be easily attributed to septic shock or metabolic encephalopathy. However, the LDH is also elevated and the possibility of hemolysis should be also considered. This patient needs to be worked up for hemolytic uremic syndrome (HUS) also (altered mentation, thrombocytopenia, fever, hemolysis and deranged RFT) and if in doubt plasma exchange needs to be considered. Unless there are obvious causes for other thrombotic microangiopathies, the presence of hemolytic anemia as evidenced by schistocytes on peripheral smear, elevated LDH, and indirect hyperbilirubinemia) and thrombocytopenia is a justification for plasma exchange. In the absence of any bleeding manifestations, correction of platelets or INR is not warranted, as it leads to unnecessary exposure to blood products and more complications. Presence of respiratory distress with basilar crackles could be a sign of early fluid overload secondary to AKI and needs close monitoring. Eculizumab, a monoclonal antibody blocks the cleavage of C5 to C5a and C5b if initiated early may improve renal and non-renal recovery in cases of atypical HUS.

Jokiranta TS. Clinical platelet disorders HUS and atypical HUS. 2017;129(21):2847-57.

Azoulay E, Knoebl P, Garnacho-Montero J, et al. Expert Statements on the Standard of Care in Critically Ill Adult Patients With Atypical Hemolytic Uremic Syndrome. Chest. 2017;152(2):424-34.

K Type Answers

Q1. Answer TFFTT

Chemotherapeutic agents for cancer can have severe cardiac side effects including acute heart failure, myocardial ischemia, pericardial effusion, arrhythmias, also ECG abnormalities. Knowledge of chemotherapeutic agents and their side effects mandates careful screening, evaluation and dose modification of these agents in high risk patients undergoing chemotherapy with these agents. Agents commonly implicated with myocardial ischemia are 5-FU, Cisplatin, cyclophosphamide, Capecitabine, paclitaxel and docetaxel. Vinca alkaloids like vincristine also cause Prinzmetal's angina that are relieved by rest. The incidence of myocardial ischemia secondary to 5 FU is approximately 2-7%.

Monsuez JJ, Charniot JC, Vignat N. Cardiac side-effects of cancer chemotherapy. Int J Cardiol. 2010;144(1):3-15.

Q2. Answer FTTF

Hypercalcemia is not a rare phenomenon in oncologic critical care. It is estimated to occur in up to 20 to 30% of oncologic patients. Hypercalcemia is caused by systemic secretion of a PTH like hormone (PTHrP), or due to the secretion of 1,25-dihydroxy vitamin D (1,25(OH) D) as in case of lymphomas, or due to osteolysis and rarely by ectopic PTH secretion. Measured ionised calcium is recommended as total calcium levels may vary depending upon hypoalbuminemia or hypergammaglobulinemia. If a malignant cause of hypercalcemia is not evident, non-malignant causes such as primary hyperparathyroidism, thiazide diuretics, sarcoidosis etc. have to be ruled out. Primary work up will include serum PTH assessment, Plasma 1, 25(OH) D levels and a skeletal survey. The rise of serum calcium is more important clinically rather than the absolute value of calcium. The development of symptoms depend on how acute is the change in serum calcium. The symptoms of hypercalcemia can be recalled with the mnemonic – stones, bones, abdominal moans and psychic groans.
Renal - Dehydration, renal stones, Skeleton Nephrocalcinosis
Skeletal – Osteoporosis, Arthritis
GI - Anorexia, Nausea, vomiting, Constipation and abdominal pain
CNS – altered sensorium, Lethargy, fatigue
CVS - Shortened QT interval, arrhythmias hypertension.

Carroll MF, New E. A Practical Approach to Hypercalcemia - American Family Physician. 2003;1959-66.

Q3. Answer TTFF

Metastatic malignancy eroding into the epidural space or direct metastasis to the epidural or intradural tissue causing compression of the spinal cord is the most common cause of MSCC. Acute compression causes occlusion of venous stasis of the batson plexus, leading to vasogenic oedema. This later progress to arterial occlusion and irreversible cord infarct. Patients may be involved at multiple regions although the thoracic lumbosacral region is commonly affected. Patients present with pain, weakness, paraesthesia, and autonomic dysfunction, urinary retention, and overflow incontinence are usually indicative of cauda equina syndrome. The Frankel grading system and Barthel index are scores for assessing severity and prognostication. Radiographs of spine lack sensitivity and specificity and MRI spine is the investigation of choice. Because of an element of vasogenic edema, high dose dexamethasone is considered first-line treatment for MSCC. Radiation to the involved segments and surgery in a select group of patients satisfying Patchell criteria, surgery might be beneficial.

Jacobsen NEB, Beck SDW, Foster RS. Oncologic emergencies. Emergencies Urol. 2007;26:142-71.

Q4. Answer FTTF

Increase in intra-cranial pressure reduces the blood flow to brain leading to the typical response known as Cushing's reflex. It is characterized as an increase in systolic and decrease in diastolic pressure (widened pulse pressure), bradycardia and irregular respiration. It is considered to be a sign of imminent cerebral herniation with associated brainstem compression. This was first described by Harvey Cushing in 1901. Uncal herniation causing compression of the contralateral Crus cerebri leads to pupillary asymmetry with contralateral pupillary dilation. This is called Kernohan sign. It is not included in Cushing's reflex.

Fodstad, Kelly HJ, Buchfelder P, Michael. History of the Cushing reflex. Neurosurgery. 2006;59(11):32-7.

Q5. Answer TTTT

Hyperviscosity syndrome occurs in many hematologic disorders such as Waldenstrom macroglobulinemia, multiple myeloma, and leukemia, etc. The triad of symptoms include neurologic abnormalities, visual changes, and bleeding. Increased paraproteinemia can lead to rouleaux formation and intra-vascular stasis. Fundoscopic examination reveals dilated and engorged retinal veins (fundus paraproteinemic). Platelet dysfunction tends to occur due to protein coating on platelets that prevent aggregation. Lab studies will reveal a (pseudo) hyponatremia and hypercalcemia. Urgent plasmapheresis is the treatment of such condition and might be able to prevent blindness from retinal vein occlusion.

Jacobsen NEB, Beck SDW, Foster RS. Oncologic emergencies. Emergencies Urol. 2007;26:142-71.

Stone MJ, Bogen SA. Evidence-based focused review Evidence-based focused review of management of hyperviscosity syndrome Case presentations. 2015;119(10):2205-9.

Q6. Answer TFFT

Following HSCT, patients are at risk of infectious and non-infectious pulmonary complications that have a similar clinical presentation. A National Institutes of Health workshop defined IPS as "diffuse lung injury occurring after bone marrow transplant for which an infectious aetiology is not identified". The diagnostic criteria for IPS includes: (1) Widespread alveolar damage manifested by multilobar infiltrates, clinical features of pneumonia, and increased alveolar-arterial gradient with pulmonary function tests suggestive of restriction. (2) Exclusion of lower respiratory tract infection (BAL that is negative for bacterial and non-bacterial pathogens), no clinical improvement with broad spectrum antibiotics, and a repeat confirmatory test within 2 weeks. (3) Histopathology that reveals diffuse alveolar damage or interstitial pneumonitis. There is no proven therapy for IPS, and progressive respiratory failure ensues. The response to steroids is not beneficial. Prognosis is usually poor though there have been case reports with good response to eternacept.

Soubani AO, Pandya CM. The spectrum of noninfectious pulmonary complications following hematopoietic stem cell transplantation.Hematol Oncol Stem Cell Ther. 2010;3(3):143-57.

Clark JG, Hansen JA, Hertz MI, et al. Idiopathic Pneumonia Syndrome after Bone Marrow Transplantation. Am Rev Respir Dis. 1993;147(61):1601-6.

Q7. Answer FTTF

This patient is having a trachea esophageal fistula complicated with pneumonia. Tracheoesophageal fistula occurs late in malignancy and patients are usually inoperable due to local infiltration or metastasis. If left untreated, these patients have a median survival time of only 1 to 6 weeks. The best management is palliative, aimed at relieving dysphagia while maintaining nutrition and protecting the airway. Any surgical intervention will not be tolerated and carries undue risk. Hence esophageal stent placement and tube feeding will be appropriate measures for such patients.

Chauhan SS, Long JD. Management of Tracheoesophageal Fistulas in Adults. Curr Treat Options Gastroenterol. 2004;7(1):31-40.

Q8. Answer TTTT

Hypercalcemia due to malignancy is usually due to systemic secretion of a PTH like hormone (PTHrP) from tumour cells, or due to osteolysis and release of calcium from the bone, or due to the secretion of 1,25-dihydroxyvitamin D (1,25(OH) D) as in case of lymphomas, and rarely by ectopic PTH secretion.

Stewart AF. Hypercalcemia Associated with Cancer. Available from: http://dx.doi.org.ez.statsbiblioteket.dk:2048/101056/NEJMcp042806 (Accessed 9 November 2017).

Q9. Answer TTFF

The child has presented with obstruction of the superior vena cava (SVC) and respiratory distress. SVC syndrome is associated with venous congestion and upper airway edema that can cause respiratory embarrassment. Symptomatic management will include head end elevation, high flow oxygen while preparing for a difficult intubation. In cases of SVC obstruction due to solid tumor malignancy, steroids are being used though the efficacy is not documented. However, in patients with leukemia, administration of steroids might interfere with the diagnosis and also precipitate rapid lysis of cells causing tumor lysis syndrome. Adrenalin nebulization has no role in reducing the vasogenic edema, secondary to venous congestion and might even increase the tachycardia and untoward events.

Wilson LD, Detterbeck FC, Yahalom J. Clinical practice.Superior vena cava syndrome with malignant causes. N Engl J Med. 2007;356(18):1862-9.

Q10. Answer TFFT

This child is suffering from mucormycosis. Mucormycosis is usually occurs in immunocompromised states like patients with hematological malignancies, organ transplant recipients, diabetes mellitus etc. Commonly affected sites include lungs and sinus. The role of PCR for early diagnosis is still under evaluation and tissue biopsy with culture is essential for diagnosis of mucor. On microscopy, presence of broad, non-septate hyphae with right angles and a ribbon-like appearance with angioinvasion or tissue invasion is adequate to confirm the diagnosis. Mucor does not secrete galactomannan nor beta glucan. Hence, they cannot be used in screening for the same. Surgery remains the key element in the management and liposomal amphotericin B, is the treatment of choice for mucormycosis. Voriconazole has poor action on mucormycosis and does not protect against mucor.

Bassetti M, Bouza E. Invasive mould infections in the ICU setting: Complexities and solutions. J Antimicrob Chemother. 2017;72:i39-47.

Q11. Answer FFFTT

Radiation pneumonitis is typically seen 1 to 6 months after completion of radiotherapy. A mild non-productive cough, low-grade fever, and dyspnoea on exertion characterize symptomatic radiation pneumonitis.

10–15% of patients with large mediastinal tumors who receive a combination of chemotherapy and mantle field radiation therapy develop radiation pneumonitis. Radiographically, pneumonitis is characterized by the formation of infiltrates confined to the original radiation fields.

Infection rather than pneumonitis is more likely if the infiltrates extend into areas of the lung initially protected from radiation. Severe pneumonitis may require treatment with steroids. Underlying COPD does not appear to potentiate radiation damage. Mediastinal or hilar adenopathy and cavitation are almost always due to causes other than radiation pneumonitis. Pneumothorax in radiation pneumonitis seldom occurs with fractionated total doses of less than 20 Gy but is more likely when doses exceed 60 Gy.

DeVita, Hellman, and Rosenberg's Cancer: Principles & Practice of Oncology. 10th edition. 2014. Chapter 138 Pulmonary Toxicity.

Q12. Answer FTFFT

Neutropenic Enterocolitis is also observed in patients with solid tumors receiving taxane-containing chemotherapy. Positive CT scan findings are present in about 80% of cases. More extensive involvement of the large bowel and disease of the terminal ileum may occur. The indications for surgery are persistent gastrointestinal bleeding after resolution of neutropenia, thrombocytopenia, and clotting abnormalities; free intraperitoneal perforation; uncontrolled sepsis despite fluid and vasopressor support; and an intra-abdominal process.

DeVita, Hellman, and Rosenberg's Cancer: Principles & Practice of Oncology. 10th edition. 2014. Chapter 156: Infections in the Cancer Patient 2287.

Q13. Answer FTFTF

Prophylactic use of myeloid CSFs has been shown to reduce the incidence of neutropenic fever in a variety of studies and in meta-analyses was shown to be associated with reductions in infection related mortality and all-cause mortality. Prophylactic use of myeloid colony-stimulating factors (CSFs; also referred to as hematopoietic growth factors) should be considered for patients in whom the anticipated risk of fever and neutropenia is >20%. CSF prophylaxis should be especially considered for older patients or if the presence of additional risk factors, including prior fever and neutropenia, poor nutritional or performance status, no antibiotic prophylaxis, comorbid medical conditions, or other modifying disease characteristics, suggests that there is substantial risk of fever and/or severe infection during neutropenia. CSFs are not generally recommended for treatment of established fever and neutropenia.

IDSA febrile neutropenia 2010: Clinical Practice Guideline for the Use of Antimicrobial Agents in Neutropenic Patients with Cancer: 2010 Update by the Infectious Diseases Society of America. Clinical Infectious Diseases 2011;52(4):e56-e93.

Q14. Answer FFTT

DeVita, Hellman, and Rosenberg's Cancer: Principles & Practice of Oncology. 10th edition. 2014. Chapter 136: Plasma Cell Neoplasms. 2007

Q15. Answer TTTFF

Q16. Answer TTTF

Corticosteroids should be avoided if CNS lymphoma is suspected before a tissue diagnosis has been established. Dexamethasone and related drugs induce lymphocytic apoptosis and may obscure morphologic diagnosis. Although lung cancer is the most common primary tumor leading to hemorrhagic brain seeding, the relative incidence of hemorrhagic transformation of a cerebral metastasis is highest in melanoma, choriocarcinoma, renal cell carcinoma, and papillary thyroid cancer. Systemic intravenous anticoagulation with heparin or fractionated heparinoid are used in dural sinus thrombosis. When l-asparaginase therapy is involved in the pathogenesis of the prothrombotic stage, substitution with fresh-frozen plasma and antithrombin III is often administered prior to anticoagulant use.

Leukostasis in leukemic diseases responds to hydration, leukapheresis, systemic chemotherapy, and low-dose whole-brain irradiation

DeVita, Hellman, and Rosenberg's Cancer: Principles & Practice of Oncology. 10th edition. 2014. 120. Increased Intracranial Pressure.

Q17. Answer FTTF

This patient has fever, persisting for more than 3 days in spite of being on broad spectrum antibiotics. He is at considerable risk to have fungemia which is substantiated by the positive blood culture. In the neutropenic patient, other sources of candidiasis like GI source predominate than CRBSI. An Echinocandin is the recommended drug as initial therapy. In the absence of hemodynamic instability or recent azole exposure, fluconazole may be tried, although the evidence is weak. Ophthalmological findings of metastatic infection can be detected only after full recovery of neutropenia. Therefore, there is no role for an urgent fundoscopic examination currently. Blood culture should be taken on alternate days, and in the absence of metastatic fungemia, the antifungals should be continued for 2 more weeks after the last positive blood culture.

    Pappas PG, Kauffman CA, Andes DR, et al. Clinical Practice Guideline for the Management of Candidiasis: 2016 Update by the Infectious Diseases Society of America. Clin Infect Dis. 2015;62(4):e1–50.

Q18. Answer TFTF

Patients with malignancy can develop hyponatremia due to the effects of the tumor or also due to the effect of the chemotherapeutic agents. Patients undergoing chemotherapy develop hyponatremia either due to an inappropriate ADH secretion, or by potentiating the effects of ADH. The common agents implicated in inducing hyponatremia are platinum compounds (cisplatin, carboplatin), alkylating agents like cyclophosphamide, ifosfamide and vinca alkaloids (vincristine, vinblastine). Cisplatin might also induce a renal tubulopathy causing excess salt loss resulting in acute hyponatremia.

    Castilllo J, Vincent M JE. Diagnosis and management of hyponatremia in cancer patients. Oncologist. 2012;17:756-65.

CHAPTER 10

Environmental Hazard, Poisoning and Acute Pharmacology

Nita George, Jaya Susan Jacob

A Type Questions
(One best answer)

1. The indications for referral to a transplant center in paracetamol poisoning include:
   a. Arterial pH<7.3
   b. INR> 2.0
   c. Serum paracetamol levels > 100 mg/L
   d. Sr. Bilirubin level > 3 mg/dL
   e. Urine output < 0.5 mL/kg/hr

2. A 36-year-old lady under treatment for schizophrenia for the last 10 years was admitted with a history of fever (Temp-103°F) and unconsciousness. She had a history of change in her medications 2 weeks back. On examination her GCS was 3/15, heart rate 120/min, BP 190/100 mm Hg, RR 40/min and she had muscle rigidity. Her most likely diagnosis is:
   a. Malignant hyperthermia
   b. Meningitis
   c. Hysterical reaction
   d. Neuroleptic malignant syndrome
   e. Heat stroke

3. A 60-year-male was admitted in a comatose state. He was rescued from his car, which was left running with its engine switched on in a closed garage. On examination his GCS was 3/15 and oxygen saturation was 100%. The most likely cause of his condition is:
   a. Stroke
   b. Drug overdose
   c. Myocardial infarction
   d. Hypoxia
   e. Alcohol intoxication

4. A 22-year-old male was admitted with relapse of Hodgkin's lymphoma and was started on a chemotherapeutic regimen of Cyclophosphamide, Oncovin, Prednisone, Procarbazine, Adriamycin, Bleomycin and Vinblastine. He was previously treated 5 years back with the Adriamycin, Bleomycin, Vinblastine, and Dacarbazine (ABVD) regimen. Two weeks after the last chemotherapy cycle, the patient presented with complaints of breathlessness on exertion, which was insidious and progressive and hence was admitted in ICU. High Resolution Computed Tomography (HRCT) thorax showed septal thickening with interspersed areas of ground glass attenuation with an associated impression of interstitial lung disease. He was having a saturation (SpO_2) of 85% on room air and RR of 40/min. One of the following is good strategy to prevent deterioration of pulmonary function:
   a. 100% Oxygen by nonrebreathing mask
   b. Restarting the same chemotherapy regimen when the patient's condition improves
   c. NIV with minimal FiO_2 to maintain a $SpO_2 \approx 90\%$
   d. Avoiding steroids
   e. Switching to radiation therapy at the earliest

5. A 25-year-female was admitted with a history of taking 70 × 50 mg tablets of Amitryptilline. She was comatose, hypotensive and tachycardic.

ECG shows tachycardia with broad QRS complex. Which of the following is correct?
a. Gastric lavage should be given
b. This condition is associated with miosis
c. Sodium bicarbonate is the treatment of choice
d. Amiodarone should be given to treat arrhythmias
e. Glucagon is contraindicated

6. In a poisoned patient with increased anion gap metabolic acidosis, which etiology is most likely to cause optic atrophy and blindness?
a. Ethylene glycol
b. Arsenic poisoning
c. Methanol poisoning
d. Carbon monoxide poisoning
e. Cocaine poisoning

7. Treatment of cyanide toxicity includes all the following *except*:
a. Sodium nitrite
b. Thiamine
c. Sodium thiosulphate
d. Amyl Nitrite
e. Hydroxycobalamin

8. IV lipid emulsion may be used to treat toxicity due to all of the following *except*:
a. Verapamil
b. Bupivacaine
c. Clomipramine
d. Atenolol
e. Lamotrigine

9. A 45-year-old male was admitted to your ICU with agitation, confusion, diarrhea, shivering and myoclonus. He was sweating profusely and his temp was 40°C and was found to have hyper reflexia. He has a history of depression on multiple antidepressant medication. His Fluoxetine dose had been increased 6 hours ago. His treatment may include all of the following *except*:
a. Activated charcoal
b. Cyproheptadine
c. Antipyretics
d. Nondepolarizing muscle relaxants
e. Risperidone

10. Metformin intoxication causes:
a. Normal anion gap acidosis
b. Type A lactic acidosis
c. Type B lactic acidosis
d. Alkalosis
e. High anion gap acidosis due to uremia

11. A 2-year-old child suffered second degree burns to the legs. The mother who is a nurse applied Prilox cream (Prilocaine + Lignocaine) to the burnt area for pain relief. 2 hours later she found the child blue and unresponsive. Treatment options include:
a. IV Methylene Blue
b. Disulphiram
c. N acetyl cysteine
d. Sodium Citrate
e. Deferoxamine mesylate

12. A 20-year-old male with suspected drug overdose was admitted to the emergency department with decreased level of consciousness, pin point pupils and a respiratory rate of 8/min. What is the most likely diagnosis?
a. Tricyclic antidepressant overdose
b. Benzodiazepine overdose
c. Alcohol intoxication
d. Cocaine toxicity
e. Heroin overdose

13. Regarding digoxin toxicity:
a. 'Reverse tick' sign on the ECG is pathognomonic of digoxin toxicity
b. Digoxin-specific Fab fragments (digibind) is the definitive treatment
c. Treatment success after digibind is measured by checking for decreasing digoxin levels
d. Digoxin toxicity cannot occur if digoxin levels are within the therapeutic range
e. Atrial tachyarrhythmias with a rapid ventricular response is common

14. Regarding Acute Radiation Syndrome (ARS) all the following are true *except*:
a. ARS can occur with exposure of more than 30 rads of radiation
b. Is more common when fractionated doses are given over a long period of time
c. Sequential changes in absolute lymphocyte count over time can be a guide to the degree of radiation exposure
d. The patient may look and feel healthy for up to a few weeks after radiation exposure
e. Human Leucocyte Antigen (HLA) typing has to be done prior to any initial transfusion

15. **Regarding Paraquat poisoning:**
    a. Is commoner in the developed world
    b. Paraquat is metabolized into toxic byproducts and then excreted in urine
    c. A positive sodium dithionite test on urine indicates a poor prognosis
    d. The concentration is lowest in the lung due to reduced uptake by the cells
    e. Gastric lavage should be done within one hour of ingestion

16. **A 10-year-old child was admitted to the hospital with accidental kerosene ingestion:**
    a. Activated charcoal should be given through a wide gauge orogastric tube
    b. Induced vomiting is indicated
    c. A bowel wash should be given
    d. Early intubation and ventilation is warranted
    e. Early corticosteroid therapy is indicated

17. **A 20-year-old male was brought by ambulance with a history of suicide attempt by eating the fruit of the plant Cerbera odollam. Which of the following is correct?**
    a. Its effects are caused by an atropine like effect
    b. Eating 1 fruit is not fatal
    c. The most common ECG abnormality is sinus tachycardia
    d. The only available antidote is digoxin immune FAB
    e. It cannot be detected by any means and hence is called the perfect murder weapon

18. **Regarding Aluminum phosphide (Celphos) poisoning all the following statements are true *except*:**
    a. There is no known antidote
    b. Gastric lavage with coconut oil is useful
    c. Potassium permanganate is used for gastric lavage
    d. The lethal dose for an adult is 10 mg
    e. Activated Charcoal should be given

19. **The antidote for beta blocker overdose is:**
    a. Atropine
    b. Adrenaline
    c. Glucagon
    d. Calcium chloride
    e. Isoprenaline

20. **Dialyzable toxins include all the following *except*:**
    a. Lithium
    b. Ethylene glycol
    c. Carbamazepine
    d. Paraquat
    e. Digoxin

21. **All of the following may be associated with methanol intoxication *except*:**
    a. Pancreatitis
    b. Absent light perception
    c. Putaminal necrosis
    d. Crystalluria
    e. High anion gap metabolic acidosis

22. **N-acetylcysteine (NAC) is NOT useful in the management of:**
    a. Paracetamol toxicity
    b. Bronchial asthma
    c. Contrast nephropathy
    d. Idiopathic pulmonary fibrosis
    e. Acute pancreatitis

23. **Most likely cause of persistent abdominal pain in a patient with organophosphorus poisoning and low pseudocholinesterase level is:**
    a. Intestinal obstruction
    b. Mesenteric ischemia
    c. Acute pancreatitis
    d. Hepatitis
    e. Gallbladder calculi

24. **Which of the following is TRUE regarding medication errors in critically ill patients?**
    a. Account for less than half of the errors reported
    b. May be influenced by large volume resuscitation in these patients
    c. Prescription errors are more common than administration errors
    d. Transdermal drug delivery is an effective and safe alternative to subcutaneous route
    e. Are more likely to be reported than those occurring in patients admitted in wards

25. **High priority investigations in patients with inhalational injury include all of the following *except*:**
    a. Arterial blood gas analysis
    b. RBC cyanide levels
    c. Bronchoscopy
    d. Chest X ray
    e. Flow volume loops on pulmonary function tests

26. **Acute kidney injury occurring as a consequence of snake bite is caused by all of the following *except*:**

a. Severe persistent hypotension leading to acute tubular necrosis
b. Rhabdomyolysis and subsequent myoglobinuria
c. Vasculitis
d. Volume overload from transfusions
e. Acute extracapillary proliferative glomerulonephritis

27. Noise pollution in ICU can be managed by all of the following methods *except*:
    a. Use of noise level monitors
    b. Behavior modification programs for nurses
    c. Headsets for patients
    d. Music therapy
    e. Sound absorbent surface coverings

28. Treatment that is unnecessary in the treatment of insect bite/sting is:
    a. Antihistamines
    b. Oral corticosteroid
    c. Antibiotics
    d. Cold compresses
    e. Analgesics

29. Scorpion envenomation:
    a. Causes coagulopathy
    b. Results in tetany
    c. Causes hypophosphatemia
    d. Results in 'adrenergic storm'
    e. Should be treated primarily with corticosteroids

30. Dehydration that is common in hot environments results in maximal utilization of endogenous:
    a. Corticosteroids
    b. Vasopressin
    c. Melatonin
    d. Thyroxin
    e. None of the above

31. The gold standard for measurement of body temperature in heat related illness in the field setting is:
    a. Aural thermometry
    b. Temporal temperature
    c. Axillary thermometry
    d. Esophageal temperature
    e. Rectal thermometry

32. Ethanol administration to treat methanol poisoning:
    a. Adversely affects mortality
    b. Is considered the 'first aid' antidote
    c. Should be considered only in unconscious victims
    d. May hasten the onset of visual sequelae
    e. Should only be administered in a hospital environment

33. Tissue damage from viper bites:
    a. Results from the accompanying DIC
    b. Often occurs in sites remote from site of bite
    c. Cannot be prevented by early administration of Anti Snake Venom (ASV)
    d. May be minimized by early and radical wound debridement
    e. Is related to the amount of venom injected with the bite

34. Most common etiology for insect related anaphylaxis comes from:
    a. Culicidae
    b. Hymenoptera
    c. Periplaneta
    d. Schistocerca
    e. Latrodectus

35. Most common vascular injury reported with central venous cannulation is:
    a. Right atrial perforation
    b. Vena caval injury
    c. Arterial puncture
    d. Mediastinal perforation
    e. Pericardial tamponade

36. The role of damage control surgery in blast injuries is:
    a. Early recognition of patients likely to benefit from surgery
    b. Relies on resuscitation first and subsequent surgery
    c. Emphasizes the importance of early correction of the altered anatomy
    d. Is ineffective in preventing development of the 'lethal triad'
    e. Indicated in less severe or non-life threatening injuries only

37. Regarding the use of Bispectral Index (BIS) monitor for measurement of sleep in agitated patients:
    a. It is regarded as the gold standard for sleep measurement
    b. Of the values from 0 to 100, higher values indicate deeper plane of sleep
    c. Is complicated by the use of minimally invasive electrodes

d. Is prone to error from movement induced artifacts
   e. Maybe falsely elevated in deeply sedated patients

38. **Clinical effects of muscarinic receptor stimulation by organophosphorus (OP) compounds include:**
   a. Fasciculations
   b. SLUDGE symptoms
   c. Tachycardia
   d. Paralysis
   e. Hypertension

39. **The medication that is ineffective in preventing delirium in the critically ill patients is:**
   a. Risperidone
   b. Haloperidol
   c. Rivastigmine
   d. Dexmedetomidine
   e. Low dose ketamine

40. **Highly water soluble occupational chemical irritants include:**
   a. Chlorine
   b. Sulphur dioxide
   c. Phosgene
   d. Mustard gas
   e. Ozone

K Type Questions
[Marked True (T)/False (F)]

1. **With regards to salicylate intoxication:**
   a. Respiratory alkalosis occurs as a compensatory phenomenon in response to metabolic acidosis
   b. Patient commonly presents with hypothermia
   c. Acetazolamide is used in treatment of salicylate overdose
   d. On initiating mechanical ventilation the settings should be adjusted to induce respiratory alkalosis
   e. Forced alkaline diuresis is the treatment of choice

2. **Regarding acetaminophen overdose:**
   a. Oral activated charcoal avidly adsorbs acetaminophen
   b. There is no need for treatment if the patient is asymptomatic and liver function tests are normal
   c. If patients present late following overdose (beyond 8 hours) treatment with N acetyl-cysteine is not indicated
   d. Renal failure occurs secondary to liver failure
   e. Toxic doses are 10 g in adults and 200 mg/kg bodyweight in children

3. **Toxins associated with an elevated oxygen saturation gap include:**
   a. Cyanide
   b. Iron
   c. Carbon monoxide
   d. Hydrogen sulphide
   e. Methemoglobin

4. **Drugs associated with an increased anion gap metabolic acidosis include:**
   a. Lithium
   b. Ethanol
   c. Acetaminophen
   d. Polymyxin B
   e. Metformin

5. **A 70/F with bipolar disorder on treatment with lithium for many years was admitted with seizures, renal failure and hypotension.**
   a. She should be treated with activated charcoal
   b. Treatment of choice is renal replacement therapy
   c. Is associated with a decreased anion gap
   d. Whole bowel irrigation with polyethylene glycol is indicated
   e. Treatment includes forced alkaline diuresis

6. **A 7-year-old boy accidentally drank a bottle of antifreeze (radiator coolant) and was brought to your hospital. He was unconscious and was having seizures with tachycardia and tachypnea:**
   a. The patient should be given activated charcoal down a nasogastric tube immediately
   b. Oxalic acid crystals in urine are pathognomonic for this condition
   c. Initially high osmolar gap is common
   d. Associated with normal anion gap metabolic acidosis
   e. Fomepizole (4-methylpyruvate) is used for treatment

7. **A 47-year-old male who is a cocaine abuser was admitted with severe agitation, hyperthermia, tachycardia and hypertension. His creatinine**

kinase levels were elevated. His initial treatment includes:
a. Benzodiazepines
b. Haloperidol
c. Beta blockers
d. Restrict fluids
e. Cooling measures

8. Which of the following drugs/conditions are associated with hyperthermia?
a. Cocaine
b. Alcohol
c. Lithium
d. Monoamine oxidase inhibitors
e. Salicylates

9. Activated charcoal should be given for the treatment of overdose with:
a. Lithium
b. Digoxin
c. Amitryptiline
d. Methanol
e. Phencyclidine

10. Overdoses causing rhabdomyolysis include:
a. Phencyclidine
b. Opioids
c. Cocaine
d. Alcohol
e. Lithium

11. Drugs that can cause hyponatremia due to SIADH include:
a. Ecstasy
b. Cocaine
c. Carbamazepine
d. Fluoxetine
e. Lithium

12. Regarding Gamma Hydroxybutyrate (GHB) also called the date-rape drug:
a. It cannot be detected by toxicological analysis
b. Its antidote is naloxone
c. It acts as an inhibitory neurotransmitter to GHB and GABA receptors
d. Recovery is usually rapid
e. It does not cause tolerance or dependence

13. Regarding acute alcohol intoxication:
a. Death can occur at lower blood alcohol levels in "non-tolerant" subjects
b. Toxicity is not related to the person's body weight
c. Can cause new onset atrial and ventricular arrhythmias
d. It may cause Zieve Syndrome (hemolytic anemia, jaundice, and hypertriglyceridemia)
e. Alcohol levels cannot be detected from urine

14. Antidotes to heavy metal poisoning are:
a. Lead—2,3-dimercaptosuccinic acid (DMSA or succimer)
b. Mercury—Deferoxamine
c. Iron—D-penicillamine
d. Gold—Dimercaprol
e. Arsenic—Calcium chloride

15. A 20-year-old female who is a known drug user was admitted in an unconscious state with history of having consumed a handful of Lorazepam tablets. The treatment includes:
a. IV Flumazenil
b. Activated Charcoal
c. Gastric Lavage
d. Intubation and ventilation
e. IV Naloxone

16. Calcium channel blocker (CCB) overdose:
a. Manifests as hyperglycemia
b. Tachyarrhythmias are common
c. Atrial pacing is sufficient to treat CCB toxicity
d. Treatment with IV Atropine is very effective
e. Hyperinsulinemic Euglycemia (HIE) is used for treatment

17. A postoperative patient on an epidural bupivacaine infusion suddenly developed ventricular arrhythmias and seizures followed by unconsciousness. The bupivacaine syringe was found to be connected to the IV cannula. The treatment includes:
a. IV 20% intralipid
b. Continuing the bupivacaine infusion epidurally
c. Vasopressin
d. IV Metaprolol
e. IV Midazolam

18. Phencyclidine (PCP) overdose:
a. Manifests as delirium, agitation and hyperthermia
b. The most common clinical features are hypertension and nystagmus

c. Activated charcoal should not be given
d. It is effectively removed by hemodialysis
e. Treatment with Benzodiazepines are contraindicated

19. **Conditions causing a high osmolar gap include:**
    a. Propylene glycol
    b. Ethanol
    c. Chronic renal failure
    d. Mannitol

20. **Poisonings that can be treated by extracorporeal membrane oxygenation include:**
    a. Aluminum phosphide
    b. Tricyclic antidepressants
    c. Paraquat
    d. Calcium channel blockers
    e. Cocaine

21. **With respect to cold exposure injuries:**
    a. Trench foot is a kind of freezing injury
    b. Alcohol use is linked to risk of developing frostbite
    c. Re-warming of frostbitten extremity should be done by submersion in hot water
    d. Debridement of necrotic tissues should be carried out as soon as possible
    e. Repeated freeze-thaw cycles may be beneficial.

22. **The intermediate syndrome associated with organophosphorus poisoning:**
    a. Occurs 1-4 days after resolution of acute intoxication
    b. Is seen in all patients with organophosphorus poisoning
    c. Affects only lower cranial nerves
    d. Is likely caused by recirculation of cholinesterase inhibitors sequestrated in the lung
    e. May be prevented by oxime therapy

23. **When dealing with lightning related injuries:**
    a. Eyes and ears of the victims are usually spared of injury
    b. Kidneys are likely to suffer anoxic damage
    c. Thermal injury to lungs is a common event
    d. Early institution of CPR has shown equivocal results
    e. The cardiac arrhythmia resulting in arrest is asystole

24. **The 'big four' poisonous snakes in India are:**
    a. Echis carinatus
    b. Daboia russelii
    c. Bungarus caeruleus
    d. Zamenis longissimus
    e. Naja naja

25. **The following statements are true with regard to the '20 minute whole blood clotting test':**
    a. The reliability is inconsistent
    b. Fresh venous blood is drawn to perform the test
    c. Accuracy is improved when the test samples are maintained at body temperature
    d. Plastic tubes and syringes may give false readings
    e. The test should be carried out every 6 hours after admission of a patient with suspected envenomation

26. **In victims of drowning:**
    a. The most important factor that determines the outcome is the temperature of water.
    b. Outcomes are better with salt water drowning
    c. Increased pulmonary capillary permeability may result in delayed onset of pulmonary complications
    d. Hypothermia may be protective if the temperature is less than 28°C
    e. The primary insult is circulatory arrest

27. **The most frequent complication seen during resuscitation of a drowning victim is:**
    a. Asystole
    b. Hypothermia
    c. Regurgitation of stomach contents
    d. Cervical spine injury
    e. Ventricular fibrillation

28. **In a suspected case of ethylene glycol poisoning:**
    a. Metabolism causes production of toxic substrates
    b. Ethanol may be used in treatment
    c. Inhibition of alcohol dehydrogenase enzyme is life-threatening
    d. Fomepizole is recommended as antidote
    e. Hemodialysis is ineffective

29. **Venom immunotherapy (VIT):**
    a. Is recommended for all patients who have experienced a systemic reaction to an insect sting and who have specific IgE to venom allergens
    b. Is advisable in patients who have experienced large local reactions to stings

c. Might be considered in those who have frequent unavoidable exposure
d. Is necessary in children 16 years of age and younger who have experienced cutaneous systemic reactions
e. is an extremely effective form of treatment for subjects at risk of insect sting anaphylaxis

30. **Heat related illness that is often benign and self-limiting is:**
    a. Heat cramps
    b. Heat syncope
    c. Heat edema
    d. Heat exhaustion
    e. Heat stroke

31. **Treatment modalities that have been successful in the management of heat stroke include:**
    a. Body cooling units
    b. Dantrolene
    c. Cold water immersion
    d. Whole body ice packs
    e. Antipyretics

32. **Acute kidney injury may occur with bites from:**
    a. Cobra
    b. Russel's viper
    c. Krait
    d. Hump nosed viper
    e. Saw scaled viper

33. **Domestic cat and dog bite wounds cause infections from:**
    a. Pasteurella
    b. Streptococcus
    c. Fusobacterium
    d. Capnocytophaga
    e. Methicillin resistant Staphylococcus

34. **Management of patients with blast lung injury may require:**
    a. Supplemental high flow oxygen via noninvasive continuous positive airway pressure or endotracheal tube
    b. High inspiratory pressure and volume
    c. One lung ventilation in severe hemoptysis or significant air leak
    d. Hyperbaric oxygen therapy for patients with arterial gas embolism
    e. Permissive hypercapnia, high-frequency jet ventilation and extracorporeal membrane oxygenation for patients with ARDS

35. **Inhalational manifestation of disease is likely with these agents of biowarfare:**
    a. Anthrax
    b. Botulism
    c. Plague
    d. Smallpox
    e. Tularemia

36. **Management of crush syndrome utilizes:**
    a. Isotonic saline
    b. Hypotonic saline
    c. Mannitol
    d. Sodium bicarbonate
    e. Restrictive fluid resuscitation

37. **Mortality in avalanche victims is most commonly due to:**
    a. Starvation
    b. Asphyxia
    c. Trauma
    d. Hypothermia
    e. Stress induced cardiac failure

38. **Medications that have been effectively used in the management of organophosphorus compound toxicity include:**
    a. Magnesium sulphate
    b. Pralidoxime
    c. Atropine
    d. Calcium chloride
    e. Hypertonic saline

39. **The top five substance classes most frequently involved in exposures in children of 5 years or less are:**
    a. Cosmetics/personal care products
    b. Household cleaning substances
    c. Analgesics
    d. Foreign bodies/toys/miscellaneous
    e. Sedative/hypnotics

40. **Ingestion of 'Magic mushrooms':**
    a. Causes sensory distortions
    b. Is endemic to Asia
    c. Causes toxic symptoms due to psilocin and psilocybin
    d. Is treated by liver transplantation
    e. Leads to multiorgan failure

ANSWERS

A Type Answers

Q1. Answer a
King's College Criteria for referral for liver transplantation in paracetamol toxicity include pH<7.3 despite fluid resuscitation or all of the following criteria INR>6.5 (Prothrombin Time>100 sec), Sr. Creatinine >3.5 mg/dL (>300 µmol/L) and hepatic encephalopathy grade 3 or 4.

O' Grady JG, et al. Early indicators of prognosis in fulminant hepatic failure. Gastroenterology. 1989;97:439-45.

Q2. Answer d
Neuroleptic malignant syndrome (NMS) is a rare, but life-threatening, idiosyncratic reaction to neuroleptic medications that is characterized by fever, muscular rigidity, altered mental status, and autonomic dysfunction. It has been associated with virtually all neuroleptics, including newer atypical antipsychotics, as well as a variety of other medications that affect central dopaminergic neurotransmission. NMS can be precipitated by the abrupt cessation or reduction in dose of dopaminergic medications, rapid switching from one type of dopamine receptor agonist to another or within hours or days after exposure to a causative drug, with most exhibiting symptoms within 2 weeks and nearly all within 30 days.

Berman BD. Neuroleptic malignant syndrome. A review for neurohospitalists. Neurohospitalist. 2011;1(1):41-7.

Q3. Answer d
Carbon monoxide (CO) poisoning occurs in the setting of attempted suicide from automobile exhaust, smoke inhalation, poorly ventilated charcoal or gas stoves. CO binds to hemoglobin with an affinity that is 240 times greater than oxygen to form carboxyhemoglobin and it decreases oxyhemoglobin saturation. Its toxicity results from a combination of tissue hypoxia and direct inhibition of cellular respiration by blocking cytochrome oxidase.

Because O_2Hb and COHb absorb red light (660 nm) similarly and COHb absorbs very little near-IR light (940 nm), the photodiode of standard pulse oximeters that only emit red and near-IR light cannot differentiate between O_2Hb and COHb.

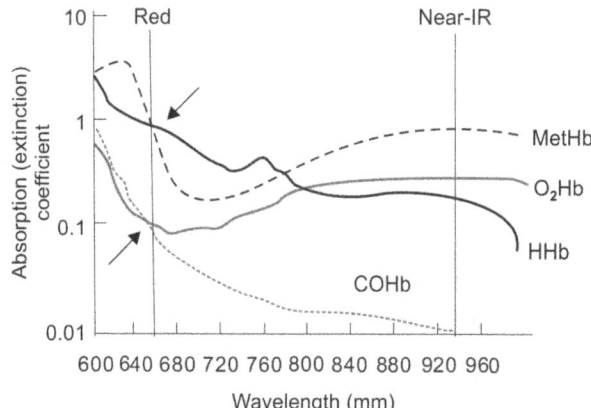

As O_2Hb and COHb have a similar absorptive property for red light, patients with carboxyhemoglobinemia appear bright red and not cyanotic. Arterial blood gas will show a normal PaO_2 and SaO_2. SaO_2 is accurate only if directly measured but not if calculated from PaO_2, which is common in many blood gas analyzers. The clinical diagnosis of acute carbon monoxide (CO) poisoning should be confirmed by demonstrating an elevated level of carboxyhemoglobin (HbCO) which can be measured by co-oximetry (direct spectrophotometric measurement in specific blood gas analyzers). Bedside, pulse carbon monoxide (CO)-oximetry is now available but requires a special unit and is not a component of routine pulse oximetry.

Mokhlesi B et al. Adult toxicology in critical care. Part II: Specific poisonings. Chest 2003;123:897-922.

Chan ED, et al. Pulse oximetry: Understanding its basic principles facilitates appreciation of its limitations. Respiratory Medicine. 2013;107:789-99.

Q4. Answer c

The patient most probably has bleomycin induced lung toxicity. Some of the risk factors associated with bleomycin induced lung fibrosis include: repeated systemic administration of bleomycin, total cumulative dose more than 450 units, elderly and in patients receiving oxygen therapy, those with a history of previous thoracic irradiation, renal insufficiency, smoking history, any underlying lung disease and supplementation G-CSF. The development of bleomycin induced pulmonary toxicity has been reported up to two years after discontinuation of bleomycin therapy. Oxygen therapy can induce and exacerbate bleomycin lung injury. A lower FiO_2 decreases the risk. The treatment includes steroids, administering minimal oxygen to maintain a SpO_2 of ≈90% and avoiding bleomycin from subsequent chemotherapy.

> Reinert T et al. Bleomycin induced lung injury. Journal of Cancer Research. 2013;2(13):1-9.
>
> Navin P et al. Pulmonary Toxicity of Bleomycin – A Case Series from a Tertiary Care Center in South India. Journal of Clinical and Diagnostic Research. 2016;10(4):FR01-FR03.

Q5. Answer c

Gastric lavage in tricyclic antidepressant (TCA) overdose may be useless as the administration of lavage fluid into the stomach only serves to propel some tricyclic tablets into the small bowel, facilitating absorption. TCA overdose is associated with mydriasis due to its anticholinergic effects. Sodium bicarbonate is the specific antidote and should be given if there is widening of the QRS interval, hypotension or cardiac arrest. It acts by increasing protein binding and decreasing the fraction of free drug. QRS prolongation in TCA overdose seems to result from voltage-gated sodium channel blockade. Increased availability of sodium reverses this effect. An alkaline environment permits TCA molecules to be in a non-ionized lipid-soluble state which diffuses away and unblocks the sodium channels. Amiodarone prolongs the QT interval and should be avoided. In general all antiarrhythmic drugs should be avoided and the correction of hypotension, hypoxia and acidosis will reduce the cardiotoxic effects of tricyclics. 10 mg intravenous glucagon may be given to treat life-threatening hypotension or arrhythmias refractory to other measures.

> Kerr GW et al. Tricyclic antidepressant overdose: a review. Emerg Med J. 2001;18:236-41.
>
> Rick B et al. Guideline for the Management of Tricyclic Antidepressant Overdose. Available at: https://www.rcem.ac.uk/docs (Accessed 6th August 2017).

Q6. Answer c

Methanol is metabolized to formic acid, which is neurotoxic and can cause visual disturbances and blindness.

> Kruse JA. Methanol and Ethylene Glycol Intoxication. Crit Care Clin. 2012;28:661-711.

Q7. Answer b

Antidotes to cyanide include nitrites, which induce methehemoglobin in red blood cells that combines with cyanide, thus releasing cytochrome oxidase enzyme. Sodium thiosulfate donates a sulfur atom necessary for the transformation of cyanide to thiocyanate by rhodanese, thus increasing the activity of the endogenous detoxification system. The thiocyanate is then renally excreted. Hydroxocobalamin is the drug of choice for treating known or suspected cyanide poisoning. Hydroxocobalamin combines with cyanide to form cyanocobalamin (vitamin B-12), which is renally cleared. Alternatively, cyanocobalamin may dissociate from cyanide at a slow enough rate to allow for cyanide detoxification by the mitochondrial enzyme rhodanese.

> Holstege CP, Kirk MA. Cyanide and Hydrogen Sulfide. Goldfrank's Toxicologic Emergencies. 10th ed. New York, NY: McGraw-Hill Education; 2015. Chapter 126.

Q8. Answer d

The exact mechanism of IV Lipid Emulsion (ILE) is unknown, but it likely involves decreasing the toxin's volume of distribution by shifting lipophilic drugs into the vascular compartment and limiting target tissue concentration. Other theories include inhibition of mitochondrial metabolism of lipids, impairment of fatty acid delivery to mitochondria, and activation of potassium and calcium channels involved with local anesthetic toxicity. Use of ILE should be considered for patients with severe toxicity due to a lipophilic drug who does not respond to standard measures.

> Levine M et al. Toxicology in the ICU Part 1: General overview and approach to treatment. Chest. 2011;140(3):795-806.

Q9. Answer c

Serotonin toxicity is most likely to develop following the initiation of a new serotonergic medication or the increase in dosage of a previously prescribed SSRI. Most reported cases are in patients taking multiple serotonergic agents or who have had considerable exposure to a single serotonin-augmenting drug. Treatment includes withdrawal of the offending serotonergic drugs and provision of supportive care. Administer activated charcoal if a potentially lethal amount or combination of pro-serotonergic agents have been ingested and if the presentation is within 1 to 2 hours. Cyproheptadine, a serotonin 2A antagonist, is usually recommended and is the most widely used antidote. The mainstays of therapy in managing hyperthermia and increased muscle rigidity in severely ill patients are neuromuscular paralysis, sedation, and possible intubation. Treat hyperthermia with cooling blankets, fans, ice packs, and IV fluids. Antipyretics are not indicated, as the mechanism for temperature alteration is centrally mediated. Risperidone is a 5-HT2a antagonist and has been shown to prevent the onset of Serotonin Syndrome.

Boyer EW, Shannon M. The serotonin syndrome. N Engl J Med. 2005;352(11):1112-20.

Ables AZ et al. Prevention, Diagnosis, and Management of Serotonin Syndrome. American Family Physician. 2010;81(9):1139-42.

Q10. Answer c

Metformin causes type B lactic acidosis due to its blockage of the metabolism of lactate and alanine to pyruvate. Metformin suppresses the enzyme pyruvate carboxylase. Patients present with a high anion-gap metabolic acidosis, related to high serum lactate levels. Treatment is by hemodialysis or CVVH and the endpoint for dialysis should be resolution of the lactic acidosis.

Jagia M et al. Metformin poisoning: A complex presentation. Indian J Anaesth. 2011;55(2):190-2.

Abramson S. Pharmacology and Toxicology: Treatment of Poisons - Metformin Intoxication. Available from: http://www.renalandurologynews.com/nephrology-hypertension/pharmacology-and-toxicology-treatment-of-poisons--metforminintoxication/article/616875/ (Accessed 11 June, 2017).

Q11. Answer a

Local anesthetics such as benzocaine and Prilocaine are common causes of methemoglobinemia. The risk of methemoglobinemia increases when the area of application is large and when applied over raw surfaces for a prolonged period of time. Initial care includes administration of supplemental oxygen and removal of the offending agent. The skin should be washed thoroughly. Intravenous (IV) methylene blue is the first-line antidotal agent. Exchange transfusion and hyperbaric oxygen treatment are second-line options for patients with severe methemoglobinemia whose condition does not respond to methylene blue or who cannot be treated with methylene blue (e.g. G6PD deficiency).

Denshaw-Burke M. Methemoglobinemia. Available from: http://emedicine.medscape.com/article/204178-overview (Accessed 6th August, 2017).

Q12. Answer e

Opioid overdose presents with the triad of decreased consciousness, respiratory depression and miosis. Opioid based drugs include morphine, heroin, oxycodone, and synthetic opioid narcotics. Tricyclic antidepressants and cocaine causes mydriasis. Alcohol and benzodiazepines do not cause any effect on pupil size.

Mokhlesi B et al. Adult toxicology in critical care. Part I: General approach to the intoxicated person. Chest. 2003;123:577-92.

Q13. Answer b

Reverse tick' T-wave inversion is a sign of digoxin effect and not a sign of toxicity. Serum digoxin concentration is of no use in diagnosis, because it measures the digoxin in the complexes with antibody fragments as well as unbound digoxin. The concentration therefore rises many folds after digoxin-specific antibody fragments are given. Toxicity can occur even when the serum digoxin concentration is within the therapeutic range. Conditions such as hypokalemia, hypomagnesemia, hypercalcemia, myocardial ischaemia, and hypoxemia and acid–base disturbances increase sensitivity to digoxin. They at least partly account for patients who develop toxicity when their serum digoxin concentration is within the therapeutic range. Atrial tachyarrhythmias with a rapid ventricular response require intact conduction through the AV node. Except for this all other arrhythmias can develop.

Mathew P et al. Management of digoxin toxicity. Aust Prescr. 2016;39(1):18-20.

Q14. Answer b

ARS is more common if large doses of radiation are given over a short period of time. ARS occurs with doses over 70 rads but mild symptoms may occur as low as 30 rads. Repeat CBC analysis, with special attention to the lymphocyte count, every 2 to 3 hours for the first 8 to 12 hours following exposure (and every 4 to 6 hours for the following 2 or 3 days). Monitoring the decrease in absolute lymphocyte count has been found to be the most practical method to assess the radiation dose within hours or days following a radiation exposure.

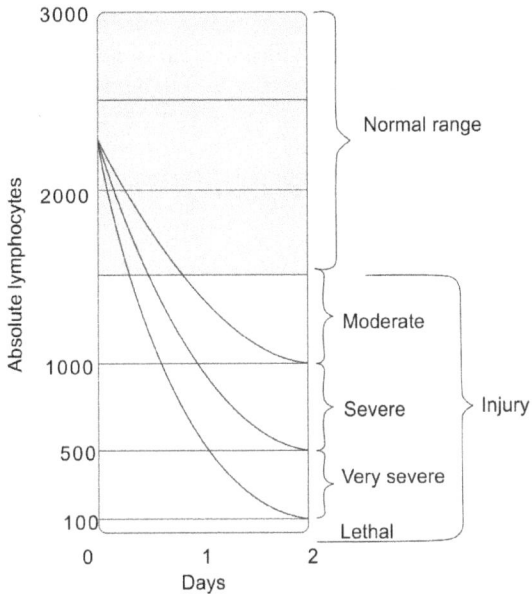

The Andrews lymphocyte normogram

Since hematopoietic stem cell (HSC) transplantation may be required to treat radiation accident victims a sample for HLA typing should be taken immediately and the search for potential donor initiated early.

<small>Acute Radiation Syndrome: A Fact Sheet for Clinicians. Available from: https://emergency.cdc.gov/radiation/arsphysicianfactsheet.asp (Accessed 6th August 2017).</small>

Q15. Answer c

Paraquat is a highly toxic herbicide and is a common agent for suicide in 3rd world, especially Asia. Paraquat is rapidly but incompletely absorbed and then largely eliminated unchanged in urine. Paraquat generates reactive oxygen species, which cause cellular damage via lipid peroxidation, activation of NF-κB, mitochondrial damage and apoptosis in many organs. It is actively taken up against a concentration gradient into lung tissue leading to pneumonitis and lung fibrosis. Sodium dithionite test on urine if positive (color changes to blue) confirms urine paraquat concentration >1 mg/L which indicates a very poor prognosis. Avoid gastric lavage as it causes caustic injury and is unlikely to provide any benefit.

<small>Gawarammana IB, Buckley NA. Medical management of paraquat ingestion. Br J Clin Pharmacol. 2011;72(5):745-57.</small>

Q16. Answer d

Highly volatile hydrocarbon compounds with low viscosity such as kerosene are more likely to be inhaled or aspirated. The hydrophobic nature of hydrocarbons allows them to penetrate deep into the tracheobronchial tree, producing inflammation and bronchospasm. Treatment by induced vomiting is contraindicated, as risk for aspiration is high. Gastric lavage should not be attempted since the risk and complications of aspiration generally outweigh the benefits. Charcoal poorly adsorbs most hydrocarbons. Furthermore, charcoal tends to distend the stomach and causes vomiting, increasing the aspiration potential. These volatile chemicals can displace alveolar oxygen, leading to hypoxia. Corticosteroid therapy is also not beneficial, and may be harmful in some cases. Early intubation for protection of the airway and mechanical ventilation, and use of positive end-expiratory pressure may be warranted in a patient with inadequate oxygenation, severe respiratory distress, or a decreased level of consciousness.

> Tormoehlen LM et al. Hydrocarbon toxicity: A review. Clin Toxicol (Phila). 2014;52(5):479-89.

> Ramnarine M. Hydrocarbons Toxicity. Available from: http://emedicine.medscape.com/article/1010734-overview (Accessed 6th August 2017).

Q17. Answer d

The seed inside the fruit of C. Odollam is highly poisonous. It contains the powerful alkaloid, cerberin, which is similar to digoxin. Eating the core of one fruit is sufficient to cause death. The minimum lethal dose is half a kernel of C. Odollam. The most common ECG abnormality is sinus bradycardia. Treatment modalities include temporary cardiac pacing and atropine administration. Survival has been reported after administration of digoxin immune FAB which is very expensive. It is very difficult to detect as it can be concealed in spicy dishes. It can be detected only if samples are subjected to liquid chromatography and mass spectrometry, hence it is said to be the perfect murder weapon.

> David Kassop et al. An unusual case of cardiac glycoside toxicity. International Journal of Cardiology. 2014;170:434-44.

> Menon MS, Kumar P, Jayachandran Cl. Clinical profile and management of poisoning with suicide tree: An observational study. Heart Views 2016; 17:136-9.

Q18. Answer d

Aluminum phosphide (Celphos/Quickphos) is a highly toxic fumigant for stored cereal grains. Lethal dose of ALP is 1–1.5 g but deaths have been reported even with a dose of 150–500 mg. After ingestion, effectiveness of gut decontamination primarily depends on the duration of exposure of poison and should be done as early as possible. Potassium permanganate (1:10000) is used for gastric lavage as it oxidizes phosphine to nontoxic phosphate. Slurry of activated charcoal also helps to adsorb phosphine from the gastrointestinal (GI) tract. The mechanism by which coconut oil reduces the toxicity of phosphides was proposed that it forms a protective layer around the gastric mucosa, thereby preventing the absorption of phosphine gas. Secondly, it helps in diluting the HCl and again inhibiting the breakdown of phosphide from the pellet. There is no known antidote and the treatment is mainly supportive. It is common in northern India, particularly in Haryana and Rajasthan. The treatment is supportive particularly cardiac like inotropes, IABP and ECMO.

> Agarwal VK et al. Aluminum phosphide poisoning: Possible role of supportive measures in the absence of specific antidote. Indian J Crit Care Med. 2015;19(2):109-12.

Q19. Answer c

For cases of β-blocker poisoning where symptomatic bradycardia and hypotension are present, high-dose glucagon is considered the first-line antidote.

> Shepherd G. Treatment of poisoning caused by β-adrenergic and calcium-channel blockers. American Journal of Health-System Pharmacy. 2006; 63(19):1828-35.

Q20. Answer e

Hemodialysis effectively enhances elimination of any drug that:
- Is a small molecule
- Has a small volume of distribution
- Has rapid redistribution from tissues and plasma
- Has slow endogenous elimination

> Cadogan M. Enhanced Elimination. Available from: https://lifeinthefastlane.com/ccc/enhanced-elimination/ (Accessed 8th August 2017).

> Levine M et al. Toxicology in the ICU Part 1: General Overview and Approach to Treatment. Chest. 2011;140(3):795-806.

Q21. Answer d

Visual disturbances, including decreased visual acuity, photophobia, and blurred vision, and abdominal pain are the most common symptoms of methanol intoxication one or both being found in 37% to 72% of patients. Abdominal pain can be present in both the presence and the absence of pancreatitis. Neurologic abnormalities including confusion, stupor, and coma are often present. The most severe neurologic dysfunctions are found in patients with the most severe metabolic acidosis. A rare complication of methanol intoxication is putaminal necrosis, which presents with rigidity, tremor and masked faces.

> Kraut JA, Kurtz I. Toxic Alcohol Ingestions: Clinical Features, Diagnosis, and Management. Clin J Am Soc Nephrol. 2008;3:208-25.

Q22. Answer b

Because of the highly favorable risk/benefit ratio and the low rate of adverse events, physicians might consider use of NAC in select patients to diminish exacerbation of COPD symptoms; reduce the risk of contrast-induced nephropathy; attenuate influenza illness; decrease the rate of deterioration of pulmonary function in idiopathic pulmonary fibrosis; and serve as an adjunct to clomiphene in the treatment of infertility in women with polycystic ovary syndrome. In addition, an intravenous preparation to treat acetaminophen overdose is available. NAC may attenuate oxidative-stress-induced cell injury and other pathological events at early stages of acute pancreatitis and potentially reduce the severity of disease.

> Millea PJ. N-acetylcysteine: multiple clinical applications. Am Fam Physician. 2009;80(3):265-9.

Q23. Answer c

Organophosphate insecticides are the potent inhibitors of the acetylcholinesterase enzyme which lead to an increased acetylcholine activity, responsible for symptoms such as abdominal pain, diarrhoea, vomiting and hypersalivation. Acute pancreatitis (toxic pancreatitis) is a rare complication of organophosphorus poisoning. It is mainly caused by acetylcholine release from the pancreatic nerves and the prolonged hyper stimulation of the acinar cells.

> LV, Rao VD, Rao MS, YM. Toxic Pancreatitis with an Intra-Abdominal Abscess which was caused by Organophosphate Poisoning (OP). J Clin Diagn Res. 2013;7(2):366-8.

Q24. Answer b

Medication errors are estimated to account for 78% of all medical errors in ICUs, with an average of 1.75 medication errors per patient per day. Large volume resuscitations, positive pressure ventilation, surgical procedures, systemic inflammatory response, and changes in protein binding, all common in ICU patients, affect the pharmacokinetics of many drugs. Administration is vulnerable to error because it is the last step in the process before the patient receives the medication. Transdermal drug delivery is erratic in critically ill patients. Because perfusion to epidermal and subcutaneous tissue is often lower than normal, it can cause unpredictable and often less-than-optimal absorption. The transdermal route should not be a target for novel drug delivery in the critically ill patient population. Fear of negative consequences can be a major barrier to accurate reporting of errors, with as many as 50% to 96% going unreported.

> Kruer RM, Jarrell AS, Latif A. Reducing medication errors in critical care: a multimodal approach. Clinical Pharmacology: Advances and Applications. 2014;6:117-26.

Q25. Answer c

Laboratory studies include arterial blood gas analysis with Carboxyhemoglobin, methemoglobin, and lactate levels; RBC Cyanide levels if persistent acidosis occurs; electrocardiographic (ECG) monitoring; and chest X-ray. For severe inhalation exposure or suspected pulmonary aspiration, chest radiography and arterial blood gas analysis are strongly recommended. The presence of hypoxemia despite a normal arterial partial pressure of oxygen suggests carbon monoxide toxicity. Carboxyhemoglobin levels should be obtained for all fire and explosion victims. Metabolic acidosis may indicate cyanide or hydrogen sulfide intoxication. Pulmonary edema, atelectasis or infiltrates may be detected on chest radiographs. As the final step, baseline pulmonary function should be determined through pulmonary function tests. Flow volume loops are the most sensitive noninvasive indicators of upper and lower airway obstruction. On the other hand, the utility of diagnostic bronchoscopy for inhaled toxin exposure remains controversial.

> Gorguner M, Akgun M. Acute Inhalation Injury. EAJM. 2010;42:28-35.

Q26. Answer d

The acute renal failure which occurs due to snake bite are multifactorial. (1) Severe and persistent hypotension leading to acute tubular necrosis, (2) Hb and other cellular parts of RBC and others (myoglobin and rhabdomyolysis, (3) Part of DIC, (4) Vasculitis (5) Acute diffuse interstitial nephritis, (6) Extracapillary proliferative glomerulonephritis.

Ghosh S, Mukhopadhyay P, Chatterjee T. Management of snake bite in India. JAPI. 2016;64:11-14.

Q27. Answer d

Because noise may be the most aversive effect of the ICU environment, efforts need to be directed to limiting the sounds of the ICU. Paying attention to the behavior of health care providers is the key to noise control. Behavior modification programs have had positive effects on altering the routines of staff related to noise in the ICU setting. Using headsets for patients, making periodic assessment of noise through noise level monitors, and selecting sound absorbent surface coverings in the ICU are recommended interventions.

Morton PG, Fontaine DK (eds.). Essentials of Critical Care Nursing: A Holistic Approach. Impact of the Critical Care Environment on the Patient. 2012 Page 42.

Q28. Answer c

Usually large local reactions should be treated symptomatically, with antihistamines, cold compresses, and analgesics as needed. In severe cases a short course of oral corticosteroids may be useful. Antibiotics are usually not necessary.

Golden DBK, Demain J, Freeman T, et al. Stinging insect hypersensitivity: A practice parameter update 2016. Ann Allergy Asthma Immunol. 2017;(118):28-54.

Q29. Answer d

Overstimulation of the sympathetic system increases blood levels of catecholamines, resulting in a characteristic "adrenergic (autonomic) storm" which consists of cardiac (tachycardia, peripheral vasoconstriction, hypertension, diaphoresis), metabolic (hyperthermia, hyperglycemia), urogenital (bladder dilatation, urinary retention, ejaculation in males), respiratory (bronchial dilation, tachypnea), and neuromuscular (mydriasis, tremor, agitation, convulsions) complications. It is indeed easy to treat pain with analgesics having an anti-inflammatory effect, such as salicylates.

Chippaux JP. Emerging options for the management of scorpion stings. Drug Des Devel Ther. 2012;6:165-73.

Q30. Answer b

Sometimes, injury may result from the pathophysiologic end points of normal processes used to maintain homeostasis rather than elevated core temperature. The dehydration that is common in hot environments can result in maximal utilization of endogenous vasopressin to reclaim free water. Although the goal is to maintain euvolemia, prolonged reclamation of free water out of proportion to sodium with the additional consumption of free water may result in dilutional hyponatremia.

Lipman GS, Eifling KP et al. Wilderness Medical Society Practice Guidelines for the Prevention and Treatment of Heat-Related Illness: 2014 Update. Wilderness & Environmental Medicine. 2014;(25):S55-S65.

Q31. Answer e

When possible, obtaining an accurate core body temperature is a critical diagnostic step in differentiating heat stroke from less severe heat injuries. Rectal temperature is widely considered the gold standard because it is the most reliable and practical measurement of core temperature and is more accurate than temporal, axillary, oral, or aural thermometry in the field setting. Esophageal and ingestible thermistors have been validated but are impractical in the wilderness setting.

Lipman GS, Eifling KP et al .Wilderness Medical Society Practice Guidelines for the Prevention and Treatment of Heat-Related Illness: 2014 Update. Wilderness & Environmental Medicine. 2014;(25):S55-S65.

Q32. Answer b

Ethanol, the active ingredient in alcoholic beverages, acts as a competitive inhibitor by more effectively binding and saturating the alcohol dehydrogenase enzyme in the liver thus blocking the binding of methanol. No patients with positive serum ethanol level on admission died compared with 21 with negative serum ethanol level (0% versus 36.2%). Patients receiving out-of-hospital ethanol survived without visual and central nervous system sequelae more often than those not receiving it (90.5% versus 19.0%). A positive association was present between out-of-hospital ethanol administration by paramedic or medical staff, serum ethanol concentration on admission, and both total survival and survival without sequelae of poisoning.

Zakharov S, Pelclova D et al. Use of out-of-hospital ethanol administration to improve outcome in mass methanol outbreaks. Ann Emerg Med. 2016;68(1):52-61.

Q33. Answer e

If the victim receives timely management with resuscitation and ASV administration, it can significantly reduce the local swellings and complications, curbing the need for surgical management. Most often, surgical intervention will be needed in late presentations or if the degree of envenomation was high. Huang et al. have used excisional treatment in the management of snake bite based upon the finding that bulk of deposited venom will remain in the area of bite and much removal of the tissue containing injected venom can eliminate the local tissue toxicity and reduce the magnitude of systemic toxicity.

Sheeja Rajan TM. Surgical Management of Snake Envenomation in India Current Perspective. Public health Rev: Int J Public health Res. 2017;4(1):13-9.

Q34. Answer b

Stinging insects of the order Hymenoptera are the main cause of insect-related anaphylaxis. There are 3 families of Hymenoptera with clinical importance: the bees (honeybees, bumblebees), vespids (yellow jackets, hornets, wasps), and stinging ants (genus Solenopsis and others). Exposure to these insects is affected by environmental and ecological factors.

Golden DBK. Insect sting anaphylaxis. Immunology and allergy clinics of North America. 2007;27(2):261-7.

Q35. Answer c

While arterial injuries are more common, lacerations of the vena cava, mediastinal vessels, and right atrium have been reported. The proposed mechanism of these injuries is that the guide wire becomes trapped against a vessel wall, and subsequent insertion of dilator or catheter causes injury.

Kornbau C, Lee KC, Hughes GD. Central line complications. International Journal of Critical Illness and Injury Science. 2015;5(3):170-8.

Q36. Answer a

Damage control surgery (DCS) is indicated when a person sustains an injury of such severity that it impairs their ability to maintain homeostasis. Severe hemorrhage then leads to triad of metabolic acidosis, hypothermia and increased coagulopathy. This form of surgery puts more emphasis on preventing the above-mentioned trauma triad of death, rather than correcting the anatomy. A major component of the surgery is early recognition of a person who could benefit from it and thus patients are transported to the operating room upon arrival, and resuscitation ensues concurrently with surgery. Goals of DCS are to stop the bleeding, remove contaminants and leave the wound open to avoid abdominal compartment syndrome.

Samra T, Pawar M, Kaur J. Challenges in management of blast injuries in Intensive Care Unit: Case series and review. Indian J Crit Care Med. 2014;18(12):814-8.

Q37. Answer d

BIS integrates EEG data to provide a scaled numerical value from 0 to 100, with a larger value representing a higher degree of consciousness. It utilizes a single foam sensor containing several EEG electrodes and is sometimes used in monitoring the depth of anesthesia in the operating room. Unlike actigraphy, BIS has the potential to estimate sleep depth, although significant overlap and variability in inter-rater cutoffs for sleep stages can lead to inaccurate characterization of sleep architecture. Furthermore, studies employing BIS in the ICU have been complicated by detachment of electrodes and artifact due to patient movement. BIS has not yet shown clinical benefit in ICU care.

Kamdar BB, Needham DM, Collop NA. Sleep deprivation in critical illness: Its role in physical and psychological recovery. J Intensive Care Med. 2012;27(2):97-111.

Q38. Answer b

Receptor-based manifestations were categorized as nicotinic and muscarinic receptor manifestations. Irreversible binding of OP to acetylcholinesterase in the cholinergic synapses in the CNS and peripheral nervous system (PNS) results in high concentrations of acetylcholine in the synaptic clefts that cause initial excessive stimulation and later, blockade of synaptic transmission. The peripheral muscarinic SLUDGE symptoms are due to actions on the relevant glands whilst central muscarinic effects result in symptoms such as confusion, coma and convulsions. Nicotinic effects are motor and sympathetic and result in fasciculations, muscle weakness, tachycardia and hypertension.

Peter JV, Sudarsan TI, Moran JL. Clinical features of organophosphate poisoning: A review of different classification systems and approaches. Indian Journal of Critical Care Medicine. 2014;18(11):735-45.

Q39. Answer c

There is some evidence that delirium can be prevented. Outside the ICU, repeated reorientation, noise reduction, cognitive stimulation, vision and hearing aids, adequate hydration, and early mobilization can reduce the incidence of delirium in hospitalized patients. Haloperidol prophylaxis in patients undergoing hip surgery reduced the severity and duration of delirium. Four placebo-controlled trials have evaluated pharmacologic prophylaxis of delirium; low-dose haloperidol and low-dose risperidone both reduced the incidence of delirium, as did a single low dose of ketamine during the induction of anesthesia. In contrast, the cholinesterase inhibitor rivastigmine was ineffective in preventing delirium. Sedation with dexmedetomidine rather than benzodiazepines appears to reduce the incidence of delirium in the ICU.

Reade MC, Finfer S. Sedation and Delirium in the Intensive Care Unit .N Engl J Med. 2014;370:444-54.

Q40. Answer b

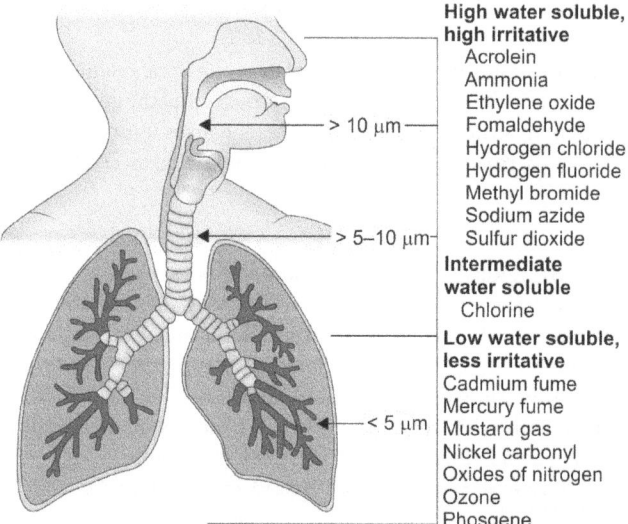

Distribution of the irritant gases and the site of injury in the respiratory tract according to their particle size and water solubility

Gorguner M, Akgun M. Acute Inhalation Injury. EAJM 2010;42:28-35.

K Type Answers

Q1. Answer FFFTF

In salicylate overdose, there is a mixed acid-base response with respiratory alkalosis and anion gap metabolic acidosis. The initial response is hyperpnea due to direct stimulation of the respiratory center in the brain stem. This is followed by uncoupling of oxidative phosphorylation with accumulation of lactate and pyruvate and the release of energy as heat resulting in hyperthermia and diaphoresis.

Sodium bicarbonate is used to increase serum pH and raise urine pH to > 7.5. Salicylates are ionized in alkaline pH and gets excreted unchanged. In acidic pH, salicylate are nonionized and therefore cross the blood-brain barrier and are responsible for increasing CNS toxicity and also gets re-absorbed into the renal tubules. Acetazolamide should not be used since it can increase the risk of systemic acidosis.

Forced diuresis does not appear to increase clearance and may lead to volume overload and worsen electrolyte disturbances.

Patients with salicylate intoxication benefit from their salicylate induced hyperventilation and subsequent respiratory alkalosis. Rapid neurologic deterioration and death has been described in patients who became more acidemic in the setting of initiation of mechanical ventilation.

Abramson S. Pharmacology and Toxicology: Treatment of Poisons - Salicylate Intoxication. Renal and Urology News. Available from: http://www.renalandurologynews.com/nephrology-hypertension/pharmacology-and-toxicology-treatment-of-poisons--salicylate-intoxication/article/616622/ [Accessed 14th July 2017].

Q2. Answer TFFFT

Activated charcoal should be given to all cooperative adults presenting early with paracetamol overdose. In the first 24 hours the patient may be asymptomatic clinically and biochemically. The best surrogate marker which indicates the potential for liver injury is a timed serum paracetamol level which is plotted on a nomogram. If the time since ingestion is beyond eight hours, infusion of N acetylcysteine should commence immediately, and serum paracetamol concentration and alanine aminotransferase (ALT) level determined to ascertain if the treatment should be continued. Renal injury may also occur through tubular necrosis, and this is thought to be a result of local production of NAPQI. Direct injury to organs other than the liver and kidney is rarely reported.

Guidelines from Australia and New Zealand. https://www.nzdoctor.co.nz/in-print/2017/march-2017/15-march-2017/paracetamol-toxicity,-overdose-and-associated-treatment-an-update.aspx

Nambiar N J. Management of Paracetamol Poisoning: The Old and the New. Journal of Clinical and Diagnostic Research. 2012;6(6):1101-04.

Q3. Answer TFTTT

An oxygen saturation gap is present when there is more than 5% difference between the saturation calculated from an arterial blood gas and the saturation measured by co-oximetry. Co-oximetry determines oxygen saturation by detecting the absorption of 4 different wavelengths of light enabling it to directly measure the levels of oxyhemoglobin, reduced hemoglobin, carboxyhemoglobin and methemoglobin. Arterial blood gas analysis calculates the oxygen saturation from the measured oxygen tension.

Mokhlesi B et al. Adult toxicology in critical care. Part I: General approach to the intoxicated person. Chest. 2003;123:577-92.

Q4. Answer FTTFT

Lithium and polymyxin B causes a decreased anion gap.

Mokhlesi B et al. Adult toxicology in critical care. Part I: General approach to the intoxicated person. Chest. 2003;123:577-92.

Q5. Answer FTTTF

Lithium is adsorbed poorly by activated charcoal and is not indicated. Lithium is a prototypical dialyzable toxin because of its low molecular weight, lack of protein binding, water solubility, low volume of distribution and prolonged half-life. Lithium is a monovalent cation and therefore causes a decreased anion gap if serum levels are severely elevated and may be a clue to the diagnosis. Whole bowel irrigation with polyethylene glycol is used to decrease absorption of sustained release lithium. Altering the urine pH with bicarbonate does not enhance lithium excretion.

Mokhlesi B et al. Adult toxicology in critical care. Part II: Specific poisonings. Chest. 2003;123:897-922.

Q6. Answer FTTFT

The gastrointestinal tract rapidly absorbs alcohols and they do not bind to activated charcoal.

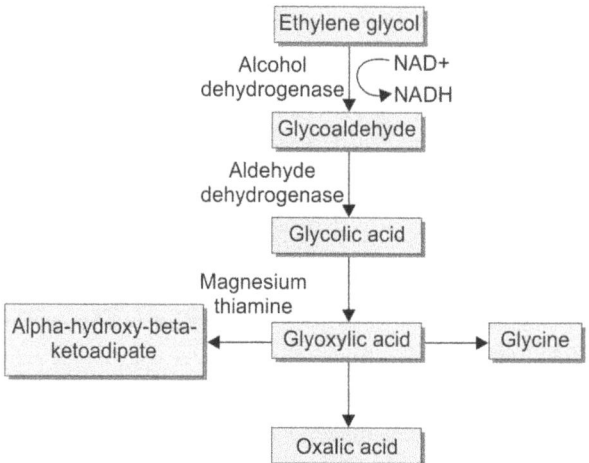

Ethylene glycol is metabolized in the liver by alcohol dehydrogenase to glycoaldehyde, which is then metabolized to glycolic acid by aldehyde dehydrogenase. Glycolic acid is further metabolized to glyoxylic acid and oxalic acid. Oxalic acid complexes with calcium lead to crystal formation in the renal tubules, renal failure and hypocalcemia. There is a high osmolar gap due to the presence of ethylene glycol. A high anion-gap metabolic acidosis develops due to the formation of glycolic acid and its metabolites, as well as hyperlactemia (increased NADH suppresses the conversion of lactate to pyruvate). Fomepizole is competitive antagonist that prevents ethylene glycol from being converted into its toxic metabolites by alcohol dehydrogenase. Ethanol also competes with ethylene glycol for metabolism by alcohol dehydrogenase

    Chris Nickson. Ethylene glycol inebriation. Available from: https://lifeinthefastlane.com/toxicology-conundrum-035/ (Accessed 7th August 2017).

    James A. Kruse. Methanol and Ethylene Glycol Intoxication. Crit Care Clin. 2012;28:661-711.

Q7. Answer TFFFT

The mainstay of treatment for manifestations related to the acute sympathomimetic effects of cocaine is sedation with benzodiazepines. Haloperidol may lower the seizure threshold and hence is not a first line drug. Administration of β-blockers may cause an unopposed α-adrenergic–mediated vasoconstriction leading to elevated blood pressures. It is prudent to initiate treatment of possible rhabdomyolysis and prevent renal tubular damage by providing aggressive intravenous hydration with crystalloids.

    Janice L. Zimmerman. Cocaine Intoxication. Crit Care Clin. 2012;28(1):517-26.

Q8. Answer TFFTT

Drugs, which have an anticholinergic or sympathomimetic effect, increases temperature. In contrast, organophosphates, opiates, barbiturates, β-blockers, benzodiazepines, alcohol, and clonidine cause hypothermia. Salicylates cause hyperthermia by uncoupling of oxidative phosphorylation.

    Mokhlesi B et al. Adult toxicology in critical care. Part I: General approach to the intoxicated person. Chest. 2003;123:577-92.

Q9. Answer FTTFT

The mechanism by which charcoal accomplishes enhancement of elimination is either by interrupting the enterohepatic/enterogastric circulation of drugs or through the binding of any drug that diffuses from the circulation into the gut lumen (called GI dialysis). However, it has limited application because the toxin must have a low volume of distribution, low protein binding, prolonged elimination half-life, and low pKa, which maximizes transport across mucosal membranes into the GI tract.

    Mokhlesi B et al. Adult toxicology in critical care. Part I: General approach to the intoxicated person. Chest 2003;123:577-92.

Q10. Answer TTTTT

Ethanol-induced rhabdomyolysis may develop from direct toxic effects on the sarcoplasmic reticulum by increasing sodium permeability and disrupting calcium homeostasis, disintegration of the cell membrane, and alterations in intracellular energy sources. The secondary effects of alcohol pertain to the altered mental status, loss of consciousness, and coma that can lead to prolonged immobilization and muscle compression. Ethanol ingestions can present with a history of poor nutrition, hypokalemia, and hypophosphatemia, which can predispose the patient to rhabdomyolysis. Cocaine can cause a direct effect on the muscle tissue, inducing vasoconstriction and tissue ischemia. Cocaine associated rhabdomyolysis may also contribute to the state of hyperthermia and hyperactivity. Phencyclidine can produce agitation and prolonged muscular activity that may contribute to muscle damage. It can also be due to seizures, hyperthermia, and delirium requiring restraints. Drugs that induce central nervous system depression such as opioids can cause prolonged immobilization, muscle compression, and tissue ischemia that result in myocyte injury. Lithium causes hyperthermia induced rhabdomyolysis.

Teresa J. Coco and Ann E. Klasner. Drug-induced rhabdomyolysis. Current Opinion in Pediatrics. 2004;16:206-10.

Huerta-Alardín AL, et al. Bench-to-bedside review: Rhabdomyolysis – an overview for clinicians. Critical Care. 2005;9:158-16.

Q11. Answer TFTTF

Drug-induced SIADH

The proposed mechanism by which some drugs induce SIADH may be broadly divided into three categories: (i) Stimulation of the release of ADH from the posterior pituitary: Nicotine, Phenothiazines, Tricyclics etc. (ii) Potentiation of the renal action of ADH: Desmopressin, Oxytocin, Prostaglandin synthesis inhibitors etc. (iii) Mixed or uncertain mechanism of action: Chlorpropamide, Carbamazepine, Cyclophosphamide, Vincristine, Ecstasy [3,4 methylene dioxymethamphetamine (MDMA)] etc.

A Brief Review of Drug-Induced Syndrome of Inappropriate Secretion of Antidiuretic Hormone - *Medscape* - Jan 24, 2002. http://www.medscape.com/viewarticle/420687_6 (Accessed 6th August, 2017).

Q12. Answer FFTTF

GHB is also known as liquid ecstasy or fantasy. It is derived from GABA and acts as an inhibitory neurotransmitter to GHB and GABA receptors in the brain. The clinical manifestations depend on the dose and range from euphoria to deep coma and death. Regular use produces tolerance and dependence. Treatment is mainly supportive which may be required only for a short time since rapid recovery is the norm. Naloxone is not helpful. Although normal toxicological screens do not include GHB, specialized laboratories can detect GHB in both urine and blood by gas chromatography- mass spectroscopy. GHB can also be detected by hair analysis.

Mokhlesi B et al. Adult toxicology in critical care. Part II: Specific poisonings. Chest. 2003;123:897-22.

Q13. Answer TFTTF

Alcohol toxicity depends on the amount of alcohol ingested, individual body weight and tolerance to alcohol, the percentage of alcohol in the beverage, and the period of alcohol ingestion. Symptoms are usually related to blood alcohol concentration. Alcohol levels can also be determined by breath analysis, with a saliva dipstick and levels of free ethanol and ethanol conjugates can be measured in urine. Acute alcohol ingestion can cause "holiday heart syndrome", characterized by atrial or ventricular tachyarrhythmias and new-onset atrial fibrillation.

Vonghia L et al. Acute alcohol intoxication. European Journal of Internal Medicine. 2008;19:561-67.

Q14. Answer TFFTF

Antidotes for Mercury, arsenic and copper is D-penicillamine, for Iron it is deferoxamine, for lead, mercury, arsenic and gold is dimercaprol, for Lead is Ca-EDTA and succimer.

Rusyniak DE et al. Heavy metal poisoning: management of intoxication and antidotes. EXS. 2010;100:365-96.

Q15. Answer FFFTF

Flumazenil is an antidote for benzodiazepines (BZD). It reverses CNS depression but does not reliably reverse respiratory depression. It is contraindicated in BZD-dependent patients because of the risk of provoking seizures. It should also be avoided in those patients known to be taking drugs that can increase the risk of seizures. The first step is to assess the patient's airway, breathing, and circulation and to address these rapidly as needed. The cornerstone of treatment in BZD overdose is good supportive care and monitoring. Gastric lavage should not be employed because of the risk of hypoxia, laryngospasm, and aspiration pneumonia. Because

BZD overdose is rarely dangerous and most patients do not present within an hour or so of overdose, activated charcoal to reduce absorption is not generally recommended. Naloxone does not reverse the effect of BZD.

Gresham C. Benzodiazepine Toxicity Treatment & Management. Available from: http://emedicine.medscape.com/article/813255-treatment (Accessed 6th August 2017).

Q16. Answer TFFFT

Hyperglycemia can occur and is a marker of severity. It is multifactorial in origin. (i) hypoinsulinaemia, as insulin release is dependent on calcium influx into islet beta cells through L-type calcium channels (ii) calcium channel blocker-induced insulin resistance (iii) During CCB toxicity, the myocardial cells change their preferred energy substrate from free fatty acids to glucose due to: impaired uptake of glucose and free fatty acids by cardiac myocytes inhibition of calcium-dependent mitochondrial activity required for glucose catabolism. High-dose insulin therapy has been shown to promote cellular uptake of glucose into adipose and muscle tissue, reduce cytosolic calcium concentration, and promote intracellular potassium movement. It may increase myocardial contractility and mean arterial pressure.

Cardiovascular manifestations of toxicity are usually bradycardia and first degree heart block and hypotension. IV atropine is usually not effective in treatment. If pacing is used, ventricular pacing to bypass the AV node should be used.

Levine M et al. Toxicology in the ICU Part 1: General Overview and Approach to Treatment. Chest. 2011;140(3):795-806.

Q17. Answer TFFFT

Bupivacaine infusion should be stopped immediately and no other local anaesthetic should be given. Treatment is supportive. Resistant ventricular arrhythmias are common with bupivacaine. IV 20% Intralipid should be given in a dose of 1.5 mL/kg bolus over 1 min, repeated up to 2 times, followed by 15 mL/kg/hr increased to 30 mL/kg/hr until cardiovascular stability. Benzodiazepines are the drugs of choice for seizure control. Vasopressin is not recommended in the treatment of hypotension. Calcium channel blockers and beta blockers should be avoided.

Neal JM, Mulroy MF, Weinberg GL. American Society of Regional Anesthesia and Pain Medicine checklist for managing local anesthetic systemic toxicity: 2012 version. Reg Anesth Pain Med. 2012;37(1):16-8.

Q18. Answer TTFFF

Activated charcoal (1 g/kg) may be administered and repeated every 4 hours for several doses in most symptomatic patients. Activated charcoal adsorbs PCP and increases its nonrenal clearance.

Because of its large volume of distribution, PCP is not effectively removed with hemodialysis or hemoperfusion.

Benzodiazepines are usually effective in managing aggressive behavior and in treating seizures.

Stephan Brenner. PCP Toxicity Treatment & Management. Available from: http://emedicine.medscape.com/article/1010821-treatment (Accessed 7th August 2017).

Q19. Answer TTFT

The difference between the measured and calculated osmotic concentrations is the osmolar gap. If a significant elevation of the osmolar gap is discovered, the difference in the two values may represent presence of foreign substances in the blood.

Christopher PH, Heather AB. Toxidromes. Crit Care Clin. 2012;28(1):479-98.

Q20. Answer TTFTT

VV-ECMO can be considered in patients with type I and II respiratory failure. In patients with life-threatening hemodynamic instability, VA-ECMO can be considered when shock persists despite volume administration, inotropes and vasoconstrictors, and (sometimes) intra-aortic balloon counter pulsation.

Typical examples include poisoning due to calcium channel antagonists, beta-blockers, tricyclic antidepressants, chloroquine and colchicine. Absolute contraindications are uncontrolled coagulopathy and severe intracranial bleeding, which precludes the use of anticoagulation therapy. In Paraquat poisoning

ECMO can be used as a bridge to lung transplantation but not as a treatment as generation of highly reactive oxygen species results in severe lung toxicity as paraquat is taken up against a concentration gradient into the lung. Oxygen will worsen oxidative stress and increase mortality.

    Hassanian-Moghaddam H et al. Successful Treatment of Aluminum Phosphide Poisoning by Extracorporeal Membrane Oxygenation. Basic Clin Pharmacol Toxicol. 2016;118(3):243-6.

    de Lange DW, Sikma MA, Meulenbelt J. Extracorporeal membrane oxygenation in the treatment of poisoned patients, Clinical Toxicology. 2013; 51(5):385-93.

    Gawarammana IB, et al. Medical management of paraquat ingestion. Br J Clin Pharmacol. 2011;72(5):745-57.

Q21. Answer FTFFF

Cold exposure injuries comprise nonfreezing injuries that include chilblain (aka pernio) and trench, or immersion, foot, as well as freezing injuries that affect core body tissues resulting in hypothermia of peripheral tissues, causing frostnip or frostbite. The risk of frostbite is influenced by host factors, particularly alcohol use and smoking, and environmental factors, including ambient temperature, duration of exposure, altitude, and wind speed. Rewarming for frostbite should not begin until definitive medical care can be provided to avoid repeated freeze-thaw cycles, as these cause additional tissue necrosis. Rewarming should be rapid and for an affected limb should be performed by submersion in warm water at 104° to 107.6°F (40° to 42°C) for 15 to 30 minutes. Debridement of necrotic tissues is generally delayed until there is a clear demarcation from viable tissues, a process that usually takes from 1 to 3 months from the time of initial exposure. Immediate escharotomy and/or fasciotomy is necessary when circulation is compromised.

    Golant A, Nord RM, Paksima N; et al. Cold exposure injuries to the extremities. J Am Acad Orthop Surg. 2008;16(12):704-15.

Q22. Answer TFFFF

Intermediate Syndrome (IMS) was first described as a syndrome of muscular paralysis occurring in conscious patients 24-96 hours following ingestion, after their acute cholinergic syndrome was treated with atropine. Muscle weakness affected predominantly the proximal limb muscles and those supplied by the cranial nerves. IMS was often associated with respiratory failure. More recent work suggest that IMS could occur before 24 hours and even after 96 hours. The pathophysiology of IMS is not clearly understood but is generally believed to result from a persistent excess of acetylcholine (ACh) at the neuromuscular junction. Recent studies have shown that intermediate syndrome is accompanied by the excretion of cholinesterase inhibitor metabolites in the urine and by severe depression in cholinesterase levels. Incidence: Estimates are that 10-68% of those poisoned with organophosphorus agents will develop intermediate syndrome.

    Reddy NG, Kahlekar, Priyanka L. Anesthetic management of a ectopic pregnancy patient with organophosphorus poisoning. J of evolution of med and dent sci. 2015;4(2):285-95.

Q23. Answer FTFFT

Lightning acts as a massive cosmic counter shock that causes cardiac standstill. Although respiratory arrest is one of the common causes of acute death in serious electrical injuries, there are no specific injuries to the lungs or the airways. Although direct injury from electric current is unusual, the kidneys are very susceptible to anoxic/ischemic injury that accompanies severe electrical injury. Because of its inherent automaticity, it is possible for the heart to recover spontaneously. Considering that the majority of lightning victims tend to be relatively young and previously healthy individuals, the possibility of successful resuscitation is high if proper care is instituted immediately.

    Koumbourlis AC. Electrical injuries. Crit Care Med. 2002;30(11):S424-30.

Q24. Answer TTTFT

In India, more than 200 species of snakes have been identified but only 52 are poisonous; the common krait (Bungarus caeruleus), Indian cobra (Naja naja), Russell's viper (Daboia russelii), and saw-scaled viper (Echis carinatus) are the most poisonous ("the big four").

    Ahmed SM, Ahmed M, Nadeem A. Emergency treatment of a snake bite: Pearls from literature. Journal of Emergencies, Trauma and Shock. 2008;1(2):97-105.

Q25. Answer FTFTF

Considered the most reliable test of coagulation and should be carried out at the bedside by treating physician. It can also be carried out in the most basic settings. A few milliliters of fresh venous blood is placed in a new, clean and dry, glass vessel and left at ambient temperature for 20 minutes. The vessel ideally should be a small glass test tube. The use of plastic bottles, tubes or syringes will give false, readings and should not be used. The test should be carried out every. 30 minutes from admission for three hours and then hourly after that. If incoagulable blood is discovered, the 6 hourly cycle is then be adopted to test for the requirement for repeat doses of ASV.

Ghosh S, Mukhopadhyay P, Chatterjee T. Management of snake bite in India. JAPI. 2016;64:11-14.

Q26. Answer FFTFF

Early basic and advanced life support is the most important factor to improve the outcome. Hypothermia associated with drowning can provide a protective mechanism that allows persons to survive prolonged submersion episodes. Hypothermia can reduce the consumption of oxygen in the brain, delaying cellular anoxia and ATP depletion. Aspiration of salt water and aspiration of fresh water cause similar degrees of injury. Cardiac arrest from drowning is due primarily to lack of oxygen. It is usually best not to initiate weaning from mechanical ventilation for at least 24 hours, even when gas exchange appears to be adequate. The local pulmonary injury may not have resolved sufficiently, and pulmonary edema may recur. Hypoxemia quickly leads to loss of consciousness and apnea followed by cardiac rhythm deterioration such as tachycardia, bradycardia, pulseless electrical activity, and finally, asystole.

Szpilman D, Bierens J, Handley AJ, et al. Drowning. N Engl J Med. 2012;366:2102-10.

Q27. Answer FFTFF

Injuries to the cervical spine occur in less than 0.5% of persons who are drowning, and immobilization of the spine in the water is indicated only in cases in which head or neck injury is strongly suspected (e.g. accidents involving diving, waterskiing, surfing, or watercraft). The most frequent complication during a resuscitation attempt is the regurgitation of stomach contents, which occurs in more than 65% of persons who require rescue breathing alone and in 86% of those who require CPR.

Szpilman D, Bierens J, Handley AJ, et al. Drowning. N Engl J Med. 2012;366:2102-10.

Q28. Answer TTFTF

Ethylene glycol exerts most of its toxicity by conversion to its metabolites. Ethylene glycol itself may cause some alteration of mental status but it is a relatively nontoxic compound before it is metabolized. It is metabolized by the enzyme alcohol dehydrogenase to form glycoaldehyde and glycolic acid. A profound acidosis often ensues with this intoxication which is attributable to the glycolic acid in circulation. Ethanol acts by competing with ethylene glycol for alcohol dehydrogenase, the first enzyme in the degradation pathway. Either ethanol or fomepizole may be used to inhibit alcohol dehydrogenase. Hemodialysis has also been an important treatment in ethylene glycol poisoning, especially in patients with severe metabolic acidosis and acute kidney injury. Hemodialysis removes glycolate (metabolite of ethylene glycol) and ethylene glycol from the blood effectively and corrects the acidosis.

McMartin K, Jacobsen D, Hovda KE. Antidotes for poisoning by alcohols that form toxic metabolites. Br J Clin Pharmacol. 2016; 81(3):505-15.

Q29. Answer TFTFT

Recommendations for VIT in Insect stings:

Recommend and initiate VIT in all patients who have experienced an anaphylactic reaction to an insect sting and who have specific IgE to venom allergens. (Strong Recommendation; A evidence)

Avoid VIT based solely on in vivo and in vitro testing for venom IgE, without a history of systemic reaction to a sting. (Strong Recommendation; A evidence)

Counsel patients who have experienced only large local reactions to stings that VIT is generally not required but might be considered in those who have frequent unavoidable exposure. (Recommendation; B evidence)

In a change from previous recommendations, advise both children and adults who have experienced only cutaneous systemic reactions without other systemic manifestations after an insect sting that VIT is generally not required but may be considered when there are special circumstances.

Golden DBK, Demain J, Freeman T, et al. Stinging insect hypersensitivity A practice parameter update 2016. Ann Allergy Asthma Immunol. 2017;(118):28-54.

Q30. Answer TFTFF

Heat-related illness can be manifested as a spectrum of disease from minor to severe, such as heat cramps, heat syncope, heat exhaustion, and life-threatening heat stroke. (i) Heat Edema is a benign condition that is often seen in nonacclimatized and elderly individuals when presented with a heat stress and is described as a mild edema that develops in dependent areas. This condition will resolve once the individual acclimates, though symptomatic treatment includes rest, lower extremity elevation, and possibly compression stockings. Interstitial fluid accumulates in dependent extremities as a result of hydrostatic pressure, vascular leak, and cutaneous vaso dilation. (ii) Heat cramps are fleeting painful spasms commonly involving the thighs, calves, abdominal wall and shoulder that occur after strenuous exertion. The condition is thought to be secondary to large amounts of sweat that is subsequently replaced by hypotonic solutions, resulting in a dilutional hyponatremia. Elevated core temperature is not a required feature as the cramps may present several hours after the exertion.

Lipman GS, Eifling KP et al. Wilderness Medical Society Practice Guidelines for the Prevention and Treatment of Heat-Related Illness: 2014 Update. Wilderness & Environmental Medicine. 2014;25:S55-S65.

Q31. Answer TFTTF

Ice packs have been shown to be more efficacious when covering the entire body. Antipyretic drugs are ineffectual and should be avoided. The larger studies using a specially constructed device, termed a body cooling unit (BCU), have produced cooling rates ranging from 0.041°C/min to 0.111 C/min, with an average cooling time of 68 to 78 minutes and 10% mortality. A well-designed randomized clinical trial of dantrolene vs placebo in classic heat stroke showed no difference in cooling rates or outcome, concluding that this pharmacologic treatment should not be used in heat- stroke patients.

Lipman GS, Eifling KP et al .Wilderness Medical Society Practice Guidelines for the Prevention and Treatment of Heat-Related Illness: 2014 Update. Wilderness & Environmental Medicine 2014;25:S55-S65.

Q32. Answer FTFTF

Hemostatic abnormalities are the prima facie evidence of a viper bite. Cobras and kraits do not cause hemostatic disturbances. Saw scaled vipers do not cause renal failure whereas Russell's viper and hump-nosed pit viper do. Russell's viper can also manifest with neurotoxic symptoms in a wide area of India which can cause confusion.

Singh S, Singh G. Snake Bite: Indian Guidelines Protocol, Toxicology 2013. Available at: www.apiindia.org/medicine - update - 2013/Chap.94 (Accessed 6th August 2017).

Q33. Answer TTTTT

Bite infections can contain a mix of anaerobes and aerobes from the patient's skin and the animal's oral cavity, including species of Pasteurella, Streptococcus, Fusobacterium, and Capnocytophaga. Domestic cat and dog bite wounds can produce substantial morbidity and often require specialized care techniques and specific antibiotic therapy. Bite wounds can be complicated by sepsis. Disseminated infections, particularly those caused by Capnocytophaga canimorsus and Pasteurella multocida, can lead to septic shock, meningitis, endocarditis, and other severe sequelae. An emerging syndrome in veterinary and human medicine is methicillin-resistant Staphylococcus aureus (MRSA) infections shared between pets and human handlers, particularly community-acquired MRSA disease involving the USA300 clone. Skin, soft-tissue, and surgical infections are the most common. MRSA-associated infections in pets are typically acquired from their owners and can potentially cycle between pets and their human acquaintances.

Oehler RL, Velez AP, Mizrachi M, et al. Bite-related and septic syndromes caused by cats and dogs. Lancet Infect Dis. 2009; 9(7):439.

Q34. Answer TFTTT

Management of patients with blast lung injury
- Supplemental high flow oxygen via noninvasive continuous positive airway pressure or endotracheal tube
- Avoidance of high inspiratory pressure and volume; (upper limit of inspiratory pressures < 40 cm H_2O)
- One lung ventilation in severe hemoptysis or significant air leak (Bronchopleural fistula)
- Chest tubes for pneumothorax and hemothorax
- Hyperbaric oxygen therapy for patients with arterial gas embolism
- Permissive hypercapnia, high-frequency jet ventilation and extracorporeal membrane oxygenation for patients with ARDS
- Pneumomediastinum, persistent pneumothorax, subcutaneous emphysema, fallen lung sign (collapse of the lung away from hilum) should raise suspicion of tracheobronchial injury.

Samra T, Pawar M, and Kaur J. Challenges in management of blast injuries in Intensive Care Unit: Case series and review. Indian J Crit Care Med. 2014;18(12):814-8.

Q35. Answer TTTFT

Table 1: Selected features of the conditions discussed.

Condition	Contagious	Clinical form or forms	Vaccine available	Treatment
Anthrax	No	Three primary forms: cutaneous, inhalational, and gastrointestinal	Yes	Combination anti-microbials, effusion drainage, monoclonal antibody
Smallpox	Yes	Centrifugal rash with same-stage lesions	Yes	Supportive treatment
Plague	Yes	Pneumonic or bubonic	No	Antimicrobials
Botulism	No	Inhalational or gastro-intestinal	No	Antitoxin
Tularemia	No	Inhalational or ulceroglandualr	No	Antimicrobials

Adalja AA, Toner E, and Inglesby TV. Clinical Management of Potential Bioterrorism-Related Conditions. N Engl J Med. 2015; 372:954-62.

Q36. Answer TTTTF

Medical professionals living in disaster-prone regions should learn about the pathophysiology, complications, and treatment of crush-related acute renal failure. Impaired kidney perfusion and intratubular obstruction by myoglobin and uric acid contribute to the pathogenesis. Early fluid resuscitation (within the first six hours, preferably before the victim is extricated) is essential. The preferred fluid is isotonic saline, given at a rate of 1 liter per hour (10 to 15 mL/Kg of body weight per hour), while the victim is under the rubble, followed by hypotonic saline soon after rescue. Adding 50 mEq of sodium bicarbonate to each second or third liter of hypotonic saline (usually a total of 200 to 300 mEq the first day) will maintain urinary pH above 6.5 and prevent intratubular deposition of myoglobin and uric acid. If urinary flow exceeds 20 ml per hour, 50 mL/hour of 20% mannitol (1 to 2 g per kilogram per day [total, 120 g], given at a rate of 5 g per hour) may be added to each liter of infusate.

Sever MS, Vanholder R, and Lameire N. Management of Crush-Related Injuries after Disasters. N Engl J Med. 2006;354:1052-63.

Q37. Answer FTTTF

Completely buried victims suffer a mortality rate of roughly 50%, while the mortality rate of non-buried victims drops to 3-4%. The vast majority of deaths in completely buried victims are caused by asphyxiation, trauma and hypothermia. Of these, asphyxia is the predominant mechanism, causing 80% of avalanche related deaths. Obviously, these mechanisms frequently coexist, further augmenting lethality.

Kornhall DK, Martens-Nielsen J. The prehospital management of avalanche victims. J R Army Med Corps. 2016;162:406-12.

Q38. Answer TFTFF

Incremental dose administration of atropine as the standard of care is recommended. The role of glycopyrrolate alone or in combination with atropine is not clear. Overall null effect or potential harm with oximes was found on meta-analysis of trials. The largest oxime study tends to harm. Blood alkalinization with high dose $NaHCO_3$ in OP poisoning was shown to be useful. Intravenous $MgSO_4$ (4 g) given in the first day after admission has been shown to decrease hospitalization period and improve outcomes in patients with OP poisoning Intravenous $MgSO_4$ (4 g) given in the first day after admission has been shown to decrease hospitalization period and improve outcomes in patients with OP poisoning.

Palaniappen V. Current concepts in the management of organophosphorus compound poisoning. Medicine Update. Mumbai, India: The Association of Physicians of India. 2013:427-33.

Q39. Answer TTTTF

The top five substance classes most frequently involved in all human exposures were analgesics (11.5%), cosmetics/personal care products (7.7%), household cleaning substances (7.6%), sedatives/hypnotics/antipsychotics (5.9%), and antidepressants (4.2%). Sedative/hypnotics/antipsychotics exposures as a class increased most rapidly (2,559 calls/year) over the last 13 years for cases showing more serious outcomes. The top five most common exposures in children of 5 years or less were cosmetics/personal care products (13.8%), household cleaning substances (10.4%), analgesics (9.8%), foreign bodies/toys/miscellaneous (6.9%), and topical preparations (6.1%).

Mowry JB, Spyker DA, Cantilena LR. 2013 Annual Report of the American Association of Poison Control Centers' National Poison Data System (NPDS): 31st Annual Report. Clin Toxicol (Phila). 2014;52(10):1032-283.

Q40. Answer TFTFF

A second group of hallucinogenic mushrooms comes from the three genera Psilocybe, Paneolus, and Gymnopilus. Mushrooms of the Psilocybe group stain blue when handled. These small dung dependent mushrooms contain psilocybin, a lysergic acid diethylamide-like tryptophane derivative. These mushrooms, like the Amanita muscaria group, have been eaten recreationally for hundreds of years, with Mexican and Central American use of these drugs well described. In the Pacific Northwest, this group of mushrooms is avidly consumed for its hallucinogenic properties. Psilocybin effects are dose related. They are also often associated with laughter, euphoria, hallucinations, and impaired time-space perception. When unpleasant experiences or accidental ingestions occur, medical help might be sought.

Blackman JR. Clinical Approach to Toxic Mushroom Ingestion. JABFP. 1993;7(1):31-7.

CHAPTER 11

Severe Infection and Sepsis (Part I)

Rajeev Soman, Pratik Savaj

A Type Questions
(One best answer)

1. Treatment of choice for community acquired native valve infective endocarditis:
   a. Ampicillin/sulbactum with gentamicin
   b. Ceftriaxone
   c. Vancomycin
   d. Ceftriaxone/gentamicin
   e. Daptomycin

2. Treatment of life-threatening C difficile colitis is:
   a. High dose oral Vancomycin
   b. Oral Vancomycin plus intravenous Metronidazole
   c. Fecal microbiota transplantation
   d. IVIG
   e. Rifaximin

3. Which of the following is FALSE about Pyoderma Gangrenosum (PG):
   a. Rapid progression of a painful necrolytic cutaneous ulcer with an irregular, violaceous, and undermined border
   b. Worsening after debridement
   c. Commonly associated with systemic autoimmune disease
   d. Rapid response to glucocorticoids
   e. Surgical resection is the only definitive treatment

4. Following is true about H1N1 Influenza except:
   a. Throat swab for H1N1 is indicated only for category 3
   b. Close contacts should be given Tab. Oseltamivir 75 mg OD for 7 days
   c. Oseltamivir requires dose adjustment in CKD
   d. Category A requires symptomatic treatment only
   e. Influenza virus is sometimes called 'swine flu' since it is very similar to virus found in the birds

5. Laboratory Risk Indicator for Necrotizing Fasciitis (LRINEC) score for assessing severity of necrotizing soft tissue infection includes all except:
   a. WBC
   b. CRP
   c. Blood glucose
   d. Sodium
   e. PCT

6. A 45-year-male patient recently diagnosed as Human Immunodeficiency Virus (HIV) positive and started on Antiretroviral therapy (ART). After 2 months, he came with complaint of breathlessness and on evaluation was found to have creatinine of 9.0 and urine routine was showing proteinuria and glycosuria, blood sugar was 92. ABG analysis showed mixed metabolic acidosis. What could be the likely ART he was taking?
   a. Zidovudine
   b. Tenofovir
   c. Efavirenz
   d. Lopinavir/Ritonavir
   e. Atazanavir/Ritonavir

7. A 25-year-old immunocompetent male patient presented with severe headache followed by fever. CNS imaging showed multiple ring enhancing lesions in the brain. Stereotactic biopsy was done. TB MGIT culture showed MTB detected and Drug Sensitivity Test (DST) was pan susceptible. Started on weight based ATT (HRZE) and IV Dexamethasone 24 mg/day. Patient improved. IV dexamethasone was changed to oral dexamethasone 4 mg TDS and got discharged. After 2 days he had severe headache and vomiting again. Repeat imaging showed increase in the size of tuberculomas and peri-lesional edema with normal size ventricles. What could be the diagnosis of his current presentation?
   a. Hydrocephalus
   b. Paradoxical response
   c. MDR-TB
   d. TB with secondary bacterial infection
   e. None of above

8. A 55-year-old male patient, known case of DM and CKD, started developing subacute onset of cough followed by fever. CT chest revealed right upper zone consolidation with hilar adenopathy. He had visit to Ratnagiri prior to this symptoms. Blood culture revealed gram negative bacilli. What is the most appropriate treatment for this patient?
   a. Injection Ceftazidime with TMP-SMX
   b. Injection Levofloxacin
   c. Injection Ceftriaxone
   d. Injection Colistin
   e. ATT Injection (HRZE)

9. A 60-year-male patient known case of depression and taking Citalopram. He had history of fall and left humerus fracture for which plating and screw fixation was done. A few days later there was pus discharge from surgical site. Pus swab was sent which grew MRSA susceptible to TMP-SMX, Doxycycline, Linezolid and Vancomycin. He was started on Linezolid. A few days later he started having high grade fever, tremors, agitation and profuse sweating. What is diagnosis of his condition?
   a. Idiopathic hypersensitivity reaction
   b. Serotonin syndrome
   c. Drug fever
   d. Disseminated *Staphylococcus aureus* bacteremia
   e. None of above

10. Advantage of Polymyxin B over Colistin are all except:
    a. Better PK/PD features
    b. Rapid onset of action
    c. Less nephrotoxic
    d. No dose adjustment needed for low creatinine clearance
    e. Polymyxin B can be absorbed by gut

11. Antibiotics should not be given in diarrhea due to:
    a. Enteropathogenic *E. coli* (EPEC)
    b. Enteroaggregative *E. coli* (EAggEC)
    c. Enteroinvasive *E. coli* (EIEC)
    d. Enteroaggregative *E. coli* (EAEC)
    e. Enterohemorrhagic *E. coli* (EHEC)

12. What is FALSE about Vancomycin?
    a. It is a highly protein bound drug
    b. Trough level to be collected 30 minutes prior 4th dose
    c. Should not be used in MRSA
    d. Trough level of 15-20 is required for endocarditis
    e. Slow infusion is to be given to prevent red man syndrome

13. Following is true about treatment of MRSA
    a. Pneumonia can be treated with Daptomycin
    b. Linezolid is a bactericidal drug
    c. Tigecycline can be used in bacteremia due to MRSA
    d. Fosfomycin has good biofilm activity
    e. None of above

14. The following are true about Lemierre's syndrome except:
    a. Septic thrombophlebitis of the internal jugular vein
    b. Caused by Fusobacterium necrophorum
    c. Most common presentation is fever with unilateral neck pain
    d. Aminoglycoside is the drug of choice
    e. Usually has a dental source of the infection

15. A 37-year-female patient presented with sore throat followed by large joint polyarthritis and fever. Total count was normal with high ESR and high CRP. Transthoracic echo – grade 2 MR. 1 out of 3 blood culture – Methicillin

resistant Coagulase Negative Staphylococcus. ASO titre was high and ANA was awaited. What is the likely diagnosis?
   a. Infective endocarditis
   b. Rheumatic fever
   c. SLE
   d. Rheumatic fever + infective endocarditis
   e. MR-CoNS bacteremia

16. What is true about serum procalcitonin (PCT)?
   a. Interferon (IFN) released in response to viral infection can cause a down-regulation of PCT
   b. Gram-positive bacteraemias cause higher elevation of PCT than those caused by Gram-negative pathogens
   c. PCT < 2 rules out sepsis
   d. Value comes very high in localized infections
   e. All of above

17. True about management of suspected pyogenic meningitis:
   a. Brain imaging is needed prior to lumbar puncture in all the cases
   b. Steroid is indicated before or along with antibiotic in all the cases
   c. Empirical antibiotic of choice in patients with age > 65 years is Ceftriaxone
   d. Blood culture should be done
   e. All of above

18. True about Fosfomycin:
   a. Not useful for the treatment of infection due to Acinetobacter
   b. Causes hyperkalemia and hyponatremia
   c. Dose adjustment is not needed in patients with CKD
   d. Tissue penetration is very poor
   e. It is to be given in 0.9% normal saline

19. A 60-year-male patient with infective endocarditis due to Enterococcus faecalis (susceptible to Ampicillin and Gentamicin) found to have creatinine of 2.0. What is the treatment of choice?
   a. Injection Ampicillin
   b. Injection Ceftriaxone
   c. Injection Ampicillin with Gentamicin
   d. Injection Daptomycin
   e. Injection Ampicillin with Ceftriaxone

20. A 50-year-male patient with type 2 DM and atherosclerosis bioprosthetic valve presented with fever followed by sudden onset of anomic aphasia. On examination, pansystolic murmur over mitral area. 2/2 blood cultures- Streptococcus Gallolyticus subspecies pasteurianus (Penicillin MIC ≤0.12). MRI brain showed multiple embolic infarcts. The following are needed for the patient except:
   a. Transoesophageal echocardiogram
   b. Colonoscopy
   c. IV Ceftriaxone 2 g OD
   d. Carotid doppler
   e. Ceftriaxone + Gentamicin

21. A 17-year-girl, history of fall from height presented with open calcaneal fracture with soil contamination. K-wire fixation was done. 15 days later, pus discharge from the suture site, debridement done. Intraoperative pus culture grew Enterobacter Cloacae, susceptible to 3rd generation Cephalosporin, BL + BLI, Carbapenems, Polymyxins and resistant to fluoroquinolones. Antibiotic of choice in this patient is:
   a. Injection Cetriaxone
   b. Injection Piperacillin + Tazobactam
   c. Injection Cefoperazone + Sulbactam
   d. Injection Meropenem
   e. Injection Colistin

22. *Beta-D-glucan* is positive in the following infections except:
   a. Candia species
   b. Aspergillus species
   c. *Pneumocystis jiroveci*
   d. Mucor species
   e. Gram-positive and Gram-negative bacteremia

23. True about the management of MDR-TB:
   a. Should receive both 1st and 2nd line treatment
   b. Most cases are due to acquired resistance
   c. Clarithromycin is the most useful drug in the management
   d. Intensive phase should be given for 2 months
   e. Treatment should be given as per Drug-susceptibility Testing (DST)

24. Which of the following is true about drug interactions with antibiotics?
   a. Rifampicin should not be given with Tacrolimus

b. Voriconazole should not be given with phenytoin, carbamazepine
c. Proton pump inhibitors should not be given with Posaconazole
d. Calcium supplements should not be given at the same time with ciprofloxacin
e. All of above

25. Most significant biochemical abnormality associated with severe malaria is:
a. Hyponatremia
b. Hypocalcemia
c. Hypoglycemia
d. Hypokalemia
e. All of the above

26. A 10-year-girl, relapsed Acute Myeloblastic Leukemia (AML) with febrile neutropenia developed Invasive Pulmonary Aspergillosis (IPA) started on Voriconazole and improved. After few days she again started spiking fever. Serum Voriconazole level was in therapeutic range. LFT showed high ALP and high GGT. CT chest and abdomen revealed multiple hypodense lesions in spleen and liver parenchyma. Repeated blood cultures were negative. What could be the likely diagnosis?
a. Disseminated TB
b. Resistant Aspergillosis
c. Deep seated or disseminated Candidiasis
d. AML with metastasis
e. Mucormycosis

27. True about Galactomannan (GM) all except:
a. High sensitivity and specificity in neutropenic patients
b. It is a product of budding hypha
c. Level is not affected by treatment
d. It is a biomarker for diagnosis of Aspergillosis
e. Positive in Histoplasmosis

28. A 60-year-male patient known case of Acute Myeloid Leukemia (AML), developed prolonged and profound neutropenia after chemotherapy. Developed fever followed by breathlessness. High-resolution computed tomography (HRCT) chest showed multiple nodules with Halo sign. Bronchoalveolar lavage (BAL), Galactomannan was 3.1 (positive). What is the diagnosis as per EORTC/MSG criteria?
a. Possible Invasive pulmonary Aspergillosis (IPA)
b. Probable IPA
c. Proven IPA
d. Allergic Broncho-pulmonary Aspergillosis (ABPA)
e. Chronic Pulmonary Aspergillosis (CPA)

29. Antifungal agent of choice for the treatment of Candida infective endocarditis:
a. L-AMB + 5 FC
b. Fluconazole+ 5 FC
c. High dose Echinocandin
d. L-AMB + Fluconazole
e. a or c

30. Empirical antifungal of choice for candidemia in hemodynamically unstable patient is:
a. Amphotericin B
b. Echinocandin
c. Fluconazole
d. Voriconazole
e. Posaconazole

K Type Questions
[Marked True (T)/False (F)]

1. In management of candidemia in neutropenic patient:
a. Fundus examination should be done after recovery of neutropenia
b. Empirical antifungal of choice is echinocandin
c. Removal of CVC is not needed in all the cases
d. CVC is almost the source of Candida in all cases
e. Minimum duration of therapy for candidemia without metastatic complications is 4 weeks

2. About PCP infection:
a. TMP-SMX is the treatment of choice
b. BDG is a useful biomarker in the diagnosis
c. Steroids are always contraindicated
d. Caspofungin can be used in the treatment
e. Clindamycin with primaquine an alternative therapy

3. A 45-year-old male patient presented with lymphatic filariasis and started on Diethylcarbamazine (DEC). After few hours, he stared developing high grade fever, headache, nausea, and vomiting. What is the likely diagnosis?

a. DEC drug reaction
   b. Acute hypersensitivity reaction due to dying microfilaria
   c. Resistant filarial infection
   d. Viral fever
   e. All of the above

4. **Isolation of following organism from blood collected from central line requires removal of catheter even if peripheral blood culture is negative:**
   a. *Staphylococcus aureus*
   b. *Enterococcus* and *Pseudomonas*
   c. *Pseudomonas* and CoNS
   d. CoNs
   e. Candida

5. **Echinocandin can be given in the treatment of:**
   a. Trichosporon
   b. Cryptococcus
   c. Rhizopus
   d. *C. glabrata*
   e. *C. krusei*

6. **Following is true about TB meningitis in HIV:**
   a. Can occur at any CD4 cell count
   b. Causes obstructive hydrocephalus
   c. CSF drainage should be used to reduce ICP
   d. IRIS is common after tapering the dose of steroids
   e. Pathogenesis is mainly due to inflammation, exudates and vasculitis

7. **About CSF examination for post neurosurgery meningitis:**
   a. CSF cell count has very high specificity
   b. Gram-staining has low specificity
   c. Lactate concentration of 4 mmol/L or more in the cerebrospinal fluid has high sensitivity plus high specificity
   d. No growth of organism in CSF culture after 3 days should be reported as negative culture.
   e. PCR test is not very useful in diagnosis

8. **True about CNS Toxoplasmosis:**
   a. Sulfadiazine + pyrimethamine are the drug of choice
   b. Presents as ring enhancing lesion with significant peri-lesional edema in the brain on imaging
   c. IRIS is more common than TB
   d. Toxoplasma IgG has very high positive predictive value
   e. Leucovorin is given to prevent cytopenia associate with treatment

9. **A 25-year-male patient with AML underwent allogenic bone marrow transplantation, started developing fever, diarrhea followed by skin rashes all over the body. Blood investigation revealed raised AST and ALT. Most likely diagnosis is:**
   a. Acute viral hepatitis
   b. Coli bacteremia
   c. HLH
   d. Acute Graft Versus Host Disease (GVHD)
   e. Disseminated candidiasis

10. **A 45-year-female patient presented with PUO and skin rashes. Serum ferritin was 30,000. The following other investigations should be sent for the further evaluation of this patient:**
    a. Fibrinogen and triglyceride
    b. Serum PCT
    c. Bone marrow examination
    d. Anticardiolipin antibody
    e. None of the above

11. **True about drug fever:**
    a. Relative bradycadia
    b. Eosinopenia
    c. Mild elevated liver enzymes
    d. Leucopenia
    e. Rash

12. **Advantage of Minocycline over Tigecycline is:**
    a. Can be given for VAP
    b. Better CNS penetration
    c. Good serum concentration
    d. More active against MRSA
    e. More active against Enterococcus

13. **Role of fluconazole in the management of candidemia is:**
    a. Not critically ill patients
    b. No prior azole exposure
    c. Long-term suppressive therapy in prosthetic valve infective endocarditis
    d. No adjustment in renal failure
    e. Better for non *C. albicans*

14. **Consider about Zika virus:**
    a. Transmitted by same mosquito which causes dengue fever
    b. Does not transmitted by use of blood products
    c. Antenatal infections can cause microcephaly in a newborn

d. Fever, headache and joint pain are common presentations
   e. Diagnosis is done by RT-PCR
15. **Criteria for diagnosis of severe *C. difficile* infections may be the following:**
   a. WBC > 15,000
   b. Rise of creatinine >50 % above baseline
   c. Normal colon on imaging
   d. More than 10 episodes of diarrhea
   e. Bowel perforation
16. **About CMV disease in solid organ transplantation:**
   a. Less commonly associated with lung and intestinal transplantation
   b. CMV suppresses immunity
   c. Treatment of choice is oral Ganciclovir
   d. It does not cause graft dysfunction
   e. Valganciclovir require dose adjustment in CKD
17. **All of the following are true about *Candida auris*:**
   a. It can be misidentified as Candida haemulonii or C. famata on automated identification system
   b. It has good susceptibilities to Triazoles
   c. Commonly seen in the patients with prolonged ICU stay
   d. High APACHE-II score is the risk factor
   e. I grows at 42°C but fails to grow in presence of 0.01% or 0.1% cycloheximide
18. **All of following are true about Cryptococcal infection in patients with HIV:**
   a. Meningitis is the least common presentation
   b. Treatment of choice is Amphotericin-B with 5FC
   c. Can involve lung, skin, bone
   d. Occur in the patient with CD4 <200
   e. CSF, WBC count is usually high
19. **All of the following are true about Moxifloxacin:**
   a. It requires dose adjustment in CKD
   b. Can cause QT prolongation
   c. Mechanism of action is DNA gyrase inhibition
   d. It is one of the important drug for the management of MDR-TB
   e. Achieves good level in bile
20. **Consider the following about Carbapenems:**
   a. Meropenem+ clavulanic acid can be used in the treatment of MDR TB
   b. Ertapenem has good gram antipseudomonal activity
   c. Imipenem is always combined with cilastatin
   d. Doripenem is not approved for the treatment of ventilator associated pneumonia
   e. All carbapenem has good anaerobic cover

ANSWERS

A Type Answers

Q1. Answer a

Treatment of endocarditis requires bactericidal antimicrobial therapy which should be dosed to optimize sustained bactericidal serum concentrations throughout as much of the dosing interval as possible. In vitro determination of the minimum inhibitory concentration should be performed routinely. Therapy for infective endocarditis (IE) should be targeted to the organism isolated from blood cultures; cultures are positive in over 90% of patients with IE. For patients with suspected IE who present without acute symptoms, empiric therapy is not always necessary, and therapy can await blood culture results. In general, empiric therapy should cover staphylococci (methicillin susceptible and resistant), streptococci, and enterococci.

Sexton DJ. Antimicrobial therapy of native valve endocarditis. Available from: https://www.uptodate.com/contents/antimicrobial-therapy-of-native-valve-endocarditis?(Accessed 31 October, 2016).

Q2. Answer b

Vancomycin delivered orally (500 mg four times per day) and per rectum (500 mg in a volume of 500 ml four times a day) plus intravenous metronidazole (500 mg three times a day) is the treatment of choice for patients with complicated clostridium difficile. infection (CDI) with ileus or toxic colon and/or significant abdominal distention.

Surawicz CM, Brandt LJ, Binion DG, et al. Guidelines for Diagnosis, Treatment, and Prevention of Clostridium difficile Infections. Available from: https://gi.org/guideline/diagnosis-and-management-of-c-difficile-associated-diarrhea-and-colitis/ (Accessed 22 August 2017).

Q3. Answer e

PG has an unpredictable and highly variable course from its onset and during its progression. Some patients develop lesions of sudden onset associated with progressive increase followed by pain and fever. Others have chronic lesions with ulcerations that progress slowly. Regardless of the variant, most lesions are self-limiting and progress to spontaneous healing in a short time. Some patients have recurrent lesions periodically. Also some do not respond to the medications commonly used which then have to be empirically replaced, while other drugs are added to ensure PG cure or retrogression. The main objective of PG treatment is to limit tissue destruction, promote wound healing and obtain a good esthetic result. Surgical debridement and skin grafts should be avoided because of the potential risk of deterioration.

Konopka CL, Padulla GA, Ortiz MP, et al. Pyoderma Gangrenosum: A Review Article. J Vasc Bras. 2013;12(1):25-33.

Q4. Answer e

Influenza virus was originally referred to as 'swine flu' because laboratory testing showed that many of the genes in the virus were very similar to influenza viruses that normally occur in pigs (swine). The influenza viruses circulating are very much human flu now.

Pandemic Influenza A h1n1. World Health Organization. Available from: http://www.who.int/csr/resources/publications/swineflu/h1n1_donor_032011.pdf.

Q5. Answer e

Laboratory Risk Indicator for Necrotizing Fasciitis (LRINEC) Score

Variable (units)		Score points
C-Reactive Protein (CRP) (mg/L)	<150	0
	>150	4
White blood cell count (per mm^3)	<15	0
	15-25	1
	>25	2

Contd...

Contd...

Variable (units)		Score points
Hemoglobin (g/dL)	>13.5	0
	11-13.5	1
	<11	2
Serum sodium (mmol/L)	≥135	0
	<135	2
Serum creatinine (mg/dL)	≤1.6	0
	>1.6	2
Serum glucose (mg/dL)	≤180	0
	>180	1
Types of NF based on microorganisms	Type I	NF comprised of synergistic polymicrobial infection
	Type II	NF is caused by monomicrobial Gram-positive organisms
	Type III	NF involves Gram-negative monobacteria usually marine-related organisms
	Type IV	NF is caused by fungal infection

Menyar AEL, Asim M, Mudali IN, et al. The laboratory risk indicator for necrotizing fasciitis (LRINEC) scoring: the diagnostic and potential prognostic role. Scandinavian Journal of Trauma, Resuscitation and Emergency Medicine. 2017;25:28.

Q6. Answer b

The main clinical presentations of tenofovir nephrotoxicity are (a) proximal tubular dysfunction with preserved renal function and (b) proximal tubular dysfunction associated with decreased renal function. Recent guidelines from the HIV Medicine Association of the Infectious Diseases Society of America (IDSA) recommend at least biannual monitoring of renal function, serum phosphorus, proteinuria, and glycosuria in HIV patients receiving tenofovir with glomerular filtration rate (GFR) <90mL/min/1.73m_2, other comorbid diseases or cotreated with protease inhibitors due to the potential risk of nephrotoxicity.

Fernandez BF, Ferrer AM-Sanz AB, et al. Tenofovir nephrotoxicity: 2011 Update. AIDS Res Treat. 2011;1-12

Q7. Answer b

Paradoxical response is now increasingly being recognized as a cause of subsequent deterioration in cases of CNS tuberculosis despite adequate and appropriate therapy. This phenomenon complicates the decision about the therapy of CNS tuberculosis. It is not possible to clearly differentiate between paradoxical deterioration and development of secondary resistance in the absence of positive tests of culture and sensitivity for *Mycobacterium tuberculosis*.

Gupta M, Bajaj BJ, Khwaja G. Paradoxical response in patients with CNS tuberculosis. JAPI. 2003;51:257-60.

Q8. Answer a

Melioidosis caused by the Gram-negative bacterium *Burkholderia pseudomallei* is endemic in Southeast Asia but may be under-diagnosed and underreported in the Indian subcontinent. Melioidosis is an emerging infection in India especially in males from rural areas with diabetes and alcoholism being the most common risk factors. Both sepsis with bacteremia and localized disease involving joints or focal abscess were common presentations. Diagnosis is readily made by culturing the organism from appropriate clinical specimens and identifying non-fermenting Gram negative bacteria to the species level. As there was an excellent response in 75% of patients, early suspicion, culture confirmation and therapy is warranted in India.

Patients with severe or bacteraemic melioidosis is treated either with ceftazidime alone or ceftazidime plus co-trimoxazole for at least 14 days. They are then switched to oral treatment with a combination of oral co-trimoxazole and doxycycline for a total duration of 24 weeks.

Gopalakrishnan R, Sureshkumar D, Thirunarayan MA, et al. Melioidosis: An emerging infection in India. Journal of the association of physicians of India. 2013;61(9):612-4.

Q9. Answer b

Linezolid is an oxazolidinone antibiotic that is widely used and has mild reversible nonselective inhibition of monoamine oxidase (MAO). In patients taking linezolid along with serotonin agonists, there is a small but documented risk for serotonin syndrome. The syndrome is characterized by mental status changes, autonomic hyperactivity, and neuromuscular abnormalities that may range in severity from almost imperceptible to lethal.

On the basis of this risk, clinicians often have to decide whether to discontinue either linezolid or a selective serotonin reuptake inhibitor (SSRI) in situations in which both medications are present.

Quinn DK, Stern TA, Linezolid and Serotonin Syndrome. Prim Care Companion J Clin Psychiatry. 2009;11(6):353-6.

Q10. Answer e

None of the polymyxin are absorbed when given orally, and oral usage is reserved for selective gut decontamination. Pharmacokinetic parameters of intravenous CMS and polymyxin B from the 'old' literature are poorly described, and this poor description is one of the major reasons that current dosing regimens are difficult to understand and in many cases they are inappropriate and inadequate. CMS package insert dosing recommendations differ significantly with regard to which preparation is selected and are based on levels obtained by nonspecific microbiologic assays of biologic fluids. These assays were unable to differentiate the inactive prodrug, CMS, from the active moiety, colistin. Recent evidence has shown that only approximately 20% of the sum of CMS and colistin in serum is active colistin.

Kaye KS, Pogue JM, Kaye D Polymyxins/Polymyxin Bond Colistin) in Bennett JE, Dolin R, Mandell, Douglas, and Bennett's Principles and Practice of Infectious Diseases, 8th edition Philadelphia, Saunders. 2015;31:401-5.e1.

Q11. Answer e

Enterohemorrhagic *Escherichia coli* (EHEC) infection- Due to the potential for undesirable release of verotoxin (VT)/Stx by dying and dead bacterial cells, antibiotics are usually avoided.

Wong CS, Jelacic S, Habeeb RL, Watkins SL, et al. The risk of the hemolytic-uremic syndrome after antibiotic treatment of *Escherichia coli* O157:H7 infections. N Engl J Med. 2000;342(26):1930-6.

Q12. Answer c

Vancomycin is a bactericidal glycopeptide antibiotic that inhibits cell wall synthesis; it is the antibiotic agent for which there is the greatest cumulative clinical experience for the treatment of bacteremia caused by methicillin-resistant *S. aureus*. Tissue penetration is highly variable and depends on the degree of inflammation. Vancomycin kills staphylococci more slowly than do beta-lactam antibiotics in vitro and is clearly inferior to beta-lactams for the treatment of methicillin-susceptible *S. aureus* (MSSA) bacteremia and infective endocarditis.

Lowy FD. Methicillin-resistant Staphylococcus aureus (MRSA) in adults: Treatment of bacteremia. Available from: https://www.uptodate.com/contents/methicillin-resistant-staphylococcus-aureus-mrsa-in-adults-treatment-of-bacteremia (Accessed 29 August 2018).

Q13. Answer d

Microcalorimetry showed synergistic activity of fosfomycin and rifampin at sub inhibitory concentrations against planktonic and biofilm MRSA.

Mihailescu R, Tafin UF, Corvec S, Oliva A, et al. High activity of Fosfomycin and Rifampin against methicillin-resistant staphylococcus aureus biofilm in vitro and in an experimental foreign-body infection model. Antimicrob Agents and Chemother. 2014;58(5):2547-53.

Q14. Answer d

Empiric therapy for peripheral vein suppurative thrombophlebitis should include an agent with activity against staphylococci such as Vancomycin (15 to 20 mg/kg/dose every 8 to 12 hours, not to exceed 2 g per dose) plus an agent with activity against Enterobacteriaceae such as ceftriaxone (1 g IV daily). Antibiotics should be tailored accordingly to culture and sensitivity data when available.

Spelman D. Suppurative (septic) thrombophlebitis. Available from: https://www.uptodate.com/contents/suppurative-septic-thrombophlebitis?(Accessed 23 August 2017).

Q15. Answer b

Revised Jones criteria, low-risk populations: Major and minor criteria are as follows:
- Major criteria: Carditis (clinical and/or subclinical), arthritis (polyarthritis), chorea, Erythema marginatum, and subcutaneous nodules
- Minor criteria: Olyarthralgia, fever (≥38.5° F), sedimentation rate ≥60 mm and/or C-reactive protein (CRP) ≥3.0 mg/dL, and prolonged PR interval (unless carditis is a major criterion)

Two major manifestations or one major plus two minor are sufficient for diagnosis of an initial episode of Acute Rheumatic Fever (ARF) in a patient with evidence of a preceding GAS infection.

> Bach DS. Revised Jones Criteria for Acute Rheumatic Fever | Ten Points to Remember. Available from: http://www.acc.org/latest-in-cardiology/ten-points-to-remember/2015/05/08/15/22/revision-of-the-jones-criteria-for-the-diagnosis-of-acute-rheumatic-fever (Accessed 3 September 2017).

Q16. Answer a

In this diagnostic dilemma, PCT has stimulated great interest as a potentially more specific marker for bacterial infection. PCT is produced ubiquitously in response to endotoxin or mediators released in response to bacterial infections (that is, interleukin (IL) - 1b, tumor necrosis factor (TNF)-a, and IL-6) and strongly correlates with extent and severity of bacterial infections. Up-regulation of PCT is attenuated by interferon (INF)-g, a cytokine released in response to viral infections, PCT is more specific for bacterial infections and may help to distinguish bacterial infections from viral illnesses.

> Schuetz P, Albrich W, Mueller B. Procalcitonin for diagnosis of infection and guide to antibiotic decisions: past, present and future BMC Medicine. 2011;9:107.

Q17. Answer d

Brain imaging is needed prior to lumbar puncture in cases with signs of raised ICP. The benefit of adjunctive dexamethasone for all or any subgroup of patients with bacterial meningitis thus remains unproven. To initiate the definitive identification of a bacterium responsible for meningitis, CSF and blood culture specimens should be obtained from patients with clinical signs and symptoms of meningitis and should be transported to the laboratory without delay. Empiric antibiotics should be chosen based on patient history, review of patient's known illnesses and risk factors, results of CSF Gram-stain, and local institution antibiotic resistance patterns. Clinicians should remember that Streptococcus pneumoniae may be resistant to penicillin and cephalosporins, so vancomycin is usually also administered until the bacterial resistance pattern is known.

> Gray LD, Fedorko DP. Laboratory Diagnosis of Bacterial Meningitis. Clinical Microbiology Reviews. 1992;130-145.

Q18. Answer a

Studies have demonstrated that fosfomycin is a promising drug, particularly in combination with other antimicrobials for the treatment of infections due to multidrug-resistant (MDR) Gram-negative bacilli. However, there is concern about its use against *Acinetobecter baumannii*, due to intrinsic resistance to fosfomycin.

> Leite GC, Oliveira MS, Perdigão-Neto LV, et al. Antimicrobial Combinations against Pan-Resistant *Acinetobacter baumannii* Isolates with Different Resistance Mechanisms. PLoS One. 2016;11(3):e0151270.

Q19. Answer e

Enterococci have a narrower spectrum of susceptibility than streptococcal species. In particular, members of the genus *Enterococcus* are all resistant to low concentrations of penicillin. They are also relatively resistant to expanded-spectrum penicillins, resistant to cephalosporins, and typically resistant to aminoglycosides at concentrations achieved with standard dosing regimens. However, many strains of enterococci are killed both in vitro and in vivo if penicillin, ampicillin, or vancomycin is given in synergistic combination with an aminoglycoside such as gentamicin. Ampicillin plus ceftriaxone is as effective as ampicillin plus gentamicin for treating enterococcus faecalis infective endocarditis.

> Fernández-Hidalgo N, Almirante B, Gavaldà J, Gurgui M, et al. Ampicillin plus ceftriaxone is as effective as ampicillin plus gentamicin for treating enterococcus faecalis infective endocarditis. Clin Infect Dis. 2013;56(9):1261-8.

Q20. Answer e

Bactericidal activity against enterococci requires the synergistic interaction of a cell wall active agent (penicillin, ampicillin, or vancomycin) and an aminoglycoside (gentamicin or streptomycin). Treatment regimen for enterococcal PVE that includes the synergistic interaction of a cell wall active agent (penicillin, ampicillin, or vancomycin) and an aminoglycoside (gentamicin or streptomycin) if possible. When these combinations are precluded by the resistance pattern of the organism or the patient's risk for aminoglycoside nephrotoxicity, the high-dose ceftriaxone-ampicillin is a reasonable alternative regimen.

Karchmer AW. Antimicrobial therapy of prosthetic valve endocarditis. Available at: https://www.uptodate.com/contents/antimicrobial-therapy-of-prosthetic-valve-endocarditis (Accessed 24 August 2017).

Q21. Answer d

Enterobacter cloacae is a clinically significant Gram-negative, facultative anaerobic, rod-shaped bacterium. Carbapenems display superb activity against a wide variety of enteric Gram-negative pathogens-including *Enterobacter*. Strains of *Enterobacter*, *Citrobacter*, and *Pseudomonas aeruginosa* which are resistant to extended-spectrum cephalosporins on the basis of hyperproduction of type I beta-lactamase typically remain susceptible to carbapenems. Resistance to carbapenems in *Enterobacter* is rare (1% of NNIS isolates in 1999), presumably because *Enterobacter* isolates require two separate mutations to acquire carbapenem resistance: Loss of porin proteins plus hyperproduction of beta-lactamase. Carbapenem resistance among *Enterobacter* isolates does not appear to be increasing over time. In the series of Chow et al. none of seventeen patients receiving imipenem for *Enterobacter* bacteremia had resistant organisms emerge during therapy. Meropenem has activity comparable to imipenem against *Enterobacter* and has proven effective in the therapy of these infections.

Villegas MV, Quinn JP, Enterobacter **species.** Availanle from: http://www.antimicrobe.org/b97.asp (Accessed 2 Septemebr 2017).

Q22. Answer d

β-d-Glucan is an attractive antigen in that it is found in a broad range of fungal agents including the commonly encountered agents *Candida* spp., *Aspergillus* spp., and *Pneumocystis jirovecii*. Cross-reactions with certain hemodialysis filters, beta-lactam antimicrobials, and immunoglobulins, which raise concerns about false-positive tests, have also been described. As a result, the use of this testing must be closely monitored. It is generally observed that 1,3 beta-D glucan detection test is negative in Mucorales infections.

Theel ES, Doern CD. β-d-Glucan Testing Is Important for Diagnosis of Invasive Fungal Infections. J Clin Microbiol. 2013; 51(11):3478-83.

Q23. Answer e

The WHO estimates that 5% of all TB cases worldwide harbor a multidrug-resistant *Mycobacterium tuberculosis* (MDR-TB) strain. MDR-TB is defined as resistance against, at least, rifampicin (RMP) and isoniazid (INH). Extensively drug-resistant TB(XDR-TB) is defined as MDR-TB plus resistance to any fluoroquinolone, and to at least one out of three injectable second-line anti-TB drugs (capreomycin, kanamicin and amikacin). For patients with MDR-TB, second-line drug treatment is mandatory and based on DST.

Richter Y, Rüsch-Gerdes S, Hillemann D. Drug-susceptibility Testing in TB: Current Status and Future Prospects. Expert Rev Resp Med. 2009;3(5):497-510.

Q24. Answer a

The calcineurin inhibitor tacrolimus is used to prevent organ rejection following renal transplant. This drug is metabolized through the hepatic cytochrome P450 (CYP450) 3A enzymes, in particular, CYP3A4 and CYP3A5. A strong relationship between CYP3A5 genetic polymorphisms and the pharmacokinetics of tacrolimus has been demonstrated in kidney, heart, and liver graft recipients. Rifampin is known to affect the metabolism of tacrolimus through induction of CYP3A4 and, to a far lesser extent, CYP3A5.

Naylor H. Decreased Tacrolimus levels after administration of rifampin to a patient with renal transplant. Can J Hosp Pharm. 2013;66(6):388-92.

Q25. Answer c

Hypoglycemia is the most significant biochemical abnormality and a common feature in patients with severe malaria. It may be overlooked because all clinical features of hypoglycemia (anxiety, dyspnea, tachycardia, sweating, coma, abnormal posturing, and generalized convulsions) are also typical of severe malaria itself. Hypoglycemia may be caused by quinine- or quinidine-induced hyperinsulinemia, but it may be found also in patients with normal insulin levels.

Trampuz A, Jereb M, Muzlovic I, Prabhu RM. Clinical review: Severe malaria. Crit Care. 2003;7(4):315-23.

Q26. Answer c

Chronic disseminated candidiasis (also called hepatosplenic candidiasis) is seen almost entirely in patients with hematologic malignancies who have just recovered from an episode of neutropenia. Very few cases, some of which were not well documented have been reported in patients who did not have leukemia or neutropenia. The classic presentation of chronic disseminated candidiasis consists of persistent fever that is frequently high and spiking in a patient who was previously neutropenic and whose neutrophil count has returned to normal. Contrast-enhanced computed tomography (CT) scanning, ultrasonography, magnetic resonance imaging (MRI), and positron emission tomography-CT during neutrophil recovery reveal characteristic multiple lesions which represent microabscesses, in the liver, spleen, and sometimes the kidney.

Q27. Answer c

Serum galactomannan and (1→3)-β-D-glucan in treatment groups demonstrate therapeutic responses with similarly lower levels in comparison to untreated (P < .01).

Petraitiene R, Petraitis V, Bacher JD, Finkelman MA, et al. Effects of host response and antifungal therapy on serum and BAL levels of galactomannan and (1→3)-β-D-glucan in experimental invasive pulmonary aspergillosis. Med Mycol. 2015;53(6):558-68.

Q28. Answer b

Diagnostic criteria for invasive pulmonary aspergillosis according to the European organization for the research and treatment of cancer/mycosis study group and the clinical algorithm
- Proven invasive pulmonary aspergillosis:
  - Microscopic analysis on sterile material: Histopathologic, cytopathologic, or direct microscopic examination of a specimen obtained by needle aspiration or sterile biopsy in which hypha are seen accompanied by evidence of associated tissue damage. Culture on sterile material: Recovery of Aspergillus by culture of a specimen obtained by lung biopsy
- Probable invasive pulmonary aspergillosis (all three criteria must be met)
  1. Host factors (one of the following)
     Recent history of neutropenia (<500 neutrophils/mm^3) for 110 days
     Receipt of an allogeneic stem cell transplant
     Prolonged use of corticosteroids at a mean minimum dose of 0.3 mg/kg/d of prednisone equivalent for 13 weeks.
     Treatment with other recognized T-cell immunosuppressants
     Inherited severe immunodeficiency
  2. Clinical features (one of the following three signs on CT)
     Dense, well-circumscribed lesion(s) with/without a halo sign
     Air-crescent sign
     Cavity
  3. Mycological criteria (one of the following)
     Direct test (cytology, direct microscopy, or culture) on sputum, BAL fluid, bronchial brush indicating presence of fungal elements or culture recovery
     Aspergillus spp.
     Indirect tests (detection of antigen or cell-wall constituents): Galactomannan antigen detected in plasma, serum, or BAL fluid.
- Possible invasive pulmonary aspergillosis
  - Presence of host factors and clinical features (cf. probable invasive aspergillosis) but in the absence of or negative mycological findings.

Blot SI, Taccone FS, Van den Abeele AM, et al. A clinical algorithm to diagnose invasive Pulmonary Aspergillosis in Critically Ill Patients. Am J Respir Crit Care Med. 2012;186(1):56-64.

Q29. Answer e

For native valve endocarditis, lipid formulation AmB, 3–5 mg/kg daily, with/without flucytosine, 25 mg/kg 4 times daily, OR high-dose echinocandin (caspofungin 150 mg daily, micafungin 150 mg daily, or anidulafungin 200 mg daily) is recommended for initial therapy.

> Pappas PG, Kauffman CA, Andes DR, Clancy CJ, et al. Clinical Practice Guideline for the Management of Candidiasis: 2016 Update by the Infectious Diseases Society of America University of Alabama at Birmingham, Division of Infectious Disease, 2015; AL 35294-0006.

Q30. Answer b

Widespread use of antifungal agents must be balanced against the cost, the risk of toxicity, and the emergence of resistance. None of the existing clinical trials have been adequately powered to assess the risk of the emergence of azole or echinocandin resistance. Empiric antifungal therapy should be considered in critically ill patients with risk factors for invasive candidiasis and no other known cause of fever. Preference should be given to an echinocandin in hemodynamically unstable patients, those previously exposed to an azole, and in those colonized with azole-resistant Candida species. Fluconazole may be considered in hemodynamically stable patients who are colonized with azole-susceptible Candida species or who have no prior exposure to azoles.

> Pappas PG, Kauffman CA, Andes DR, Clancy CJ, et al. Clinical Practice Guideline for the Management of Candidiasis: 2016 Update by the Infectious Diseases Society of America University of Alabama at Birmingham, Division of Infectious Disease, 2015;AL 35294-0006.

K Type Answers

Q1. Answer TTTFF

Ophthalmological findings of choroidal and vitreal infection are minimal until recovery from neutropenia; therefore, dilated fundoscopic examinations should be performed within the first week after recovery from neutropenia. An echinocandin is recommended as initial therapy. In the neutropenic patient, sources of candidiasis other than a CVC (e.g. gastrointestinal tract) predominate. Catheter removal should be considered on an individual basis. Minimum duration of therapy for candidemia without metastatic complications is 2 weeks.

> Pappas PG, Kauffman CA, Andes DR, Clancy CJ, et al. Clinical Practice Guideline for the Management of Candidiasis: 2016 Update by the Infectious Diseases Society of America University of Alabama at Birmingham, Division of Infectious Disease, 2015; AL 35294-0006.

Q2. Answer TTFTT

Anti-pneumocystis treatment should be started as soon as the diagnosis is suspected. Treatment of choice is trimethoprim plus sulfamethoxazole (co-trimoxazole) 20 mg/kg/day + 100 mg/kg/day for 3 weeks plus prednisolone 40 mg orally twice daily for 5 days followed by 20 mg twice daily for 5 days and then 20 mg per day until the end of PCP treatment. Caspofungin may improve outcomes from PCP, with favorable comparative mortalities in confirmed cases of PCP. Side-effects of co-trimoxazole are common in HIV patients (nausea, vomiting, skin rash, myelotoxicity). The dose should be reduced by 25% if the WBC count falls. Patients who are intolerant of co-trimoxazole should be treated with: (i) pentamidine 4 mg/kg/day i.v. or (ii) primaquine with clindamycin or (iii) trimetrexate with leucovorin (±oral dapsone).

> Sax PE, Clinical presentation and diagnosis of Pneumocystis pulmonary infection in HIV-infected patients. Available from: https://www.uptodate.com/contents/clinical-presentation-and-diagnosis-of-pneumocystis-pulmonary-infection-in-hiv-infected-patients? (Accesed 24 August 2017).

Q3. Answer TFFFF

Diethylcarbamazine adverse effects: Among uninfected persons, GI upset, characterized by anorexia and nausea are is the most common side effect. Among infected persons, adverse reactions to DEC are common and proportional to the dose administered and intensity of infection. In patients with onchocerciasis, DEC can precipitate a typical side effect termed the Mazzotti reaction, characterized by pruritus, fever, and arthralgia. The inflammatory response occurring in both the anterior (cornea) and posterior (retina) segments of the eye can result in permanent visual damage. In persons with lymphatic filariasis, similar but generally less severe systemic adverse reactions may occur, characterized by fever, headache, malaise, myalgia, and microscopic hematuria. Localized effects in patients with lymphatic filariasis can include pain, adenitis, lymphangitis, epididymitis, or lymphedema. As for ivermectin, life-threatening encephalitis can develop in patients with loiasis and high-burden parasitemia.

> McCarthy JS, Moore TA. Drugs for Helminths. In: Mandell, Douglas, and Bennett's Principles and Practice of Infectious Diseases, Updated Edition, 42;519-527.e4.

Q4. Answer TFFFT

Infection is a serious delayed complication associated with central venous access that can lead to sepsis, shock, and death. Infections become established on the catheter through the production of biofilm. *Staphylococcus aureus* and *Staphylococcus epidermidis* are the two most common pathogens. Catheter infection sources include contamination from skin flora, contamination from infused substance, or from hematogenous spread from an unrelated site. Femoral catheters have the highest rate of infection, and non-cuffed catheters have higher risk than cuffed catheters. Catheters with greater number of lumens have been associated with a greater risk of infection. Antimicrobial impregnated catheters can also aid in decreasing central line infection rates.

> Craig Kornbau, Kathryn C Lee,[1] Gwendolyn D Hughes,[1] and Michael S Firstenberg Central line complications Int J Crit Illn Inj Sci. 2015;5(3):170-8.

Q5. Answer TTFTT

No prospective comparative studies of the primary treatment of mucormycosis have been performed, largely because of the rarity of this disease. In current practice, amphotericin B and isavuconazole are the two antifungal agents licensed by the US Food and Drug Administration (FDA) for the primary therapy of mucormycosis. First-line treatment is with an amphotericin derivative, preferably the liposomal form of amphotericin B to minimize nephrotoxicity. Other options include amphotericin B deoxycholate, isavuconazole, and posaconazole.

The Echinocandin are preferred over azoles for the initial treatment of candidemia if *C. glabrata* or *C. krusei* is identified or suspected or if the patient has been previously treated with an azole agent.

> McDonald PJ, Mucormycosis (Zygomycosis) Treatment & Management. Available from: http://emedicine.medscape.com/article/222551-treatment#d9 (Accessed 25 Aug 2017).

Q6. Answer TTFTT

Infection with HIV is associated with increased risk of activation of latent infection, as well as increased risk of rapid progression of primary infection, without an intervening period of latency. Without HIV infection, individuals with latent infection have a lifetime risk of developing tuberculosis that ranges between 10% and 20%. In contrast, the HIV-infected individual will carry a 10% annual risk of progression to active infection, with increasing risk as the CD4+ count declines. Surgical intervention should not be undertaken unless obstructive hydrocephalus or brainstem herniation is impending otherwise it may precipitate severe meningitis. Initiation of antiretroviral therapy (ART) may be complicated by the immune reconstitution inflammatory syndrome (IRIS), which can manifest as reactivation of latent TB, progression of active TB disease, or clinical deterioration in patients previously improving on antituberculous therapy. Adjunctive corticosteroids reduce death and disability from tuberculous meningitis by about 25 percent.

> Leonard JM. Central nervous system tuberculosis. Available from: https://www.uptodate.com/contents/central-nervous-system-tuberculosis? (Accessed 27th August 2017).

Q7. Answer FFTFF

CSF lactate concentration has relatively high sensitivity and specificity for the diagnosis of post-neurosurgical bacterial meningitis and thus has relatively good efficacy.

> Xiao X, Zhang Y, Zhang L, Kang P, Ji N. The diagnostic value of cerebrospinal fluid lactate for post-neurosurgical bacterial meningitis: a meta-analysis. BMC Infect Dis. 2016;16(1):483.

Q8. Answer TTFFT

Standard therapy consists of pyrimethamine, sulfadiazine, and folinic acid in combination. Single or multiple hypodense or hypointense lesions in white matter and basal ganglia with mass effects may be observed on CT or MRI scans. Lesions may enhance in a homogeneous or ring pattern with contrast. Imaging studies may be normal in diffuse toxoplasmosis.

Anti-*Toxoplasmagondii* IgG detection may be unreliable in immunodeficient individuals who fail to produce significant titers of specific antibodies. In one study, 16% of patients with a clinical diagnosis and 22% of patients with a histologic diagnosis of toxoplasmosis had undetectable anti-*T gondii* IgG levels. Causes of false-negative results also include recent infection and insensitive assays. Leucovorin (i.e. folinic acid) should be administered concomitantly to prevent bone marrow suppression. Unless circumstances preclude using more than 1 drug, a second drug (eg, sulfadiazine, clindamycin) should be added.

Uppal G. CNS Toxoplasmosis in HIV. Available from: http://emedicine.medscape.com/article/1167298-overview (Accessed 27 August 2017).

Q9. Answer FFFTF

GVHD remains a source of significant morbidity and mortality in the setting of allogeneic stem cell transplantation. Improving outcomes in stem cell transplant recipients will require additional therapeutic modalities for GVHD especially for those patients who fail to respond to initial therapy with steroids.

Komanduri KV, Couriel D, Champlin RE. Graft-versus-host disease after allogeneic stem cell transplantation: evolving concepts and novel therapies including photopheresis. Biol Blood Marrow Transplant. 2006;12(1 Suppl 2):1-6.

Q10. Answer TTTTF

Increased serum ferritin may be a useful index for differentiation of infectious and noninfectious (hematologic disease or NIID) diseases. During chronic inflammation such as hematologic malignancy or autoimmune diseases, the body produces hepcidin in the liver as a defense mechanism so that neither pathogens nor tumor cells can utilize serum iron by suppressing intestinal absorption and sequestration of iron in the macrophage producing a relatively iron-deficient state which is reflected by an increase in serum ferritin. Reactive hemophagocytic syndrome patients showed higher frequencies of leukopenia, anemia, thrombocytopenia, hypoalbuminemia, hypofibrinogenemia, hypertriglyceridemia, and elevated LDH levels. Procalcitonin as a marker of sepsis. Anti-cardiolipin antibodies (ACA) are antibodies often directed against cardiolipin and found in several diseases, including syphilis, antiphospholipid syndrome, livedoid vasculitis, vertebrobasilar insufficiency, Behçet's syndrome, idiopathic spontaneous abortion, and systemic lupus erythematosus (SLE).

Kima SE, Kima UJ, Janga MO, Kanga SJ, et al. Diagnostic use of serum ferritin levels to differentiate infectious and noninfectious diseases in patients with fever of unknown origin. Disease Markers. 2013;34:211-8

Q11. Answer TFTFT

Most medications can cause fever, with/without concomitant clinical manifestations. The fever may arise from the drug's pharmacologic action, its effects on thermoregulation, a local complication following parenteral administration, or an idiosyncratic response. The most common mechanism is probably an immunologic reaction mediated by drug-induced antibodies. Drug fever may have any pattern; it typically occurs after seven to ten days of treatment and usually resolves within 48 hours of discontinuing the administration. Failure to diagnose drug fever may lead to inappropriate and potentially harmful diagnostic and therapeutic interventions. In suspected cases, it is necessary to discontinue administration of all potentially causative medicines, together or sequentially. Rechallenge with the offending agent will usually cause recurrence of fever within a few hours, confirming the diagnosis.

Lipsky BA, Hirschmann JV, Drug Fever. JAMA. 1981;245(8):851-4.

Q12. Answer TTTFF

Minocycline is a broad-spectrum tetracycline antibiotic, and has a broader spectrum than the other members of the group. It is a bacteriostatic antibiotic, classified as a long-acting type. As a result of its long half-life it generally has serum levels 2-4 times that of the simple water-soluble tetracyclines. Minocycline is the most lipid-soluble of the tetracycline-class of antibiotics, giving it the greatest penetration into the prostate and brain, but also the greatest amount of central nervous system (CNS)-related side effects, such as vertigo. Minocycline remains more active than Tigecycline against methicillin-susceptible *Staphylococcus aureus* and *Staphylococcus epidermidis,* while tigecycline is more active against the methicillin-resistant strains of these organisms. Tigecycline has demonstrated improved activity against *Streptococcus* species, including penicillin-susceptible, penicillin-intermediate, and penicillin-resistant strains of *Streptococcus pneumoniae.* Tigecycline also has improved activity against *Enterococcus* species when compared with the other tetracycline agents. Tigecycline, minocycline, and doxycycline have better activity against *Listeria monocytogenes* when compared with tetracycline.

    Aronson JK. Minocycline. In: Meyler's Side Effects of Drugs. 16th Ed. Elsevier. 2016; p 1042-1052.

Q13. Answer TTTFF

Preferred empiric therapy for suspected candidiasis in non neutropenic patients in the intensive care unit (ICU) is an echinocandin. Fluconazole may be considered in hemodynamically stable patients who are colonized with azole-susceptible Candida Species or who have no prior exposure to azoles. Azoles are also used for Long term suppressive therapy in prosthetic valve infective endocarditis. It is renally excreted. Most non albicans have intrinsic resistance to Fluconazole.

    Pappas PG, Kauffman CA, Andes DR, et al. Clinical practice guideline for the management of candidiasis: 2016 Update by the Infectious Diseases Society of America. Available from: http://www.life-worldwide.org/assets/uploads/files/Pappas%20Candidiasis%20IDSA%20guidelines%20Clin%20Infect%20Dis2015(1).pdf (Accessed 30 August, 2017).

Q14. Answer TFTTT

Zika virus disease is caused by a virus transmitted primarily by *Aedes* mosquitoes. To date, there have been no confirmed transfusion-transmission cases of Zika virus in the United States. However, cases of Zika virus transmission through platelet transfusions have been documented in Brazil. There is scientific consensus that Zika virus is a cause of microcephaly and Guillain-Barré syndrome. Links to other neurological complications are also being investigated. People with Zika virus disease can have symptoms including mild fever, skin rash, conjunctivitis, muscle and joint pain, malaise or headache. These symptoms normally last for 2-7 days. The Trioplex rRT-PCR is a laboratory test designed to detect Zika virus, dengue virus, and chikungunya virus RNA. The Food and Drug Administration (FDA) has authorized the use of this test under an Emergency Use Authorization (EUA).

    Zika virus. Available from: http://www.who.int/mediacentre/factsheets/zika/en/(Accessed 30 August 2017).

Q15. Answer TTFFT

Patients with acute *C. difficile* infection (CDI) may develop signs of systemic toxicity with/without profuse diarrhea warranting admission to an intensive care unit or emergency surgery. There is no consensus definition for severe CDI nor is there agreement as to the most important clinical indicators that should be used to differentiate severity. The following illustrate some definitions that have been described in the literature: (i) White blood cell count of >15,000 cells/microL (ii) Serum albumin <3 g/dL (iii) Serum creatinine level ≥1.5 times the premorbid level (iv) Evidence of severe colitis on imaging (v) Bowel perforation etc.

    Kelly CP, Lamont JT, Clostridium difficile in adults: Treatment. Available from: https://www.uptodate.com/contents/clostridium-difficile-in-adults-treatment (Accessed 22 August 2017).

Q16. Answer FTFFT

Lung and small bowel transplant recipients carry a higher risk of acquiring CMV disease compared to kidney and liver transplant recipients. During acute infection CMV suppresses the cellular arm of immune system. The two main drugs used for treating CMV disease are intravenous (IV) ganciclovir (5-mg/kg every 12 hours) and oral valganciclovir (900-mg twice daily). CMV infection may also have indirect effects that influence graft dysfunction, accelerate coronary artery atherosclerosis and increase the risk of other opportunistic infections. The dosage of valganciclovir has to be adjusted to the degree of renal impairment.

    Ramanan P, Razonable RR. Pharmacokinetics of valganciclovir and ganciclovir in renal impairment. Infect Chemother 2013;45(3):260-71.

Q17. Answer TFTFT

Candida albicans remains the most frequently isolated *Candida* species in the clinical setting, in some countries, a marked shift towards species of *Candida* that have increased resistance to azoles such as fluconazole (FLU), the standard antifungal drug of choice in many countries, and to echinocandins. Several species of non-*albicans Candida*, such as *C. tropicalis*, *C. glabrata*, and *C. parapsilosis*, are well-recognized pathogens in bloodstream infections (BSIs) in different geographic locations. More recently, *Candida auris*, multidrug-resistant (MDR) yeast that exhibits resistance to FLU and markedly variable susceptibility to other azoles, amphotericin B (AMB), and echinocandin, has globally emerged as a nosocomial pathogen. Alarmingly, in a span of only 7 years, this yeast which is difficult to treat and displays clonal inter- and intra-hospital transmission has become widespread across several countries, causing a broad range of healthcare-associated invasive infections. It can be misidentified as C. haeumuloni or C. famata on automated identification system.

> Chowdhary A, Sharma C, Meis JF. Candida auris: A rapidly emerging cause of hospital-acquired multidrug-resistant fungal infections globally. PLoS Pathog. 13(5):e1006290.

Q18. Answer FTTTF

The parasite *Toxoplasma gondii* and the fungus *Cryptococcus neoformans* are the most common causes of opportunistic brain infections in patients with HIV/AIDS. Treatment often consists of fluconazole or amphotericin B (or one of its lipid derivatives). In the setting of HIV infection, both meningoencephalitis and isolated encephalitis may occur, usually in patients in whom CD4+ T cell counts are lower than 200/μL. It can involve lung, skin, bone.

> Nicholas MK, Collins J. Lukas RV. Acquired Immunodeficiency Syndrome. In: Youmans and Winn Neurological Surgery, 7th Ed. Elsevier, Inc. 2017; 41,e223-e241.

Q19. Answer FTTTT

Moxifloxacin is a recently developed fluoroquinolone antibiotic. It is rapidly absorbed following oral administration, reaching a mean peak drug plasma concentration (C max) of approximately 3.56 mg/L within 2 hours after a 400 mg dose. The rate and extent of absorption are not significantly affected by food or elevated gastric pH. Moxifloxacin binds weakly to plasma proteins and penetrates well into most tissue and fluid compartments with generally higher drug concentrations in tissue and fluid compartments than those observed in plasma. Moxifloxacin is metabolized to an N-sulfate conjugate and an acyl glucuronide in humans. The N-sulfate and the unchanged moxifloxacin are detected in plasma, urine and feces. The acyl-glucuronide is detected in plasma and urine, but not in feces. The plasma elimination half-life ranges from 8.2-15.1 hours in healthy individuals. The urinary excretion of the unchanged drug accounts for 19-22% of the given dose. Neither renal nor hepatic impairment significantly affect the pharmacokinetics of moxifloxacin.

> Moise PA, Birmingham MC, Schentag JJ. Pharmacokinetics and metabolism of moxifloxacin. Drugs Today (Barc). 2000; 36(4):229-44.
>
> Moxifloxacin. Available from: http://www.globalrph.com/moxifloxacin_renal.htm (Accessed 31 August, 2017).

Q20. Answer TFTTT

Clavulanic acid is β-lactamase inhibitor. The spectrum of activity of ertapenem is more limited primarily because it lacks activity against Pseudomonas aeruginosa and Enterococcus spp. Dehydropeptidase is an enzyme found in the kidney and is responsible for degrading the antibiotic imipenem. Cilastatin can therefore be combined intravenously with imipenem in order to protect it from dehydropeptidase and prolong its antibacterial effect. Carbapenems (imipenem, meropenem, doripenem) possess broad-spectrum in vitro activity, which includes activity against many Gram-positive, Gram-negative and anaerobic bacteria; carbapenems lack activity against Enterococcus faecium, methicillin-resistant Staphylococcus aureus and Stenotrophomonas maltophilia.

> Zhanel GG, Wiebe R, Dilay L, Thomson K, Rubinstein E, Hoban DJ, Noreddin AM, Karlowsky JA. Comparative review of the carbapenems. Drugs. 2007;67(7):1027-52.

Severe Infection and Sepsis (Part II)

Bala Prakash, Babu K Abraham

A Type Questions
(One best answer)

1. A 49-year-old male presented to the ER with complaints of (c/o) abdominal pain. His comorbidities include Diabetes and HTN. He was recently admitted to the hospital 50 days ago for the c/o sudden onset severe abdominal pain radiating to his back. During that hospital stay, he was diagnosed to have gallstone induced pancreatitis and cholecystitis. ERCP was done with sphincterotomy and stent placement. After interval resolution of symptoms, he underwent lap cholecystectomy. Patient was discharged to home 3 weeks ago and was doing well until 2 days ago. Initially treated with meropenem and was deescalated appropriately. All started again with nausea and vomiting followed by diarrhea and now severe abdominal pain and distention. No hematochezia or melena. In the ER, he is mildly hypotensive, tachycardic and hypoxic with SPO$_2$ 80% noted on room air. Initial volume resuscitation is attempted. Oxygen mask is initiated.

    CXR is suggestive of B/L basal infiltrates.

    AKI with metabolic acidosis is noted. LA level is high.

    TLC is 32,000/cmL with a left shift.

    What antibiotics should be initiated next after cultures are sent?

    Abdominal X-ray:

    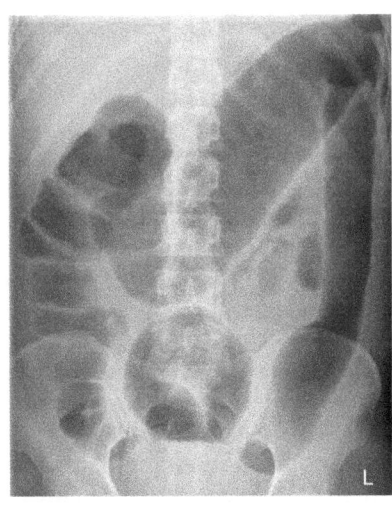

    a. Pip + Tazo with vancomycin
    b. Meropenem with vancomycin IV and oral
    c. Colistin with Pip + Tazo with PO vancomycin
    d. Poly B with meropenem with IV metronidazole

2. A 52-year-old male presented with fever, chills and rigors. His previous medical history was significant for uncontrolled DM, and peripheral vascular disease. 2 days ago he noticed a small freckle on his left hand, which he had tried to remove. Following day he developed pain and swelling at the site of the freckle which now worsened with fever, chills

and rigors. So family brought him to the ER. In the ER, he was noted to be tachycardic and hypotensive. Aggressive fluid resuscitation was initiated. On exam, the L arm appeared to be pale with delayed capillary refill and swelling. Labs revealed elevated WBC counts, AKI with elevated CPK levels. After fluid resuscitation and C X-ray, broad-spectrum antibiotic with anti-toxin action was initiated.

Within the next few hours, his pain worsened and he could not even perform any passive action on the limb. Next step should be:
a. CT Angio of the LUE
b. MRI of the LUE
c. Add crystalline penicillin to treat against gas gangrene
d. Surgical evaluation for debridement and fasciotomy

3. A 42-year-old male with no comorbidities was brought in by family when he started to have complaints of severe abdominal pain with nausea/vomiting and obstipation. In the ER, he was noted to be tachycardic and hypotensive. Aggressive fluid resuscitation was initiated, CT abdomen with contrast was performed which revealed a paraduodenal hernia. Immediate laparotomy was conducted; incarcerated and gangrenous bowel segment was visualized and resected. Pus was drained. Abdomen was closed with drain placement. He was left intubated and mechanically ventilated. On arrival, in the ICU, he was noted to have an HR 130/min, MAP 56 mm Hg. Minimal dark urine was noted in the urinary bag. Blood loss during surgery was around 500 mL; he received a total of 2L crystalloids and 2 Units of PRBC. 4 Units FFP was administered to correct coagulopathy, INR was 1.8 preoperative. Esophageal Doppler was done which revealed a Pk velocity of 55 with a corrected flow time (FTc) of 280. What next?
a. 500 mL RL bolus
b. Initiate norepinephrine drip
c. Initiate phenylephrine drip
d. Initiate dobutamine drip

4. Patient condition significantly improves over the next few days. Antibiotics against secondary peritonitis is working, with good urine output. Patient started to tolerate pressure support ventilation (PSV) and RT feeds. Within the next 12–18 hours, he is noted to have increased abdominal distention and decreased bowel sounds. Dilated bowel loops were noted on X-ray. Ileus is suspected. RT feeds are held. Electrolytes are checked and replaced, but condition deteriorated with decrease in BP. He also started to become hypoxic with decreased tidal volume and increased PK pressures on the ventilator, and so was placed on volume control ventilation (VCV). Sedation could not be initiated due to hypotension. What should be suspected now?
a. Recurrent intestinal obstruction, so CT abdomen/pelvis w/o contrast
b. Intestinal ischemia, so CT abdomen/pelvis w/contrast
c. Abdominal hypertension, so measure intra-abdominal pressure (IAP) and girth
d. Ileus, hold feed and continue current resuscitation and broaden antibiotics

5. A 48-year-old south Indian house wife with known diabetes and hypertension (HTN) here with new sudden onset of headache and fever, which was followed by change in mental status. In the ER, she was febrile to 102°F and hypotensive. After initial resuscitation, CT brain without contrast was performed which revealed no acute findings. When no other obvious source of infection was observed, LP was performed. Gram stain of cerebrospinal fluid (CSF) revealed:

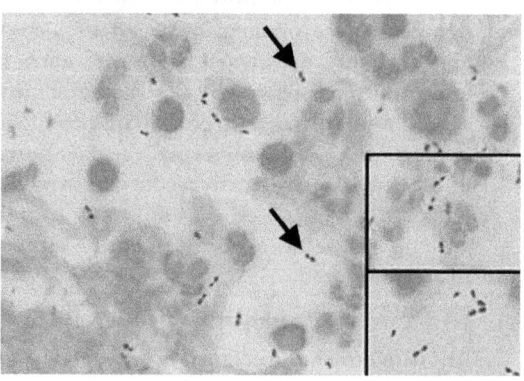

Now the treatment should include?
a. Isoniazid, rifampicin, ethambutol and pyrazinamide
b. Amphotericin B
c. Voriconazole

d. Vancomycin + ceftriaxone with dexamethasone
e. Vancomycin + meropenem with dexamethasone

6. A 42-year-old male with prior alcohol abuse, congenital mitral valve prolapse with atrial fibrillation on coumadin presents to the ER with profuse bleeding from all mucosal surfaces including hematuria and melena. Hypotensive in the ER, initial resuscitation is done. Initial lab results reveal positive for NS1 antigen. BUN 72, Cr 5.04, Hg 6.2, INR 7, Plt 85,000, PTT 62, PT 89, Fibrinogen 210, AST/ ALT 208/ 162, Alk Phos 260. PT and PTT corrected to normal when mixing studies was performed. Other than thrombocytopenia, cause for bleeding in this patient is:
   a. Alcohol induced liver disease
   b. Warfarin treatment
   c. Uremia
   d. Disseminated intravascular coagulation
   e. All of the above

7. A 41-year-old male with DM, HTN had a root canal treatment of his teeth 4 days ago. Since that night he has been complaining of pain at the local site but that has progressed to his entire face and also the same side of the neck with swelling. Now he is having dysphagia and some scanty hemoptysis. On arrival in the ER, patient was looking very toxic. After initial resuscitation, ENT opinion is obtained. CT face/neck with contrast showed this:

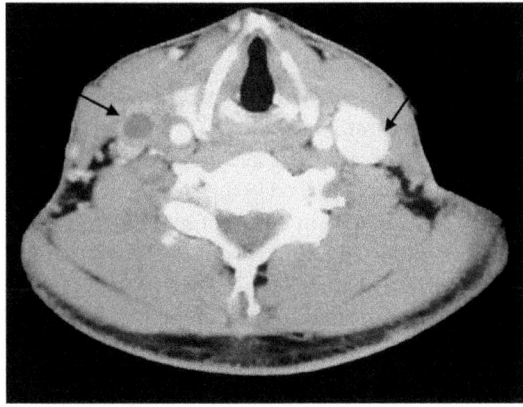

Treatment should include:
   a. Crystalline penicillin
   b. Doxycycline
   c. Piperacillin/tazobactam with heparin
   d. Ampicillin/sulbactam
   e. Piperacillin/tazobactam with vancomycin.

8. A 56-year-old female with past medical history of myasthenia gravis and chronic respiratory failure needing noninvasive ventilatory support during sleep presented with complaints of fevers and shortness of breath. His home care nurse was recently sick from URI and had taken antibiotics. In the ER, she was noted to be hypoxic with SPO_2 80% on room air which improved to 95% on 4L nasal cannulla and also some lethargy. ABG done was 7.28/64/88. She was not able to manage her secretions and so eventually was intubated for better secretion clearance. CXR revealed bilateral basal airspace disease. Appropriate antibiotic treatment should include:
   a. Ceftriaxone and azithromycin
   b. Colistin and tigecycline
   c. Ceftriaxone and doxycycline
   d. Amoxicillin + sulbactum and azithromycin
   e. Piperacillin + tazobactam

9. A 68-year-old male with HTN, DM, old history of treated pulmonary TB and some residual bronchiectasis presented with new onset fever, chills and rigors. Patient had excessive cough compared to his baseline with increased sputum production. In the ER, he is hypotensive and tachycardic. CXR reveals right lower lobe consolidation with tram track sign. Now on O_2 50% by venturi mask, his oxygen saturation was about 90%. Antibiotic regimen should include:
   a. Ceftriaxone and azithromycin
   b. Vancomycin
   c. Isoniazid, rifampicin and ethambutol
   d. Ciprofloxacin
   e. Ceftazidime

10. A 62-year-old male with uncontrolled DM presented with right periorbital pain and swelling. He also noticed that his vision has been worsening. On physical exam, he had blackish discharge from nostril of the same side. ENT after examination sent biopsies to the lab which revealed some fungus. Beta D glucan testing in this patient was negative. Likely infection is from:
   a. Candida
   b. Aspergillosis
   c. Mucormycosis

d. Cryptococcal infection
e. Histoplasmosis

11. A 36-year-old healthy male comes to the emergency room in September with c/o fever and chills, generalized body aches for the past 2-3 days. His office coworkers had similar symptoms. In the ER, he is hypoxic SPO$_2$ 79% on room air with improvement to low 90s on non-rebreathing masks. His RR > 35/min, is hypotensive and tachycardic with a fever of 102°F. H1N1 infection is suspected and pharyngeal swab is sent for testing. On admission to the ICU, what kind of infection prevention measure should be followed?
    a. Contact precaution
    b. Droplet precaution
    c. Negative pressure isolation
    d. Reverse isolation
    e. Universal patient precaution

12. On admission to the ICU, he becomes progressively hypoxic. ABG is 7.24/52/58 on NRB mask 15 L/min. Intubation and mechanical ventilation was required. CXR reveals bilateral diffuse air space disease and good endotracheal tube position. Which mode of ventilation would be ideal?
    a. Low PEEP low tidal volume
    b. High PEEP high tidal volume
    c. High PEEP low flow low tidal volume
    d. High PEEP low flow high tidal volume
    e. Low PEEP high flow low tidal volume

13. Patient is treated with ceftriaxone, azithromycin and oseltamivir. H1N1 swab is positive. With appropriate ventilation, after a significant radiological and clinical improvement, on day 6 of ICU stay, patient develops worsening oxygenation, increased secretions with fevers and worsening hemodynamics. All are risk factors to develop multidrug resistant ventilator associated pneumonia except:
    a. IV antibiotic use within the previous 90 days
    b. Septic shock at the time of VAP
    c. Acute respiratory distress syndrome (ARDS) preceding VAP
    d. ≥5 days of hospitalization prior to the occurrence of VAP
    e. Oliguric acute kidney injury

14. During the third week of his sickness, he develops some hemoptysis. CXR is suggestive of new findings and so CT chest is performed.

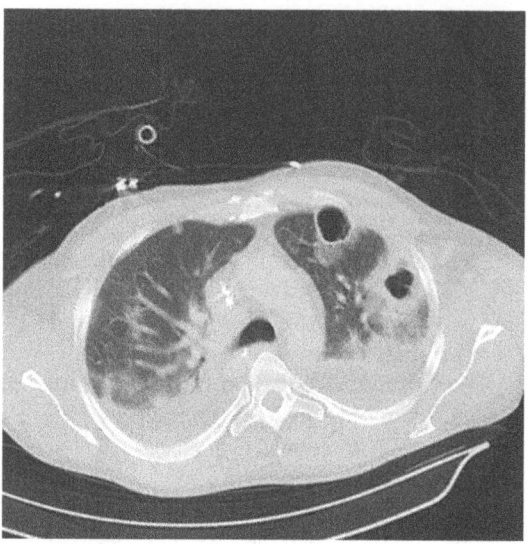

If hemoptysis worsens, next step in the management would be:
    a. Ventilation with the affected lung above
    b. CT pulmonary angiogram
    c. Bronchial artery angiogram with embolization
    d. Lobectomy

15. Which of the following statements is false?
    a. Community acquired MRSA has higher incidence of panton-valentine leukocidin (PVL) toxin
    b. Daptomycin **cannot** be used to treat pneumonia because it does not achieve sufficiently high concentrations in the respiratory tract
    c. Tigecycline has activity against MRSA but is not indicated in the treatment of VAP
    d. Vancomycin does not need to be renally adjusted
    e. Linezolid is noninferior to vancomycin to treat MRSA pneumonia and has better tissue penetration

16. Poor prognostic factors of sepsis include all except:
    a. Hypothermia
    b. Leukocytosis

c. Nonurinary source of infection
d. Nosocomial infection
e. Late or inappropriate antibiotic coverage

17. Which of the following statement about sepsis is incorrect?
    a. Systemic inflammatory response syndrome criteria (SIRS) is no longer included in the sepsis definition for this can also be caused by noninfectious etiology
    b. Infection is defined as the invasion of normally sterile tissue by organisms resulting in infectious pathology
    c. Bacteremia is the presence of viable bacteria in the blood
    d. The qSOFA score is easy to calculate with these 3 components, respiratory rate ≥22/minute, altered mentation and a heart rate > 120/min
    e. Secondary MODS is organ failure that is not in direct response to the insult itself, but is a consequence of the host's response

18. A 38-year-old female with ALL post chemotherapy given 3 weeks ago now awaiting bone marrow transplant was noted to have fevers and chills, and was referred to the ER by the hematologist. No other localizing symptoms were reported. After initial evaluation and resuscitation, blood and urine cultures are obtained. The nurse asks you about which antibiotics to be given next?
    a. Ceftriazone and azithromycin
    b. Cefepime
    c. Piperacillin and tazobactum with metronidazole
    d. Meropenem and vancomycin
    e. Colistin and tiegcycline

19. A 52-year-old male with past history of DM was found to have an infected pustule along his right nostril. After surgical drainage under conscious sedation and appropriate IV antibiotics, he significantly improved. Patient has chronic pain syndrome and treats himself with fentanyl patches changed every 24 hrs. Culture results from the pus revealed MRSA infection and his antibiotics was deescalated to linezolid oral for ease of administration and discharged to home. 5th day post discharge, patient was brought back to the ER by his family with complaints of being extremely agitated and febrile, temperatures up to 103°F was noted at home. In the ER, haloperidol was given for he was uncontrollable. On physical exam, he was noted to be diaphoretic and have clonus. Likely diagnosis includes:
    a. Serotonin syndrome
    b. Malignant hyperthermia
    c. Worsening cellulitis with meningeal extension
    d. Central venous thrombosis
    e. Neuroleptic malignant syndrome

20. A 28-year-old female with past history of bipolar disorder on fluoxetine and alprazolam develops low grade fevers and significant weight loss over a period of two months. Then over the last 2–3 days because she became extremely aggressive, she was brought to the ER. In the ER, temp was 100.5°F w/ WBC of 16. Routine CT head was negative for any acute findings. LP is performed which was exudative with lymphocyte predominance. Gene Xpert was positive for tuberculosis. 4 drug antituberculosis regimen was initiated along with dexamethasone. By the end of the 1st week of treatment, significant improvement was noted. On day 9, she started complaining of some headache. But as the day progressed, she started having difficulty speaking followed by altered mentation, she was very agitated. CT head done revealed.

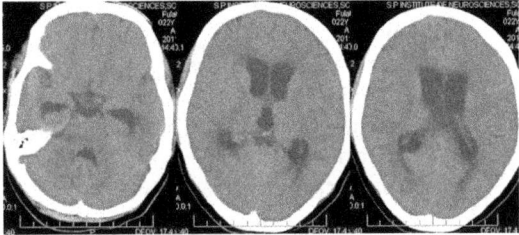

The next best step should be?
    a. Continue the current management
    b. Obtain urgent psychiatric evaluation
    c. Drug serum level testing
    d. Obtain urgent neurosurgical evaluation
    e. Initiate antiepileptics medications

21. A 61-year-old male with history of DM was brought to the emergency department with complaints of fevers, chills and severe lower abdominal pain. Patient has had recurrent urinary retention due to benign prostatic hypertrophy needing urinary catheter

drainage once. In the ER, he was hypotensive. Intravenous fluids for resuscitation was started. An arterial line was placed. ABG was 7.24/68/102 on 5L nasal canulla. Patient was intubated for increased work of breathing. Now sedated with propofol and is comfortable.

BP from the A line was 80s/60 mm Hg with an MAP of about low 65s.

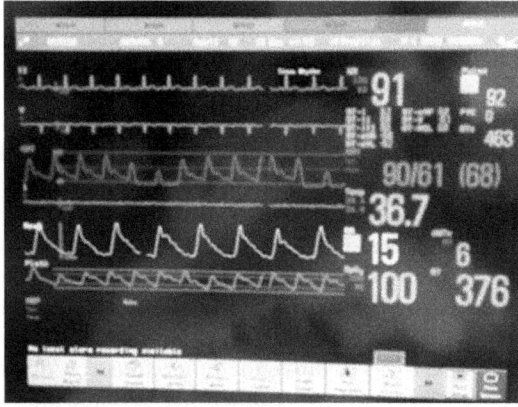

Next best step would be to:
a. Start vasopressors
b. Start inotropic agents
c. Intravenous fluids
d. Stress dose steroids
e. Broad-spectrum antibiotics

22. Risk factor for invasive candidemia includes all except:
a. Central venous catheter
b. Abdominal surgery
c. Recent broad-spectrum antibiotics usage
d. Enteral feeding
e. Acute renal replacement therapy

23. On day 4 of hospitalization, it was noted that the patient's blood cultures were positive for fungus, later identified as *Candida albicans*. Patient was on fluconazole which was escalated to caspofungin for it was azole resistant, but he continued to be febrile and repeat blood cultures were sent. Day 6, these cultures also grew Candida species. Transthoracic echocardiogram was done which was positive for endocarditis involving the mitral valve. Next action should include:
a. Transesophageal echocardiogram
b. Retinoscopy
c. Add liposomal amphotericin
d. Cardiothoracic surgical review for valve replacement
e. All of the above

24. Which of the following statement is incorrect?
a. Spontaneous bacterial peritonitis (SBP) is defined as an ascitic fluid infection without an evident intra-abdominal surgically treatable source
b. Diagnosis is established by a positive ascitic fluid bacterial culture and an ascitic fluid absolute polymorphonuclear leukocyte count ≥250 cells/mm^3
c. Bacterascites is when bacteria is detected in the ascitic fluid, but the PMN count is <250 cells/mm^3, and always should be treated with antibiotics
d. Most common causes of SBP are gut bacteria like *E. coli* and *Klebsiella*
e. In patients with SBP, beta blocker use is associated with worse outcomes

25. A 42-year-old male with DM presents to your hospital from West Bengal with complaints of worsening fevers, chills and rigors. Family also reported that he has been coughing with increased phlegm production. In the ER, patient looks extremely toxic and is intubated for hypoxia. CXR reveals multilobar pneumonia with effusions. Blood, tracheal and urine cultures are obtained. They later reveal gram negative organisms. Which one of the following is untrue?
a. This organism is a widely distributed environmental saprophyte in soil and surface water in endemic regions
b. Predominant mode of transmission is percutaneous inoculation during exposure to wet season soils or contaminated water
c. Most important risk factors include diabetes, hazardous alcohol use, and chronic renal disease
d. *Burkholderia cepacia*, facultative intracellular gram-negative bacterium causes this infection
e. This organism can be latent in our body, cause reactivation and infection later like tuberculosis

26. A 46-year-old female with history of HTN, DM, hypothyroidism presented with increasing

cough and yellow phlegm production with fevers and chills at home. Symptoms started 10 days ago when she went on a picnic with some friends. Initially had runny nose with fevers and chills, which gradually worsened to this now. On arrival in the ER, she was hypotensive and tachycardic. Febrile to 39°C. After some fluid hydration, her oxygenation worsened to 80% non-rebreathing O_2 needing to be urgently intubated. Chest XR and ultrasonogram of the chest was suggestive of right middle and lower lobe pneumonia while diffuse pulmonary congestion was also noted. CVP from the RIJ central line was about 14. Bedside echocardiography demonstrates basal akinesis and apical ballooning with systolic anterior movement of the mitral valve. The vasopressor to be initiated next would be:
a. Norepinephrine
b. Vasopressin
c. Epinephrine
d. Dobutamine
e. Phenylephrine

27. A 36-year-old male smoker and alcohol abuser with no significant medical history here with ARDS secondary to H1N1 pneumonia and secondary bacterial pneumonia on prolonged mechanical ventilation, day 8 now. Patient has been extremely agitated needing high amounts of sedation, including dexmedetomidine, midazolam and propofol. He was also given IV methyl prednisolone to help with ventilation and prevent ARDS induced lung fibrosis. Patient has been on hemodialysis to help with fluid removal for he was in acute kidney injury induced anuria and acidosis. Given the above picture, which single factor may be associated with decreasing his risk of developing postintensive care syndrome (PCIS)?
a. Benzodiazepam use
b. IV methyl prednisolone
c. Severity of illness
d. Prolonged ICU stay with mechanical ventilation
e. Hemodialysis

28. A 42-year-old female with past medical history of hyperlipidemia, rheumatoid arthritis on chronic prednisone therapy presents with abdominal pain and distention. She has been nauseous and vomited multiple times during the same day. On arrival in the ER, she is noted to be hypotensive at 70/50 mm Hg, started on aggressive fluid resuscitation. Ultrasonogram abdomen is suggestive of gallstone cholecystitis with pancreatitis. Lipase was elevated at 2000. During this time, she has a large bout vomiting followed by acute hypoxia, saturation down to the 60s.

Rapid sequence intubation is immediately attempted. Anesthetic drug that should be avoided here would be:
a. Propofol
b. Midazolam
c. Lorazepam
d. Etomidate
e. Ketamine

29. Patient was found to have emphysematous cholecystitis and pancreatitis, drifted to severe sepsis in shock even after multiple fluid boluses. Currently on triple vasopressors and still hypotensive. Based on the available data, which of the following statements would be true?
a. An immediate random serum cortisol should be sent
b. ACTH low dose stimulation test should be performed immediately
c. Serum free cortisol level is less informative compared to total cortisol level
d. Etomidate given to this patient will not affect ACTH stimulation testing
e. Initiation of hydrocortisone injection should be done immediately

30. A 36-year-old male active smoker with congenital hypothyroidism on replacement thyroxine was brought in by family for worsening fevers/chills/rigors at home with extensive cough and yellow phlegm production. On arrival in the ER, he was noted to be in type 2 respiratory failure (7.28/60/54 on 50% venturi mask in the ER) and was intubated by rapid sequence intubation with ketamine and rocuronium. Patient had refused care for more than 2–3 days for he might not be able to smoke in the hospital. Chest X-ray postintubation was

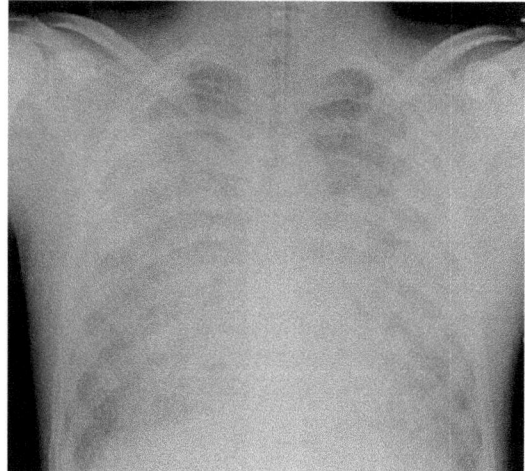

ARDS was suspected and PEEP was titrated to 14 in PCV with the most ideal tidal volume. Which subsequent observation after PEEP titration is associated with decreased mortality?

a. Increased PaO₂
b. Decreased PaCO₂
c. Increase in plateau to PEEP pressure gradient
d. Improved mixed venous oxygen saturation
e. Decrease in plateau to PEEP pressure gradient

31. A 43-year-old male with history of alcohol abuse presented to the ER 7 days ago with complaints of bloody vomitus. Patient was admitted to the regular wards, kept nil by mouth, pantoprazole infusion and IV fluid were given. Upper GI endoscopy performed was suggestive of peptic ulcer disease; appropriate treatment was initiated and discharged to home. Patient returned now with family for he was minimally responsive at home. He had been coughing extensively at home with excessive yellow phlegm production. Initial ABG revealed type 1 respiratory failure and he was intubated. Also he had severe metabolic acidosis with potassium of 6.9 for which immediate CRRT was initiated. Dual vasopressors were on flow. Now on the ventilator, Plateau pressures recorded were more than 34. Severe ARDS was documented with a P/F ratio of 80. Which of the following is indicative of good prognosis with Extracorporeal Membrane Oxygenation (ECMO)?

a. Multiorgan dysfunction syndrome
b. Severe ARDS resistant to all forms of ventilation
c. Late ARDS, > 10 days of hypoxic respiratory failure
d. Disseminated intravascular coagulation
e. Plateau pressure of 22 with good lung compliance

32. A 56-year-old male with past medical history of DM and HTN is here with c/o fevers/chills and rigors. Productive cough with green phlegm was noted. After initial aggressive fluid resuscitation with 2 L crystalloids, patient hemodynamics improved and was admitted to the ICU for further care, and given ceftriaxone and azithromycin. Right IJ triple lumen catheter was placed followed by significant drop in BP and raised HR. Bedside USG R chest along the midclavicular and anterior axillary line revealed this with good pleural sliding. Bedside ECHO revealed preserved LV function with normal RA and RV. Immediate chest X-ray was pending.

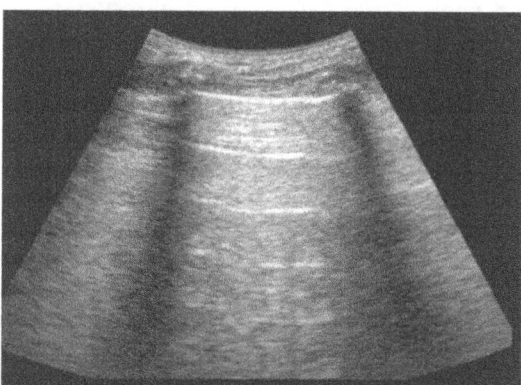

TLC was noted as $16 \times 10^3/\mu L$ with neutrophil predominance. What caused this acute worsening?

a. Pneumothorax
b. Pulmonary edema
c. Sepsis
d. Large pleural effusion
e. Pulmonary embolism

33. A 44-year-old male with past medical history of HTN and DM was admitted to the hospital due to urosepsis from nephrolithiasis. While having septic shock and being mechanically ventilated for ARDS his blood sugars should be:

a. A tight intensive insulin therapy regimen to achieve a target blood glucose range of 80 to 110 mg/dL
b. Blood glucose target of 140 to 180 mg/dL rather than a more stringent target
c. Always intravenous fluids (IVF) that contain glucose should be administered
d. High dose intravenous insulin therapy should be given continuous
e. Hypoglycemia has hardly been noted during intensive insulin therapy

34. A 62-year-old male ex-smoker with past medical history of DM, HTN, chronic respiratory failure status post tracheostomy due to CVA on 2L oxygen via T piece at home was brought to the hospital for he developed fever and chills at home. The home care nurse mentioned that there was increase amount of yellow secretions from the trachy site on suctioning. Chest XR in the ER was suggestive for bibasilar pneumonia. Patient was admitted to the hospital. Initial ABG was 7.3/62/54 on 2L O_2. He was placed on the ventilator to assist his breathing, A/VC 450/+6/16/50% settings. Oxygenation stayed the same for next 2–3 days and he needed to be on the ventilator. Tracheal aspirate culture sent from the ER grew MDR pneumococcus, antibiotics were deescalated as per sensitivities pattern. What is his diagnosis?
    a. Ventilator associated tracheitis (VAT)
    b. Ventilator associated pneumonia (VAP)
    c. No ventilator associated condition (VAC)
    d. Infection related ventilator associated condition (IVAC)

35. A 42-year-old male with past medical history HTN, CAD post stenting on aspirin and clopidogrel came to the ER with complains of fever and productive cough. Chest XR was suggestive of pneumonia. He had not taken his flu shot this year. He is a respiratory therapist by profession. Patient was started on ceftriaxone and azithromycin to treat for health care associated pneumonia. Given his increased work of breathing, he was placed on high flow nasal oxygen therapy. He was admitted to the high dependency unit. Nasal swab polymerase chain reaction (PCR) assay came positive for Rhino virus. What would be the next step?
    a. Add vancomycin to help treat post viral Staph infection
    b. Add ribavirin
    c. Continue current therapy with droplet isolation
    d. Start oseltamivir
    e. Stop antibiotics with droplet isolation

K Type Questions
[Marked True (T)/False (F)]

1. A 25-year-old gentleman, who had a road traffic accident and sustained traumatic brain injury requiring a neurosurgical intervention to evacuate an intracerebral hematoma with intraventricular extension with an external ventricular drain (EVD) placement, seven days ago, has become febrile and less responsive. State which of the following statement are true or false about the diagnosis of possible healthcare related meningitis/ventriculitis in this patient?
    a. CSF analysis with normal cell count, glucose and protein rules out a meningitis/ventriculitis
    b. An elevated CSF lactate may be useful in the diagnosis
    c. CSF cultures are essential to establish the diagnosis
    d. Neuroimaging with MRI with gadolinium enhancement and diffusion weighted imaging gives no added information and is not recommended
    e. Empirical antibiotics are to be withheld until the culture reports are available, unless the patient is hemodynamically unstable

2. The available data in literature, at the moment suggest that qSOFA:
    a. Is validated to diagnosis sepsis in patients in ICU with suspected infection
    b. Has a superior diagnostic accuracy compared to SIRS in diagnosis of sepsis
    c. Is superior to SOFA in predicting in hospital mortality
    d. Is superior to MEWS in predicting ICU mortality

3. As per the Surviving Sepsis Campaign 2016 recommendations, in patients with sepsis and septic shock:

    a. The initial mean arterial pressure (MAP) is to be maintained at 65 mm Hg
    b. With signs of organ hypoperfusion the initial resuscitation recommended is at least 30 mL/kg of intravenous crystalloid over the first three hours
    c. After the initial resuscitation intravenous fluids should be given as a continuous infusion as long hemodynamic factors continue to improve
    d. Appropriate routine microbiological cultures should be obtained without any delay before starting antibiotics
    e. Intravenous antimicrobials should be administered within 1 hour of recognition of the condition

4. **State which of the following statements are true or false about a suspected *Cryptococcus neoformans*' pneumonia in an immunocompetent host.**
    a. *Cryptococcus neoformans* never causes pneumonia in immune competent hosts
    b. Serum cryptococcal antigen assay being negative rules out the possibility of the pneumonia being due to *Cryptoccocus neoformanns*
    c. If the cryptococcal antigen assay is positive, serial monitoring of its titers will help with deciding the duration of therapy
    d. Culturing the organism in the sputum or bronchial-alveolar lavage confirms the diagnosis
    e. Drug of choice for treatment of mild to moderate pulmonary disease is fluconazole

5. **A 35-year-old lady who has discharged from hospital 5 days ago following a laparoscopic hysterectomy is brought into the ER in a delirious state. She is warm to touch and her heart rate on arrival is 120/min with a blood pressure of 80/30 mm Hg. An ultrasound abdomen done shows a pelvic collection. State which of the following statements are true/false about her management.**
    a. The initial volume of fluid she should be resuscitated with is 30 mL/kg of crystalloid given intravenous over the first three hours
    b. After collecting appropriate samples for microbiological cultures she should be initiated on empiric combination antibiotic therapy
    c. There is no indication for the drainage of the collection in her pelvis
    d. Vasopressin is the drug of choice if hypotension persists despite initial fluid resuscitation
    e. There is no role for hydrocortisone if hemodynamic stability has been achieved with fluid resuscitation and vasopressor therapy

6. **An 85-year-old gentleman, who is on regular maintenance dialysis, is admitted from a retirement home with complaints of altered mental status and confusion since two days. Which of the following statements are true about his care?**
    a. His altered mental status and confusion can be a sign of sepsis
    b. Immune senescence improves his immunity
    c. Initiation of inappropriate therapy can increase mortality compared to younger population
    d. He is at a higher risk for developing bloodstream infection with drug resistant bacteria

7. **A 65-year-old man with diabetes mellitus is admitted to the ICU with history of fever, headache and severe myalgia since last 7 days and petechiae over his body since the last 2 days. His family noticed him to be breathless since a day and confused since few hours. On examination, he is febrile, tachycardic, has visible ecchymosis over both forearms and is confused and agitated. His blood pressure is 110/90 mm Hg. A chest X-ray done shows bilateral pleural effusion and an ultrasound abdomen confirms ascites. His laboratory investigations show a hematocrit of 55, platelet count of 50,000/mm^3. Dengue serology done returns IgM positive. Which of the following statements are true/false about his condition?**
    a. His clinical features are consistent with the criteria to make a diagnosis of dengue hemorrhagic fever
    b. Viral antigen NS1 cannot be detected in blood this late in the disease
    c. Single blood specimen dengue serology IgM positivity can confirm the diagnosis
    d. High titers of IgG positivity in this patient are more indicative of a secondary dengue infection

e. Features of encephalitis rules out dengue infection

8. A 25-year-old lady is admitted to the ICU with history of fever, headache and severe myalgia since last 7 days and petechiae over her body since the last 2 days. She complains of intense abdominal pain and breathless since a day. On examination she is afebrile but tachycardic with low volume pulse, blood pressure of 110/90 mm Hg and is restless. There is visible ecchymosis over both forearms. A chest X-ray done shows bilateral pleural effusion and an ultrasound abdomen confirms ascites. Her laboratory investigations show a hematocrit of 55, platelet count of 50,000 cells/mm^3. Dengue serum antigen test is positive for NS1 and the serology for IgM antibodies.

   Which of the following symptoms/signs should alert the physician to impending dengue shock syndrome?
   a. Tachycardia with low volume pulse
   b. Narrow pulse pressure
   c. Severe abdominal pain
   d. Restlessness
   e. Platelet count of 50,000 cells/mm^3

9. Which of the following statements are true/false about severe dengue infection (WHO classification 2009) in the adult patients?
   a. Age greater than 50 years is associated with increased incidence of both need for ICU admission and ICU mortality
   b. High SOFA or APACHE II scores are associated with high mortality
   c. High arterial lactate levels are associated with high mortality
   d. Among patients with multiple organ failure hematological complications predict risk of in ICU mortality the best
   e. SOFA score at ICU discharge has no predictive value

10. Which of the following statements are true/false about solid organ transplant recipients?
    a. Generally the 28 and 90 day mortality from bacteremic sepsis is lower than that in non-transplant patients
    b. The first month after the transplantation is the period where the patients are at risk for opportunistic infections
    c. Infections that happen between 1 and 6 months after the transplantation are usually caused by community micro-organisms
    d. Prophylactic antimicrobial therapy completely prevents opportunistic infections
    e. The most common presentation of a CMV infection is fever, malaise, leukopenia, thrombocytopenia and elevated liver enzymes

11. A 55-year-old gentleman who had a renal transplant done 6 months ago is admitted to the ICU with history of fever and shortness of breath of 7 days duration. On arrival he is found to be tachypneic with a respiratory rate of 40 breaths/ minute, tachycardic with a pulse rate of 130/min and hypoxic with a room air saturation of 82%. A chest X-ray done shows bilateral interstitial opacities. Which of the following statements are true/false about his condition?
    a. *Pneumocystis jirovecii* pneumonia (PCP) is the most common opportunistic infection that can be the cause for his acute respiratory failure
    b. It is less likely to be PCP infection as the period for the highest risk for PCP infection is after 1 year of transplantation surgery
    c. Elevated serum LDH confirms the diagnosis of PCP
    d. Elevated serum beta –D – glucan rules out the clinical suspicion for PCP
    e. Irrespective of the severity of the illness the drug of choice for the treatment of PCP is tablet trimethoprim – sulfamethoxazole (TMP – SMX)

12. Which of the following statements are true/false about severe *Pneumocystis jirovecii* pneumonia (PCP) in non-HIV patients?
    a. The treatment of choice is tablet trimethoprim – sulfamethoxazole (TMP–SMX)
    b. Atovaquone is the preferred drug if the patient does not tolerate TMP- SMX
    c. The total duration of antimicrobial therapy is for 21 days
    d. Lack of clinical improvement despite appropriate therapy for more than 7 days should be considered as treatment failure
    e. Despite appropriate therapy the outcome is worse than in HIV patients with PCP

13. A 35-year-old farmer was brought to the hospital with history of fever since 5 days, associated with headache, anorexia, malaise and myalgia. He had noticed red, non-pruritic rash over his body which started on the abdomen and spread to his arms and legs. On examination, he is febrile, with a temperature of 101°F, pulse rate of 90/min, blood pressure of 120/60 mm Hg and room air saturation is 90%. An eschar is noticed on his abdomen. State which of the following statements are true/ false about scrub typhus.
    a. During the early phase of illness, scrub typhus can be diagnosed only clinically based on epidemiological clues, clinical features and laboratory findings
    b. Relative bradycardia rules out a diagnosis of scrub typhus
    c. The presence of eschar is a must to confirm the diagnosis of scrub typhus
    d. Weil- Felix test in neither specific nor sensitive to help with the diagnosis
    e. Indirect fluorescent antibody (IFA) test is the gold standard serological test to be used for diagnosis

14. State which of the following statements are true or false about scrub typhus infection:
    a. It is an infection caused by a gram negative coccobacillus
    b. The infection occurs 7 to 10 days after the bite of an infected mite
    c. Classically described eschar that occurs at the site of the mite bite is seen in all patients
    d. Serological tests that confirm the diagnosis requires demonstration of fourfold increase in antibody titer in a paired blood sample drawn at least 14 days apart
    e. The antibiotic of choice for treatment is doxycycline

15. Previously healthy 26-year-old lady who is a cine actor by profession is brought to the hospital with history of fever, sore throat and loose stools of 1 week duration, painful deglutition of 5 days duration, extensive maculopapular rash all over her body of 5 days duration and cough with breathlessness of 1 day duration. She was started on oral augmentin by her GP about 6 days ago. On examination, she is febrile with a temperature of 39°C, tachycardic with a heart rate of 120/min and tachypneic with a respiratory rate of 34/min. Her blood pressure is 120/70 mm Hg and room air oxygen saturation is 90%. She has extensive mucocutaneous ulcers involving her oropharyngeal and urogential tract, which bleeds to touch. Which of the following statements are true or false?
    a. A clinical differential diagnosis that can be considered in this lady is acute retroviral infection
    b. A negative retroviral serology completely rules out HIV infection in her
    c. CD4 counts would remain unchanged if she has acute retroviral infection
    d. Virological markers will be positive if she has retroviral infection
    e. Antiretroviral therapy (ART) has no role in the acute retroviral infection phase

16. State which of the following statements are true/false about acute retroviral syndrome:
    a. The clinical presentation can mimic infectious mononucleosis
    b. The presence of heterophile antibody test positive mononucleosis rules out the diagnosis
    c. The time from exposure to the development of symptoms of acute retroviral syndrome is generally 2-4 weeks
    d. Opportunistic infections never occur during this phase of the illness.
    e. There is no role for antiretroviral therapy (ART) in this phase of illness

17. State which of the following factors have been found to be associated with increased in hospital death in a patient admitted to the ICU with community acquired pneumonia (CAP):
    a. Diastolic blood pressure less than 60 mm Hg
    b. Respiratory rate greater than 30 breaths/min
    c. Bacteremia
    d. Arterial blood gas analysis showing a pH less than 7.35
    e. Need for mechanical ventilation

18. A 50-year-old lady with no premorbid condition is brought to the emergency room with complaints of fever, cough with expectoration and breathlessness of three day duration. She is tachypneic (RR – 35/min), tachycardic (Pulse – 130/min), hypoxic

(SpO$_2$ – 80%), hypotensive (BP – 80/40 mm Hg) and disoriented on arrival. There are bilateral crackles in her chest on auscultation. Her chest X-ray shows bilateral mid zone consolidations. She is moved to the ICU with oxygen therapy and an infusion of dopamine where her sputum and blood are send for culture. State which of the following statements are true/false about her.

a. The combination of her clinical signs, symptoms and chest radiological findings has a very good sensitivity in diagnosing community acquired pneumonia (CAP)
b. The decision to continue her treatment in the ICU is medically correct
c. There is no added benefit in doing microbial cultures of her respiratory secretions and blood
d. The most likely pathogen to cause her CAP is *Streptococcus pneumonia*
e. There is no role for urinary pneumococcal antigen assay in her

ANSWERS

A Type Answers

Q1. Answer c

Give broad-spectrum antibiotics to treat likely healthcare associated pneumonia Vs aspiration pneumonia. As per the guidelines issued after 2010, recommendation is oral vancomycin is the first-line therapy for severe *Clostridium difficile* infection (CDI). This practice reflects reports of frequent metronidazole failures in CDI and studies showing the superiority of oral vancomycin in severe disease. The major pharmacologic advantage of vancomycin over metronidazole is that vancomycin is not absorbed, so maximal concentrations of the drug can act intracolonically at the site of infection.

> Cohen SH et al. Clinical practice guidelines for *Clostridium difficile* infection in adults: 2010 update by the society for healthcare epidemiology of America (SHEA) and the infectious diseases society of America (IDSA). Society for Healthcare Epidemiology of America; Infectious Diseases Society of America. Infect Control Hosp Epidemiol. 2010;31(5):431-55.

Q2. Answer d

Although patients with necrotizing soft tissue infection (NSTI) may appear quite well during the early part of their clinical course, deterioration within hours of presentation frequently occurs, with the infection having the potential to cause extensive soft tissue necrosis. As such, a suspicion of NSTI is all that is required to prompt surgical exploration, particularly in high-risk patients (e.g. immunocompromised, diabetic, or postsurgical patients). Delays in surgical treatment correlate with worse outcomes and higher mortality rates.

> Hadeed GJ, et al. Early surgical intervention and its impact on patients presenting with necrotizing soft tissue infections: A single academic center experience. J Emerg Trauma Shock. 2016;9(1):22-7.

Q3. Answer c

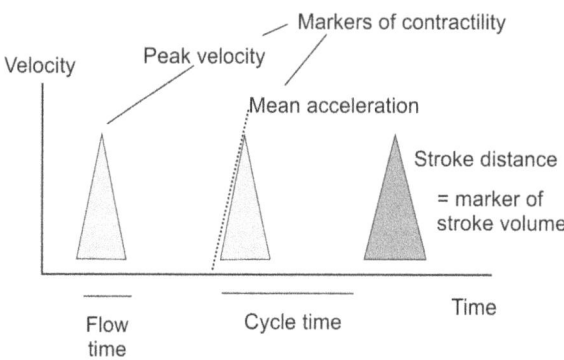

- Stroke volume (SV) is dependent on preload, afterload and contractility.
- Corrected (systolic) flow time (FTc)
  - Indicates preload
  - Normal = 0.33–0.36s
- Peak velocity (PV)
  - Indicates contractility
  - Normal range is age related. (20 yrs 90–120 cm/sec, 90 yrs 30–60 cm/sec).
- Interpretation of FTc and PV helps determine afterload related issues.
- Considerable actions based on readings in the right clinical context:
- Low SV → IV fluid
- Low FTc → IV fluid
- Low PV → Inotrope
- Low PV + Low FTc → Decrease afterload.

> Morris C, et al. Oesophageal Doppler monitoring, doubt and equipoise: evidence based medicine means change. Anaesthesia. 2013;68(7):684-8.

Q4. Answer c

Increased IAP is called intra-abdominal hypertension (IAH). Abdominal compartment syndrome (ACS) refers to organ dysfunction caused by IAH. ACS can impair the function of nearly every organ system causing physiologic consequences like impaired cardiac function, decreased venous return, hypoxemia, hypercarbia, renal impairment, diminished gut perfusion, and elevated intracranial pressure. Diagnosis of ACS requires that IAP be measured. Management initially consists of careful observation and supportive care. In some cases abdominal compartment surgical decompression may be required.

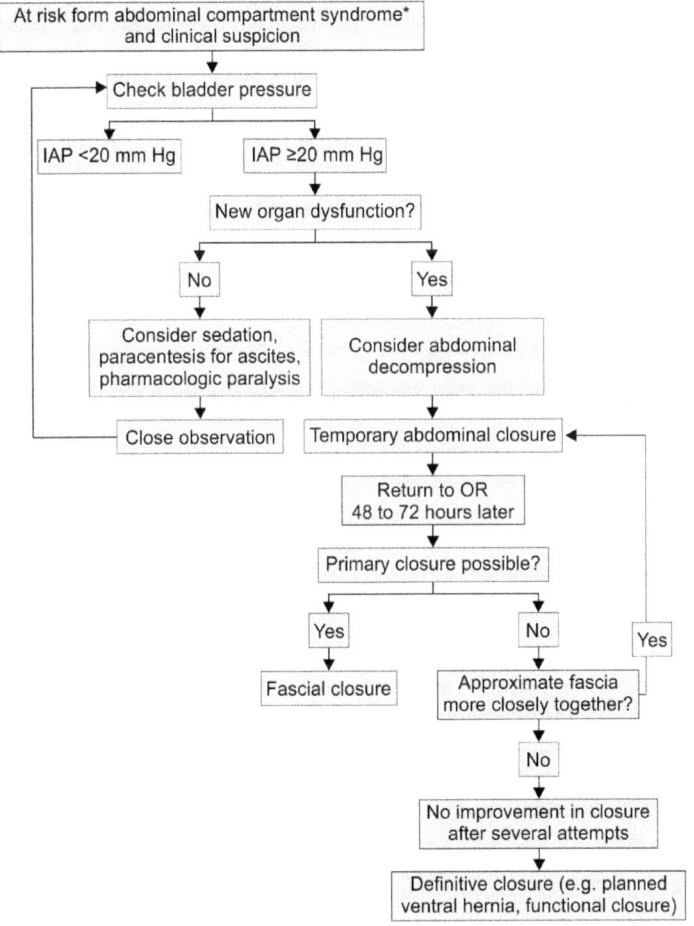

Malbrain ML, et al. Results from the International Conference of Experts on Intra-abdominal Hypertension and Abdominal Compartment Syndrome. I. Definitions. Intensive Care Med. 2006;32(11):1722-32.

Q5. Answer d

Cerebrospinal fluid (CSF) Gram stain image here is suggestive of *Streptococcus pneumonae* infection. Initial empiric therapy in patients with normal renal function includes vancomycin (15 to 20 mg/kg IV every 8 to 12 hours) plus either ceftriaxone (2 g IV every 12 hours) or cefotaxime (2 g IV every 4 to 6 hours). If the isolate is susceptible to third-generation cephalosporins (MIC <1.0 mcg/mL), ceftriaxone or cefotaxime is continued but combination with vancomycin is needed if there is penicillin resistance (MIC ≥0.12 mcg/mL) and an MIC ≥1.0 mcg/mL to third-generation cephalosporins. Early intravenous administration of dexamethasone has been evaluated as adjuvant therapy in an attempt to diminish the rate of hearing loss and other neurologic complications as well as mortality in selected patients with bacterial meningitis. The rationale for this approach is provided by animal studies showing that hearing loss is temporally associated with severe inflammatory changes induced by bacterial meningitis and that dexamethasone reduces CSF concentrations of cytokines (such as tumor necrosis factor [TNF]-alpha and interleukin [IL]-1), CSF inflammation, and cerebral edema.

Lutsar I, et al. Factors influencing the anti-inflammatory effect of dexamethasone therapy in experimental pneumococcal meningitis. J Antimicrob Chemother. 2003;52(4):651.

Q6. Answer e

Mixing studies help when PT and PTT are prolonged outside the upper limit of the laboratory's established normal range. Helps determine if this is due to a factor deficiency or circulating anticoagulant (inhibitor). Factor deficiencies that cause these prolongations can be congenital or acquired. A deficiency of coagulation factors II, V, X or fibrinogen will cause a prolongation of both the PT and aPTT (common pathway). The PT is prolonged with a deficiency of VII and the aPTT with a deficiency of VIII, IX, XI, or XII. Acquired factor deficiencies can be attributed to liver disease, warfarin therapy (II, VII, IX, and X) and DIC. If mixing study does not correct the PT or PTT, then it is due to an inhibitor like heparin and direct thrombin inhibitors (DTI) or nonspecific inhibitors such as lupus anticoagulants.

Chang S, Tillema V, Scherr D. A 'percent correction' formula for evaluation of mixing studies. Am J Clin Pathol. 2002;117:62-73.

Q7. Answer d

Jugular vein suppurative thrombophlebitis (Lemierre's syndrome) is characterized by infectious involvement of the carotid sheath vessels with bacteremia. Jugular vein suppurative thrombophlebitis can also be associated with intravenous catheter insertion. Septic emboli to the lung are common. The causative organism is usually anaerobe *Fusobacterium necrophorum*. Catheter associated jugular vein suppurative thrombophlebitis can be associated with skin flora/ nosocomial pathogens including methicillin resistant *Staphylococcus aureus* (MRSA). Acceptable regimens include ampicillin/sulbactam, piperacillin/tazobactam or carbepenem monotherapy. If it is catheter associated, vancomycin can be added. The role of anticoagulation for jugular vein suppurative thrombophlebitis is controversial; there are no controlled studies. Some authors favor anticoagulation only if there is evidence for extension of thrombus. We suggest not administering anticoagulation in the absence of evidence for extension of thrombus.

Golpe R, et al. Lemierre's syndrome (necrobacillosis). Postgrad Med J. 1999;75(881):141.

Q8. Answer d

Most patients with aspiration pneumonia acquired in the community have a mixed infection that includes aerobes and anaerobes. For hospital-acquired or healthcare-associated aspiration pneumonia, aerobic bacteria, especially gram-negative bacilli and *S. aureus*, are more important than the anaerobes. However, in patients with poor dentition, we generally use a regimen with activity against both aerobes and anaerobes. This patient given the history of sick contact from the community should also have adequate coverage for atypical bacteria.

Bartlett JG, et al. Bacteriology of hospital-acquired pneumonia. Arch Intern Med. 1986;146(5):868.

Q9. Answer e

Initial inpatient treatment of an exacerbation is appropriate for patients with characteristics such as increased respiratory rate ≥25/minute, hypotension, temperature ≥38°C, hypoxemia (pulse oxygen saturation <92%), or failure to improve after oral antibiotics (and no facilities for home intravenous therapy). Initial antibiotic of choice should be based on the sensitivity profile from culture data and history of allergy to antibiotics of the patient.

If sputum culture data are not available, local antibiotic resistance patterns and responses to recent antibiotics should guide empiric antibiotic selection. We typically use a single agent (e.g. antipseudomonal penicillin like ceftazidime or aztreonam). If the patient is extremely sick, then adding a second agent like fluoroquinolone or aminoglycoside may be appropriate, but monotherapy with these agents may be inadequate. There is no role for aerosol antibiotics as sole agents or in addition to intravenous administration.

Pasteur MC, et al. British Thoracic Society guideline for non-CF bronchiectasis. British Thoracic Society Bronchiectasis non-CF Guideline Group. Thorax. 2010;65(Suppl 1):i1.

Q10. Answer c

1, 3-Beta-D-glucan, a cell wall component of many fungi, is detected by the beta-D-glucan assay. The beta-D-glucan assay is not specific but can be positive if infected by *Aspergillus* species, Candidiasis and *Pneumocystis jirovecii*. But this test is clearly negative in patients with mucormycosis or cryptococcosis. Given the clinical setting and symptoms, Mucor infection is more likely.

> Odabasi Z, et al. Beta-D-glucan as a diagnostic adjunct for invasive fungal infections: validation, cutoff development, and performance in patients with acute myelogenous leukemia and myelodysplastic syndrome. Clin Infect Dis. 2004;39(2):199.

Q11. Answer b

Isolation precautions are used to interrupt or reduce the risk of transmission of pathogens. Contact precautions are used for with multidrug-resistant bacteria (MRSA, VRE, drug-resistant gram-negative organisms), Enteric infections (Norovirus, *Clostridium difficile, Escherichia coli* O157:H7), Viral infections (HSV, VZV, RSV, parainfluenza, enterovirus), scabies, impetigo, noncontained abcesses or decubitus ulcers (especially for *Staphylococcus aureus* and group A *Streptococcus*). Medical equipment should be dedicated to a single patient when possible in order to avoid transfer of pathogens via fomites. Droplets are particles of respiratory secretions ≥5 microns. Droplets remain suspended in the air for limited periods. Transmission is associated with exposure within three to six feet (one to two meters) of the source. Droplet precautions are used for the care of patients with suspected or confirmed infections with *Neisseria meningitidis, Bordetella pertussis*, influenza, parainfluenza, adenovirus, *Haemophilus influenzae* type b, *Mycoplasma pneumoniae*, rubella. In some situations like parainfluenza infection, both droplet and contact isolation may be necessary. Airborne droplet nuclei are particles of respiratory secretions <5 microns. Droplet nuclei can remain suspended in the air for extended periods and thus can be a source of inhalational exposure for susceptible individuals. Airborne precautions are warranted for the care of patients with suspected or confirmed tuberculosis (TB), measles, varicella, smallpox, and severe acute respiratory syndrome (SARS). Patients on airborne isolation precautions should be placed in a private room with negative air pressure that has a minimum of 6 to 12 air changes per hour. Reverse isolation is for patients with neutropenia or who are post bone marrow transplant.

> Siegel JD, et al. Healthcare Infection Control Practices Advisory Committee 2007 Guideline for Isolation Precautions: Preventing Transmission of Infectious Agents in Healthcare Settings, June 2007.

Q12. Answer c

As per ARMA trial, Low tidal volume ventilation (LTVV) should be used to achieve an inspiratory plateau airway pressure ≤30 cm H_2O. This is referred to as lung protective ventilation. Mostly noted adverse effects are Auto-PEEP due to higher respiratory rates and need for high levels of sedation to achieve synchrony with the ventilator. A reasonable oxygenation goal during LTVV is an arterial oxygen tension (PaO_2) between 55 and 80 mm Hg or oxyhemoglobin saturation (SpO_2) between 88% and 95%. Permissive hypercapnia may happen due to the ventilatory strategy that accepts alveolar hypoventilation in order to maintain a low alveolar pressure and minimize the complications of alveolar over distension (e.g. ventilator-associated lung injury). Hypercapnia and respiratory acidosis are a consequence of this strategy.

> Brower RG, et al. Ventilation with lower tidal volumes as compared with traditional tidal volumes for acute lung injury and the acute respiratory distress syndrome. Acute Respiratory Distress Syndrome Network. N Engl J Med. 2000;342(18):1301.

Q13. Answer e

Recognized risk factors to develop MDR VAP include:
- IV antibiotic use within the previous 90 days
- Septic shock at the time of VAP
- ARDS preceding VAP
- ≥5 days of hospitalization prior to the occurrence of VAP
- Acute renal replacement therapy prior to VAP onset.

In a meta-analysis that included 15 studies, the above factors were associated with an increased risk of MDR VAP while coma present at the time of ICU admission was associated with lower risk of MDR VAP. In a meta-analysis of observational studies of patients with VAP and bacteremia, inappropriate therapy significantly increased patients' odds of mortality.

Kalil AC, et al. Management of Adults with Hospital-acquired and Ventilator-associated Pneumonia: Clinical Practice Guidelines by the Infectious Diseases Society of America and the American Thoracic Society. Clin Infect Dis. 2016;63(5):e61.

Q14. Answer c

Blood traversing the lungs can arrive from one of two sources: low-pressure pulmonary arteries or the bronchial arteries which are under higher systemic pressure. Bleeding from a bronchial artery is the cause of massive hemoptysis in 90% of cases. The initial steps in managing massive hemoptysis are to ensure adequate gas exchange and to determine which lung is likely bleeding by CT imaging or bronchoscopy. Patients should be immediately placed into a position in which the lung that is presumed to be bleeding is in the dependent position. Arteriographic embolization successfully stops the pulmonary hemorrhage in more than 85% of attempted embolizations, especially if the bronchial, pulmonary, and/or systemic arterial circulations are well defined during the procedure.

Yoon W, et al. Bronchial and nonbronchial systemic artery embolization for life-threatening hemoptysis: a comprehensive review. Radiographics. 2002;22(6):1395.

Q15. Answer d

The 2016 IDSA/ATS guidelines on HAP and VAP and the 2011 IDSA guidelines for the treatment of MRSA infections recommended either linezolid or vancomycin to treat MRSA infection. There is an absolute difference in nephrotoxicity risk between vancomycin and linezolid. Linezolid needs no renal dosing and is preferred in patients with renal insufficiency. PVL is a cytotoxin that causes leukocyte destruction and tissue necrosis commonly isolated in community acquired MRSA strains.

Boyle-Vavra S, et al. Community-acquired methicillin-resistant *Staphylococcus aureus*: the role of Panton-Valentine leukocidin. Lab Invest. 2007;87(1):3.

Q16. Answer b

Mortality associated with sepsis is ≥10% while that associated with septic shock was ≥40%. Anomalies in the host's inflammatory response may indicate increased susceptibility to severe disease and mortality like failure to develop a fever (or hypothermia), leukopenia, thrombocytopenia, hyperchloremia, > 40 years of age, hyperglycemia, hypocoagulability, and failure of procalcitonin to fall have all been associated with poor outcomes. Other identified risk factors for mortality include new-onset atrial fibrillation, and comorbidities such as AIDS, liver disease, cancer, alcohol dependence, and/or immune suppression. The site of infection in patients with sepsis may be an important determinant of outcome, with sepsis from a urinary tract infection generally being associated with the lowest mortality rates. Sepsis due to nosocomial pathogens has a higher mortality than sepsis due to community-acquired pathogens. Failure to aggressively try to restore perfusion early and an elevated lactate is associated with poor outcomes. Studies have shown that the early administration of appropriate and adequate antibiotic therapy has a beneficial impact on bacteremic sepsis. In contrast, prior antibiotic therapy (i.e. antibiotics within the past 90 days) may be associated with increased mortality, at least among patients with gram negative sepsis. Likely because they are increased risk for resistant bacteria.

Krieger JN, et al. Urinary tract etiology of bloodstream infections in hospitalized patients. J Infect Dis. 1983;148(1):57.

Q17. Answer d

The 2016 SCCM/ESICM task force have described an assessment score for patients outside the intensive care unit as a way to facilitate the identification of patients potentially at risk of dying from sepsis. Modified version of the Sequential (Sepsis-related) Organ Failure Assessment score (SOFA) called the quick SOFA (qSOFA) score was made. A score ≥2 is associated with poor outcomes due to sepsis. Three components include respiratory rate ≥22/minute, altered mentation and a systolic blood pressure ≤100 mm Hg. The qSOFA score was originally validated in 2016 as most useful in patients suspected as having sepsis **outside** of the ICU. It has since been prospectively validated in the emergency department (ED) and confirmed to be less valuable in the ICU setting. In addition, qSOFA was superior to the systemic inflammatory response syndrome criteria (SIRS). In contrast, a retrospective analysis defined that qSOFA is inferior to SOFA in predicting in hospital mortality. Multiple organ dysfunction syndrome (MODS) refers to progressive organ dysfunction in an acutely ill patient, such that homeostasis cannot be maintained without intervention. It is at the severe end of the severity of illness spectrum of both infectious (sepsis, septic shock) and noninfectious conditions (e.g. SIRS from pancreatitis). MODS can be primary if it is the result of a well-defined insult in which organ dysfunction occurs early and can be directly attributable to the insult itself or secondary if the organ failure is not in direct response to the insult itself, but is a consequence of the host's response.

> Singer M, et al. The Third International Consensus Definitions for Sepsis and Septic Shock (Sepsis-3). JAMA. 2016;315(8):801-10.

Q18. Answer b

The choice of antibiotics is driven by multiple factors, including the degree of immunocompromise, prior antibiotic and infection history, local patterns of antibiotic resistance, and whether an agent is bactericidal or not. Initiation of monotherapy with an antipseudomonal beta-lactam agent is preferred. Ceftazidime monotherapy has also been shown to be effective but many experts avoid this due to the rising resistance rates among gram-negative bacteria and its limited activity against gram-positive bacteria, such as streptococci. Although anaerobic bacteria are present in abundance in the gastrointestinal tract, it is usually not necessary to include specific anaerobic antibiotic coverage in the initial empiric regimen. Numerous combination antibiotic regimens have been studied as initial empiric therapy in neutropenic fever, but none has been shown to be clearly superior to monotherapy. Monotherapy has fewer adverse events generally and is well tolerated. Vancomycin is not recommended as a standard part of the initial regimen, but gram-positive coverage should be added in patients if they are hemodynamically unstable, have pneumonia, positive blood cultures for gram-positive bacteria while awaiting speciation and susceptibility results, have suspected central venous catheter (CVC)-related infection or skin or soft tissue infection. If severe mucositis is noted in patients who were receiving prophylaxis with a fluoroquinolone, if ceftazidime monotherapy is initiated, then vancomycin is added to help its lack of adequate *Streptococcus* coverage.

> Freifeld AG, et al. Clinical practice guideline for the use of antimicrobial agents in neutropenic patients with cancer: 2010 update by the infectious diseases society of america. Infectious Diseases Society of America. Clin Infect Dis. 2011;52(4):e56.

Q19. Answer a

Serotonin syndrome (i.e. serotonin toxicity) is a potentially life-threatening condition associated with increased serotonergic activity in the central nervous system, seen with therapeutic medication use, inadvertent interactions between drugs, and intentional self-poisoning. This is observed in all age groups. The Hunter Toxicity Criteria includes spontaneous clonus, inducible clonus PLUS agitation or diaphoresis, ocular clonus PLUS agitation or diaphoresis, tremor PLUS hyperreflexia or hypertonia PLUS temperature above 38ºC PLUS ocular clonus or inducible clonus. Presence of one these symptoms should suggest the diagnosis. Management includes discontinuation of all serotonergic agents, supportive care aimed at normalization of vital signs, sedation with benzodiazepines, administration of serotonin antagonists like cyproheptadine, which is a histamine-1 receptor antagonist with nonspecific 5-HT1A and 5-HT2A antagonistic properties.

> Boyer EW, et al. The serotonin syndrome. Engl J Med. 2005;352(11):1112.

Q20. Answer d

Patients with hydrocephalus may require surgical decompression of the ventricular system in order to effectively manage the complications of raised intracranial pressure. In such patients with clinical stage II disease, the combination of serial lumbar puncture and steroid therapy may suffice while judging the early response to chemotherapy. However, surgical intervention should not be delayed in patients with stupor and coma or when the clinical course of therapy is marked by progressive neurologic impairment.

> Kingsley DP, et al. Tuberculous meningitis: role of CT in management and prognosis. J Neurol Neurosurg Psychiatry. 1987;50(1):30.

Q21. Answer c

Variation in pulse pressure is thought to be an indicator of a patient's position on the Frank-Starling Curve that denotes a response to pre-load (i.e. fluid responsiveness). Patients operating on the flat part of the curve are insensitive to changes in preload induced by mechanical ventilation and thus have a low variation in the pulse pressure, indicating a lack of fluid responsiveness. In contrast, patients operating on the steep portion of the curve, are sensitive to the cyclic changes in preload induced by mechanical ventilation and hence, exhibit greater variation in the pulse pressure (i.e. fluid responsive).

$$PPV = 100 \times (PP_{max} - PP_{min})/PP_{mean}$$

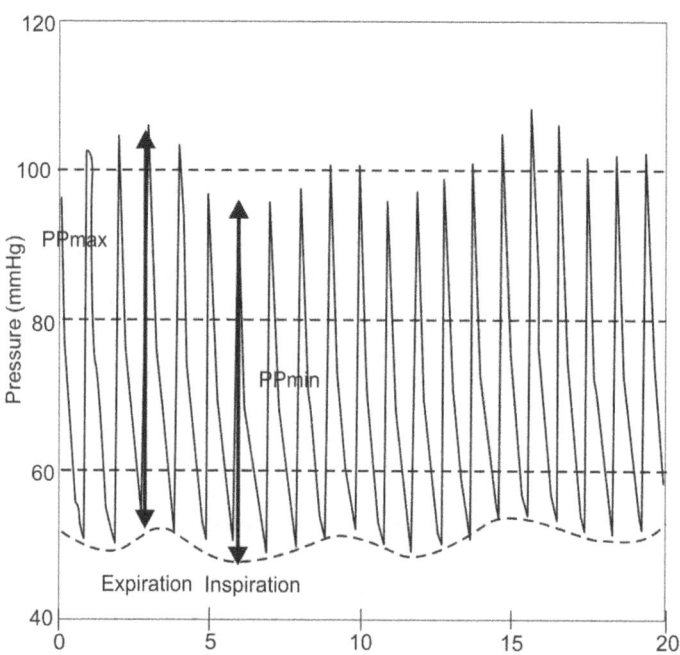

(PPV- Pulse pressure variation; PPmax: Maximum pulse pressure; PPmin: Minimum pulse pressure; PPmean: Mean pulse pressure)

While encouraging, this technique is limited to patients who are mechanically ventilated, receiving ≥8 mL/kg of tidal volume, in sinus rhythm, and **not** spontaneously triggering the ventilator. Although patients with intra-abdominal hypertension often have markedly abnormal respiratory system compliance, PPV is thought to be accurate in this setting.

Michard F, et al. Pulse pressure variation: beyond the fluid management of patients with shock. Crit Care. 2007;11(3):131.

Pinsky MR, et al. Functional haemodynamic monitoring. Curr Opin Crit Care. 2014;20(3):288-93.

Q22. Answer d

Patients in ICUs account for the greatest number of episodes of candidemia in most hospitals, especially surgical, trauma, neonatal and burns units. Risk factors include central venous catheters, total parenteral nutrition, broad-spectrum antibiotics, high APACHE scores, acute renal failure, particularly if requiring hemodialysis, prior surgery, particularly abdominal surgery and gastrointestinal tract perforations and anastomotic leaks. Immunocompromised patients like those with hematologic malignancies, recipients of solid organ or hematopoietic stem cell transplants, those on chemotherapeutic agents or steroids, especially those associated with extensive gastrointestinal mucosal damage are at increased risk for invasive candidemia. Fluconazole prophylaxis in these patients' places at them at increased rise for non-*Candida albicans* infection.

Chow JK, et al. Risk factors for albicans and non-albicans candidemia in the intensive care unit. Crit Care Med. 2008;36(7):1993.

Q23. Answer e

Candidemia management should mainly include these 2 aspects:
1. Evaluation for *Candida* endophthalmitis. Most cases of *Candida* endophthalmitis are endogenous. Most common is with *C. albicans,* often seen in hospitalized patients with indwelling central venous catheter. Treatment is systemic therapy.

2. Evaluation and management of Infective endocarditis. More common with prosthetic valves than native valve to develop endocarditis. Combined medical and surgical approach may be better in terms of outcomes. Initial antifungal therapy for native or prosthetic valve endocarditis would be either lipid formulation of amphotericin B with or without flucytosine or an echinocandin at a higher dose. Resection of the valve and any associated abscesses is essential for cure in most, but not all, patients. Following surgery, antifungal therapy should be continued for at least 6 weeks. After the patient's condition has stabilized and the blood cultures have remained negative, therapy can be changed to oral fluconazole if the organism is susceptible to complete the course of therapy or with oral voriconazole or delayed-release posaconazole if resistant.

Arnold CJ, et al. Candida infective endocarditis: an observational cohort study with a focus on therapy. Antimicrob Agents Chemother. 2015;59(4):2365-73.

Q24. Answer c

Bacterascites happens when bacteria are present in the ascitic fluid, but the PMN count is <250 cells/mm^3. Patients with bacterascites who progress to SBP commonly have signs or symptoms of infection (usually fever) at the time of the paracentesis. Treatment should be started for patients with bacterascites who are symptomatic. For patients who are asymptomatic, a repeat paracentesis should be obtained after 48 hours (or if the patient develops symptoms) and treatment initiated if the PMN count has risen to ≥250 cells/mm^3. Culture-negative neutrocytic ascites is when the ascitic fluid PMN count ≥250 cells/mm^3 but have negative ascitic fluid cultures. Most patients actually have SBP. These patients should receive empiric broad-spectrum antibiotics. However, because the cultures are negative, the antibiotic regimen cannot subsequently be tailored based on the results of sensitivity testing.

Runyon BA. Monomicrobial non neutrocytic bacterascites: a variant of spontaneous bacterial peritonitis. Hepatology. 1990;12(4 Pt 1):710.

Asymptomatic bacterascites: is it spontaneous bacterial peritonitis? Palletier G, et al. Hepatology. 1991;14(1):112.

Q25. Answer d

Melioidosis is an infection caused by the facultative intracellular gram-negative bacterium, *Burkholderia pseudomallei*. This organism is a widely distributed environmental saprophyte in soil and fresh surface water in endemic regions. Most *B. pseudomallei* infections are subclinical. The most common clinical manifestations are pneumonia and localized skin infection. The reported latent periods between exposure in an endemic region and the development of melioidosis in a non-endemic region can be in decades. The organism can reach the lung via the hematogenous route or, rarely, via aspiration of contaminated water. Gram stain of sputum and abscess pus may reveal gram-negative bacilli with a characteristic bipolar staining with a "safety pin" appearance. Serologic testing alone is not a reliable method of diagnosis.

Cheng AC, et al. Melioidosis: epidemiology, pathophysiology, and management. Clin Microbiol Rev. 2005;18(2):383.

Q26. Answer e

This Echocardiogram is suggestive of Takotsubo (stress induced) cardiomyopathy with left ventricular outflow obstruction related to the systolic anterior motion of the mitral valve (SAM). SAM complicates as many as 20% of cases of takotsubo cardiomyopathy. Hypovolemia, inotropes, and vasodilators worsen the obstruction. Therapy consists of fluids and beta-adrenergic blockers to slow the heart rate and decrease contractility. In patients with hypotension not responding to fluids, phenylephrine is preferred because it has no beta activity and thus no inotropic or chronotropic effect. Indeed, it frequently decreases heart rate, and increases afterload, which decreases the outflow obstruction. Similar considerations apply to the management of patients with hypertrophic cardiomyopathy and hypotension. An intra-aortic balloon can be considered, but may worsen the obstruction by decreasing afterload. Dobutamine, dopamine, and norepinephrine, to a lesser extent, all have beta activity, which could exacerbate the patient's outflow obstruction related to both the increase in contractility and the increase in heart rate. Other situations where SAM may occur are in myocardial infarction and following mitral valve surgery.

Villareal RP, et al. Anteroapical stunning and left ventricular outflow tract obstruction. Mayo Clin Proc. 2001;76(1):79.

Q27. Answer b

Risk factors for the development of PICS have not been clearly defined. Commonly cited risk factors can be divided as pre-existing factors, e.g. neuromuscular disorders, dementia, psychiatric illness, comorbid conditions like alcohol abuse, smoking and ICU-specific factors, e.g. mechanical ventilation, acute delirium, sepsis, acute respiratory distress syndrome. Whether ICU-related factors unmask pre-existing illness and to what degree critical illness accelerates pre-existing neuropsychological or functional decline is unclear, although some of this morbidity is likely also entirely new. Duration of delirium seem to be more important than the sedating medications. Glucocorticoids are associated with a reduced risk for PICS. Reduced levels of cortisol are thought to play a role in the development of post-traumatic stress disorder (PTSD) and it has been hypothesized that the administration of glucocorticoids during a critical illness may replenish cortisol levels thereby reducing the risk of developing PICS as well.

Schelling G, et al. The effect of stress doses of hydrocortisone during septic shock on posttraumatic stress disorder and health-related quality of life in survivors. Crit Care Med. 1999;27(12):2678-83.

Q28. Answer d

Etomidate can cause transient acute adrenal insufficiency by inhibiting cortisol biosynthesis. Only administering multiple bolus doses or infusions seem to increase this risk. Although in patients with suspected adrenal insufficiency, such as those on chronic glucocorticoid therapy this can be more pronounced causing more hemodynamic instability. In critically ill patients undergoing emergency tracheal intubation, a 2015 systematic review of eight randomized trials concluded that etomidate was not associated with increased mortality compared with any other induction agent but use of etomidate in patients with frank septic shock is controversial and we usually select an alternative anesthetic induction agent in this circumstance. If etomidate has been used in a septic patient who subsequently develops refractory hypotension, a stress dose of a glucocorticoid should be administered.

Jackson WL. Should we use etomidate as an induction agent for endotracheal intubation in patients with septic shock?: a critical appraisal. Chest. 2005;127(3):1031.

Q29. Answer e

Assessing adrenal insufficiency or relative adrenal insufficiency in critically ill patients is challenging. In critically ill patients, loss of cortisol binding globulin (CBG) results in decreased protein-bound cortisol and increased free cortisol. Therefore, for any given amount of serum total cortisol, there is a shift from inactive protein-bound cortisol to physiologically active free cortisol. This suggests that standard assays for plasma cortisol (which measure total plasma cortisol) underestimate hypothalamic-pituitary-adrenal (HPA) axis activity. It has been proposed that free cortisol more accurately reflects HPA axis activation. In patients without shock, or patients with less severe septic shock (defined as those in whom fluid resuscitation and pressor therapy have restored hemodynamic stability), glucocorticoid therapy does not appear to be beneficial. Some studies suggest that glucocorticoid therapy is most likely to be beneficial in patients who have severe septic shock (defined as a systolic blood pressure <90 mm Hg for more than one hour despite adequate fluid resuscitation and vasopressor administration). Until data from ongoing clinical trials confirm that benefit, we typically administer hydrocortisone, pharmacologic form of cortisol for refractory septic shock. The ACTH stimulation test has failed to consistently identify patients with septic shock who benefit from glucocorticoid use. This, together with the unreliability of available plasma cortisol assays, suggests that ACTH stimulation testing is not clinically useful in distinguishing responders from not responders. An observational study of 62 patients found that the use of etomidate for intubation was associated with increased likelihood of having a poor response to ACTH stimulation 24 hours later.

Sprung CL, et al. Hydrocortisone therapy for patients with septic shock. CORTICUS Study Group. N Engl J Med. 2008;358(2):111.

Q30. Answer e

Plateau pressure (Pplat) minus PEEP pressure gradient referred to as "delta P" or driving pressure has now shown to be very important. According to this retrospective meta-analysis of more than 3500 patients who had acute respiratory distress syndrome (ARDS) enrolled in trials of low-tidal-volume ventilation indicated that improved survival is strongly correlated with a decrease in this driving pressure. This significance was similar to that of Simplified Acute Physiologic Scale (SAPS) or the Acute Physiology and Chronic Health Evaluation (APACHE) score. An important requirement for accurate assessment of driving pressure is the absence of active inspiratory efforts. Reductions in tidal volume (Vt) or inspiratory plateau pressure (Pplat) during lung-protective mechanical ventilation correlated with improved survival only if they were associated with a reduction in driving pressure. These data suggest that PEEP increments are protective when associated with an improvement in respiratory system compliance, so that the same Vt can be delivered with a lower delta P. An increase in delta P and increase in physiologic dead-space ventilation (Vd/Vt) have been associated with worse ARDS survival. If plateau pressure increases after the application of an increment of PEEP, oxygenation may improve, but ventilator-induced lung injury may occur.

Amato MB, et al. Driving pressure and survival in the acute respiratory distress syndrome. N Engl J Med. 2015;372:747-55.

Q31. Answer b

Extracorporeal membrane oxygenation (ECMO) is best applied when patients are suffering from a single organ disease, only with acute hypoxic respiratory failure from a poorly compliant lung due to an acute infection with high plateau pressures not responding to the usual modes of ventilation. ECMO should be considered if expected mortality is greater than 50% and there is a likelihood of responding to the treatment. Parameters that suggest high mortality are failure of conventional management as evidenced by severe hypoxia despite a high FIO_2 and PEEP, the development of hypercapnia, and high plateau pressures despite lung-protective strategies. Duration of ARDS greater than 7 days, associated multiple organ failure, and development of ARDS late in a patient's course are associated with increased mortality and are indicative of patients who are less likely to benefit from ECMO.

Combes A, et al. Extracorporeal membrane oxygenation for respiratory failure in adults. Curr Opin Crit Care Med. 2012;18:99-104.

Q32. Answer c

This patient had a right internal jugular catheter placed and because of her hypotension, a pneumothorax needed to be excluded. On ultrasound images, lung sliding is a very important sign. The pleura is scanned in the longitudinal axis. Two adjacent ribs are identified on ultrasound scan, and about 0.5 cm below the two ribs is the pleural line, seen as a hyperechoic shimmering horizontal line with lung movement during the respiratory cycle. The advantage of ultrasound scanning for evaluation of pneumothorax includes immediate availability of the equipment at bedside, ability to do repeated measurements, and the noninvasive radiation free test. A pleural sliding sign demonstrated on different views excludes pneumothorax in the scanned area. Since the anterior chest is nondependent in the supine position, a pneumothorax is excluded with lung sliding. Signs of pneumothorax include the barcode sign, the lung point sign, and the absence of lung sliding. The A lines present on this ultrasound scan are reverberation artifact seen as multiple horizontal lines at multiplicative distances from the skin to the pleural surface in a normal lung. B lines are usually seen in pulmonary edema; they start at the pleural surface and extend to the bottom of the screen. Pleural effusion is seen as anechoic black shadow on the ultrasound scan. Pulmonary embolism is unlikely with normal RA and RV seen in the ECHO.

Mayo PH, Doelken P. Pleural ultrasonography. Clin Chest Med. 2006;27(2):215-27.

Q33. Answer b

Hyperglycemia is associated with poor clinical outcomes in all critically ill patients. The optimal blood glucose range is a blood glucose target of 140 to 180 mg/dL. Studies recommend against using a tight intensive insulin therapy regimen to achieve a target blood glucose range of 80 to 110 mg/dL due to harmful effects of hypoglycemia which occurred often. Minimizing IVF that contain glucose and administer insulin only when necessary is widely accepted. Sliding scale with subcutaneous short acting insulin administration is preferred.

The NICE-SUGAR Study Investigators. Hypoglycemia and risk of death in critically ill patients. N Engl J Med. 2012;367:1108.

Q34. Answer b

The National Health Safety Network (NHSN) in America has utilized new definitions for tracking ventilator-associated events (VAEs) for surveillance of ventilator-associated conditions (VAC) since 2013. These definitions were updated in January 2016. Prior to this change in surveillance definitions, VAP was the only VAE tracked. These new surveillance definitions are more objective. In order to diagnose a VAE, patients must have stable oxygenation (FIO_2 and PEEP) for 2 or more calendar days followed by a persistent worsening of oxygenation for 2 or more calendar days, as marked by an increase of PEEP of 3 cm H_2O or more, or an increase of FiO_2 of 0.20 or more. If patients meet those criteria, they have a VAC. If the VAC is associated with a fever or increased leukocyte count and the start of a new antibiotic, the patient is said to have an infection-related VAC (IVAC). If patients have an IVAC and meet one of three criteria for lung infection (combination of cultures, secretions, tissue or pleural fluid culture), they are diagnosed with possible ventilator-associated pneumonia (VAP). This is how the patient in this scenario has VAP.

CDC Device-associated module. Ventilator-Associated Event (VAE). (For use in adult locations only) January 2016. http://www.cdc.gov/nhsn/PDFs/pscManual/10- AE_FINAL.pdf (11 February 2018).

Q35. Answer c

Viral pneumonias are increasingly being diagnosed with the utilization of PCR assay for viral agents performed on sputum samples. In a majority of patients with viral pneumonias, there is no associated bacterial infection. In a recent study, patients who had pure viral pneumonia by culture did not appear to benefit from prolonged antibacterial therapy. Other than medications for pneumonias caused by influenza virus or respiratory syncytial virus, there are no proven effective drug therapies, although ribavirin has been used in some cases of pneumonia caused by parainfluenza virus or metapneumovirus.

Rhinovirus has been associated with pneumonia, particularly in immunocompromised hosts, and may play an important role in exacerbations of chronic obstructive pulmonary disease. In the case presented in this question, it is difficult to determine the role of the rhinovirus in the respiratory failure without additional culture information. Regardless, in the case of pneumonia caused by rhinovirus, only supportive care is recommended. Although viral pneumonias can be complicated by *Staphylococcus* superinfections, such infections occur in the minority of cases and do not require an immediate antibiotic change.

Crotty MP, et al. Impact of antibacterials on subsequent resistance and clinical outcomes in adult patients with viral pneumonia: an opportunity for stewardship. Crit Care. 2015;19:404.

K Type Answers

Q1. Answer FTTFF

The diagnosis of healthcare related infectious meningitis/ventriculitis in patients who have had neurosurgery or head trauma is difficult. Elicitation of the usual symptoms and signs of meningitis can be difficult. In the ICU many noninfectious causes can mimic many of these signs and symptoms. Most of the patients have multiple risk factors like subarachnoid bleed, cranial fracture with CSF leak, craniotomy and external ventricular drain for extended durations, all of which predispose them to infection. Under these circumstances diagnosis of a new healthcare related infection becomes difficult. Although high CSF white blood cell counts correlate with the presence of infection, in this situation a normal CSF white blood cell count cannot reliably rule out an infection. Standard laboratory parameters, like CSF glucose and CSF protein too are not reliable predictors. An elevated CSF lactate concentration of more than 3.5 to 4.2 mmol/L occurs more frequently in bacterial than in aseptic meningitis and an elevated CSF lactate in this situation may be useful in the diagnosis. CSF cultures are the most important tests for establishing the diagnosis of infection in this situation. In patients with infected devices, the culture can be positive even when there is no pleocytosis or alterations in CSF chemistries. A negative CSF culture does not exclude the possibility of infection completely especially if they have had antibiotic therapy previously. Cultures should then be repeated especially if infection is considered likely. Neuroimaging is useful in determining the source of infection (e.g. local extension from an adjacent infection) and in identifying complications from the infection (e.g. hydrocephalus, vasculitis, or thrombosis of vessels). Magnetic resonance imaging is more sensitive than CT for detecting ventriculitis. Fluid attenuation inversion recovery and post-contrast T1 weighted images may be most useful. Diffusion weighted imaging may be used to detect pus in the ventricular system and to differentiate a brain abscess from malignancy. The general principles of antimicrobial therapy are the same as those for acute bacterial meningitis. If there is a suspicion of infection and there is CSF pleocytosis, antimicrobial therapy should be initiated after appropriate cultures are obtained without waiting for the culture results.

Tunkel AR, Hasbun R, Bhimraj R, et al. 2017 Infectious Diseases Society of America's Clinical Practice Guidelines for Healthcare-Associated Ventriculitis and Meningitis. Clinical Infectious Diseases. Clinical Infectious Diseases. 2017;1-32.

Q2. Answer FTFF

A large retrospective analysis published in 2016 validated qSOFA, initially, as a useful tool for the diagnosis of sepsis in patients who were suspected to have infection and were admitted outside the ICU. Subsequently prospective a study has validated this in patients in the emergency room (ER). However, this study clearly showed that qSOFA was less valuable in the ICU setting and that it had better diagnostic accuracy than systemic inflammatory response syndrome (SIRS) area under receiver operative curve (AUROC) [0.80 vs 0.65]. Another retrospective study showed qSOFA to be inferior to SOFA when it comes to predicting in hospital mortality (AUROC 0.75 vs 0.60). These studies have their limitations and cannot be generalized to all EDs and ICUs. Early identification scores like modified early warning scores (MEWS) and the national early warning scores (NEWS) have been shown to be superior to qSOFA for predicting ICU mortality.

    JAMA 2016;315:762.
    JAMA 2017;317:310.
    JAMA 2017;317:290.
    AJRCCM 2017;195:906.

Q3. Answer TTFTT

Maintaining the initial MAP at 65 mm Hg in patients with sepsis and septic shock is a strong recommendation with moderate quality of evidence. Targeting an MAP of 65 mm Hg initially, before a better understanding of patient's condition is obtained reduced risk of atrial fibrillation and lowered the doses of vasopressors with no difference in mortality. Once a better handle of patient's condition is obtained then the target need to be individualized. The initial resuscitation fluid and volume is a strong recommendation with low quality of evidence. There is little data in literature to support this volume of fluid. The aim of giving this fixed volume of fluid initially is to enable clinicians to initiate resuscitation while obtaining more specific information. Many patients will require more fluid than this initial bolus and this is titrated with functional/ dynamic hemodynamic measurements. After the initial resuscitation fluid challenge technique and not a continuous infusion of fluid is to be applied where fluid administration is required as long as hemodynamic factors continue to improve. Obtaining cultures before administration of antibiotics enhances the yield of cultures and this helps with tailoring of antibiotic therapy. It has been seen that cultures can become sterile within minutes to hours of appropriate antibiotic administration. However, in the process of aiming to obtain cultures prior to initiating antimicrobial therapy other key therapies like initiation of antimicrobials should not be delayed. If it is not possible to obtain cultures promptly the risk/benefit ratio favors rapid administration of antimicrobials. The timing of intravenous antimicrobial administration is a strong recommendation with moderate quality of evidence. In sepsis and septic shock every hour of delay in administration of appropriate antimicrobial is associated with increasing mortality and worsening organ dysfunction. Available data in literature shows that appropriate antimicrobial should be administered the earliest and 1 hour is being recommended as a minimal target.

    Rhodes A, Evans LE, Alhazzani W, et al. Surviving Sepsis Campaign: International Guidelines for Management of Sepsis and Septic Shock: 2016. Intensive Care Med. 2017;43(3):304-77.

Q4. Answer FFFTT

Exposure to *Cryptococcus neoformans* is not uncommon. In the immunocompetent patient most infections are subclinical and asymptomatic. However, seldom symptomatic pulmonary cryptococcosis can present as a pneumonia. The diagnosis of the disease is established by culturing the organism in the sputum, bronchioalveolar lavage or tissue. Serum cryptococcal antigen assay should be performed, but has a very low sensitivity to confirm the diagnosis. It is seldom positive in the immunocompetent host and there is no role for monitoring the assay titers to decide on the duration of antimicrobial therapy. The optimal treatment for pulmonary cryptococcosis is uncertain, but in mild to moderate disease the treatment recommended is fluconazole 400 mg daily (6 mg/kg) for 6 to 12 months. (Grade 2B recommendation).

    Clin Infect Dis. 2010;50(3):291.

Q5. Answer TTFFT

As per the Surviving Sepsis Campaign 2016 the initial resuscitation fluid and volume is a strong recommendation with low quality of evidence. There is little data in literature to support this volume of fluid. The aim of giving this fixed volume of fluid initially is to enable clinicians to initiate resuscitation while obtaining more specific information. Many patients will require more fluid than this initial bolus and this is titrated with functional hemodynamic measurements. The recommendation on empiric antibiotic is a weak recommendation with low quality evidence. In the initial management of septic shock, the recommendation is to use at least two antibiotics of different classes ("combination therapy") empirically. "Combination therapy" in this situation means use of two different classes of antibiotics which are sensitive against a particular pathogen (e.g. β lactam and aminoglycoside) and do not mean the use of multidrug therapy to cover multiple organisms. The recommendation also suggests against use of combination therapy if there is no shock. The evidence for combination therapy providing a higher survival benefit is only in severely ill patients with septic shock. If the foci of infection are amenable to source control then it should be done as soon as possible following initial resuscitation. Prolonged efforts at stabilization prior to source control are not warranted. Nor adrenaline is the vasopressor of choice to be used if hypotension persists despite adequate fluid resuscitation. (Strong recommendation with a moderate quality of evidence). Vasopressin is to be added to noradrenaline if the target MAP is not achieved or to help with decreasing the dose of noradrenaline. (Weak recommendation with moderate quality of evidence). Vasopressin in low doses has been shown to be effective in raising the blood pressure in conditions refractory to other vasopressors. It may also have other physiological benefits. Hydrocortisone at a dose of 200 mg/day is indicated only in patients with septic shock who's hemodynamic stability cannot be achieved with adequate fluid resuscitation and vasopressor therapy.

    Rhodes A, Evans LE, Alhazzani W, et al. Surviving Sepsis Campaign: International Guidelines for Management of Sepsis and Septic Shock: 2016. Intensive Care Med. 2017;43(3):304-77.

Q6. Answer TFTT

The elderly lack the ability to mount the classical signs and symptoms with sepsis – fever, leukocytosis, tachycardia, and hypothermia. Sepsis should be considered when they present with mental confusion, respiratory distress, multiorgan failure and shock. Immune senescence that sets in with aging, affects the adaptive immune system causing defects in both cellular and humoral immune response. This leads to an impaired ability to rapidly and effectively respond to a pathogen which increases susceptibility to systemic infection. Recognizing sepsis and initiating early appropriate antibiotics have been shown to reduce mortality. However, inappropriate initial therapy has been shown to increase mortality by up to four folds in the elderly when compared to the young. Repeated visits to hospital for procedures like dialysis and being in a nursing home have been shown to predispose the patients to infection with pathogens resistant to common antibiotics.

    Ther Adv Infectious Dis. 2017;4(6):171-91.
    Clin Infect Dis. 2005;41(Suppl. 7):S504-S12.
    J Hepatol. 2014;60(6):1310-24.

Q7. Answer TFFTF

WHO's classification (1997) of Dengue hemorrhagic fever diagnostic criteria consists of fever or history of acute fever lasting for 2 to 7 days that can occasionally be biphasic; hemorrhagic tendencies, as evidenced by at least one of the following – a positive tourniquet test, petechiae/ecchymosis/purpura, bleeding from mucosa or melena/ hematemesis; thrombocytopenia (counts less than 100,00 cell/mm^3) and evidence of plasma leakage, as evidenced by any one of the following – a raise in hematocrit by equal or greater than 20%, a fall in hematocrit following fluid resuscitation by equal to or greater than 20%, hypoproteinemia or development of ascites/pleural effusion.

    The NS1 antigen test is one that directly detects viral components in the serum. This is highly specific and has about 90% sensitivity in primary dengue viral infections. It can remain positive for up to 7 days since onset of infection.

    The dengue serological test for IgM antibodies can become positive as early as 4 days after onset of the infection. Single specimen IgM positivity establishes only a presumptive diagnosis of the viral infection. To confirm the diagnosis demonstration of a fourfold or greater rise in antibody titer between a paired acute and convalescent phase serum specimen is necessary.

The IgG antibodies start to rise by seven days after the onset of the illness. However, initially it is detected in low titers and rises very slowly. If high titers are seen by day four to seven it indicates a secondary dengue infection.

Dengue viral infection has been reported to cause neurological symptoms in about 1% of the infections and of this encephalitis is one of the presentations.

> Dengue haemorrhagic fever Diagnosis, treatment, prevention and control. Available from: http://apps.who.int/iris/bitstream/10665/41988/1/9241545003_eng.pdf (Accessed 11 February 2018).

Q8. Answer TTTTF

Dengue shock syndrome (DSS) is a severe form of dengue viral infection and follows the initial febrile phase. It usually occurs about 3 to 7 days after the onset of the infection. Thrombocytopenia can occur even in the febrile phase and is not a hallmark of DSS, even though it could get worse during the critical phase. During this phase, there is defervescence and signs of severe systemic vascular leak set in (increase in the hematocrit by 20%, hypoproteinemia, pleural effusion/ ascites). The severe systemic vascular leak along with thrombocytopenia induced bleed leads to a hypovolemic shock, which in its early phase presents with tachycardia, low volume pulse and narrow pulse pressure, even before hypotension sets in. Tissue hypoperfusion results in lethargy, restlessness, cool peripheries and intense abdominal pain. These signs and symptoms should be recognized as early features of impending shock and appropriate resuscitation initiated.

> Dengue haemorrhagic fever Diagnosis, treatment, prevention and control, SECOND EDITION Available from: http://apps.who.int/iris/bitstream/10665/41988/1/9241545003_eng.pdf (Accessed 15 February 2018).

Q9. Answer TTTFF

Predictors of mortality in the ICU for patients with severe dengue are not well studied. Age greater than 50 years was seen to be associated with higher incidence of admission to the ICU and also higher mortality in the ICU. Higher SOFA score, higher APACHE II score and higher arterial lactate level were all independent predictors of mortality in adult patients admitted to ICU with severe dengue infection. Three or more organ failure on ICU admission was associated with 67% mortality. It was non-hematological organ failure that significantly predicted mortality and presence of respiratory failure was the best in discriminating survivors from non-survivors and hematological complications the weakest. It was seen that SOFA score at ICU discharge predicted both mortality and survival after ICU discharge.

> Perkins ZB, Lendrum RA, Brohi K. Resuscitative endovascular balloon occlusion of the aorta: promise, practice, and progress? Curr Opin Crit Care. 2016;22(6):563-71.

Q10. Answer TFFFF

The bacteremia sepsis induced mortality (both 28 and 90 days) have been seen to be lower in all solid organ transplant recipients, other than in lung and heart transplant recipients, than in non transplant patients. This is postulated to be due to the blunted inflammatory response to infection from the immunosuppressive therapy. The first month after transplantation surgery, called the early post transplant period is one during which the effects of immunosuppression is not fully evident. Infections happening during this period are usually from microorganisms harbored in the donor/recipient and from the complications of surgery or prolonged hospitalization. 1 to 6 months period after the transplantation surgery is when the immunosuppressive effects are at the peak. During this period infections that happen are mostly due to opportunistic organisms. Prevention of these infections is by appropriate prophylactic antibiotic therapy. Prophylactic antibiotics have been successful in delaying these infections. The most common presentation of CMV infection in a transplant recipient is a viral syndrome, characterized by fever and malaise as well as leukopenia, thrombocytopenia and elevated liver enzymes. These signs can appear from the 3rd to 4th week, but generally peaks in the 6th to 16th week to become rare after the 6th month.

> Clin Infect Dis. 2016;63:186.
> Am J Transplant. 2013;13 Suppl 4:3-8.
> Clinics. 2015;70:515-23.

Q11. Answer TFFFT

PCP is the most common opportunistic infection in post renal transplant recipients that are admitted to the ICU with acute respiratory failure.

The highest risk for opportunistic infection following solid organ transplantation is around 6 months after the surgery when the immunosuppressive therapy is most intense and the risk is higher if the patient is not on any antimicrobial prophylaxis. Elevated serum LDH does not confirm the diagnosis of PCP. It is an indicator of possible PCP infection in HIV patients, but its utility in non-HIV patients with suspected PCP is not clear. It is seen to be elevated in all causes of acute lung injury. Even in non HIV patients elevated LDH in the presence of pulmonary infiltrates without any apparent cause should raise the suspicion of PCP. Beta – D glucan is a cell wall component of most fungi. It can be used as a screening test for a variety of invasive fungal infections. It has been best studied for Candida and Aspergillus specie. An increase in serum beta – D – glucan in a patient with the risk factors and clinical features suggestive of PCP heightens the clinical suspicion for the disease and can be used as an adjunct to the diagnosis of PCP.

TMP – SMX is the most effective regimen for the treatment of PCP and is the treatment of choice for any severity of the disease. Due to its excellent bioavailability oral preparation of the drug is appropriate for all patients. It is given at a dose of 15 to 20 mg/kg/day of TMP component in three to four divided doses for patients with normal renal function for duration of 21 days.

Chest. 2016;149:1546-55.

Transpl Infect Dis. 2003;5(2):84.

Clin Microbiol Infect. 2013;19(1):39.

Q12. Answer TFTTT

TMP – SMX is the most effective regimen for the treatment of PCP and is the treatment of choice for any severity of the disease. Due to its excellent bioavailability oral preparation of the drug is appropriate for all patients. It is given at a dose of 15 to 20 mg/kg/day of TMP component in three to four divided doses for patients with normal renal function for duration of 21 days.

Alternative regimens are only considered if TMP – SMX cannot be given for any reason. These regimens are usually based on the severity of PCP. Atovaquone is the drug recommended in mild form of PCP and not the severe form. The duration of antimicrobial therapy in non HIV patients with PCP has not been studied separately. The recommendation for 21 days therapy is an extrapolation from HIV patients with PCP, who have a greater organism burden, slower clinical response and show greater risk for relapse if duration of therapy is less than 21 days. Similarly non-HIV patients with PCP start showing clinical improvement with seven days of therapy. Not achieving clinical improvement even after 7 days of therapy should be considered as failure of therapy. The outcomes of non-HIV patients with PCP, despite adequate therapy are around 35–50%, compared to that of HIV patients with PCP, which is 10–20%.

AJRCCM. 2011;183(1):96.

Am Rev Respir Dis. 1989;140(5):1204.

Clin Infect Dis. 2002;34(8):1098.

Q13. Answer TFFTT

During the early phase of the infection no laboratory tests are diagnostic of scrub typhus as many of the tests are nonspecific and share results that are common to many tropical infective illnesses. During this phase the diagnosis is arrived at mainly from a combination of epidemiological clues, clinical features and laboratory findings. The illness can be insidious with headache, anorexia, malaise and myalgia or acute with fever and chills. The fever can be prolonged (9–19 days), especially if not treated. About 50% of patients develop a non-pruritic macular- maculopapular rash that begins on the abdomen and then spreads to the limbs. Relative bradycardia is quite common in scrub typhus. The eschar that forms at the site of the chigger bite has been shown in studies to be seen in up to 80% of patients. So the absence of an eschar does not rule out scrub typhus. Weil Felix test is not sensitive or specific for scrub typhus and recommendations are to not use it as a diagnostic tool. The IFA test, even though fraught with lack of clarity, is the gold standard serological test available at the moment for diagnosis of scrub typhus.

Koh GCKW, Maude RJ, Paris DJ, et al. Diagnosis of Scrub Typhus. Source: The American Journal of Tropical Medicine and Hygiene. 2010;82(3):368-70.

PLoS Negl Trop Dis. 2015;9(8):e0003971.

Clin Infect Dis. 2007;44(3):391.

Q14. Answer TTFTT

Scrub typhus is a mite-borne infectious disease caused by *Orientia tsutsugamushi,* a gram-negative coccobacillus which has features that are common to and distinct from other rickettsiae. The infection generally occurs 7-10 days (can range from 6 to 19 days) after a bite of an infected mite. The eschar that forms at the site of the chigger bite has been shown in studies to be seen in up to 80% of patients. So the absence of an eschar does not rule out scrub typhus. Serological diagnosis of acute scrub typhus infection can be made only if a fourfold increase in the antibody titer in paired samples of blood drawn at least 14 days apart is demonstrated. A single blood sample antibody titer may be suggestive of an acute infection when there are locally validated criteria for positive test. The antibiotic of choice for treatment is Doxycycline given orally or intravenous at a dose of 100 mg twice a day.

Am J Trop Med Hyg. 2001;65(6):899.

Cochrane Database Syst Rev. 2000.

Am J Trop Med Hyg 2010;82(3):368-70.

PLoS Negl Trop Dis. 2015;9(8):e0003971.

Clin Infect Dis. 2007;44(3):391.

Q15. Answer TFFTF

Acute retroviral infection presents with a constellation of nonspecific symptoms. A good history with high degree of suspicion is required for making the diagnosis. The severity and duration of symptoms vary from patients to patients and up to 60% of early HIV infection can be asymptomatic. The common symptoms and signs of acute retroviral syndrome are fever, lymphadenopathy, sore throat with odynophagia, generalized rash, painful mucocutaneous ulcers, myalgia/arthralgia, diarrhea and weight loss. The usual time from HIV exposure to development of these symptoms is 2 to 4 weeks. The sensitivity of retroviral serological tests to detect HIV antigens/antibodies have improved over the years. The 4th generation serological assays have the shortest window period and can become positive within 14 days of exposure. So there is an initial period during which time serological tests can be negative. CD4 counts are unpredictable during the acute retroviral infection phase. It can drop transiently to pick up again. Clinical symptoms happen at the peak of viremia and RNA RT – PCR viral load testing will confirm the diagnosis when symptoms are present. HIV RNA or DNA becomes detectable by nucleic acid tests around 12-14 days postexposure. Early and prompt ART is recommended during this phase and this has been shown to reduce likelihood of viral transmission, reduce the size of latent HIV reservoir and improve symptoms related to acute retroviral syndrome.

WHO - Consolidated guidelines on HIV testing services, 2015.

Clin Infect Dis. 2015;61(6):1013-21.

N Engl J Med. 2016;374(22):2120.

Q16. Answer TFTFF

The acute HIV infection can be mistaken for infectious mononucleosis. In fact one of the first descriptions in literature of acute HIV infection termed it as "mononucleosis like illness". The initial presentation of acute retroviral syndrome is very nonspecific and high degree of suspicion is needed for its diagnosis. A positive heterophile antibody test is not uncommon during this phase of illness and a heterophile positive mononucleosis in an unusual host should raise suspicion of this condition. From the time of exposure it generally takes 2-4 weeks for the development of acute HIV infection symptoms and this happens at the peak of viremia. There have been reports of incubation periods of as long as 10 months and as high as 10-60% of the early infection can be asymptomatic. Even though not common, opportunistic infections can rarely occur during this phase of illness too, when there is a transient drop in CD4 lymphocytes. Early and prompt ART is recommended during this phase and this has been shown to reduce likelihood of viral transmission, reduce the size of latent HIV reservoir and improve symptoms related to acute retroviral syndrome.

Lancet. 1985;1(8428):537.
J Infect Dis. 2013;208(8):1202.
Clin Infect Dis. 2015;61(6):1013-21.
N Engl J Med. 2016;374(22):2120.

Q17. Answer TTTTT

A large retrospective study looking at the mortality in patients greater than 65 years of age admitted to hospital with CAP found the overall mortality to be 12.1%, within 30 days of admission. Of this 52.4% died during the hospital stay and the remaining 47.6% died after discharge. On multivariate analysis, this study found seven factors to be associated with death prior to discharge - a systolic blood pressure < 90 mm Hg, a respiratory rate > 30 breaths/min, an arterial blood gas pH < 7.35, a partial pressure of oxygen < 60 mm Hg or an arterial oxygen saturation < 90%, blood urea nitrogen (BUN) level > 11 mmol/L, presence of bacteremia and a need for mechanical ventilation. A 21 fold increase in mortality was reported by the British Thoracic Society in any patient with CAP who had two or more of the following findings – a diastolic pressure < 60 mm Hg, a respiratory rate > 30 breaths/min and a BUN level > 7 mmol/L.

Chest. 2012;142:476.
Br J Hospital Med. 1993;49:346.

Q18. Answer FTFTF

Even though the clinical approach to the diagnosis of CAP involving clinical evaluation, chest radiography with or without microbiological testing is considered the gold standard for the diagnosis, it carries a sensitivity of less than 50%. The decision about the site of care for patients with CAP entirely rests on the physician's judgment and is supplemented by certain validated clinical prediction rule for prognosis like the CRUB-65/CRB-65, Pneumonia severity Index (PSI) and the IDSA/ATS major/minor criteria. This lady qualifies for ICU admission as she already has one major criterion of the IDSA/ATS severe CAP criteria. IDSA/ATS Guidelines on management of CAP recommends that patients who are hospitalized with CAP and especially those who are admitted to the ICU would benefit from pathogen directed antimicrobial therapy. This is facilitated by sending microbial cultures of respiratory secretions and blood, prior to initiation of antibiotics. The etiology of CAP varies by geographical region. However, *Strep. pneumoniae* is the most commonly identified bacterial cause of CAP worldwide. It accounts for about 65% of bacterial CAP. Urinary pneumococcal antigen assay has been recommended by the IDSA/ATS guidelines as a means to augment standard diagnostic methods. The advantages of this test are it is quite sensitive and specific, results are quick, retain validity when done even after starting antibiotics and can be done even when it is difficult to get respiratory secretions for microbiological analysis.

Clin Infect Dis. 2007;44 Suppl2:S27.
Ann Intern Med. 2001;138:109.
Int J Antimicrob Agents. 2008;31:107.

CHAPTER 12

Surgery and Trauma

BK Rao, Saurabh Taneja

A Type Questions
(One best answer)

1. Which of the following can be a criterion for rejecting a diagnosis of infective endocarditis (IE)?
   a. Three sets of negative blood cultures after five days of incubation and subculturing
   b. Fever – Temperature ≥38.0°C
   c. Echocardiography showing vegetation or abscess
   d. New valvular regurgitation
   e. Resolution of fever and other clinical manifestations occurs in ≤4 days of antibiotic therapy

2. The sign least likely to be present in tension pneumothorax with massive blood loss:
   a. Tachycardia
   b. Hypotension
   c. Hemoglobin desaturation
   d. Jugular venous distention (JVD)
   e. Absent breath sounds on the ipsilateral side

3. As per 'American Society of Anesthesiologists (ASA) physical status classification system' which of the following is wrong?
   a. ASA I: a normal healthy patient
   b. ASA II: a patient with mild systemic disease
   c. ASA III: a patient with severe systemic disease
   d. ASA IV: a patient with controlled severe systemic disease
   e. ASA V: a moribund patient not expected to survive without operation

4. A 72-year-old female presented with dyspnea, hypoxia and altered mental status within 24 hours of admission for femur fracture. Invasive mechanical ventilation was initiated for severe hypoxia. Chest X-ray was relatively clear. An Echocardiogram revealed right ventricular strain and MRI of the brain showed multiple acute/subacute infarcts. Pulmonary thromboembolism was deemed less likely with a negative CT Chest Angiogram and US Doppler of Legs. A diagnosis of fat embolism syndrome (FES) can be confirmed by one of the following:
   a. Getsalt fat embolism score combining thrombocytopenia, anemia, and hypofibrinogenemia
   b. Urinary fat stain
   c. Fat globules on cytology of pulmonary capillary blood obtained from a wedged pulmonary artery catheter
   d. Genotyping for polymorphisms associated with increased susceptibility to inflammatory stimuli
   e. None of the above

5. Which of the following is not true for rhabdomyolysis?
   a. Rhabdomyolysis and myoglobinuria can develop in patients with significant muscle injury including crush injuries
   b. Rhabdomyolysis presents with elevated serum muscle enzymes and red to brown urine and electrolyte abnormalities
   c. Peak serum creatine kinase levels does not depend upon the volume of muscle breakdown and the muscle mass of the patient

d. A brisk urine output should be maintained with intravenous fluid therapy until the creatine kinase value starts to decrease
e. The urine dipstick can be used as a screening test for rhabdomyolysis

6. **The best sign on chest ultrasonography to negate the diagnosis of pneumothorax:**
   a. Stratosphere or barcode sign
   b. Lung point sign
   c. Absence of lung sliding
   d. Seashore sign
   e. Presence of 'A-lines'

7. **In acute cholangitis (also called ascending cholangitis); one of the following is not TRUE:**
   a. Acute cholangitis is caused primarily by bacterial infection in a patient with biliary obstruction
   b. The most common symptoms are fever, abdominal pain and jaundice (Charcot's triad)
   c. Empiric broad-spectrum parenteral antibiotics should aim to cover colonic bacteria
   d. Over 50% patients respond to conservative management with antibiotic therapy
   e. In patients who respond well to antibiotics, the biliary drainage procedures should be delayed by at least 3 weeks

8. **As per 2012 Infectious Diseases Society of America clinical practice guideline for the diagnosis and treatment of diabetic foot infections, which of the following is not TRUE for empiric therapy?**
   a. A wound swab before the wound has been cleansed and debrided makes a good specimen for culture
   b. Empiric antibiotic coverage for aerobic gram-positive cocci (GPC) including methicillin-resistant *Staphylococcus aureus* (MRSA) is enough in mild infections in patients with no recent previous antibiotic intake
   c. Empiric antibiotic coverage for aerobic gram-negative pathogens is required for severe infection, chronic infection, or infection that fails to respond to recent antibiotic therapy
   d. Empiric antianaerobic therapy is usually required for necrotic, gangrenous, or foul-smelling wounds
   e. Empiric antipseudomonal antibiotic is usually required for patients with risk factors for true infection with this organism

9. **Which of the following is not a cause of nonocclusive mesenteric ischemia (NOMI)?**
   a. Sepsis
   b. Congestive heart failure
   c. Vasopressors
   d. Cocaine
   e. Factor V Leiden mutation

10. **In the immediate postoperative period following thyroidectomy, which of the following conditions is least likely to cause respiratory distress?**
    a. Injury to recurrent laryngeal nerve
    b. Injury to external branch of superior laryngeal nerve
    c. Injury to the vocal folds from intubation
    d. Large hematoma
    e. Tracheomalacia

11. **A 75-year-old man, known case of coronary artery disease and congestive heart failure, is operated for a fracture neck femur. On 3rd postoperative day he started developing abdominal distension which was increasing every day. He stopped passing stool or gas. Stopping oral feed, starting nasogastric suctioning, rectal tube decompression and correction of serum potassium did not help over the next 48 hours. A plain semi-reclining abdomen X-ray showed marked dilation of the right hemicolon. A CT abdomen confirmed the diagnosis of acute colonic pseudo-obstruction. Cecum was 12 cm in diameter.**
    Now the best course of treatment is:
    a. Continue nasogastric suction and intravenous fluid; review every 24 hours
    b. Intravenous neostigmine
    c. Intravenous erythromycin
    d. Colonoscopy decompression
    e. Exploratory laparotomy

12. **In a frontal chest X-ray the least likely causes of opacification of all or most of unilateral hemithorax is:**
    a. Collapse of the entire lung with pleural effusion
    b. Large pleural effusion with lung collapse
    c. Large pneumothorax with hemothorax
    d. Large pneumonia involving entire lung
    e. Previous pneumonectomy

13. The most common cause of ureteral injury in gynecologic, urologic procedures is:
    a. Cauterisation
    b. Transection/avulsion
    c. Ligation/ kinking by suture
    d. Crush
    e. Devascularization with delayed necrosis/stricture

14. In patients with urinary tract infection (UTI) and neurogenic bladder (NGB), which of the following is least possible?
    a. NGB is seen in spina bifida (SB), spinal cord injury (SCI)
    b. UTIs are the most common infection in this population
    c. UTI in NGB typically presents with symptoms of dysuria, urgency, and frequency
    d. Urinary catheters are a mainstay management strategy
    e. Clean intermittent catheterization (CIC) is the preferred method of bladder drainage

15. World Society of the Abdominal Compartment Syndrome (WSACS) grades of intra-abdominal hypertension (IAH) in adults include all but one:
    a. Grade 0: IAP 0-11 mm Hg
    b. Grade I: IAP 12 to 15 mm Hg
    c. Grade II: IAP 16 to 20 mm Hg
    d. Grade III: IAP 21 to 25 mm Hg
    e. Grade IV: IAP greater than 25 mm Hg

16. In imaging assessment of GI tract perforations which one of the following is FALSE?
    a. Rupture of hollow abdominal organs can cause pneumoperitoneum
    b. On a plain X-ray films direct finding of perforation is free intraperitoneal gas
    c. Ultrasonography is not sensitive in identifying free gas in the peritoneal cavity
    d. Computed tomography (CT) is most sensitive modality for detecting pneumoperitoneum
    e. Free air above the diaphragm can be used for quick diagnosis in upright chest X-ray

17. Which procedure should be avoided in patients with fracture base of skull with CSF leak?
    a. Nasogastric tube placement
    b. Oral intubation
    c. Laryngeal mask airway
    d. Cricothyroidotomy
    e. Tracheostomy

18. Which of the following is against the class 1 recommendation of the American Heart Association/American Stroke Association "Guidelines for the Management of Spontaneous Intracerebral Hemorrhage (ICH)"?
    a. Rapid neuroimaging with CT or MRI is recommended to distinguish ischemic stroke from ICH
    b. For ICH patients presenting with systolic blood pressure (SBP) between 150 and 220 mm Hg and without contraindication to acute BP treatment, acute lowering of SBP to 140 mm Hg is safe
    c. Coagulation factor deficiency or severe thrombocytopenia, raised INR should be treated with appropriate measures
    d. Blood sugar must be targeted below 220 mg/dL by plain insulin
    e. Clinical seizures should be treated with antiseizure drugs

19. Which adult patient is most suitable for non-operative management of traumatic acute subdural hematoma (SDH)?
    a. SDH thickness >10 mm irrespective of patient's GCS score
    b. Midline shift >5 mm irrespective of patient's GCS score
    c. A comatose patient with a SDH thickness <10 mm and a midline shift < 5 mm and the GCS score has not deteriorated between the time of injury and hospital admission
    d. A comatose patient with a SDH thickness <10 mm and a midline shift < 5 mm who develops asymmetric or fixed and dilated pupils
    e. A comatose patient with a SDH thickness <10 mm and a midline shift < 5 mm whose ICP is consistently above 20 mm Hg

20. A 50-year-old man will be considered to have a low risk for cervical spine injury if any one of the following is present except:
    a. Involved in a minor rear-end motor vehicle collision
    b. Comfortable in a sitting position
    c. Ambulatory at any time since the injury
    d. No midline cervical spine tenderness
    e. Paresthesia in the upper or lower limbs

21. Which of the following patients with trauma will most likely not require an urgent definite secured airway?

a. GCS ≥13
b. Unstable facial trauma
c. High aspiration risk
d. Airway injuries
e. Upper cervical spinal cord trauma

22. **In blunt thoracic trauma causing aortic injury, which of the following statement is not true?**
    a. Classic radiological finding in aortic injury is a widened mediastinum
    b. A normal aorta morphology with no mediastinal hematoma on contrast CT has a 100% negative predictive value
    c. Aortic injury can occur with no overt clinical sign of thoracic trauma
    d. Most blunt aortic injuries occur in the ascending aorta
    e. Ascending aorta injuries are frequently associated with significant cardiac damage

23. **Which of the following is not correct in acute phase of burn?**
    a. The primary focus of early burn treatment is fluid resuscitation
    b. Burn patients can develop abdominal compartment syndrome with excessive crystalloid administration during resuscitation
    c. During the first 8 to 12 hours after burn, crystalloid solutions should be the sole fluids used for burn resuscitation
    d. Acute airway obstruction can occur during the first 24 hours of injury, even in the absence of smoke inhalation
    e. Hallmark hypermetabolic response seen in severe burns causes repeated episodes of hypoglycemia

24. **Regarding acute spinal cord injury (ASCI), what is not TRUE?**
    a. The majority of traumatic ASCI involve the lumbosacral spine
    b. Delayed neurologic deterioration may be seen from hours to days following the onset of injury
    c. The use of methylprednisolone is controversial
    d. The neurogenic shock following cervical results from loss of vasoconstrictor tone in peripheral arterioles and pooling of blood within the peripheral vasculature.
    e. Pharmacologic thromboprophylaxis should be started as soon as possible

25. **One of the following is FALSE in cases of suspected renal injury in blunt abdominal trauma:**
    a. The kidneys are the most commonly injured genitourinary organs
    b. The majority of blunt renal injuries are low-grade injuries, not requiring any intervention
    c. Ipsilateral lower rib fracture can increase the incidence of significant renal trauma
    d. Radiological evaluation of kidney is indicated for patients with hypotension < 90 mm Hg and hematuria
    e. There is a strong relationship between the presence, absence or degree of hematuria and the severity of renal injury

26. **Which of the following is FALSE concerning pulmonary contusion?**
    a. Classically pulmonary contusion opacities and consolidations do not cross segmental and fissure boundaries
    b. Pulmonary parenchymal contusion can usually be seen in X-ray chest within 24 hours of the injury
    c. The pulmonary parenchymal contusion usually disappears within 14 days of injury
    d. Thoracic ultrasound will show a sub-pleural hypo-echoic blurred lesion and multiple B-lines
    e. Clinical manifestations include hypoxemia and dyspnea

27. **In an adult male who has sustained abdominal and pelvic trauma in a high-velocity motor vehicle accident, the following findings usually suggest urethral injury except:**
    a. Blood at the urethral meatus
    b. Inability to void
    c. High-riding prostate on rectal examination
    d. Perineal swelling or hematoma
    e. Intraperitoneal free fluid on FAST

28. **Which of the following findings is confirmatory for traumatic cardiac tamponade?**
    a. Large cardiac silhouette on chest X-ray
    b. Low-voltage QRS complexes in the ECG
    c. Electrical alternans in the ECG
    d. Presence of increased pericardial fluid on CT
    e. Increased pericardial fluid with diastolic collapse of right atrium and right ventricle on echocardiography

29. **In an adult head injury patient in emergency unit, which of these conditions may not require a CT head within 1 hour?**
    a. GCS score less than 11 on initial assessment
    b. Suspected open or depressed skull fracture
    c. Focal neurological deficit
    d. Patient taking anticoagulant medication but with no signs or risk factors for brain injury
    e. More than three episodes of vomiting

30. **Fixed and dilated pupils may be a reliable indicator of brain death in one of the following conditions:**
    a. Lightning strike victim
    b. Muscle relaxant administration
    c. Ocular trauma
    d. Cerebellar tonsillar herniation
    e. Barbiturate poisoning

K Type Questions
[Marked True (T)/False (F)]

1. **Regarding acute mediastinitis:**
   a. Most cases are due to the spread of infection from other sites or direct inoculation resulting from trauma or surgery
   b. Esophageal perforation is the most common cause of mediastinitis
   c. Computed tomography is the preferred diagnostic imaging for all forms of mediastinitis
   d. Post sternotomy mediastinitis is most frequently due to gram-positive cocci, especially staphylococci
   e. Mediastinitis mostly recovers with conservative management only

2. **The following are characteristic of pulmonary arterial hypertension (PAH):**
   a. PAH primarily affects the small pulmonary arterioles
   b. Loud P_2 (second pulmonic closure sound) and tricuspid regurgitation murmur are frequently heard on chest auscultation
   c. Pulmonary artery wedge pressure (PAWP) is more than 20 mmHg
   d. Electrocardiogram (ECG) frequently shows changes suggesting right ventricular hypertrophy
   e. Echocardiography is the gold standard for diagnosing PAH

3. **The following statements are apropos to heparin induced thrombocytopenia (HIT):**
   a. HIT incidence is more with use of unfractionated heparin (UFH) than with use of low molecular weight heparin (LMWH)
   b. HIT type I (nonimmune HIT) are more common than HIT type II (immune-mediated HIT)
   c. Thrombosis has not been reported in HIT type II
   d. Intravenous heparin catheter flushes are safe in presence of HIT
   e. The risk of HIT is negligible with the use of Fondaparinux

4. **Regarding End-tidal CO_2 ($EtCO_2$) monitoring which of the following is TRUE or FALSE:**
   a. $EtCO_2$ can detect apnea, upper airway obstruction, laryngospasm
   b. $EtCO_2$ is used for confirming tracheal placement of the endotracheal tube (ETT)
   c. An $EtCO_2$ <10 mm Hg after 20 min of cardiopulmonary resuscitation (CPR) is associated with very high mortality
   d. $EtCO_2$ allows indirect assessment of ventilation, circulation, and metabolism.
   e. Normal difference between arterial $PaCO_2$ and $EtCO_2$ is 2–5 mm Hg

5. **The following is TRUE about *Clostridium difficile* infection (CDI):**
   a. CDI ranges from mild diarrheal illness to pseudomembranous colitis
   b. CDI is often associated with antibiotic use
   c. Clinical presentation and features of diarrhea are classical and laboratory confirmation is not required for establishing diagnosis
   d. Vancomycin and metronidazole are currently the most important drugs for treating *Clostridium difficile* associated diarrhea (CDAD)
   e. Recurrence of CDAD is very rare after initial treatment

6. **Which of the following features of transfusion related acute lung injury (TRALI) is TRUE or FALSE?**
   a. TRALI has been reported only after administration of whole blood or packed red blood cells
   b. The pulmonary edema seen in TRALI is usually due to fluid overload and responds well to diuretics

c. Respiratory distress symptoms appears within 6 hours from the relevant blood transfusion
d. Radiographic evidence of bilateral pulmonary infiltrates, may progress to "white out"
e. $PaO_2/FiO_2 \leq 300$ or pulse oximetry <90% on room air or other clinical evidence

7. **Transesophageal echocardiography (TEE) is contraindicated in the following conditions:**
   a. Esophageal perforation
   b. Suspicion about stability of cervical spine
   c. Extensive radiation to the mediastinum
   d. Tracheal intubation
   e. Implanted pacemaker

8. **The Hounsfield units (HU) used to express CT image attenuation is correctly matched as follows:**
   a. Air: −1000
   b. Air: +1000
   c. Dense bone: +1000
   d. Dense bone: −1000
   e. Water: ±100

9. **Regarding hemorrhagic infarct (HI):**
   a. HI is a hemorrhagic transformation of ischemic stroke
   b. HI must be differentiated from primary intracerebral hemorrhage (ICH)
   c. HI typically happens within 1–2 weeks and less commonly in the first 24 hours after ischemic stroke onset
   d. Usually the intrainfarct hematoma is very dense
   e. Spontaneous intrainfarct hematoma does not happen in the absence of thrombolysis therapy

10. **Vascular intestinal ischemia may be characterized as:**
    a. Acute vascular intestinal ischemia can be arterial or venous in origin
    b. Thrombotic intestinal ischemia is more common than embolic intestinal ischemia
    c. The source of embolism is usually a leg deep vein thrombosis
    d. Hemodynamic events led low-flow states in ICU patients can provoke intestinal ischemia
    e. The outcome of acute intestinal ischemia has greatly improved over time with more aggressive treatment

11. **In patients of acute acalculous cholecystitis (AAC) which of the following is TRUE or FALSE:**
    a. It is more common in women than in men
    b. Incidence of gallbladder gangrene and perforation in ICU patients is higher than the non-ICU patients
    c. Right upper quadrant tenderness and Murphy sign is a reliable sign in most of the intubated and sedated patients in ICU
    d. It should be suspected in ICU patients with unexplained fever, leukocytosis, and an undefined source of sepsis
    e. Absence of gallstones in AAC decreases the sensitivity of bedside abdominal ultrasonography

12. **Partial pressures of CO_2 levels in a healthy adult are TRUE as shown below:**
    a. Inspired: 0.2 mm Hg
    b. Alveolar: 50 mm Hg
    c. Arterial: 40 mm Hg
    d. Venous: 46 mm Hg
    e. Expired: 50 mm Hg

13. **Concerning direct oral anticoagulants (DOAs):**
    a. DOAs include inhibitors of thrombin or factor-Xa
    b. Vitamin K is a specific antagonist of DOAs
    c. DOAs can be easily monitored by simple standardized laboratory assays
    d. DOAs pharmacokinetics vary significantly between patients
    e. DOAs have a lower bleeding risk compared to warfarin

14. **The following are immediate complications associated with massive blood transfusion:**
    a. Dilutional coagulopathy
    b. Citrate toxicity
    c. Hypokalemia
    d. Metabolic alkalosis
    e. Hypomagnesemia

15. **Trauma in pregnancy is associated with:**
    a. Chance of injury to uterus are more at 12 weeks than at 20-week of gestation
    b. X-rays and CT scans are not contraindicated if used judiciously
    c. The most common cause of fetal death after blunt injury is abruptio placentae
    d. Risk of hypoperfusion to fetus happens only after the mother develops hypotension

e. Left lateral uterine displacement by tilting the whole maternal body 25 to 30 degrees improve the effectiveness of cardiopulmonary resuscitation

16. **In patients with maxillofacial trauma with CSF leak factors influencing the technique used for securing airway in emergency unit are:**
    a. Urgency of securing airway
    b. Anticipated difficult airway
    c. Possibility of cervical spine fracture
    d. Possibility of concurrent base skull fracture
    e. Availability of airway devices

17. **The following is correct about a case of abdominal trauma:**
    a. Spleen and liver are the most commonly injured abdominal organ
    b. A normal serum amylase rules out pancreatic injury
    c. Hemodynamically stable patients with free abdominal fluid on FAST examination should undergo an emergent laparotomy to control bleeding
    d. Sensitivity of CT is better for hollow viscera injury than solid organ injury
    e. Presence of more than 500 white blood cells/mm^3, amylase, bilirubin, or particulate matter in the diagnostic peritoneal lavage fluid is suggestive of bowel injury

18. **In trauma patients which of the following are true or false:**
    a. Patients with major trauma are at high risk of venous thromboembolism (VTE)
    b. In most patients initial DVT after trauma is silent
    c. The positive predictive value of D-Dimer test is very high
    d. Mechanical or pharmacological thromboprohylaxis decreases the risk of DVT
    e. Inferior vena cava filter insertion effectively prevents deep venous thrombosis (DVT)

19. **The following statements about cerebral vasospasm after traumatic brain injury (TBI) seems correct:**
    a. Post-traumatic vasospasm (PTV) mainly affects posterior cerebral arteries
    b. Incidence of PTV is highest with traumatic subarachnoid hematoma (tSAH)
    c. The highest risk of developing hemodynamically significant vasospasm is the 10th day after TBI
    d. Transcranial Doppler monitoring can be used to monitor PTV
    e. PTV morphologically resembles aneurysmal vasospasm

20. **Concerning occult pneumothorax (OPTX):**
    a. An OPTX is identified on a computed tomography (CT) scan when an initial X-ray chest does not show pneumothorax
    b. Shortness of breath and chest pain are the most common presenting complaints of OPTX
    c. OPTX can be spontaneous, or caused by blunt or penetrating trauma
    d. Ultrasound sensitivity to detect OPTX is better than X-ray chest.
    e. OPTX is a benign condition which does not progress to tension pneumothorax

21. **The Wallace "rule of nine" uses which of the following for estimation the TBSA with burns in adults- answer as true or false:**
    a. Each arm – 9% TBSA
    b. Each leg - 9% TBSA
    c. Perineum – 1 % TBSA
    d. Head & Neck – 18% TBSA
    e. Anterior, posterior thorax - 18% TBSA each

22. **Regarding genitourinary injuries, which of the following statements are true or false?**
    a. Most renal injuries are secondary to blunt trauma
    b. Most ureteral and anterior urethral injuries are iatrogenic
    c. Most posterior urethral trauma injuries are from blunt mechanisms like motor vehicle collisions
    d. Pelvic ureter is involved in less than 10% of iatrogenic injuries
    e. Most blunt traumatic urinary bladder ruptures are intraperitoneal

23. **Regarding abdominal Focused assessment with sonography in trauma (FAST) which of the following is TRUE or FALSE:**
    a. It evaluates for the presence of intra-peritoneal free fluid in the abdomen and pelvis
    b. In trauma, free fluid detected by FAST is suggestive of hemoperitoneum
    c. FAST sensitivity for detecting solid organs injury is high
    d. Exploratory laparotomy should not be done in hemodynamically unstable blunt trauma patients, if the FAST is negative

e. FAST may be falsely negative if used for assessing patients with a delayed presentation after trauma

24. **Which of these are essential diagnostic criteria for traumatic brain injury (TBI) associated syndrome of inappropriate antidiuretic hormone secretion (SIADH):**
   a. Clinical hypovolemia
   b. Exclusion of hyperthyroidism and Cushing syndrome
   c. Urinary sodium excretion >30 mmol/L on normal salt and water intake
   d. Plasma osmolality < 280 mOsm/kg H_2O
   e. Urine osmolality (Uosm) >100 mOsm/kg H_2O and normal renal function

25. **Neurological examination in head injury is characterized by:**
   a. GCS score of 15 excludes the possibility of brain injury
   b. Pupillary examination for localization of an intracranial lesion is very sensitive and specific
   c. In the severely head-injured patient, the cranial nerves usually examined are (CN III), (CNs IX and X), and (CNs V and VII)
   d. Decorticate posturing implies injury above the midbrain
   e. Decerebrate posturing is suggestive of a midbrain lesion

26. **Which of the following statements about traumatic diffuse axonal injury (DAI) is TRUE or FALSE?**
   a. Depends on the mechanism of injury; it is more common in higher energy trauma
   b. Results primarily from a secondary brain injury
   c. A frequent cause of persistent vegetative state
   d. CT classically shows several >2 cm size lesions in cerebral gray matter
   e. MRI sensitivity for diagnosing DAI is better than CT

27. **Regarding the traumatic acute epidural hematoma (EDH), which of the following statement is true or false?**
   a. A lucid interval following a brief loss of consciousness or period of confusion is pathognomonic of epidural hematoma (EDH)
   b. EDH have a biconvex or lens hyperdense shape collection which typically do not cross suture lines
   c. The low density in the hematoma indicates active extravasation of fresh unclotted blood (swirl sign)
   d. Middle meningeal artery or one of its branches is the common source of hematoma
   e. Compared to adults, children have higher incidence of EDH

28. **The lethal triad of trauma includes the following:**
   a. Hypothermia
   b. Acidosis
   c. Decreased cardiac output
   d. Coagulopathy
   e. Tachycardia

29. **Consider the following about Glasgow Coma scale (GCS):**
   a. It ranges from a minimum of 2 to a maximum of 15
   b. It has three components namely, motor response, eye opening and memory
   c. A patient with severe head injury has a GCS of 13 or below
   d. The motor response component has six grades ranging from 1 to 6.
   e. Eye opening component has four grades ranging from 1 to 4

30. **Which of the following are TRUE or FALSE about a patient of flail chest?**
   a. Flail chest occurs when three or more adjacent ribs are each fractured in two places
   b. The treatment of flail chest is operative in the vast majority of cases
   c. All flail chest patients should be intubated and given ventilator support
   d. Unstable section of chest wall will exhibit paradoxical motion
   e. Pulmonary contusion, pneumothorax and hemothorax are commonly associated injuries

ANSWERS
A Type Answers

Q1. Answer e

Blood culture—negative IE is defined as endocarditis with no definitive microbiologic etiology following inoculation of at least three independently obtained blood samples in a standard blood-culture system, with negative cultures after five days of incubation and subculturing.

Echocardiography showing vegetation or abscess, new valvular regurgitation; and Fever – Temperature ≥38.0°C are major and minor diagnostic criteria of Infective endocarditis as per Modified Duke criteria.

The diagnosis of IE may be rejected if any of the following are present- A firm alternate diagnosis; Resolution of clinical manifestations occurs in ≤4 days of antibiotic therapy.

> Durack DT, Lukes AS, Bright DK. New criteria for diagnosis of infective endocarditis: utilization of specific echocardiographic findings. Duke Endocarditis Service. Am J Med. 1994;96(3):200-9.
>
> Sexton DJ, Fowler VG. Clinical manifestations and evaluation of adults with suspected native valve endocarditis. Uptodate, 2017. Available from: https://www.uptodate.com/contents/clinical-manifestations-and-evaluation-of-adults-with-suspected-native-valve-endocarditis (Accessed 12th August 2017).

Q2. Answer d

Patients with tension pneumothorax become acutely ill within minutes and develop severe cardiovascular and respiratory distress. They are dyspneic, agitated, restless, cyanotic, tachycardic, and hypotensive and display decreasing mental activity. The cardinal signs of tension pneumothorax are tachycardia, hypotension, oxyhemoglobin desaturation, jugular venous distention (JVD), and absent breath sounds on the ipsilateral side. However, JVD may not reliably be present with massive blood loss. This patient may be hypovolemic with a normal or low jugular venous pressure.

> Gaieski DF, Mikkelsen ME. Evaluation of and initial approach to the adult patient with undifferentiated hypotension and shock. Available from: https://www.uptodate.com/contents/evaluation-of-and-initial-approach-to-the-adult-patient-with-undifferentiated-hypotension-and-shock?source=search_result&search=tension%20pneumothorax%20with%20massive%20blood%20loss&selectedTitle=1~150 (Accessed 12th August 2017).

Q3. Answer d

The correct ASA physical status classification is: (1) ASA I: a normal healthy patient (2) ASA II: a patient with mild systemic disease, (3) ASA III: a patient with severe systemic disease, (4) ASA IV: a patient with severe systemic disease that is a constant threat to life, (5) ASA V: a moribund patient not expected to survive without operation, (6) ASAVI: a declared brain dead patient whose organs are being removed for donor purposes.

> Woodfield JC, Beshay NM, Pettigrew RA, et al. American Society of Anesthesiologists classification of physical status as a predictor of wound infection. ANZ J Surg. 2007;77(9):738-41.

Q4. Answer e

An otherwise unexplained increase in pulmonary shunt fraction alveolar-to-arterial oxygen tension difference, especially if it occurs within 24–48 hours of a sentinel event associated with fat embolism syndrome (FES), is strongly suggestive of the syndrome. No single test or imaging can confirm the diagnosis. The following was described in the past in this connection: (1) Thrombocytopenia, anemia, and hypofibrinogenemia are indicative of FES; however, they are nonspecific. (2) Urinary fat stains are not considered to be sensitive or specific enough for diagnosing FES or for determining the risk of it. Fat globules in the urine are common after trauma. (3) Preliminary investigations of the cytology of pulmonary capillary blood obtained from a wedged pulmonary artery catheter revealed fat globules in patients with FES and showed that this method may be beneficial in early detection of patients at risk. (4) Genotyping for polymorphisms associated with increased susceptibility to inflammatory stimuli may help identify those at risk for FES. Specific antibody therapy targeting inflammatory molecules has not been useful. (5) Radiography and computed tomography—serial chest radiographs reveal increasing diffuse bilateral pulmonary infiltrates within 24–48 hours of the onset of clinical findings. CT brain may reveal diffuse white-matter petechial hemorrhages consistent with microvascular injury. (6) Parenchymal changes consistent with lung contusion, acute lung injury, or acute respiratory distress syndrome (ARDS) may be evident. (7) Bronchoalveolar lavage with staining for fat have been evaluated in trauma patients and sickle-cell patients with acute chest syndrome, and the results have been mixed.

Bulauitan CS, Gupta R. Fat Embolism Workup. Available from: http://emedicine.medscape.com/article/460524-workup (Accessed 13th August 2017).

Q5. Answer c

Rhabdomyolysis and myoglobinuria can develop in patients with significant muscle injury including crush injuries, prolonged immobilization and compartment syndrome. Rhabdomyolysis presents with elevated serum muscle enzymes (including creatine kinase), red to brown urine due to myoglobinuria if there is persistent renal function, and electrolyte abnormalities. Peak serum creatine kinase levels depend upon the volume of muscle breakdown and the muscle mass of the patient. Creatine kinase values should be measured if there is a suspicion for rhabdomyolysis until decreasing levels are observed. A brisk urine output should be maintained with intravenous fluid therapy until the creatine kinase value starts to decrease.

Adams BD, Arbogast CB. Rhabdomyolysis. In: Adams GJ (Ed.). Emergency Medicine: Clinical Essentials. Philadelphia, USA, Elsevier, 2013. pp.1429-38.

Q6. Answer d

The presence of pleural sliding is the most important finding in normal aerated lung. Lung sliding corresponds to the to-and-fro movement of the visceral pleura on the parietal pleura that occurs with respiration and is seen as a hyperechoic pleural line shimmering back and forth.

The use of M-mode, which detects motion over time, provides more evidence that the pleural line is sliding. The M-mode cursor is placed over the pleural line and two different patterns are displayed on the screen: The motionless portion of the chest above the pleural line creates horizontal 'waves,' and the sliding below the pleural line creates a granular pattern, the 'sand'. The resultant picture is one that resembles waves crashing in onto the sand and is therefore called the 'seashore sign' and is present in normal lung.

Husain LF, Hagopian L, Wayman D et al. Sonographic diagnosis of pneumothorax. J Emerg Trauma Shock. 2012;5(1):76-81.

Q7. Answer e

Acute cholangitis is a clinical syndrome characterized by fever, jaundice, and abdominal pain that develops as a result of stasis and infection in the biliary tract. It is also referred to as ascending cholangitis.

The organisms typically ascend from the duodenum; hematogenous spread from the portal vein is a rare source of infection.

About 70 to 80% of patients with acute cholangitis will respond to conservative management with antibiotic therapy.

Therapeutic endoscopic retrograde cholangiopancreatography (ERCP) must be expediently pursued in all cases of acute cholangitis. Patients should undergo biliary drainage as soon as possible, but if they respond to antibiotics, the procedure can be done within 24 to 48 hours.

Hui CK, Lai KC, Yuen MF, et al. Acute cholangitis-predictive factors for emergency ERCP. Aliment Pharmacol Ther. 2001;15: 1633-37.

Jochen SJ, Hapfelmeier A, Thöres S et al. Mortality risk for acute cholangitis (MAC): a risk prediction model for in-hospital mortality in patients with acute cholangitis. BMC Gastroenterol. 2016;16:15.

Q8. Answer a

A specimen for culture should be from deep tissue, obtained by biopsy or curettage after the wound has been cleansed and debrided. Avoid swab specimens, which provide less accurate results. 2012 Infectious Diseases Society of America clinical practice guideline for the diagnosis and treatment of diabetic foot infections: Parentheses show level of evidence, recommendation of empiric therapy:
1. For mild to moderate infections in patients who have not recently received antibiotic treatment, therapy just targeting aerobic GPC is sufficient (weak, low).
2. For most severe infections, starting broad-spectrum empiric antibiotic therapy, pending culture results and antibiotic susceptibility data (strong, low).
3. Empiric therapy directed at Pseudomonas aeruginosa is usually unnecessary except for patients with risk factors for true infection with this organism (strong, low).

Lipsky BA, Berendt AR, Cornia PB, et al. 2012 Infectious Diseases Society of America clinical practice guideline for the diagnosis and treatment of diabetic foot infections. Clin Infect Dis. 2012;54(12):e132-73.

Q9. Answer e

NOMI occurs as a result of mesenteric vasospasm in the absence of a physical obstruction. This vasospasm is triggered by mesenteric hypoperfusion or excessive sympathetic nervous system activity. Mesenteric hypoperfusion can result from sepsis, severe dehydration, pancreatitis, or hemorrhagic shock. Excessive sympathetic activity can result from congestive heart failure, or the use of medications and drugs such as vasopressors, cocaine, or digoxin.

Factor V Leiden mutation causes a hypercoagulable state and is the most common cause of mesenteric venous thrombosis which cause mesenteric ischemia by occluding the superior mesenteric vein and its branches.

Roline CE, Reardon RF. Disorders of the Small Intestine. In: Walls RM, Hockberger RS, Gausche-Hill M (Eds.). Rosen's Emergency Medicine: Concepts and Clinical Practice, 9th edn. Philadelphia, USA: Elsevier; 2018. pp. 1112-20.

Q10. Answer b

Respiratory distress in immediate postoperative period following thyroidectomy can be a possibility with:
1. Vocal cord paresis or paralysis due to iatrogenic injury of the recurrent laryngeal nerve.
2. Tracheal intubation can cause paresis or paralyses of the vocal, temporary or definitive folds.
3. Tracheomalacia, especially in patients with a large long-standing goiter.

The external branch of the superior laryngeal nerve (SLN) is probably the nerve most commonly injured in thyroid surgery, resulting in an inability to lengthen a vocal fold, change of voice but not respiratory distress.

Orestes MI, Chhetri DK. Superior laryngeal nerve injury: effects, clinical findings, prognosis, and management options. Curr Opin Otolaryngol Head Neck Surg. 2014;22(6):439-43.

Mota LAA, de Cavalho GB, Brito VA. Laryngeal complications by orotracheal intubation: Literature review. Int Arch Otorhinolaryngol. 2012;16(2):236-45.

Findlay JM, Sadler GP, Bridge H, Mihai R. Post-thyroidectomy tracheomalacia: minimal risk despite significant tracheal compression. Br J Anaesth. 2011;106(6):903-6.

Q11. Answer d

Nasogastric suction or decompression can be helpful in some cases. This patient was already on nasogastric suction and not improving.

Neostigmine has been tried in patients who fail to show improvement after 24 to 48 hours of conservative management, or in patients who initially have cecal dilation greater than 12 cm in diameter preferably avoided in patients with heart ailments.

Erythromycin is effective for acute episodes of ileus and chronic symptoms in some patients with chronic intestinal pseudo-obstruction.

His dilated cecum necessitated an urgent cecal decompression to prevent chance of a catastrophic perforation. Decompression can be best attempted with colonoscopy before any surgical intervention is contemplated.

Emmanuel AV, Shand AG, Kamm MA. Erythromycin for the treatment of chronic intestinal pseudo-obstruction: description of six cases with a positive response. Aliment Pharmacol Ther. 2004;19(6):687-94.

Chudzinski AP, Thompson EV, Ayscue JM. Acute colonic pseudoobstruction. Clin Colon Rectal Surg. 2015;28(2):112-7.

Q12. Answer c

Both collapse and effusion look white, they can be differentiated by looking at the side towards which mediastinum is displaced.

A hemothorax is usually associated with a pneumothorax secondary to the injury of the lung, chest wall, and associated vasculature. Hemopneumothorax are characterized by an air-fluid level on the chest radiograph. Unless the pneumothorax is small or occult, the air will appear as black.

Though less common, an extensive lobar pneumonia can affect all the lobes of the lung. An air bronchogram may be visible initially, which may disappear as the bronchi get filled with pus and exudates.

Lacey GD, Morley S, Berman L. Analysis: White out. Chest X-Ray: A Survival Guide. Pensilvenia USA, Elsevier, 2008. pp. 264-7.

Q13. Answer c

Gyenocologic surgery accounts for greater than half of all iatrogenic ureteric injuries. The pelvic ureter is involved in 80% of iatrogenic ureteral injuries, making it by far the most commonly involved segment. The most common types of ureteral injury, in decreasing order of frequency, are ligation, kinking by suture, transection/avulsion, partial transection, crush, and devascularization with delayed necrosis/stricture.

Brandes S, Coburn M, Armenakas N, et al. Diagnosis and management of ureteric injury: an evidence-based analysis. BJU Int. 2004;94:277-89.

Q14. Answer c

Estimates of NGB in the United States include approximately 400,000 people with diagnoses of spina bifida (SB), spinal cord injury (SCI), cerebral palsy, multiple sclerosis (MS), and Parkinson disease.

UTIs are the most common infection in this population; 31% of patients with a new diagnosis of SCI were diagnosed with a UTI within the first year, and 21% required hospitalization.

The typical symptoms of UTI in the general population, such as dysuria, urgency, and frequency, are rarely present in the NGB population.

Urinary catheters are a mainstay management strategy for patients with NGB.

CIC is the preferred method of drainage in patients with NGB as long as their dexterity or caretaker support and body habitus allow access.

McKibben MJ, Seed P, Ross SS, et al. Urinary tract infection and neurogenic bladder. Urologic Clinics of North America. 2015;42(4):527-36.

Q15. Answer a

Normal intra-abdominal pressure (IAP) in an adult is between 0 and 5 mm Hg. IAH is defined as IAP greater than or equal to 12 mm Hg. There is no Grade 0 in WSACS grades.

Malbrain ML, Cheatham ML, Kirkpatrick A, et al. Results from the International Conference of Experts on Intra-abdominal Hypertension and Abdominal Compartment Syndrome Definitions. *Intensive Care Med.* 2006;32(11):1722-32.

Q16. Answer e

Except for part of the bowel and the duodenum that are retroperitoneal, the rupture of hollow organs causes pneumoperitoneum.

Ultrasonography is not sensitive in identifying free gas in the peritoneal cavity but it is a noninvasive, relatively simple, and repeatable examination, which can identify indirect findings of bowel perforation as intraperitoneal free fluid and intestinal paresis.

On plain films, a direct finding of perforation is free intraperitoneal gas; indirect diagnostic findings are intraperitoneal free fluid and paralytic ileus.

Computed tomography (CT) is considered as the most sensitive modality for the diagnosis of pneumoperitoneum owing to its high spatial resolution and capability to detect even the smallest amount of free intraperitoneal air. Free air under the right diaphragm from a perforated bowel can be seen in upright Chest X-ray.

Picone D, Rusignuolo R, Midiri F, et al. Imaging assessment of gastroduodenal perforations. Seminars in Ultrasound, CT, and MRI. 2016;37(1):16-22.

Q17. Answer a

Nasogastric tube placement should not be performed because of the risk of inadvertent intracranial placement through a fracture in the cribriform plate. The small size and flexibility of the nasogastric tube allow it to be misdirected through such a fracture into the brain.

Roka YB, Shrestha M, Puri RR, Aryal S. Fatal inadvertent intracranial insertion of a nasogastric tube. Neurology India. 2010;58(5):802-804.

Q18. Answer d

According to the AHA/ASA guideline:

Rapid neuroimaging with CT or MRI is recommended to distinguish ischemic stroke from ICH.

For ICH patients presenting with SBP between 150 and 220 mm Hg and without contraindication to acute BP treatment, acute lowering of SBP to 140 mm Hg is safe and can be effective for improving functional outcome. Measures to control BP should begin immediately after ICH onset.

Patients with a severe coagulation factor deficiency or severe thrombocytopenia should receive appropriate factor replacement therapy or platelets, respectively.

Glucose should be monitored. Both hyperglycemia (< 180 mg/dL) and hypoglycemia (< 70 mg/dL) should be avoided.

Clinical seizures should be treated with antiseizure drugs.

<small>Hemphill JC, Greenberg SM, Anderson CS, et al. Guidelines for the Management of Spontaneous Intracerebral Hemorrhage. Stroke. 2015;46:2032-60.</small>

Q19. Answer c

Guidelines from an expert panel published in 2006 recommend surgical evacuation for patients with acute SDH who have clot thickness >10 mm or midline shift >5 mm, regardless of the Glasgow coma scale (GCS) score. All patients with acute SDH in coma (GCS score less than 9) should undergo intracranial pressure (ICP) monitoring. A comatose patient (GCS score less than 9) with an SDH less than 10-mm thick and a midline shift less than 5 mm should undergo surgical evacuation of the lesion if the GCS score decreased between the time of injury and hospital admission by 2 or more points on the GCS and/or the patient presents with asymmetric or fixed and dilated pupils and/or the ICP exceeds 20 mm Hg.

<small>Bullock MR, Chesnut R, Ghajar J et al. Surgical management of traumatic brain injury author group. Neurosurgery. 2006;58 (3 Suppl):S16.</small>

Q20. Answer e

Adults and children who have sustained a head injury and in whom there is clinical suspicion of cervical spine injury, range of movement in the neck can be assessed safely before imaging only if no high-risk factors and at least 1 of the low-risk features is present. The low-risk features include Involvement in a minor rear-end motor vehicle collision, patient comfortable in a sitting position, was ambulatory at any time since the injury and has no midline cervical spine tenderness is present.

According to the Canadian C-spine rule any complaint of Paresthesia in the upper or lower limbs puts the person in the high risk for cervical spine injury.

<small>National Clinical Guideline Centre. Spinal injury: assessment and initial management. London (UK): National Institute for Health and Care Excellence (NICE); 2016 (NICE guideline; no. 41). Available from: https://www.nice.org.uk/guidance/.../spinal-injury-assessment-and-initial-management (Accessed 27th June 2017).</small>

Q21. Answer a

The fully conscious, talking patient is able to maintain his own airway and needs no further airway manipulation. However, patients' status may deteriorate at any time, and ABC's must constantly be reassessed.

The following categories of patients require a definitively secured airway:
  i. Apnea
  ii. Glasgow Coma Scale < 9 or sustained seizure activity.
  iii. Unstable mid-face trauma.
  iv. Airway injuries.
  v. Large flail segment or respiratory failure.
  vi. High aspiration risk.
  vii. Inability to otherwise maintain an airway or oxygenation.

<small>Airway Management of the Trauma Victim. Available from: http://www.trauma.org/archive/anaesthesia/airway.html (Accessed on 5th June 2017).</small>

Q22. Answer d

The classic finding in aortic injury is a widened mediastinum due to mediastinal hematoma.

CT showing morphologically normal aorta with no mediastinal hematoma has a 100% negative predictive value for exclusion of aortic injury.

Patients require prompt and accurate diagnosis to allow for timely repair of the injury, especially given that 60% may have no overt clinical sign of thoracic trauma.

Most blunt aortic injuries occur at the level of the aortic isthmus just distal to the subclavian artery origin. The ascending aorta is injured in <5% of patients with blunt aortic injury who survive transport for further treatment.

Ascending aorta injuries are frequently (80%) associated with significant cardiac damage, including valvular damage or pericardial tamponade, a lethal combination of injuries.

Statkus NJ, Hill JR, Gosselin MV, and Primack SL. Blunt Thoracic Trauma. In: Müller NL, Silva IS (Eds.). Imaging of the chest. Philadelphia USA, Elsevier: 2008. pp.1241-68.

Q23. Answer e

Following initial evaluation, the primary focus of early burn treatment is fluid resuscitation by crystalloids because of early post-burn capillary leakage. Excessive crystalloid infusion can cause abdominal compartment syndrome.

However, colloids can be used after capillary integrity restores to maintain oncotic pressure, expand plasma volume, and reduce secondary edema in unburned tissue, including possible prevention of abdominal compartment syndrome.

Acute airway obstruction can occur at any time during the first 24 hours of injury, even in the absence of smoke inhalation.

Stress-induced diabetes, with hyperglycemia and insulin resistance is a common pathophysiological phenomenon. Insulin administration to a target range of 130 to 150 mg/dL may be beneficial in terms of morbidity and mortality without the risk of hypoglycemia.

Jeschke MG. Clinical review: Glucose control in severely burned patients - current best practice. Crit Care. 2013;17(4):232.

Saffle JR. Critical care management of the severely burned patient. In: Parrillo JE, Dellinger, RP (Eds). Critical Care Medicine: Principles of Diagnosis and Management in the Adult, 4th edn. Philadelphia USA, Elsevier. 2014; p. 1177-98.

Q24. Answer a

The majority of traumatic SCIs (55%) involve the cervical spine.

Delayed neurologic deterioration is well described, with a reported incidence of 1.8% to 10%, and may be seen from hours to days following the onset of injury.

Initial support for methylprednisolone use was based on the findings of the National Spinal Cord Injury Study trials. Current guidelines advise against the use of methylprednisolone for ASCI.

The hypotension and neurogenic shock following acute SCI is a distributive process resulting from loss of vasoconstrictor tone in peripheral arterioles and pooling of blood within the peripheral vasculature.

The incidence of VTE following SCI is as high as 81%, with the most significant risk occurring between 72 hours and 2 weeks following injury. Prophylaxis and surveillance of deep venous thrombosis is paramount in individuals with SCI.

Evans LT, Lollis SS, Ball PA. Management of acute spinal cord injury in the neurocritical care unit. Neurosurg Clin N Am. 2013;24:339-47.

Q25. Answer e

Damage to the kidneys occurs quite commonly in the setting of direct blunt injury, multiple trauma, or penetrating trauma. About 80-90% of renal injuries are due to blunt trauma.

The majority of blunt renal injuries are minor and managed conservatively. In less than 10% of the cases, the injuries are serious enough to require surgery.

The degree of hematuria and the severity of the renal injury do not consistently correlate. Gross hematuria has been observed in minor renal contusions, and microscopic hematuria has been seen in some with severe renal injuries.

Gourgiotis S, Germanos S, Dimopoulos N, et al. Renal injury 5-year experience and literature review. Urol int. 2006;77:97-103.

Shariat SF, Jenkins A, Roehrborn CG, et al. Features and outcomes of patients with grade IV renal injury. BJU Int. 2008;102: 728-33.

Q26. Answer a

Pulmonary contusions opacities cross segmental and fissural boundaries and are often present at the site of impaction and adjacent to rib fractures.

The accumulation of blood and edema usually becomes apparent within 24 hours on X-ray chest. The appearance of radiopacity on chest radiography after 24 hours should raise suspicion of aspiration, pneumonia and fat embolism.

Pulmonary contusion usually resolves spontaneously in 3 to 5 days, provided no secondary insult occurs.

A lung contusion is diagnosed by the presence of: (a) an irregularly delineated tissue image, (b) multiple B-lines.

Impaired gas exchange at alveolar level, leads to decreasing blood oxygen saturation, reduced concentration of oxygen in arterial blood, cyanosis and dyspnea.

Costantino M, Gosselin MV, Primack SL. The ABC's of thoracic trauma imaging. Semin Roentgenol. 2006;41:209-25.

Ganie FA, Lone H, Lone GN, et al. Lung Contusion: A clinico-pathological entity with unpredictable clinical course. Bull Emerg Trauma. 2013;1(1):7-16.

Q27. Answer e

Free intraperitoneal fluid seen in FAST in a trauma setting is considered to be a hemoperitoneum. The utility of FAST examinations in the setting of major pelvic injury is relatively unstudied. Coincident injuries make the evaluation for source of hemorrhage in this subset of patients challenging. There is a report of sonographic intraperitoneal fluid in the setting of major pelvic injury and hemodynamic instability found to be uroperitoneum and not hemoperitoneum.

Rosenstein DI, Alsikafi NF. Diagnosis and classification of urethral injuries. Urol Clin N Am. 2006;33:73-85.

Jones AE, Mason PE, Tayal VS, et al. Sonographic intraperitoneal fluid in patients with pelvic fracture: two cases of traumatic intraperitoneal bladder rupture. J Emerg Med. 2003;25(4):373-7.

Q28. Answer e

When fluid accumulates more rapidly than can be accommodated by the distensibility of the pericardium, especially in the case of trauma, significant intrapericardial pressure results and can produce pericardial tamponade. Pericardial tamponade develops when intrapericardial fluid produces sufficient pressure to compress the cardiac chambers. Compression of the chambers impairs ventricular diastolic filling and stroke volume.

A large cardiac silhouette by radiography of the chest and low-voltage QRS complexes or electrical alternans in the ECG can suggest the presence of cardiac tamponade. CT can identify the size of an effusion but cannot confirm tamponade. Echocardiography can confirm the diagnosis of cardiac tamponade and is the test of choice

Mattu A, Martinez JP Pericarditis, pericardial tamponade, and myocarditis. In: Adams JG, Barton ED, Collings JL (Eds.). Emergency Medicine: Clinical Essentials, 2nd Edn. Philadelphia USA: Elsevier; 2013. pp. 514-23.

Q29. Answer d

According to NICE's guideline and associated quality standards of head injury, in adults with head injury, anyone of the following risk factors indicates the need for a CT head scan within 1 hour of the risk factor being identified:
- GCS score less than 13 on initial assessment in the emergency department.
- Suspected open or depressed skull fracture
- Focal neurological deficit
- More than 1 episode of vomiting

These guideline and other studies have shown that head injury patients with a history of anticoagulants medication but with no signs showing that the injury might have damaged their brain, need to be under observation and may not need CT head in emergency but need a CT head within 8 hours of the injury.

Head injury: assessment and early management (Nice Guidelines) Available from: https://www.nice.org.uk/guidance/cg176/chapter/1-recommendations (Accessed on 15th June 2017).

Gittleman AM, Ortiz AO, Keating DP, et al. Indications for CT in patients receiving anticoagulation after head trauma. Am J Neuroradiol. 2005;26(3):603-6.

Q30. Answer d

In the case of lightning strikes, fixed and dilated pupils cannot be used as an indicator of brain death or to gauge prognosis.

Muscle relaxants and barbiturate poisoning need to be ruled out before considering fixed and dilated pupils as a sign of brain death.

Pupillary involvement has been reported in around 20 % of head injury associated ocular trauma.

Stember A, Cushing T. Lightning and Electrical Injuries. In: Markovchick VJ, Pons PT, Bakes KM (Eds). Emergency Medicine Secrets, 6th edn. Philadelphia USA, Elsevier, 2016. pp. 366-76.

Thomas PD. The differential diagnosis of fixed dilated pupils: a case report and review. Critical Care and Resuscitation. 2000;2:34-37.

Helmy A, Kirkpatrick PJ, Seeley HM, et al. Fixed, dilated pupils following traumatic brain injury: historical perspectives, causes and ophthalmological sequelae. *Acta Neurochir Suppl.* 2012;114:295-9.

K Type Answers

Q1. Answer TFTTF

Essentially all cases of mediastinitis are due to the spread of infection from other sites or direct inoculation resulting from trauma or surgery.

Mediastinitis now occurs most frequently as a postoperative infection after median sternotomy. In the past it was esophageal perforation or contiguous spread from oropharyngeal foci.

X-ray chest may show signs of mediastinitis. CT imaging is necessary to diagnose mediastinitis and define the extent of the infection.

The bacteriology of mediastinitis complicating cardiovascular surgery is primarily caused by gram-positive cocci and less often by gram-negative bacilli as seen with head and neck infections or esophageal perforations.

Mediastinitis mortality is very high. Aggressive surgical intervention is essential in all forms of mediastinitis with debridement of any infected or necrotic tissues.

Schooneveld TCV, Rupp ME. Mediastinitis. In: Bennet JE, Dolin R, Blaser MJ (Eds). Mandell, Douglas, and Bennett's Principles and Practice of Infectious Diseases. Updated 8th edition. Philadelphia USA, Elsevier; 2015. pp. 1080-90.

Q2. Answer TTFTF

Pulmonary arterial hypertension (PAH) primarily affects the small pulmonary arterioles.

In all subtypes of PAH, a loud P2 (second pulmonic closure sound) is frequently heard in association with tricuspid regurgitation murmur.

By definition of PAH high pulmonary pressure is a result of elevated precapillary pulmonary resistance and normal pulmonary venous pressure and is measured as a pulmonary wedge pressure of 15 mm Hg or less.

Electrocardiogram (ECG) frequently shows changes compatible with right ventricular hypertrophy.

Echocardiography estimate of pulmonary artery pressure accuracy is low. Thus, despite echocardiography being a good screening tool to suggest PAH, it should never be used to establish a diagnosis of PAH without proceeding with a right heart catheterization.

Lai YC, Potoka KC, Champion HC, et al. Pulmonary arterial hypertension: the clinical syndrome. Circ Res. 2014;115(1):115-30.

Badesch DB, Champion HC, Sanchez MA, et al. Diagnosis and assessment of pulmonary arterial hypertension. J Am Coll Cardiol. 2009;54(1 suppl):S55-S66.

Q3. Answer TTFFT

HIT is characterized by thrombocytopenia, platelet activation, and thrombosis.

HIT type I (nonimmune HIT) is more common and more transient. It occurs in 10% to 30% of patients within a few days after exposure to heparin.

HIT type II (immune-mediated HIT) is uncommon but dangerous, that occurs in 0.3% to 5% of patients after heparin exposure. It is associated with a high risk (20-50%) of developing venous and arterial thrombotic events.

Once HIT is established, no heparin in any form or dose should be used. Fondaparinux, a, has been recognized as a new option to treat HIT. It has no cross reactivity with HIT antibodies.

Thai JN, Trinidad-Hernandez M, Mills JL. Complications of Heparin Anticoagulation Therapy. In: Stanley JC, Veith FJ, Wakefield TW (Eds.). Current Therapy in Vascular and Endovascular Surgery. 5th edn. Philadelphia USA, Elsevier; 2014. pp. 622-5.

Q4. Answer TTTTT

Capnography has made steady inroads in the ICU and is increasingly used for all patients who are mechanically ventilated. There is growing recognition that capnography is rich in information about lung and circulatory physiology and provides insight into many diseases and treatments. These include conditions of impaired matching of ventilation and perfusion, such as pulmonary embolism and obstructive lung diseases; circulatory questions, such as the adequacy of chest compressions during cardiac arrest or fluid responsiveness in patients in shock; and the safety of procedural sedation. In this review, we emphasize analysis of the entire capnographic waveform as a way to glean additional useful information. We also discuss important limitations of capnography, especially when it is considered to be a surrogate for $PaCO_2$.

Nassar BS, Schmidt GA. Capnography during critical illness. Chest. 2016;149(2):576-85.

Capnography Reference Handbook (Respironics). Available from: www.mysupplies.philips.com/.../CapnographyReferenceHandbook_OEM1220A.PDF (Accessed on 25th June 2017).

Q5. Answer TTFTF

The usual presentation is similar to that of other infectious diarrheas, and diagnosis usually requires identification of *C. difficile*-specific endotoxin A (rarely, also B) using laboratory assays.

Except for very mild CDI antibiotic treatment is advised. The main antibiotics that are recommended are metronidazole, vancomycin.

Relapse may occur in up to 10% to 65% of patients, usually within 2 weeks of discontinuation of initial therapy. It is due to either reinfection or failure to fully eradicate the retained *C. difficile* spores.

Cohen SH, Gerding DN, Johnson S, et al. Clinical practice guidelines for Clostridium difficile infection in adults: 2010 update by the society for healthcare epidemiology of America (SHEA) and the infectious diseases society of America (IDSA). Infect Control Hosp Epidemiol. 2010;31:431.

Q6. Answer FFTTT

TRALI can happen after all plasma containing blood product transfusion like whole blood, packed red blood cells, fresh frozen plasma, platelets concentrates, cryoprecipitate, and intravenous immunoglobulin.

TRALI is commonly misdiagnosed as volume overload and treated with diuretics before confirmatory diagnosis is made.

Canadian Consensus Conference, 2004 TRALI criteria is- 1) hypoxemia: $Pao_2/Fio_2 <= 300$ or pulse oximetry <90% on room air or other clinical evidence; 2) no preexisting acute lung injury or presence of risk factors for same.

European Haemovigilance Network (EHN) TRALI criteria is: 1) acute respiratory distress during or within 6 hours of transfusion; 2) absence of signs of circulatory overload; 3) radiographic evidence of bilateral pulmonary infiltrates, even a "white out."

Toy P, Popovsky MA, Abraham E, et al. Transfusion-related acute lung injury: Definition and review. Crit Care Med. 2005;33:721-6.

Breanndan MS. Transfusion-related acute lung injury (TRALI): Clinical presentation, treatment, and prognosis. Critical Care Medicine. 2006;34(5) Suppl.:S114-S117.

Q7. Answer TTTFF

According to the various guidelines the list of contraindications include esophageal pathologies, unstable spine, mediastinum radiation. TEE has been safely used in intubated patients as well as with patients having implanted pacemakers.

Hahn RT, Abraham T, Adams MS, et al. Guidelines for performing a comprehensive transesophageal echocardiographic examination: recommendations from the American Society of Echocardiography and the Society of Cardiovascular Anesthesiologists. J Am Soc Echocardiogr. 2013;26(9):921-64.

Q8. Answer TFTFF

A single CT image generated by the scanner is divided into many tiny blocks of different shades of black and white called pixels. The actual grayscale of each pixel on a CT depends on the amount of radiation absorbed at that point, which is termed an attenuation value. Attenuation values are expressed in Hounsfield units (HU). The HU scale, or attenuation value, is based on a reference scale in which air is assigned a value of −1000 HU and dense bone is assigned the value of +1000 HU. Water is assigned 0 HU.

Q9. Answer TTTFF

HI, or hemorrhagic transformation of an infarct, occurs in approximately one-third of cases of ischemic stroke.

When brain imaging is delayed after the onset of the patient's stroke symptoms, an erroneous diagnosis of ICH may be made if the hemorrhage appears confluent on CT. The immediate and long-term management of the two conditions are different and hence the importance of accurate diagnosis.

HI typically happens within 1–2 weeks after stroke onset, less commonly (~9%) in the first 24 hours. The occurrence of dense hematoma complicating HI may be even lower at approximately 3%.

Spontaneous intrainfarct hematoma have been reported in the absence of thrombolysis.

Paciaroni M, Agnelli G, Corea F, et al. Early hemorrhagic transformation of brain infarction: rate, predictive factors, and influence on clinical outcome: results of a prospective multicenter study. Stroke. 2008;39(8):2249-56.

Q10. Answer TFTFT

Acute intestinal ischemia can be mechanical, vascular nonocclusive, or vascular occlusive, with the last of these either arterial or venous in origin.

Approximately 65% of all vascular-related cases are embolic phenomena, arterial thrombosis accounts for 27%, while mesenteric venous thrombosis is the cause of acute intestinal ischemia in 3% to 5% of patients.

Embolism is the most common cause of vascular-related mesenteric ischemia, and is frequently a result of embolism from cardiac origin.

Hemodynamic events that lead to a low-flow state can ultimately occlude a stenotic arterial segment or hinder collateral blood flow, thus provoking intestinal ischemia.

Despite advances in diagnostic imaging, intensive care support, and surgical treatment, the average mortality rate from all causes of acute intestinal ischemia has not changed significantly in the past 30 years, and is still around 60% to 80%.

Rezende-Neto JB, Rotstein OD. Abdominal Catastrophes in the Intensive Care Unit Setting. Critical Care Clinics 2013;29(4): 1017-44.

Q11. Answer FTFTT

Demographically, AAC is more common in men than in women (3:1). Patients who undergo surgical procedures unrelated to trauma, 80% AAC are men.

Gallbladder gangrene incidence in ICU patients with AAC is greater than 50%, and that of perforation greater than 10%. In the non-ICU patients the incidence of gallbladder gangrene is 36%, with no reports of perforations.

The Murphy sign and right upper quadrant tenderness have high positive and negative likelihood ratios, for the diagnosis of acute cholecystitis. Unfortunately, physical examination of the intubated and sedated critically ill ICU patient is unreliable.

Although abdominal ultrasonography is considered the most accurate diagnostic imaging technique for acute cholecystitis, the absence of gallstones in AAC decreases the sensitivity of this method from 88% to approximately 67%.

Rezende-Neto JB, Rotstein OD. Abdominal catastrophes in the intensive care unit setting. Critical Care Clinics 2013;29(4):1017-44.

Q12. Answer TFTTF

Partial pressures of CO_2 levels in a healthy adult are:
Inspired: 0.03 kPa (0.2 mm Hg).
Alveolar: 5.3 kPa (40 mm Hg).
Arterial: 5.3 kPa (40 mm Hg).

Venous: 6.1 kPa (46 mm Hg).
Expired: 4 kPa (40 mm Hg).

Q13. Answer TFFTT

Unlike VKAs, which can be antagonized by vitamin K, the new DOAs have no specific antidote.

The INR performed in routine practice is standardized to measure the effect of VKAs, but not so for DOAs. For a given concentration, the results for PT and aPTT vary between individuals. The therapeutic ranges and safety thresholds of INR validated for VKAs do not apply to these new anticoagulants.

DOAs differ in their rate and extent of digestive adsorption and in the mechanisms and rate of elimination, predominantly renal or hepatobiliary.

DOAs have consistently been associated with a lower bleeding risk compared to warfarin.

Faraon D, Levy JH, Albaladejo P, et al. Updates in the perioperative and emergency management of non-vitamin K antagonist oral anticoagulants. Critical Care. 2015;19:203.

Q14. Answer TTFFT

True complications of massive blood transfusion can be classified as immediate and late.

The immediate complications include
  i. Inadequate or overzealous resuscitation
  ii. Dilutional coagulopathy
  iii. Citrate toxicity
  iv. Hyperkalemia
  v. hypothermia
  vi. hypomagnesemia
  vii. acidosis

Patil V, Shetmahajan M. Massive transfusion and massive transfusion protocol. Indian J Anaesth. 2014;58(5):590-5.

Q15. Answer FTTFT

The uterus remains protected and sheltered from abdominal injury by the pelvis until approximately 12 weeks of gestation. After that uterus becomes extra- pelvic and more vulnerable to injury.

Judicious use of X-rays and CT scans should be considered if there are no other modalities to diagnose a suspected injury.

The most common cause of fetal death after blunt injury is abruptio placentae.

Signs of blood loss such as tachycardia and hypotension may be delayed until the pregnant patient loses nearly 30% of blood volume. As a result, the fetus may be experiencing hypoperfusion long before the mother manifests any signs of hypotension.

Left tilting of gravid uterus prevents aortocaval compression syndrome and improves venous return to heart.

Dobiesz VA, Robinson DW. Trauma in Pregnancy. In: Walls RM, Hockberger RS, Gausche-Hill M (Eds). Rosen's Emergency Medicine: Concepts and Clinical Practice, 9th edn. Philadelphia, USA; Elsevier: 2018. pp. 2313-21.

Q16. Answer TTTTT

BioMed Research International. Volume 2015 (2015), Article ID 724032, 9 pages.
Available from: http://dx.doi.org/10.1155/2015/724032 (Accessed on 20th June 2017).

Q17. Answer TFFFT

The initial serum amylase test is neither a sensitive nor specific test for pancreatic injury (i.e., a normal amylase result does not exclude pancreatic injury), and an elevated amylase may be the result of an increase in salivary amylase.

Blunt trauma patients who are stable with positive FAST Exam should undergo CT exam for further evaluation.

Despite being sensitive for solid organ injury, CT is less capable of detecting injuries to the hollow viscera.

Martin RS, Meredith JW . Management of Acute Trauma. In: Townsend Jr CM, Beauchamp RD, Evers BM, et al (Eds). Sabiston Textbook of Surgery, 20th edn. Philadelphia USA; Elsivier:2017. p.407-448.

Dudeja V, Christein JD, Jensen EH, et al (Eds). Exocrine Pancreas. In: Townsend Jr CM, Beauchamp RD, Evers BM, et al (Eds). Sabiston Textbook of Surgery, 20th edn. Philadelphia USA; Elsivier. 2017. pp. 1520-55.

Q18. Answer TTFTF

An elevated D-dimer alone is insufficient to make a diagnosis of PE, but can be used to rule out PE especially in patients with low to moderate risk of pulmonary embolism. D-dimer testing is best used in conjunction with clinical probability assessment.

Inferior vena cava filter insertion does not prevent DVT and may increase the incidence of DVT; however, the filter can prevent a pulmonary embolism.

Barrera LM, Perel P, Ker K, et al. Thromboprophylaxis for trauma patients. Cochrane Database Syst Rev. 2013;(3):CD008303.

Hemmila MR, Osborne NH, Henke PK, et al. Prophylactic inferior vena cava filter placement does not result in a survival benefit for trauma patients. Ann Surg. 2015;262(4):577-85.

Q19. Answer FTFTT

PTV is most commonly detected on the large basal intracranial arteries: the internal carotid, the middle cerebral artery (MCA), and the basilar artery (BA) and less frequently on posterior cerebral arteries.

Most of the time, PTV seems to be associated with tSAH.

TCD measures cerebral blood flow velocities in major intracranial blood vessels to detect vasospasm in the first 2 to 3 weeks.

It typically develops between 12 hours and 5 days after injury and lasts anywhere between 12 hours and 30 days.

Although PTV morphologically resembles aneurysmal vasospasm, whether the former entails similar clinical significance as the latter is still under investigation.

Perrein A, Petry L, Reis A, et al. Cerebral vasospasm after traumatic brain injury: an update. Minerva Anestesiol 2015;81:1219-28.

Oertel M, Boscardin WJ, Obrist WD, et al. Posttraumatic vasospasm: the epidemiology, severity, and time course of an underestimated phenomenon: a prospective study performed in 299 patients. J Neurosurg. 2005;103(5):812-24.

Q20. Answer TFTTF

An OPTX occurs when air is trapped within the pleural space but is only identified on a CT scan after a normal chest radiograph. The gold standard for ruling out pneumothorax is a thoracic CT scan.

Approximately 2% to 10% of trauma patients will be seen with an OPTX. There are generally no associated clinical findings on presentation.

In ultrasound exam of OPTX, the abolition of lung sliding alone or with absent A line sign or lung point sign have high sensitivity and specificity.

The risk of progression of a known pneumothorax to a tension pneumothorax is significant.

Lichtenstein DA, Mezière G, Lascols N, et al. Ultrasound diagnosis of occult pneumothorax. Crit. Care Med. 2005;33(6):1231-8.

Omar HR, Abdelmalak H, Mangar D, et al. Occult pneumothorax, revisited. J Trauma Manag Outcomes. 2010;4:12.

Q21. Answer TFTFT

The "Rule of Nines" divides the body surface into areas of nine percent (%) or multiples of nine percent, with the exception that the perineum is estimated at one percent (%). This allows the extent of the burn to be estimated with reproducible accuracy.

Rule of Nine
- Head/neck—9% TBSA
- Each arm—9% TBSA
- Anterior thorax—18% TBSA
- Posterior thorax—18% TBSA
- Each leg—18% TBSA
- Perineum—1% TBSA

Hettiaratchy S, Papini R. Initial management of a major burn: II—assessment and resuscitation. BMJ. 2004;329(7457):101-3.

Q22. Answer TTTFF

In the United States, 82% to 95% of renal injuries are secondary to blunt trauma, slightly less than the 93% observed in Canada and 97% in Europe.

Most renal, bladder, and posterior urethral trauma is from blunt mechanisms, most commonly motor vehicle collisions.

Most ureteral and anterior urethral injuries are iatrogenic.

The pelvic ureter is involved in 80% of iatrogenic ureteral injuries, making it by far the most commonly involved segment.

Several large literature reviews have found that extraperitoneal bladder ruptures make up most injuries (55–78%), with the rest consisting of intraperitoneal (17–39%) and combined intraperitoneal and extraperitoneal (5–8%) ruptures.

McGeady JB, Breyer BN. Current epidemiology of genitourinary trauma. Urol Clin North Am. 2013;40(3):323-34.

Q23. Answer TTFFT

The abdominal FAST examination is designed to identify fluid within the abdomen/pelvis which is suggestive of blood in the setting of trauma.

The FAST exam is not designed to reliably detect injuries to the solid organs, intestine, mesentery, diaphragm, nor the retroperitoneal hemorrhage that may occur with pelvic fractures.

Volumes of less than 400 mL in the right upper quadrant (RUQ) may not be detected by FAST. In the presence of clear physical findings on examination, the decision for exploratory laparotomy should not be distracted by a negative FAST.

Free blood only remains echolucent, or anechoic (black), on ultrasound until it begins to clot. It can then become more echogenic (bright) and more difficult to differentiate from the surrounding tissue.

Williams SR, Perera P, Gharahbaghian L. The FAST and E-FAST in 2013: Trauma ultrasonography: Overview, practical techniques, controversies, and new frontiers. Critical care clinics. 2014;30(1):119-50.

Q24. Answer FFTTT

The minimal data set for diagnosis of SAIDH is hyponatremia in a euvolemic patient with inappropriately concentrated urine (osmolality >100 mOsm/kg), elevated urine sodium (>30 mmol/L), and exclusion of cortisol and thyroid hormone insufficiency.

Decreased plasma volume is seen in cerebral salt-wasting syndrome.

Hypothyroid patients have elevated AVP responses to subtle volume contraction. Hyponatremia in hypothyroidism is rare, but life-threatening hyponatremia has been occasionally reported.

Acute pituitary dysfunction occurs commonly following TBI and subarachnoid hemorrhage. ACTH deficiency can present as SIADH.

Grant P, Ayuk J, Bouloux PM, et al. The diagnosis and management of inpatient hyponatraemia and SIADH. Eur J Clin Invest. 2015;45(8):888-94.

Q25. Answer FFTTT

Although a decreasing GCS score suggests an expanding intracranial lesion, which may be intracerebral or subdural or epidural, a GCS score of 15 does not exclude the possibility of brain injury.

Use of the pupillary examination for localization of an intracranial lesion is neither sensitive nor specific.

In the severely head-injured patient, the CN examination is often limited to the pupillary responses (CN III), gag reflex (CNs IX and X), and corneal reflex (CNs V and VII).

Decorticate posturing implies injury above the midbrain.

The rate of decerebrate posturing increases significantly in the presence of midbrain lesions. Decerebrate posturing is the result of a more caudal injury, and therefore is associated with a worse prognosis.

Papa L, Goldberg SA. Head trauma. In: Walls RM, Hockberger RS, Gausche-Hill M (Eds). Rosen's Emergency Medicine: Concepts and Clinical Practice, 9th edn. Philadelphia, USA; Elsevier: 2018.301-29.

Q26. Answer TFTFT

Diffuse axonal injury (DAI) is a frequent result of traumatic acceleration/deceleration or rotational injuries.

In DAI, axons sustain a primary insult in which they are torn (axotomy) or stretched, and secondary insults lead to axon death.

DAI is the most common cause of posttraumatic coma, disability, and a persistent neurovegetative state.

Axons in the white matter appear to be especially vulnerable to injury. Small petechial hemorrhages located at the gray-white matter junction, as well as in the corpus callosum and brainstem, are characteristic of CT-scan findings in the acute setting.

MRI has proven to be the optimal means of detection and characterization of DAI lesions.

Liu J, Kou Z, Tian Y. Diffuse axonal injury after traumatic cerebral microbleeds: an evaluation of imaging techniques. Neural Regen Res. 2014;9(12):1222-30.

Johnson VE, Stewart W, Smith DH. Axonal pathology in traumatic brain injury. Exp Neurol. 2013;246:35-43.

Q27. Answer FTTTF

Lucid interval may be present in approximately 47% of patients with EDHs but is not pathognomonic of EDH as patients with subdural hematoma and with other mass lesions may also have lucid period.

EDH can cross the dural attachments but not the cranial sutures, because the hematoma exists in the potential space between the dura and the inner table of the skull.

The low density in the hematoma indicates active extravasation of fresh unclotted blood (swirl sign) and warrants immediate surgical attention.

The middle meningeal artery or one of its branches is the common source of hematoma.

EDH is common in young adults. Children, because of a compliant skull, and older people, because of a firm dural attachment to the skull, have lower incidences of EDH.

Bodanapally UK, Sours C, Zhuo J, Shanmuganathan K. Imaging of traumatic brain injury. Radiologic Clinics of North America. 2015;53(4):695-715.

Ganz JC. The lucid interval associated with epidural bleeding: evolving understanding. J Neurosurg. 2013;118(4):739-45.

Q28. Answer TTFTF

The deadly triad of trauma includes hypothermia, acidosis and coagulopathy. To successfully resuscitate the critically ill trauma patient, all emergency providers must have a firm understanding of the lethal triad. This understanding should serve as the cornerstone for all interventions provided to the bleeding trauma patient. Left untreated, hypothermia, acidosis and coagulopathy bring about and propagate each other, eventually resulting in a predictable but irreversible progression toward death.

Gerecht R. Trauma's Lethal Triad of Hypothermia, Acidosis & Coagulopathy Create a Deadly Cycle for Trauma Patients. Available from: http://www.jems.com/articles/print/volume-39/issue-4/features/trauma-s-lethal-triad-hypothermia-acidos.html (Accessed 11 August 2017).

Q29. Answer FFFTT

Glasgow Coma Scale (GCS) is a neurological scale to record the conscious state of a person for initial as well as subsequent assessment. A patient is assessed against the criteria of the scale, between 3 and 15. It has three elements—eye opening, best motor response and best verbal response each having score points of 1-4, 1-5 and 1-6 respectively.

Bordini AL, Luiz TF, Fernandes M, et al. Coma scales: a historical review. Arq Neuropsiquiatr. 2010;68(6):930-7.

Q30. Answer TFFTT

Flail chest represents the most severe form of chest wall injury after blunt trauma, with more than 80% of patients needing ICU admission, more than 50% requiring mechanical ventilation, and an overall mortality of 16%. The treatment of rib fractures and flail chest is nonoperative in the vast majority of cases, and patients usually can be managed successfully with aggressive pain control, early and effective pulmonary toilet, and supportive care. Use of noninvasive positive airway pressure by mask may obviate the need for endotracheal intubation in alert patients. Patients with severe injuries, respiratory distress, or progressively worsening respiratory function require endotracheal intubation and mechanical ventilatory support.

Moore MS, Pieracci FM, Jurkovich GJ. Chest Wall, pneumothorax, and hemothorax. In: Cameron JL, Cameron AM (Eds). Current Surgical Therapy. 12th edn. Philadelphia USA: Elsevier; 2017. pp.1151-8.

CHAPTER 13

Ethics, Quality Assurance and End of Life Care

RK Mani

A Type Questions
(One best answer)

1. **Autonomy means all of the following *except*:**
   a. Respect to patient's wishes and values
   b. Patient should be regarded as a person
   c. Patient has the right to refuse any proposed medical treatment
   d. Patient has the right to complete information about his condition
   e. Patient has the right to dictate treatment

2. **Substituted judgment by surrogate means:**
   a. Deciding on behalf of the patient
   b. Acting in the best interests of the patient
   c. Deciding according to one's own wishes and values
   d. Deciding according to patient's wishes and values
   e. Negotiating a decision with caregivers

3. **Beneficence is all of the following *except*:**
   a. Always acting in the best interests of the patient
   b. Weighing risks and benefits of a proposed intervention
   c. Acting according to the wishes of the patient
   d. Considering physical benefit over personal choices of the patient
   e. Not insisting on starting or continuing futile therapies

4. **Non-malfeasance is all of the following *except*:**
   a. To do no intended harm
   b. To ensure benefit that outweighs harm
   c. Harm is to be assessed from the physiological stand point
   d. To consider whole person concerns
   e. Protect family from preventable harm

5. **Social justice requires all of the following *except*:**
   a. Careful allocation of resources
   b. Rationing of resources in favor of salvageable patients
   c. Overriding individual right to treatment
   d. Not proposing futile therapies to curtail wastage
   e. Treating all patients equitably and fairly

6. **"Double effect" with regard to palliation means:**
   a. Analgesia and sedation should be avoided
   b. That harmful effects of these drugs should be documented
   c. Non-pharmacological means of palliation should be adopted
   d. Use of the drugs having potentially harmful side effects is illegal
   e. Use is ethically correct if freedom from pain is intended and harm is unintended

7. **The widely accepted model for end of life decision making is:**
   a. Paternalism
   b. Autonomy
   c. Family-centric
   d. Futility-based
   e. Shared decision-making

8. **Advance directives include all *except*:**
   a. Should be taken into decision making when patient loses capacity
   b. Should be strictly followed without discussion with surrogates or caregivers
   c. Becomes operative only in the event of patient's loss of capacity
   d. Can be revised anytime if the patient chooses to do so.
   e. It is one of the instruments for exercising autonomy when patient loses capacity

9. **Do not resuscitate order (DNR) is:**
   a. A form of active euthanasia
   b. It is illegal in India
   c. It is unethical as CPR is an imperative
   d. It is a refusal or withholding of the medical intervention of CPR
   e. It is a form of withdrawing of life support

10. **Foregoing of life support is none of the following *except*:**
    a. A form of active euthanasia
    b. Not acceptable in medical ethics
    c. The rule in the majority of ICU deaths in US and Northern Europe
    d. not supported by US laws
    e. Is decided unilaterally by physicians in most parts of the world

K Type Questions
[Marked True (T)/False (F)]

1. **End of life decision making involves the following:**
   a. Sending patient home through a Left Against Medical Advice (LAMA) process
   b. Truth telling or open and complete information at the earliest
   c. Prohibiting second opinion to avoid confusion
   d. Waiting for a decision until consensus of goals of care achieved among caregivers
   e. Documentation of family conferencing

2. **The following is true of legal position of EOLC in India:**
   a. Withdrawal and withholding decisions are illegal
   b. There is no consensus professional position on EOLC in India
   c. Advance Directives have legal validity in India
   d. Validation by Court is required for" involuntary passive euthanasia" for vegetative patients
   e. Indian Law does acknowledge foregoing of life support in terminal care

3. **The term Euthanasia implies:**
   a. Active ending of life of a patient by a physician with an intention of killing at the patient's request
   b. Active shortening of the dying process
   c. Withdrawal or withholding of life support
   d. DNR order or allowing natural death
   e. Physician assisting in suicide

4. **In the event of conflict in end of life decision making between family and caregivers do the following as the initial step:**
   a. Take a unilateral decision citing futility
   b. Accept family decision to continue even if futile
   c. Accept family decision to withdraw even if patient is deemed salvageable
   d. Negotiate through repeated family conferencing
   e. Refer the matter to an independent committee

5. **Palliative care:**
   a. Is not a part of ICU care
   b. Is the sole goal of care after withholding and withdrawal decision
   c. Is a part of end of life care
   d. Is instituted after an end of life decision
   e. It is a part of the entire ICU care

6. **Barriers to quality EOLC in India includes:**
   a. Public unawareness of implications of futile life support
   b. Clear law and minimum litigation
   c. Lack of professional guidelines for EOLC
   d. Lack of training at graduate and post graduate levels
   e. Social unawareness of the right to privacy as applied to medical treatment

7. **Family communication studies reveal the following:**
   a. Inadequate information about patient's condition
   b. Greater proportion of conversations occupied by family

c. Failure to address and support emotions
d. Appropriate address to patient's values and wishes
e. Failure to affirm non abandonment

8. **Regarding withholding and withdrawal of support:**
   a. Both are held to be equivalent ethically
   b. Withdrawing is ethically not equivalent to withholding
   c. Withdrawing is held to be more difficult than withholding in countries with EOLC laws
   d. Withdrawing is not needed when withholding is more easily acceptable
   e. LAMA is not equivalent to treatment withdrawal

9. **Regarding brain death:**
   a. Equivalent to circulatory death and life support should be withdrawn
   b. Not equivalent to death except for the purpose of organ donation
   c. Is equivalent to death but life support should not be withdrawn if organ donation is declined
   d. In case of brain death life support cannot be withdrawn without family consent
   e. Indian case law states brain death is equivalent to death

10. **Family satisfaction is associated with:**
    a. Consistency in goals of care among care givers
    b. Conveying of the news of death over phone
    c. Being prepared for death of the patient
    d. Advance care planning not necessarily involving the patient
    e. Having an open visitation system in the ICU

ANSWERS

A Type Answers

Q1. Answer e

Autonomy does not mean the patient can dictate medical treatment and demand interventions that are medically untenable. It is the physician's prerogative. Autonomy means respecting patient's choices and preferences. This translates in practice as the right of informed consent or refusal. For any medical intervention except in special circumstances, a consent form needs to be signed by the patient or surrogate. This would equally apply to life prolonging interventions. Physicians are by common law bound to respect patient's refusal who has received complete information even if this would lead to his or her death. The physician's approach should thus be to address the patient as a whole person than merely as a disease entity. Open and complete disclosure of information is thus an essential part of empowering the patient in taking an autonomous decision.

> Carlet J, Thijs LG, Antonelli M, et al. Challenges in end-of-life care in the ICU: Statement of the 5th International Consensus Conference in Critical Care: Brussels, Belgium, April 2003. Intensive Care Medicine. 2004;30:770-84.
>
> Truog RD, Campbell ML, Curtis JR, et al. Recommendations for end-of-life care in the intensive care unit: A consensus statement by the American College of Critical Care Medicine Crit Care Med 2008;36:953-63.

Q2. Answer d

The surrogate should be faithful to patient's wishes and values and should be careful not to project one's own opinions. To be able to exercise his/her autonomy directly the patient should be mentally competent to identify and express his/her choices. If the patient has lost capacity, the right of autonomy is maintained through other means. His/her preferences are to be elicited from the next of kin or a duly appointed legal representative and are termed as "substituted judgment".

> Crippen D, Kilcullen JK, Kelly DF, editors. Three patients: international perspectives on intensive care at the end of life. Kluver Academic Publishers, Mass: USA; 2002.

Q3. Answer d

Beneficence is not just to the physical state of the patient, but as for Autonomy it is directed at the personality of the patient and extends to protecting his whole person. Beneficence flows from the fiduciary obligation to act always in patient's best interests. While the disease can still be cured or controlled, this obligation translates as the need to carefully weigh the risks and benefits of any intervention. In terminal illness since benefits of a curative intervention are negligible, foregoing of life support (FLST) would be in patient's best interest. This is even more so when patients' values and preferences suggest that such interventions are unwanted. Best interests also include protecting him/her and the family from economic or social difficulties when these are clearly expressed. Physician's insisting on continuation of futile therapies is therefore to be regarded as violation of this principle.

> Kinsinger FS. Beneficence and the professional's moral imperative. J Chiropr Humanit. 2009;16(1):44-6.

Q4. Answer c

This is a narrow interpretation. The contemporary view is to mean no harm to the cherished interests of the patient. Non-malfeasance comes from the doctrine of "first of all do not harm". However this needs to be interpreted appropriately in terminal illness. Harm confined only to the physiological stand point would be too narrow an interpretation. A dying patient and family should be given the opportunity to prepare for death. An appropriate environment for ensuring good death should be made available. All the while whole person's interests should be safeguarded. The family too must be protected from harm that may accrue from incomplete information, financial pressure of disproportionate treatments and posttraumatic stress disorder from inadequate attention to counseling during the dying process and bereavement.

> Cook D, Rocker G, Heyland D. Dying in the ICU: strategies that may improve end-of-life care. CAN J ANESTH 2004 / 51: 3 / pp 266-72.

Q5. Answer c

Social justice can never be unjust to the individual interest. It only aims at treatment without bias or prejudice. Social justice means allocating resources appropriate to the medical condition of the patient in order to maximize their benefits and minimize wastage. Futile application of therapies would clearly violate this social obligation. Situations may arise when patient or family may insist on therapies physicians would consider inappropriate, when the principles of autonomy and justice may appear to be in conflict. In such an event repeated communication and negotiating a middle path may be the best course. It would also be worth remembering that the physician is bound to act only according to professional standards of care and not obliged to follow blindly the dictates of the patient.

>Carlet J, Thijs LG, Antonelli M, et al. Challenges in end-of-life care in the ICU: Statement of the 5th International Consensus Conference in Critical Care: Brussels, Belgium, April 2003. Intensive Care Medicine. 2004;30:770-84.

Q6. Answer e

Freedom from pain and distress is a fundamental right and withholding adequate palliative therapy would violate this principle. The doctrine of "double effect" addresses the situation when adequate analgesia and sedation may have the unintended side effect of shortening the dying process. This principle clearly sets the obligation to provide freedom from pain and distress above the principle to do no harm provided the harm is unintended. Intention is revealed in the care taken to titrate the drug dosing which would mean that protocols for palliative therapy should be in place and documentation should be meticulous. Of course doses beyond usual recommendations should be adequately justified.

>Quill TE, Dresser R, Brock DW. The role of double effect- a critique of its role in decision-making. N Engl J Med. 1997;337:1768-71.

Q7. Answer e

The model is based on the assumption that two types of expertise are being blended together: the physician is an expert at the patient's disease condition, and the family is best at representing the patient's interest. Neither of this is invariably true. The potential fallibility on the part of the physician mandates that the decision be made by a body of responsible medical persons rather than individually. An iterative process is integrated into the decision-making process. Second opinions should be sought or facilitated when family raises concerns. Determining accurate diagnosis and prognosis is not always easy and uncertainty should be shared candidly.

>Gjerberg E, Lillemoen L, Førde R, Pedersen R. End-of-life care communications and shared decision-making in Norwegian nursing homes - experiences and perspectives of patients and relatives. BMC Geriatr. 2015;15:103.

Q8. Answer b

'Should be strictly followed without discussion with surrogates or caregivers' is incorrect as patient's choices are to be integrated into a holistic and pragmatic decision in the best interests of the patient. An advance Will as permitted in US law documents patient's preferences in times of full mental capacity and is to be taken into account in EOLD by caregivers. In case patient's wishes and preferences are unknown the physician is expected to act in his/her "best interests".

>Truog RD, Campbell ML, Curtis JR, et al. Recommendations for end-of-life care in the intensive care unit: A consensus statement by the American College of Critical Care Medicine Crit Care Med. 2008;36:953-63.

Q9. Answer d

Do not resuscitate (DNR), alternatively known as 'no code' or 'allow natural death', is a legal order written either in the hospital or on a legal form to withhold cardiopulmonary resuscitation (CPR) or advanced cardiac life support (ACLS), in respect of the wishes of patients in case their heart were to stop or they were to stop breathing. Successful resuscitation is a marvel of modern medicine. But the reality is that only 5% of Cardio pulmonary resuscitation (CPR) are for sudden cardiac death. Of the rest successful resuscitation is possible in only 15-20% for shockable rhythms and even less for asystolic arrest. Outcomes of CPR in critically ill patients is beneficial in less than 5%.

>Sprung C L, Truog RD, Curtis JR, et al. Seeking Worldwide Professional Consensus on the Principles of End-of-Life Care for the Critically Ill. Am J Respir Crit Care Med. 2014;190:855-66.

Q10. Answer c

Prognostic uncertainty is real in Medicine. In India this has led to excessive caution in initiating End of Life Care (EOLC) discussions and forgoing of life supporting treatments (FLST). Despite this difficulty being the same everywhere, in developed nations 75-90% of dying patients receive an FLST decision in the ICU settings.

Learning to revise goals for the patient in response to changes in clinical status is an inescapable necessity in Medicine. Judging benefit versus harm is likewise a basic tenet termed as "acting in best interests". Evidence based medicine is rooted in such assessment. Uncertainty should be looked at both ways- in terms of likely benefit and likely harms.

> Sprung CL, Truog RD, Curtis JR, et al. Seeking Worldwide Professional Consensus on the Principles of End-of-Life Care for the Critically Ill. Am J Respir Crit Care Med; 2014;190:855-66.
>
> Prendergast TJ, Claessens MT, Luce JM. A national survey of end-of-life care for critically ill patients. Am J Respir Crit Care Med. 1998;158(4):1163-7.

K Type Answers

Q1. Answer FTFTT

LAMA certainly is not an appropriate end of life decision. A valid EOLC decision involves a deliberate algorithmic approach as outlined in the ISCCM –IAPC joint ethical Position Statement. This 12-step process integrates the end of life decision with palliative care for the patient and post bereavement care for the family. Comprehensive care of the dying is bypassed in LAMA which is ethically untenable.

> Myatra SN, Salins N, Iyer S, et al. End-of-life care policy: An integrated care plan for the dying. Ind J Crit Care Med. 2014;18: 615-635.

Q2. Answer FFTTF

There is consensus professional position on EOLC in India. The first position statement by the ISCCM was published in 2005, a revised form in 2012 and recently as a joint statement with the Indian Association of Palliative care (IAPC). There is as yet no legal or legislative position. A withdrawal or withholding decision should be implemented after completing a life support limitation form duly signed by the patient's family and the treating team. Advance directive stating the patient's preference is not a practice in India but public awareness in this regard should be encouraged. The Law Commission of India proposed that advance directives and legal powers of attorney shall be deemed invalid for decision-making as it may "create complications". In March 2011, *Aruna Shanbaug* the Supreme Court of India ruled that "involuntary passive euthanasia was allowed in principle" but must follow a strict procedure involving clearance by a High Court.

> Myatra SN, Salins N, Iyer S, et al. End-of-life care policy: An integrated care plan for the dying. Ind J Crit Care Med. 2014;18: 615-35.
>
> Mani RK, Amin P, Chawla R, et al. ISCCM position statement: limiting life-prolonging interventions and providing palliative care towards the end of life in Indian intensive care units. Indian J Crit Care Med. 2005;9:96-107.

Q3. Answer TFFFF

Active ending of life of a patient by a physician with an intention of killing at the patient's request. This is the universally accepted definition which should be followed. Otherwise there is a tendency to paint the entire FSLT with the same brush of the term "euthanasia". Terms used in common parlance serve only to confound the issue of treatment limitation. The Law Commission has also separated the term euthanasia from withdrawal and withholding decisions.

> Sprung CL, Truog RD, Curtis JR, et al. Seeking Worldwide Professional Consensus on the Principles of End-of-Life Care for the Critically Ill. Am J Respir Crit Care Med. 2014;190:855-66.
>
> Law Commission of India. 196th report (2006). Medical treatment of terminally ill patients (for the protection of patients and Medical practitioners). Available from: http://lawcommissionofindia.nic.in/reports/rep196.pdf(Accessed 23 July 2017).

Q4. Answer FFFTF

Negotiate through repeated family conferencing. This should be the first step. End of life decision making is a deliberate, iterative process and it is rooted in respecting the patient's free choice. The principle is not to enforce one's own opinion of what should be. Additionally an independent oversight committee is recommended by professional Societies for arbitration and review.

> Sprung CL, Cohen SL, Sjokvist P, et al. Ethicus Study Group. End-of-life practices in European intensive careunits: the ETHICUS study. JAMA. 2003;290(6):790-7.
>
> Mani RK, Amin P, Chawla R, et al. ISCCM position statement: limiting life-prolonging interventions and providing palliative care towards the end of life in Indian intensive care units. Indian J Crit Care Med. 2005;9:96-107.

Mani RK, Amin P, Chawla R, et al. Guidelines for end-of-life and palliative care in Indian ICUs: ISCCM consensus ethical position statement. Indian J Crit Care Med. 2012;16(3):166-81.

Q5. Answer FFTFT

Intensive care and palliative care are concurrent, not consecutive to each other. In the phase of curative treatment palliative care forms a small but integral part. As the clinical course evolves to end of life, the curative treatments give way to increasing proportions of palliative forms of care.

Myatra SN, Salins N, Iyer S, et al. End-of-life care policy: An integrated care plan for the dying. Ind J Crit Care Med. 2014;18: 615-635.

Q6. Answer TFFTT

Professional guidelines both national and international have existed since 2003. Indian case laws are scarce and dealing mainly with the issues of suicide and euthanasia. There is none directly addressing withdrawal or withholding life support, i.e., FLST. Indian Law is yet to be adequately informed on the requirements of terminally ill or incurably incapacitated patients. With a society that is increasingly strident and litigious, the fear of treatment limitation decisions being misconstrued as deficiency of service or as active euthanasia dominates the psyche of the clinician. These fears are reflected in the paper by Barnett and Aurora. The barriers to improving EOLC in India are complex involving several socio cultural and legal misperceptions.

Gursahani R, Mani RK. India: not a country to die in. Indian J Med Ethics. 2016;13(1):30-5.

Q7. Answer TFTFT

Greater proportion of speech is occupied by physicians (75%) which is associated with greater family dissatisfaction. The other factors were failure to elicit patient's values and wishes, failure to listen to and address family concerns, failure to provide empathetic support and failure to affirm non abandonment once the focus shifts to comfort care. Patient's values and wishes are inappropriately addressed.

McDonagh JR, Elliott TB, Engelberg RA, et al. Family satisfaction with family conferences about end-of-life care in the intensive care unit: Increased proportion of family speech is associated with increased satisfaction. Crit Care Med. 2004;32:1484-8.

Curtis JR, Engelberg RA, Wenrich MD, et al. Missed opportunities during family conferences about end-of-life care in the intensive care unit. Am J Respir Crit Care Med. 2005;171:844-9.

Q8. Answer TFFFT

Withholding and withdrawal of support are held to be equivalent ethically. That is the widely accepted bioethical principle. They are held to be equivalent as the underlying principle is to leave the patient alone when he has expressed a wish against the intervention. Both are founded on respect for patient's autonomy. If withdrawal were held to be unnecessary then trials of ICU care would be denied to those who may prove to be salvageable later. In view of the uncertainty in EOLC decisions the option of such trials are frequently in order.

Truog RD, Campbell ML, Curtis JR, Haas CE, Luce JM, Rubenfeld GD et. al. Recommendations for end-of-life care in the intensive care unit: A consensus statement by the American College of Critical Care Medicine. *Crit Care Med.* 2008;36:953-963.

Q9. Answer TFFFT

'Brain death is equivalent to circulatory death and life support should be withdrawn' is currently the widely accepted position. This is yet to be clarified in Indian Law although the Human Organ Transplantation Act (1994) describes brain death as a deceased state. The anomaly of brain death not being acknowledged as death outside of the context of organ donation is yet to be unequivocally rectified. In the Aruna Shanbaug judgment (2012) the bench described brain death as equivalent to death.

Aruna Ramachandra Shanbaug vs The Union of India & Ors. WRIT PETITION(CRIMINAL) NO. 115 OF 2009 (Supreme Court of India Proceedings).

Q10. Answer TFTFT

Breaking bad news should be a competency for training. Family satisfaction is a quality measure in the ICU. Inappropriate communication and lack of sensitivity in managing dying patients and their families are associated with poor quality EOLC.

Curtis JR, Engelberg RA. Measuring success of interventions to improve the quality of end-of-life care in the intensive care unit. Crit Care Med. 2006;34[Suppl.]:S341-S7.

CHAPTER 14

General Critical Care

Deven Juneja, Anish Gupta

A Type Questions
(One best answer)

1. **A 67-year-old male patient is admitted to your ICU with a diagnosis of acute ischemic stroke. On examination, he has complete paralysis of right side of the body. As he is out of the window period, thrombolysis is not considered. Which of the following statements is NOT TRUE regarding venous thromboembolism (VTE) prophylaxis in this patient?**
   a. VTE is more common in the initial few months after acute stroke
   b. VTE prophylaxis should be initiated as soon as possible
   c. Unfractionated heparin (UFH) is preferred over low molecular weight heparin (LMWH)
   d. UFH/LMWH should be withheld for at least 24 hours if thrombolysis is performed
   e. UFH/LMWH may be initiated in the immediate postoperative period, if the patient requires hemicraniectomy or endovascular procedures

2. **All the following are complications of hypervolemia *except*:**
   a. Increased demand on cardiac function
   b. Delayed wound healing
   c. Coagulation disturbances
   d. Cause acute kidney injury
   e. Increased mortality

3. **Oxygen delivery (DO2) is defined as the total amount of oxygen delivered to the body tissues by the heart per minute. It depends on all the following parameters *except*:**
   a. Heart rate
   b. Hemoglobin
   c. Arterial hemoglobin oxygen saturation
   d. Oxygen consumption (VO_2)
   e. Stroke volume

4. **Which of the following toxicities may lead to respiratory alkalosis?**
   a. Salicylates
   b. Opioid
   c. Benzodiazepine
   d. Diuretics
   e. Cyanide

5. **All of the following drugs may lead to bradycardia *except*:**
   a. Digoxin
   b. Organophosphates
   c. Ergot alkaloids
   d. Tricyclic antidepressants (TCAs)
   e. Opioids

6. **All of the following common ICU disorders may lead to dysmotility *except*:**
   a. Hyperglycemia
   b. Hypokalemia
   c. Hyperphosphatemia
   d. Intra-abdominal hypertension
   e. Intracranial hypertension

7. **Permissive hypoxemia is preferred in which of the following condition?**
   a. Paraquat poisoning
   b. Carbon monoxide poisoning

c. Myocardial infarction
d. Procedural sedation

8. The following are components of qSOFA *except*:
   a. SBP < 100 mm Hg
   b. GCS < 15
   c. Respiratory rate > 22/min
   d. Heart rate > 100/min

9. As per the American Academy of Neurology guidelines what is the level of Neuron Specific Enolase (NSE) above which it is suggestive of poor outcome?
   a. 11 ug/L
   b. 22 ug/L
   c. 33 ug/L
   d. 44 ug/L

10. The Beauchamp Childress system of medical ethics is based on all the following principles *except*:
    a. Beneficience
    b. Maleficience
    c. Autonomy
    d. Distributive justice

11. The N20 response to assess the somatosensory function in post cardiac arrest patients is assessed by stimulation of which nerve:
    a. Radial nerve
    b. Median nerve
    c. Ulnar nerve
    d. Brachial plexus

12. All the following EEG patterns are associated with poor neurological outcome in post cardiac arrest patients *except*:
    a. Generalized suppression
    b. Burst suppression
    c. Presence of reactivity
    d. Periodic epileptiform discharges

13. All the following are causes of raised A-a gradient *except*:
    a. V/Q mismatch
    b. Shunt
    c. Alveolar Hypoventilation
    d. Diffusion defect

14. All the following are measured parameters on ABG *except*:
    a. pH
    b. $PaCO_2$
    c. PO_2
    d. HCO_3

15. A Pulse oximetry measures the difference in absorption between two wavelengths of light to measure SpO_2. The wavelengths are:
    a. 660 nm and 940 nm
    b. 680 and 920 nm
    c. 640 and 960 nm
    d. 620 and 980 nm

16. All the following factors shift the oxygen-hemoglobin dissociation curve to the right *except*:
    a. Increased temperature
    b. Increase 2,3-diphosphoglycerate (2,3-DPG)
    c. Decreased H+ ion concentration
    d. Decreased pH

17. The end-tidal CO_2 ($ETCO_2$) corresponds to the highest value during which phase of the time capnogram:
    a. Phase 0
    b. Phase 1
    c. Phase 2
    d. Phase 3

18. The following capnogram represents which of the following conditions:

    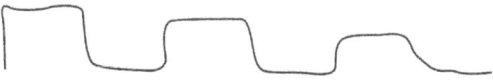

    a. Bronchospasm
    b. Cardiac arrest like situation
    c. Inadequate respiratory efforts
    d. Kinked ET tube

19. Fever in ICU is defined as a temperature more than:
    a. 38.3°C
    b. 39.3°C
    c. 38.6°C
    d. 39.6°C

20. All the following are recognized complications of metabolic alkalosis *except*:
    a. Reduced oxygen-Hb affinity
    b. Hypokalemia
    c. Neuromuscular excitability
    d. Digoxin toxicity
    e. Encephalopathy seizures

21. All the following are common causes of hypophosphatemia *except*:
    a. Refeeding syndrome
    b. Hypoparathyroidism
    c. Sepsis
    d. Vitamin D deficiency
    e. Burns

22. The cuff of an endotracheal tube having minimal effect on capillary perfusion is:
    a. High volume, High pressure
    b. Low volume, High pressure
    c. Low volume, Low pressure
    d. High volume, Low pressure

23. Continuous flush device used with arterial lines deliver fluid at:
    a. 2 ml/hr
    b. 3 ml/hr
    c. 4 ml/hr
    d. 5 ml/hr

24. All the following are causes of over damped waveform on arterial line *except*:
    a. Air bubbles
    b. Compliant tubing
    c. Low flush bag pressure
    d. Long tubing length

25. Which of the following principle was established by the declaration of Helsinki?
    a. Right to adequate medical care
    b. Ethics regarding human research and experimentation
    c. Right to die with dignity
    d. Ethical practice of medicine to treat patients

26. Beta error refers to:
    a. Type 1 error
    b. Type 2 error
    c. Type 3 error
    d. Type 4 error

27. A 24-year-female was admitted to the ICU with 60% burns following a gas cylinder leakage while cooking at home. On arrival, her vitals were as follows; HR – 136/min, RR – 36/min and BP – 124/58 mm Hg. She had labored breathing and a decision for intubation was made. Which of the following medications is contraindicated?
    a. Atracurium
    b. Succinylcholine
    c. Propofol
    d. Rocuronium

28. One of the following is a contraindication to lumbar puncture (LP):
    a. Platelet count 90,000/ul
    b. INR 1.6
    c. Bacteremia
    d. Antiplatelet therapy with Aspirin

29. Which of the following interventions helps to reduce the incidence of contrast induced nephropathy (CIN):
    a. Intravenous N-acetylcysteine
    b. IV crystalloid hydration
    c. Post contrast hemodialysis
    d. Low dose dopamine infusion

30. Which one of the following is FALSE regarding delirium in ICU?
    a. Inattention is a common feature
    b. Infections increase the risk of developing delirium
    c. The CAM-ICU model helps diagnose delirium
    d. Sedatives are safe in delirium
    e. Dexmedetomidine can prevent and treat delirium

K Type Questions
[Marked True (T)/False (F)]

1. Which of the following condition(s) interfere with the reading of pulse oximeter?
    a. Polycythemia
    b. Methemoglobinemia
    c. Shock
    d. Jaundice
    e. Nail polish

2. Comment on the following statements regarding targeted temperature management (TTM):
    a. TTM is contraindicated in patients with traumatic brain injury (TBI)
    b. In patients with severe TBI, TTM at 35–37°C should be done to improve survival with good neurological outcome
    c. In patients with TBI and refractory intracranial hypertension despite medical treatments, TTM at 34–35°C should be done with an aim to lower ICP
    d. TTM may be considered in patients with refractory or super-refractory status epilepticus, to control seizure activity
    e. Cooling upto 32°C may be required in patients with cardiogenic shock

3. Comment on the following statements regarding heparin induced thrombocytopenia (HIT):

a. Autoantibodies against the complex of platelet factor 4 bound to heparin are formed
b. Platelets generally fall by more than 50% within 5 to 10 days of exposure to heparin
c. Fall in platelet count is less rapid in patients who have been exposed to heparin previously
d. Timing and magnitude of thrombocytopenia is diagnostic of HIT
e. Medical patients are more likely to develop HIT

4. **Negative prognostic indicators post cardiac arrest includes:**
   a. Absence of axial myoclonus on day 1
   b. Absent pupillary and corneal reflex on day 3
   c. No motor response or extensor posturing on day 6
   d. Presence of N20 response on SSEP on day 2

5. **With respect to D- lactic acidosis comment on the following statements:**
   a. D- lactic acidosis is associated with short bowel syndrome
   b. It is often precipitated after a carbohydrate load
   c. Lactate levels are usually > 20
   d. Presentation is with non anion gap metabolic acidosis

6. **Drug fever:**
   a. Maculopapular rash is seen in 50% cases
   b. Associated with relative bradycardia
   c. Time interval between drug initiation to fever is 2-3 weeks
   d. B-lactam antibiotics are commonly implicated

7. **Pulmonary circulation is a:**
   a. Low pressure system
   b. Vascular pressure decreases down the lung by 1 cm H_2O for every 1 cm distance
   c. V/Q > 1 is seen in non-dependant regions
   d. Pressure difference between the top and bottom of the lung is 16-18 cm

8. **With regards to suctioning of endotracheal tube in mechanically ventilated patients, comment TRUE/ FALSE on the following:**
   a. Deep suctioning is preferred over shallow suctioning
   b. Size of suction catheter should be 60-75% of the inner diameter of endotracheal tube
   c. Duration of suctioning should be < 15 seconds
   d. Routine instillation of normal saline prior to ET suctioning is not recommended

9. **With respect to ICP waveforms comment on the following statements:**
   a. The normal ICP wave has 4 components
   b. P3 notch corresponds to closure of aortic valve
   c. Lundberg C waves are normal waves seen in health
   d. Lundberg A waves are always pathological

10. **The following are complications of lumbar puncture:**
    a. Headache
    b. Radicular pain
    c. 3rd nerve palsy
    d. Epidermoid tumor
    e. Multiple myeloma

11. **Which of the following statements apply with respect to Intra-aortic balloon counter pulsation (IABP)?**
    a. It is used as a bridge to heart transplantation
    b. Helps improve aortic regurgitation
    c. Can lead to compartment syndrome
    d. Oxygen is used to inflate the balloon
    e. Balloon inflates in diastole and deflates in systole

12. **Comment on the following statements regarding pressure sores:**
    a. NINDS scale is used to assess the risk of pressure sore development
    b. Critically ill patients are positioned every 2-3 hours to prevent pressure sore development
    c. Grade 2 score involves only epidermis
    d. Pressure scores are classified into 4 grades

13. **A 'FAST HUGS BID' to your patients daily assesses which of the following parameters:**
    a. Fever
    b. DVT prophylaxis
    c. Stress ulcer prophylaxis
    d. Position of patient
    e. Airway issues
    f. Delirium

14. **Early inflation of IABP causes the following:**
    a. Aortic regurgitation

b. Increased LVEDV, LVEDP and PCWP
c. Increased cardiac output
d. Decrease afterload

15. **Which of the following are types of ICU acquired weakness?**
    a. Critical illness myopathy
    b. Necrotizing myopathy
    c. Thick filament myopathy
    d. Critical illness polyneuropathy

16. **The following variables are directly measured by pulmonary artery catheter:**
    a. Mixed venous oxygen saturation
    b. Right atrial pressure
    c. Left atrial pressure
    d. Cardiac index

17. **An ideal scoring system should possess which of the following qualities:**
    a. Validity
    b. Feasible
    c. Should be applicable to a specific disease condition
    d. Variables used should always be simple
    e. Poor discrimination power

18. **Regarding flow through a vascular device comment on the following statements:**
    a. Directly proportional to 4th power of radius
    b. Direct proportional to pressure gradient
    c. Directly proportional to length of tube
    d. Indirectly proportional to fluid viscosity

19. **The following statements about serotonin syndrome are correct:**
    a. Cause by excessive stimulation of 5 HT1A receptors
    b. Presents with altered sensorium, ataxia, myoclonus and diarrhea
    c. Precipitated by MAO inhibitors
    d. Symptoms develop over a period of days
    e. Cyproheptadine is used for treatment

20. **The following are the physiological changes seen in pregnancy:**
    a. FRC decreases by 25%
    b. Plasma volume increases by 50%
    c. Total leucocyte count decreases by 20%
    d. Cardiac output increase by 40%
    e. Blood pressure decreases by 15%

ANSWERS

A Type Answers

Q1. Answer c

Within the first three months of development of stroke, the incidence of developing DVT and PE is 2.5 and 1.2% respectively. Hence, it is recommended that VTE pharmacoprophylaxis is initiated as soon as possible in all patients with acute ischemic stroke (AIS). In patients with AIS and restricted mobility, it is recommended that prophylactic-dose LMWH should be preferred over prophylactic-dose UFH in combination with intermittent pneumatic compression devices. VTE pharmacoprophylaxis should be continued even in those stroke patients who require hemicraniectomy or endovascular procedures. However, if the patient has received rTPA, then the initiation of UFH/LMWH should be delayed by 24 hours.

Indredavik B, Rohweder G, Naalsund E, et al. Medical complications in a comprehensive stroke unit and an early supported discharge service. Stroke. 2008;39(2):414-20.

Nyquist P, Bautista C, Jichici D, et al. Prophylaxis of Venous Thrombosis in Neurocritical Care Patients: An Evidence-Based Guideline: A Statement for Healthcare Professionals from the Neurocritical Care Society. Neurocrit Care. 2016;24(1):47-60.

Q2. Answer d

Hypervolemia may lead to several complications including increased venous pressure which may lead to pulmonary and peripheral edema causing impaired tissue oxygenation, increased demand on cardiac function, coagulation dysfunction secondary to hemodilution, decreased tissue oxygenation, delayed wound healing and an overall increase in mortality. Increased inflammatory response of the body has been reported in patients with hypovolemia. There is an increasing evidence that fluid overload and AKI are associated but the exact cause-effect relationship remains unclear. Ischemia develops with diminished GI perfusion especially in the mucosal layer of the gut. AKI is manifestation of overall multiorgan damage and not the direct renal damage.

Joosten A, Alexander B, Cannesson M. Defining Goals of Resuscitation in the Critically Ill Patient. Crit Care Clin. 2015;31(3):113-32.

Q3. Answer d

DO2 is the rate at which oxygen is transported from the lungs to the microcirculation, VO2 is the rate at which oxygen is removed from the blood for use by the tissues, and oxygen extraction is the proportion of arterial oxygen that is removed from the blood as it passes through the microcirculation. DO2 may be calculated using the following equation:

$$DO2 \text{ (mL/min)} = \text{Cardiac output (CO, L/min)} \times \text{Arterial oxygen content (CaO}_2\text{, mLO}_2\text{/dL)}$$

Which may be further expressed as:

$$DO_2 \text{ (mL/min)} = HR \times SV \times [(SaO_2 \times Hb \times 1.34) + (0.003 \times PaO_2)]$$

Wherein, HR is heart rate; SaO_2 is arterial hemoglobin oxygen saturation; Hb is hemoglobin concentration; $PaO2$ is arterial oxygen partial pressure. Hence, DO_2 may be improved by increasing either CO or CaO_2 (or both). CO is generally managed by manipulating fluids and/or inotropic agents. On the other hand, CaO_2 may be increased by augmenting SaO_2 and/or Hb concentration. VO_2 normally remains constant over a wide range of DO2 because changes in DO2 are balanced by reciprocal changes in oxygen extraction. VO_2 will decrease only if DO2 declines to such a degree that it cannot be balanced by increasing oxygen extraction.

Joosten A, Alexander B, Cannesson M. Defining Goals of Resuscitation in the Critically Ill Patient. Crit Care Clin. 2015;31:113-132.

Q4. Answer a

After salicylates toxicity, patients may develop respiratory alkalosis especially in the early phase. This is secondary to the direct stimulation of the medulla by the salicylates. This leads to increased respiratory rate and tidal volume which causes respiratory alkalosis. In the later period, patients with salicylate toxicity may develop metabolic acidosis.

Tenney SM, Miller RM. The respiratory and circulatory action of salicylate. Am J Med. 1955;19:498-508.

Wiener SW. Toxicologic Acid-Base Disorders. Emerg Med Clin N Am. 2014;32(1):149-65.

Q5. Answer d

The most commonly implicated drugs causing bradycardia are beta receptor and calcium channel blockers. However, there are several other drugs which may lead to bradycardia; these include opioids, ergot alkaloids, cholinergic agents like organophosphates, carbamates, sarin, and cardio active steroids like digoxin. TCA, on the other hand may lead to tachycardia.

> Jang DH, Spyres MB, Fox L, Manini AF. Toxin-Induced Cardiovascular Failure. Emerg Med Clin N Am. 2014;32(1):79-102.

Q6. Answer c

All of the above mentioned causes except hyperphosphatemia may lead to gut dysmotility. Other common ICU disorders or treatments which may cause gut dysmotility include hypophosphatemia, positive pressure mechanical ventilation, opioid and non-opioid sedatives, intravenous catecholamines, intraoperative intestinal manipulation and hemorrhage.

> Liu SS, Wu CL. Effect of postoperative analgesia on major postoperative complications: a systematic update of the evidence. Anesth Analg. 2007;104(3):689-702.
>
> Mutlu GM, Mutlu EA, Factor P. Prevention and treatment of gastrointestinal complications in patients on mechanical ventilation. Am J Respir Med. 2003;2(5):395-411.

Q7. Answer a

Oxygen is widely used in critical care. However, if inappropriately used the use of oxygen does come with its side effects and toxicity. There are certain conditions wherein administration of oxygen will be harmful namely paraquat poisoning, bleomycin induced lung injury and acid inhalation.

BTS guideline for oxygen use in adults in healthcare and emergency settings. BR O'Driscoll, L S Howard, J Earis, V Mak on behalf of the British Thoracic Society Emergency Oxygen Guideline Development Group.

Q8. Answer d

qSOFA was developed as a simple bedside criteria to identify patients who are likely to have a poor outcome. It encompasses 3 variables namely respiratory rate > 22/min, systolic blood pressure < 100 mm Hg and altered mental status (GCS < 15). It has been developed to help physicians investigate for organ dysfunction or initiate/ escalate therapy.

> Singer M, Deutschman CS, Seymour CW, et al. The Third International Consensus Definitions for Sepsis and Septic Shock (Sepsis-3). JAMA. 2016;315(8):801-10.

Q9. Answer c

NSE > 33 ug/L is suggestive of poor outcome in post cardiac arrest patients as per the AAN guidelines. However, these values do not apply to patients who have been treated with hypothermia.

> Daubin C, Quentin C, Allouch S et al. Serum neuron-specific enolase as predictor of outcome in comatose cardiac-arrest survivors: a prospective cohort study. BMC Cardiovascular Disorders. 2011;11:48-61.
>
> Shinokzaki K, Oda S, Sadahiro T et al. S-100B and neuron-specific enolase as predictors of neurological outcome in patients after cardiac arrest and return of spontaneous circulation: a systematic review. Critical Care. 2009;13(4):R121.

Q10. Answer b

James Childress and Tom Beauchamp in Principle of Biomedical Ethics (1978) identify beneficence as one of the core values of healthcare ethics. The four principles of Beauchamp and Childress have been extremely influential in the field of medical ethics, and are fundamental for understanding the current approach to ethical assessment in health care. The Beauchamp Childress system is based on the following four principles:
  i. Beneficence is to act with the best interest in mind
  ii. Autonomy is the right of an individual ability to make decisions for self
  iii. Distributive justice stands for equality among individuals and respect for societal values and principles.
  iv. Non-maleficence means doing no harm.

> Page K. The four principles: Can they be measured and do they predict ethical decision making. BMC Med Ethics. 2012;13:10.

General Critical Care

Q11. Answer b

The N20 response measures the response of the primary somatosensory cortex 20 msec after electrical stimulation of the median nerve. It is used as one of the prognostication markers in post cardiac arrest patients. Bilateral absence of the N20 response is indicative of poor outcome.

Tiainen M, Kovala TT, Takkunen OS, and Roine RO. Somatosensory and brainstem auditory evoked potentials in cardiac arrest patients treated with hypothermia. Critical Care Medicine. 2005;33(8):1736-40.

Q12. Answer c

EEG patterns associated with poor neurological outcome include generalized suppression, burst suppression and epileptiform discharges. Reactivity is a favorable sign signifying a change in amplitude or frequency in response to an external stimulus. Lack of reactivity is associated with a poor outcome.

Rossetti AO, Urbano LA, Delodder F et al. Prognostic value of continuous EEG monitoring during therapeutic hypothermia after cardiac arrest. Critical Care. 2010;14(5):R173.

Rossetti AO, Oddo M, Logroscino G, et al. Prognostication after cardiac arrest and hypothermia: A prospective study. Ann of Neurol. 2010;67(3):301-7.

Q13. Answer c

The Alveolar-arterial oxygen gradient (A-a gradient) is the difference between PAO_2- PaO_2 where PAO_2 is the alveolar oxygen content, while PaO_2 is the arterial oxygen saturation. Normal A-a gradient is 7–10 mm Hg. Hypoxia can be divided into two types based on the A-a gradient, i.e. Hypoxia with normal A-a gradient and Hypoxia with raised A-a gradient. Alveolar hypoventilation and low oxygen tension of inspired gas cause hypoxia with normal A-a gradient.

Lanken PN. Approach to acute respiratory failure. In: Lanken PN (ed.). The Intensive care unit manual. Philadelphia, PA:Saunders. 2001;1-12.

Q14. Answer d

pH, $PaCO_2$ and PO_2 are directly measured parameters while HCO_3, base excess and SaO_2 are derived parameters.

Schmidt C, Müller-Plathe O. Stability of pO2, pCO2 and pH in heparinized whole blood samples: influence of storage temperature with regard to leukocyte count and syringe material. Eur J Clin Chem Clin Biochem. 1992;30(11):767-73.

Burnett RW, Covington AK, et al. International Federation of Clinical Chemistry (IFCC). Scientific Division. Committee on pH, Blood Gases and Electrolytes. Approved IFCC recommendations on whole blood sampling, transport and storage for simultaneous determination of pH, blood gases and electrolytes. Eur J Clin Chem Clin Biochem. 1995;33(4):247-53.

Q15. Answer a

Pulse oximeter works on the principle of spectrophotometry. It gives a non-invasive measurement of the hemoglobin oxygen saturation. It measures the difference in absorption of red (660 nm) and infrared (940 nm) wavelengths of light to calculate SpO_2.

McMorrow RC, Mythen MG. Pulse oximetry. Curr Opin Crit Care. 2006;12(3):269-71.

Q16. Answer c

The oxyhemoglobin dissociation curve is a sigmoid shaped curve which depicts the relation between hemoglobin oxygen saturation (SaO_2) and partial pressure of oxygen in blood (PaO_2). It helps in understanding the affinity of oxygen for hemoglobin and thus oxygen availability. Factors which shift the curve to the right increase tissue oxygen availability and include hyperthermia, acidosis, hypercarbia, and increased concentration of 2,3-DPG.

West JB. Respiratory Physiology, The Essentials. 6th ed. Philadelphia Williams and Wilkins: Lippincott; 2000.

Q17. Answer d

The normal time capnogram has 4 phases:

Phase 1 - It is the beginning of expiration. During this phase, the CO_2 concentration is zero as the exhaled air comes from anatomic dead space.

Phase 2 – Upstroke of the capnogram. It represents mixing of air from alveolus with dead space.

Phase 3 – Alveolar plateau phase. It represents exhalation of pure alveolar gas. The highest value on alveolar plateau represents $ETCO_2$.

Phase 0 – Descending limb of the capnogram and initial portion of baseline. It represents the portion of capnogram corresponding to the beginning of inspiration to beginning of expiration.

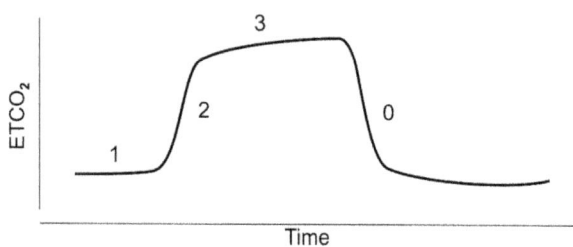

Stock MC. Noninvasive carbon dioxide monitoring. Crit Care Clin. 1988;4(3):511-26.

Q18. Answer b
The capnograph shows gradual decline in the values suggestive of worsening heart/circulation.

Kodali BS. Capnography in Cardiac Arrest. Available from: http://www.capnography.com/(Accessed11 February 2018).
Stock MC. Noninvasive carbon dioxide monitoring. Crit Care Clin. 1988;4(3):511-26.

Q19. Answer a
As per the Society of critical care medicine fever is defined as a core temperature > 38.3°C.

Laupland KB. Fever in the critically ill medical patient. Crit Care Med. 2009;37(7 Suppl):S273-78.

Q20. Answer a
Metabolic alkalosis may cause several electrolyte abnormalities which include hypokalemia, hypocalcemia, and hypophosphatemia. In addition, it can have several neurological effects like neuromuscular excitability and encephalopathy seizures. Other complications associated with metabolic alkalosis include impaired enzyme function, digoxin toxicity, decreased inotropy and increased oxy-Hb affinity.

Kellum JA. Disorders of acid-base balance. Crit Care Med. 2007;35(11):2630-6.

Q21. Answer b
Hypophosphatemia may be caused due (1) Transcellular shifts: Refeeding syndrome, respiratory alkalosis, insulin administration, (2) Renal losses: diuretic therapy, osmotic diuresis, hyperparathyroidism (primary or secondary), proximal renal tubular dysfunction: Fanconi syndrome, (3) Insufficient intestinal absorption: Malnutrition, phosphate-binding antacids, vitamin D deficiency, chronic diarrhea, nasogastric suctioning, malabsorption syndromes, (4) Extreme catabolic states: Burns, trauma, sepsis.

Amanzadeh J, Reilly RF. Hypophosphatemia: an evidence-based approach to its clinical consequences and management. Nature Clinical Practice Nephrology. 2006;2(3):136-48.

Q22. Answer d
Endotracheal tubes have a low pressure, high volume cuff so as to reduce the incidence of ischemia-related complications. Tracheal ischemia can occur if the cuff pressure exceeds 30 mm Hg.

Irwin R, Rippe J. Intensive care medicine, 7th ed. Philadelphia Williams & Wilkins: Lippincott; 2012.

Q23. Answer b
Closed blood conservation device [Venous Arterial blood Management Protection (VAMP)] decrease PRBC transfusion requirements and better handling of the lines. When the set is primed the pressure bag is fitted and inflated to 300 mm Hg, about 3 mL/hr of 0.9% sodium chloride will pass through the flush device to keep the line patent. This may be a significant volume is some cases and may be accounted.

Bedfrod RF, Shah NK. Blood pressure monitoring: Invasive and Non-invasive. In: Monitoring in anaesthesia and critical care medicine. Ed. Blitt CD, Hines RL. Third edition, Churchill Livingstone Inc.

Mcghee BH. Monitoring Arterial blood pressure: what you may not know. Critical Care Nurse. 2002.

Q24. Answer d

Both overdamped and under damped waveforms are encountered on a daily basis in the ICU. It is imperative to understand these waveforms so as to avoid any detrimental therapy based on erroneous data.

In over damped waveforms the pressure waveform is wide and slurred. It tends to under estimate the systolic and overestimate the diastolic blood pressure. Mean arterial pressure remains unchanged. Causes include air bubbles, clots, catheter kinks, overtly compliant tubing and low pressure in flush bag. Long tubing length causes an underdamped waveform.

Bedfrod RF, Shah NK. Blood pressure monitoring: Invasive and Non-invasive. Monitoring in anaesthesia and Critical care medicine. Blitt CD, Hines RL (Eds.). Third edition, Churchill Livingstone Inc.

Mcghee BH Bridges EJ. Monitoring Arterial blood pressure: what you may not know. Critical Care Nurse. 2002;22(2):60-4.

Q25. Answer b

The declaration of Helsinki was adopted in 1964. It is a document regarding human research ethics and is developed by the World Medical Association.

World Medical Association Declaration of Helsinki: ethical principles for medical research involving human subjects. JAMA. 2013;310(20):2191-4.

Q26. Answer b

Beta error is a type 2 error. It refers to the probability of a test failing to reject a null hypothesis when it is false. Alpha error refers to the probability of a test rejecting a null hypothesis when it is true.

Dawson B, Trapp RG. Basic and Clinical Biostatistics. New York: Lange Medical Books; 2004.

Q27. Answer b

Succinylcholine is the drug commonly used for rapid sequence intubation. However, it is known to cause hyperkalemia and should be avoided in situations where hyperkalemia can be precipitated such as crush injury, rhabdomyolysis, burns etc.

Martyn JA, Richtsfeld M. Succinylcholine-induced hyperkalemia in acquired pathologic states: etiologic factors and molecular mechanisms. Anesthesiology. 2006;104(1):158-69.

Q28. Answer b

Absolute contraindications to lumbar puncture: Active bleeding, Severe thrombocytopenia (Platelet < 50,000/uL), INR > 1.4, suspected spinal epidural abscess, Possible raised intracranial pressure.

Antiplatelet therapy is not clearly associated with risk of bleeding post LP. In case of elective procedure, it is considered prudent to withhold an antiplatelet. However, the effect of antiplatelets tends to wear off in 5-7 days in case of clopidogrel. Antiplatelet therapy with aspirin and nonsteroidal anti-inflammatory agents is NOT clearly associated with an increased risk of bleeding after LP. Bloodstream infection and bacteremia is not a contraindication to performing LP.

Johnson KS, Sexton DJ. Lumbar puncture: technique, indications, contraindications, and complications in adults. Available from: http://www.uptodate.com/contents/lumbar-puncture-technique-indications-contraindications-and-complications-in-adults. (Accessed 11 February 2018).

Q29. Answer b

The only intervention known to reduce the risk of CIN is intravenous hydration. There is no robust data to support the use of intravenous NAC or post contrast hemodialysis. No role of dopamine infusion to prevent CIN.

Ozcan EE, Guneri S, Akdeniz B, et al. Sodium bicarbonate, N-acetylcysteine, and saline for prevention of radiocontrast-induced nephropathy. A comparison of 3 regimens for protecting contrast-induced nephropathy in patients undergoing coronary procedures. A single-center prospective controlled trial. Am Heart J. 2007;154(3):539-44.

Hoste EA, De Waele JJ, Gevaert SA, et. al. Sodium bicarbonate for prevention of contrast induced acute kidney injury: a systematic review and meta-analysis. Nephrol Dial Transplant. 2010;25(3):747-58.

Q30. Answer d

Delirium is an acute confusional state. As per DSM-IV TR delirium is characterised by altered consciousness and cognitive impairment. One of the key features to detect delirium is inattention. There are many risk factors (modifiable and non- modifiable) which can increase the risk of developing delirium. Infections, drugs, pain, immobility, electrolyte abnormalities etc. are all risk factors for delirium. There are many delirium screening tools, the common ones used are Confusion assessment model for ICU (CAM-ICU) and Intensive Care Delirium Screening Checklist (ICDSC) model. All sedatives and opiates can potentially precipitate delirium. Dexmedetomidine has emerged as an attractive option to both prevent and treat delirium. When used as the primary sedative for intubated medical and surgical ICU patients, dexmedetomidine reduced the duration of delirium when compared to benzodiazepines.

> American Psychiatric Association: Diagnostic and Statistical Manual of Mental Disorders DSM-IV-TR. 4th ed (Text Revision) 2000 American Psychiatric Association Washington DC.
>
> Luetz A, Heymann A, Radtke FM, et al. Different assessment tools for intensive care unit delirium: which score to use? Crit Care Med. 2010;38(2):409-18.

K Type Answers

Q1. Answer FTTFT

Dyshemoglobinemia, dyes, low perfusion states, nail polish and motion artefact can all interfere in the pulse oximetry readings. Even presence of anemia may affect pulse oximetry but, polycythemia has no affect. In addition, hyperbilirubinemia does not seem to interfere in pulse oximetry as it presents a different spectrum of light absorption.

> Pretto JJ, Roebuck T, Beckert L, et al. Clinical use of pulse oximetry: Official guidelines from the Thoracic Society of Australia and New Zealand. Respirology. 2014;19(1):38-46.
>
> Crapo RO, Jensen RL, Hegewald M, et al. Arterial blood gas reference values for sea level and an altitude of 1,400 meters. Am. J. Respir. Crit. Care Med. 1999;160(5 Pt 1):1525-31.

Q2. Answer FTTTF

To achieve a good neurological outcome and to reduce intracranial hypertension, TTM is recommended in patients with severe TBI and in comatose patients with aneurysmal subarachnoid hemorrhage. In patients with refractory or super-refractory status epilepticus, TTM at 32–35°C may be advisable to control seizure activity. However, TTM below 36°C in patients with cardiogenic shock is not recommended.

> Cariou A, Payen JF, Asehnoune K, et al. Targeted temperature management in the ICU: guidelines from a French expert panel. Ann Intensive Care. 2017;7(1):70.

Q3. Answer TTFFT

In patients with HIT, there is a production of autoantibodies against the complex of platelet factor 4 bound to heparin. Typically, there is a fall in platelet levels usually to <150,000/µl, by more than 50% within 5 to 10 days of heparin exposure. It may occur even sooner in previously heparin-exposed patients. However, the timing and magnitude of thrombocytopenia can only be suggestive, but not diagnostic of HIT.

> Greinacher A. Heparin-induced thrombocytopenia. N Engl J Med. 2015;373:252-261.
>
> Salter BS, Weiner MM, Trinh MA, et al. Heparin-Induced Thrombocytopenia: a comprehensive clinical review. J Am Coll Cardiol. 2016;67(21):2519-32.

Q4. Answer FTTF

In 'post cardiac arrest patients' presence of certain signs and symptoms are suggestive of poor prognostic marker for recovery. Clinical features indicating poor outcome includes: (1) Presence of myoclonic status epilepticus on day 1, (2) Absence of pupillary responses or corneal reflexes or extensor posturing as the best motor response on day 3, (3) Bilateral absence of N20 response on somatosensory-evoked potentials (SSEPs) performed on day 1–3, (4) Serum neuron-specific enolase (NSE) >33 µg/L

> Levy DE, Caronna JJ, Singer BH et al. Predicting outcome from hypoxic-ischemic coma. Journal of the American Medical Association. 1985;253(10):1420-6.

Wijdicks EF, Hijdra A, Young GB, Bassetti CL, Wiebe S. Practice parameter: prediction of outcome in comatose survivors after cardiopulmonary resuscitation (an evidence-based review): report of the Quality Standards Subcommittee of the American Academy of Neurology. Neurology. 2006; 67(12):203-10.

Q5. Answer TTFF

D-lactic acidosis is typically seen in patients with short bowel syndrome, jejunoileal bypass or chronic pancreatic insufficiency. D-lactate is formed from anaerobic metabolism of organic acids produced in the gut from bacterial metabolism of undigested fibre, sugar and starch. As organic acids accumulate the intraluminal pH reduces thus favoring overgrowth of certain bacteria such as Lactobacillus, one of the major d-lactate producing bacteria. Normal lactate assays measure only l-lactate and not d-lactate. Hence, in d-lactic acidosis the lactate levels can be normal. Patients typically present with neurological manifestations and high anion gap metabolic acidosis following ingestion of carbohydrate load.

Oh MS, Phelps KR, Traube M, et al. D-lactic acidosis in a man with the short-bowel syndrome. N Engl J Med. 1979;301(5):249-252.

Halperin ML, Kamel KS. D-lactic acidosis: turning sugar into acids in the gastrointestinal tract. Kidney Int. 1996;49(1):1-8.

Q6. Answer FTTT

Drug fever usually manifests 2-3 weeks after the drug is started and persists for 2-3 days after the culprit drug is withdrawn. Associated with skin rash, pruritus, eosinophilia and arthralgias, mild transaminitis and raised ESR. Patients usually present with relative bradycardia. Commonly implicated drugs include b-lactams, sulphonamides, anti-convulsants, anti-arrhythmics, MAO inhibitors, tricyclic antidepressants. Treatment involves stopping the offending drug.

Wood AJ. Adverse Drug Reactions. In: Fauci AS, Braunwald E et al. (Eds.) Harrison's Principles of Internal Medicine. 14th ed. NY: McGraw-Hill; 1998. pp. 422-30.

Q7. Answer TTTF

The pulmonary circulation is a low pressure system and thus is susceptible to changes in intrathoracic pressure. Ventilation and perfusion throughout the lung is heterogeneous with ventilation highest in the apex and perfusion highest in the bases. The vascular pressure decreases in the lung by 1 cm of H_2O for every 1 cm with a pressure difference between the top and bottom of approximately 11-12 cm. As a result, V/Q is > 1 in non-dependant regions and < 1 in dependant regions.

West JB. Mechanics of breathing. In: West JB (ed.) Best and Taylor's Physiological Basis of Medical Practice. Williams and Wilkins. 1989; pp. 560-78.

Q8. Answer FFTT

Suctioning is of 2 types: (1) shallow suction and (2) deep suction. Deep suction has not shown superiority over shallow suction and is associated with more adverse effects and hence is not routinely recommended. The size of the suction catheter should be less than 50% of the internal diameter of the endotracheal tube as a large negative intrathoracic pressure can be generated during suctioning. The duration of suctioning should not exceed 15 seconds with maximum 3 passes in total. Normal saline instillation in the ET prior to suctioning is not routinely recommended as it is associated with greater harm than benefit.

American Association for Respiratory Care (AARC) Clinical Practice Guidelines. Endotracheal suctioning of mechanically ventilated patients with artificial airways 2010. Respir Care. 2010; 55(6):758-64.

Q9. Answer FTTT

The normal ICP waveform has 3 components (P1, P2, P3). P1 reflects the arterial pressure waveform transmitted to the CNS through the choroid plexus. P2 represents the cerebral compliance and P3 is the dicrotic notch which represents with closure of the aortic valve. Lundberg waves represent trends in ICP. Lundberg A waves or plateau waves are always pathological. They have amplitude of 50-100 mm Hg and last for 5-20 minutes. Lundberg B waves oscillating waves with amplitude up to 50 mm Hg and a frequency of 0.5-2/min. Lundberg C waves are oscillating waves with amplitude upto < 20 mm Hg and a frequency of 4-8/min. The significance of C waves is unknown but is usually seen in health.

Lundberg NL, Troupp H, Lorin H. Continuous recording of the ventricular-fluid pressure in patients with severe acute traumatic brain injury. A preliminary report. Journal of Neurosurgery. 1965;22(6):581-90.

Andrews PJ, Citerio G. Intracranial pressure. Part one: historical overview and basic concepts. Intensive Care Medicine. 2004;30(9):1730-3.

Q10. Answer TTFTF

Post-spinal headache is the most common complication occurring in 10–30% cases. Cerebral herniation is the most serious complication. Raised ICP is a contraindication to LP. 6th nerve palsy is seen secondary to intracranial hypotension and is associated with headache, vomiting, dizziness. Radicular pain could occur during the procedure and is a transient shock like sensation. It is uncommon for the pain to last for long periods of time. Epidermoid tumor is a rare complication occurring after years' post LP. One of the possibilities is that the epidermoid tissue that is transplanted into the spinal canal during LP without a stylet. Multiple myeloma also known as plasma cell myeloma is a cancer of plasma cells, a type of white blood cell normally responsible for producing antibodies.

Johnson KS, Sexton DJ. Lumbar puncture: technique, indications, contraindications, and complications in adults. Available from: http://www.uptodate.com/contents/lumbar-puncture-technique-indications-contraindications-and-complications-in-adults (Accessed 11 February 2018).

Q11. Answer TFTFT

IABP is a mechanical device which helps to reduce myocardial oxygen demand and increase the cardiac output. It is inserted via the femoral route. It is used in patients of left ventricular failure as a bridge to cardiac transplant. Other indications include cardiogenic shock, post cardiothoracic surgery, acute mitral regurgitation post myocardial infarction. It is contraindicated in aortic dissection, aortic regurgitation and severe aortic valve disease. Helium is used to inflate the balloon as it has a low viscosity and is easily dissolved in blood in case of balloon rupture. The balloon inflates in diastole thus improving coronary perfusion and deflates in systole thus improving cardiac output.

Krishna M, Zacharowski K. Principles of intra-aortic balloon pump counter-pulsation. Contin Educ Anaesth Crit Care and Pain. 2008;9:24-8.

Q12. Answer FTTT

Multiple scales exist to assess the risk of development of pressure sore namely Braden, Norton, Waterlow, etc. They are classified into 4 grades depending on the depth of skin involvement. Grade 1 is non blanchable erythema with intact skin. Grade 2 is skin loss involving epidermis or dermis or both. Grade 3 is full thickness skin loss which extends beyond the fascia. Grade 4 includes damage to muscle, bone or any supporting structures. Change in position of patients is one of the ways to prevent pressure sores. Patients should be repositioned at least every 6 hours while, in the critically ill, due to the higher risks, patients should be repositioned every 2–3 hours.

Keller BPJA, Wille J, van Ramshorts B, et al. Pressure ulcers in intensive care patients: a review of risks and prevention. Intensive Care Med. 2012;28(10):1379-88.

Q13. Answer FTTTFF

FAST-HUG is mnemonics which stands for feeding, analgesia/ anxiety, sedation, thromboprophylaxis, head-up position, ulcer (stress) prophylaxis, glycaemic control, spontaneous breathing trial, bowel movement, indwelling catheter removal and de-escalation of antibiotics. It is a daily bundle to apply basic intensive care to all critically ill patients.

Vincent JL. Critically ill patients need 'FAST HUGS BID' (an updated mnemonic). Crit Care Med. 2009;37(7): p. 2327.

Q14. Answer TTFF

In early inflation of the IABP, the inflation point lies before the dicrotic notch, i.e. prior to aortic valve closure. This can lead to aortic regurgitation and can lead to increased myocardial wall stress or afterload. There will be an increase in LEDV, LVEDP and PCWP with increase in myocardial oxygen demand and consumption and decrease in cardiac output.

Krishna M, Zacharowski K, Principles of intra-aortic balloon pump counter-pulsation. Contin Educ Anaesth Crit Care Pain. 2008;9:24-8.

Q15. Answer TTTT

ICU acquired weakness is seen in nearly 40-50% cases suffering from sepsis, multiorgan failure, and prolonged mechanical ventilation. The cause is not clear. ICU acquired weakness is classified on the basis of electrophysiological studies into critical illness polyneuropathy (CIP), critical illness myopathy (CIM) and critical illness neuromyopathy (CINM). CIM can be further sub classified into cachectic myopathy, thick filament myopathy and necrotizing myopathy based on histological findings.

Appleton R, Kinsella J. Intensive care unit-acquired weakness. Contin Educ Anaesth Crit Care Pain. 2012;12:62-6.

Q16. Answer TTFF

The pulmonary artery (PA) catheter is not commonly used for hemodynamic monitoring in the present era. However, it may be useful in certain clinical situation. The directly measured variables are central venous pressure (CVP), right atrial pressure (RAP), right ventricular systolic pressure (RVSP), pulmonary artery pressure (PAP), pulmonary artery occlusion pressure (PAOP) and mixed venous oxygen saturations (SVO2). PAOP is used as a surrogate of left atrial measure (LAP) which is not directly measured. Indirect variables which are calculated by thermo dilution technique using PA catheter are cardiac output (CO), cardiac index (CI), oxygen delivery, systemic vascular resistance (SVR) and pulmonary vascular resistance PVR).

Reade MC, Angus DC. PAC-Man: game over for the pulmonary artery catheter? Crit Care. 2006;10(1):303.

Q17. Answer TTFTF

An ideal scoring system should have the following qualities: (1) Validity – Ability of a score to predict the result of interest. (2) Feasible – The score should be practical. (3) Generalisability - Ability to be applied to the population at whole irrespective of race, ethnicity. (4) Well calibrated. A high level of discrimination. Discrimination power refers to the accuracy of the test. (5) Applicable to all patient populations. (6) Can be used in different countries. (7) The ability to predict functional status or quality of life after ICU discharge.

Variable if simple are always beneficial. However, if the validity and discriminative power of a score are good complex models can be used.

Bouch DC, Thompson JP. Severity scoring systems in the critically ill. Contin Educ Anaesth Crit Care and Pain. 2008;8(5):181-5.

Q18. Answer TTFT

As per Hagen-Poiseuille law flow is dependent on 4 factors namely radius of tube, length of tube, viscosity of fluid and pressure gradient. Flow is directly proportional to the fourth power of the radius and pressure gradient, and is inversely proportional to the viscosity of the fluid and the length of the tube.

Kenny G, Davis P. Basic Physics and Measurement in Anaesthesia, 5th Ed. Oxford: Butterworth-Heinemann, 2003.

Q19. Answer TTTFT

Serotonin syndrome occurs secondary to serotinergic medications. It is precipitated by MAO inhibitors, Tricyclic anti-depressants, sympathomimetic and linezolid. It is secondary to excessive stimulation of 5 HT1A receptors. Symptoms include high grade fever, altered mental status, lead pipe rigidity, autonomic instability, myoclonus and diarrhoea. It is a dose related phenomenon and has an acute presentation. Cyproheptadine is a serotonin antagonist for treatment.

Boyer EW, Shannon M. The serotonin syndrome. New Engl J Med. 2005;352:1112-20.

Q20. Answer TTFTT

There are various physiological changes that occur in pregnancy including respiratory, cardiovascular, renal, haematological and metabolic. These changes occur so as to adapt and accommodate the growing fetus. The respiratory changes include increased minute ventilation by 45%, increase oxygen consumption by 20% and reduced FRC by 25%. Cardiovascular changes include increase in plasma volume by 50%, decrease in blood pressure by 10-15%, increase heart rate by 10-15%. The white blood cell count rises in pregnancy (is in high normal range) and may make interpretation of infections difficult.

Fujitani S, Baldisseri MR. Hemodynamic assessment in a pregnant and peripartum patient. Crit Care Med 2005;33(10 Suppl): S354-361.

Guyton and hall (2005). Textbook of Medical Physiology (11 ed.). Philadelphia: Saunders. pp. 103g

CHAPTER 15

Transplantation: Heart and Liver

Rachit Saxena, Ankit Sharma, Shrikanth Srinivasan, Deepak Govil

TRANSPLANTATION: HEART
Rachit Saxena

A Type Questions
(One best answer)

1. The heart failure survival score includes all except:
   a. Coronary artery disease
   b. Resting heart rate
   c. Left ventricular ejection fraction
   d. VO_2 max
   e. NYHA class

2. Maintenance immunosuppressant in first year after heart transplant include all except:
   a. Calcineurin inhibitor
   b. Corticosteroids
   c. Antimetabolite agent
   d. Interleukine-2 receptor antagonist
   e. mTOR inhibitor

3. All of the following can be used as part of induction therapy for immunosuppression in the perioperative period of heart transplant except:
   a. Monoclonal antithymocyte antibody
   b. Polyclonal antithymocyte globulin
   c. Antimetabolite agent
   d. Corticosteroids
   e. IL-2 receptor antagonist

4. Common post heart transplant complications include all except:
   a. Infection
   b. Osteoporosis
   c. Diabetes
   d. Alopecia
   e. Graft coronary artery disease

5. Common problems in the intensive care unit following cardiac transplant include all except:
   a. Arrhythmia
   b. Right ventricular dysfunction
   c. Tricuspid regurgitation
   d. Renal dysfunction
   e. Acute hepatic failure

6. Which of the following is used for subjective assessment of cardiorespiratory function?
   a. NYHA clinical assessment
   b. 6 minute walk test
   c. Treadmill test
   d. VO_2max
   e. All of the above

7. Tacrolimus levels maintained during initiation phase is:
   a. <5 ng/mL
   b. 5–10 ng/mL
   c. 10–15 ng/mL
   d. 15–20 ng/mL
   e. >20 ng/mL

8. Management of antibody mediated rejection (AMR) include:
   a. Corticosteroids
   b. Antithymocyte globulin
   c. Photopheresis
   d. Splenectomy
   e. Antimetabolite agent

9. Which of the following provides best assessment of pulmonary vascular disease in a patient with long-standing left sided heart failure?
   a. Mean pulmonary artery pressure
   b. Pulmonary artery wedge pressure
   c. Transpulmonary gradient
   d. Diastolic pulmonary vascular pressure gradient
   e. Systolic pulmonary artery pressure

10. All the following are true regarding anesthetic managements of brain dead donors except:
    a. High filling pressure is needed to maintain hemodynamics
    b. Vasopressin infusion is frequently required.
    c. Brain dead patients develop central diabetes mellitus
    d. Brain dead patient develop neurogenic pulmonary edema
    e. Loss of central thermoregulatory mechanism

K Type Questions
[Marked True (T)/False (F)]

1. According to the ACC/AHA guidelines, analyse the following statements regarding indications for cardiac transplant:
   a. NYHA Class III or IV despite maximal medical and cardiac resynchronization therapy.
   b. Refractory cardiogenic shock requiring intra-aortic balloon pump counterpulsation or left ventricular assist device
   c. Recurrent life threatening left ventricular arrhythmia despite antiarrhythmic drugs, implantable cardiac defibrillator or ablation therapy
   d. Peak VO_2 (VO_2 max) more than 14 mL/kg/min
   e. End stage congenital heart failure with no pulmonary hypertension

2. Identify the correct and false statements about peak oxygen consumption (VO_2 max):
   a. It assesses the cardiac reserve and peripheral adaptation to reduced cardiac output
   b. Reliability is similar to the functional NYHA classification
   c. In ambulatory patients with severe left ventricular dysfunction but peak oxygen consumption (VO_2max) >14 mL/kg/min, heart transplantation can safely be deferred and medical treatment continued
   d. With the use of beta blocker, angiotensin converting enzyme inhibitors and cardiac resynchronization therapy the cut off for cardiac transplant has been decreased to VO_2 max <10 mL/kg/min
   e. It is gold standard for assessment if severity of cardiac impairment

3. Analyse the following statements regarding absolute contraindication for heart transplant:
   a. Advanced irreversible renal failure with Cr >2 or creatinine clearance <30–50 mL/min without plans for concurrent renal transplant
   b. Advanced irreversible hepatic failure
   c. Advanced irreversible pulmonary parenchymal disease or (FEV_1 <1 L/min)
   d. Advanced irreversible pulmonary artery hypertension (pulmonary artery systolic pressure >60 mm Hg, pulmonary vascular resistance >4–5 wood units despite vasodilators)
   e. Severe peripheral vascular disease

4. Analyze the following statements regarding donor selection criteria:
   a. Age cut off <25 years is acceptable in most centers.
   b. Echo radiographic confirmation of normal ventricular function
   c. Coronary angiography if age >40 years
   d. The donor recipient weight mismatch should be <30%
   e. HLA matching is essential before a cardiac transplant

5. Mark the following statements regarding cardiac transplant rejection:
   a. Acute cell-mediated rejection is a host T-lymphocyte-mediated response mounted against the allograft tissue
   b. Antibody mediated rejection (AMR) results from activation of the complement system, typically by recipient-generated antibodies directed against the allograft tissue
   c. Hyper acute rejection is a subtype of AMR, can occur within minutes to hours after transplantation

d. Cardiac allograft vasculopathy (CAV) involves concentric luminal narrowing of the epicardial and intramural coronary arteries
e. CAV is a manifestation of accelerated atherosclerosis and not an immune mediated response

6. **Assess the correctness of the following statements regarding the post-cardiac transplant patient:**
   a. Exercise capacity is less than of a non-transplanted normal individual
   b. There is rapid acceleration in the rate of the transplanted heart in response to exercise
   c. Circulation level of catecholamine is lower in transplant recipients
   d. Average resting heart rate post-transplant is 95 bpm
   e. Post-transplant there is shift to type-2 beta adrenergic receptors on cardiac myocytes

7. **Analyse the following statements in context of cardiac allograft vasculopathy:**
   a. Accelerated coronary atherosclerosis is a result of immunogenic as well non-immunogenic mechanism
   b. There is no successful medical treatment of CAV
   c. CAV can be easily diagnosed by coronary angiography or intravascular ultrasound
   d. CAV can be prevented by preventing endothelial injury just before transplantation
   e. CAV can be prevented by decreasing cold ischemia time

8. **Assess the following statements with regard to management of pulmonary arterial hypertension post-cardiac transplant:**
   a. Ketamine should be used for sedation
   b. Non-ventilated lung can be recruited by high PEEP
   c. pCO_2 should be maintained at a high normal level
   d. Phosphodiesterase III inhibitors can be used
   e. Inhaled nitric oxide should be used

9. **Left ventricular dysfunction in post-cardiac transplant patient is managed by:**
   a. Increase dose of catecholamines
   b. Maintain higher peripheral vascular resistance
   c. Maintain heart rate of less than 80 bpm
   d. Threshold for intra aortic balloon pump should be low
   e. LVAD should be used if other measures fail to maintain adequate cardiac output

10. **Analyze the following statements regarding immunosuppressants:**
    a. Tacrolimus causes hyperkalemia and renal failure
    b. Corticosteroids cause pancytopenia
    c. Mycophenolate causes pancytopenia
    d. Hypertension and diabetes are common due to high dose corticosteroids
    e. Azole group of antifungals increase the serum tacrolimus level

ANSWERS

A Type Answers

Q1. Answer e

The heart failure survival score is used to objectively assess the severity of cardiac impairment. This score has been derived from a multivariable analysis of 268 ambulatory patients referred for consideration of cardiac transplantation from 1986 to 1991 and validated in 199 similar patients from 1993 to 1995. The predictors of survival in the HFSS include:
- Presence or absence of coronary artery disease;
- Resting heart rate;
- Left ventricular ejection fraction;
- Mean arterial blood pressure;
- Presence or absence of an intraventricular conduction delay on ECG;
- Serum sodium;
- VO_2max

Scores are categorized into low-risk (score ≥8.1), medium-risk (score ≥7.2 and <8.1), and high-risk (<7.2). Patients in medium and high-risk groups (1-year survival of 72% and 43%, respectively) are most likely to die or require urgent transplant in the following year; they should be considered for cardiac transplantation if no contraindications are present. Transplantation can be safely deferred in patients in the low-risk group (1-year survival 93%).

Alraies MC, Eckman P. Adult heart transplant: indications and outcomes. J Thorac Dis. 2014;6(8):1120-8.

Q2. Answer d

Maintenance immunosuppression is routinely initiated within the first few post-operative days. Most maintenance regimens are triple therapy based and include a calcineurin inhibitor, cell cycle inhibitor and corticosteroid.

(i) Calcineurin inhibitors: Calcineurin inhibitors (CNI) are the crux of current maintenance therapy. CNIs inhibit the phosphatase action of calcineurin, a key enzyme in the production pathway of multiple cytokines including IL-2. This action inhibits the expansion of CD4+ and CD8+ cell lines and differentiation of CD4+ T-cell subsets. Currently, 2 CNIs are frequently used, cyclosporine A and tacrolimus. (ii) Cell cycle inhibitors/Antiproliferatives: Azathioprine's (AZA) active metabolite is converted into a purine analog. When incorporated into nuclear DNA, this metabolite inhibits DNA synthesis and subsequent T- and B-cell. AZA is typically used in conjunction with a CNI in maintenance therapy and is effective in preventing rejection when used in combination with CSA and steroids AZA has largely been replaced by newer agents, although it is still used by some clinicians when patients develop intolerable side effects from newer antiproliferative agents. Mycophenolate mofetil has replaced AZA in current maintenance regimens. (iii) Corticosteroids: Corticosteroids have roles in induction, maintenance therapy, and the treatment of rejection. Steroids inhibit the transcription factors activator protein-1 and nuclear factor kappa-B, which both have important roles in the production of cytokines including IL-1 and IL-2, GM-CSF, TNF-alpha, growth factors, gamma interferon, CD40 ligand, and others. These actions limit the number, function, and distribution of white blood cells and provide broad, non-specific, immune suppression. Steroids are typically initiated during and immediately after surgery in high doses and subsequently tapered to lower maintenance dosing. (iv) mTOR Inhibitors: mTOR phosphorylates cell-cycle regulatory proteins involved in the T-cell proliferation, disrupt growth and differentiation of B- and T-cell lymphocytes and inhibits vascular smooth muscle proliferation. Sirolimus is nephrotoxic, although much less so than CNIs. In adults, sirolimus has been shown to decrease CNI-induced renal insufficiency and attenuate the development of coronary vasculopathy.

Schumacher KR, Gajarski RJ. Postoperative care of the transplanted patient. Curr Cardiol Rev. 2011;7(2):110-22.

Q3. Answer c

Induction therapy refers to the administration of a special group of immunosuppressant agents in the pre and perioperative period to rapidly disable the normal host response toward the transplanted graft.
  i. Monoclonal antithymocyte antibody-Muromonab (OKT3) is a murine antibody targeting the human T-cell CD3 receptor which disrupts its ability to respond to an antigen challenge and leads to T-cell opsonization and removal by circulating macrophages.
  ii. Polyclonal antithymocyte globulin (ATG): Two polyclonal antithymocyte antibody preparations are available. Equine ATG is purified after horse immunization with human T-cells, and rabbit ATG is produced by rabbit immunization with human thymocytes.
  iii. IL-2 Receptor antagonists: Use of novel interleukin-2 receptor antagonists (IL-2Ra) has increased over the last several years. These agents bind to the alpha-subunit of the IL-2 receptor on activated T-cells preventing T-cell proliferation and attenuating the graft-directed immune response.
  iv. Corticosteroids: Corticosteroids have roles in induction, maintenance therapy, and the treatment of rejection. Steroids inhibit the transcription factors activator protein-1 and nuclear factor kappa-B, which both have important roles in the production of cytokines including IL-1 and IL-2, GM-CSF, TNF-alpha, growth factors, gamma interferon, CD40 ligand, and others.

> Schumacher KR, Gajarski RJ. Postoperative care of the transplanted patient. Curr Cardiol Rev. 2011;7(2):110-22.

Q4. Answer d

Infection, steroid induced diabetes mellitus, osteoporosis, renal failure, malignancy, lymhoproliferative disorders are primarily the side effects of immunosupressants used in post-transplant period. Graft coronary vasculopthy is a type of immune mediated reaction. Alopecia is the least common complication among the mentioned alternatives.

> Schumacher KR, Gajarski RJ. Postoperative care of the transplanted patient. Curr Cardiol Rev. 2011;7(2):110-22.

Q5. Answer e

Bradyarrhythmia and supraventricular arrhythmia are among the most frequent rhythm disturbances occurring after heart transplantation. Stable sinus rhythm is often established within the first week. Supraventricular arrhythmias are often associated with the administration of large amounts of inotropic and chronotropic substances. In the case of atrial fibrillation an acute rejection reaction should also be considered. The treatment of pulmonary hypertension after heart transplantation is an essential component of the perioperative management. Often secondarily raised pulmonary vascular resistance is found in graft recipients before the operation. Elevation of the pulmonary vascular resistance as a result of chronic heart failure with congested pulmonary circulation is one of the main risk factors for primary graft failure. Pulmonary hypertension and right ventricular failure have a considerable influence on the postoperative morbidity and mortality rates. Perioperatively the tendency toward pulmonary pressure elevation is increased by the use of the heart-lung machine, blood transfusions and protamine. Renal dysfunction can be secondary to low cardiac output or response to immunosuppression which may get exaggerated in the presence of a baseline renal dysfunction. Hepatic dysfunction is the most unlikely of the mentioned alternatives.

> Simsch O, Gromann T, Knosalla C, et al. The intensive care management of patients following heart transplantation at the Deutsches Herzzentrum. Berlin Applied Cardiopulmonary Pathophysiology. 2011;15:230-40.

Q6. Answer a

The New York Heart Association (NYHA) classification provides subjective assessment of the cardiorespiratory function whereas the 6 Minute Walk Test (6MWT), Treadmill test and VO_2 max provide an objective assessment of the cardiorespiratory function and hence are more reliable. However, all of them are indicators of the cardiorespiratory function.

> Ross RM, Murthy JN, Wollak ID, et al. The six minute walk test accurately estimates mean peak oxygen uptake. BMC Pulm Med. 2010;10:31.

Q7. Answer c

Heart transplant	Range (ug/L)
Pediatric	
0–12 months post-transplant	10–15
>12 months post-transplant	5–10
Adult	
0–3 months post-transplant	10–15
3–6 months post-transplant	8–12
6–12 months post-transplant	6–12
>12 months post-transplant	6–10

Pham MX. Induction and maintenance of immunosuppressive therapy in cardiac transplantation. Available from: http://www.uptodate.com/contents/induction-and-maintenance-of-immunosuppressive-therapy-in-cardiac-transplantation (Accessed 6th August 2017).

Q8. Answer e

The guiding principles for the management of AMR comprise removing circulating alloantibodies, reducing production of additional alloantibodies, and suppressing T-cell and B-cell responses. There are no large randomized trials evaluating therapies for AMR in heart transplant recipients. The underlying mechanisms for these therapies are based on the following:

(i) Suppression of the T-cell response (e.g., corticosteroids, mycophenolate mofetil (MMF), anti-lymphocyte antibodies, photopheresis, or total lymphoid irradiation); (ii) Elimination of circulating antibodies (e.g., plasmapheresis); (iii) Inhibition of residual antibodies (e.g., intravenous immunoglobulins); (iv) Suppression or depletion of B cells (e.g., corticosteroids, rituximab, or splenectomy); (v) Suppression or depletion of plasma cells (e.g., bortezomib); (vi) inhibition of complement (e.g., eculizumab, intravenous gamma globulin [IVIg]).

Colvin MM, Cook JL, et al. Antibody-mediated rejection in cardiac transplantation: Emerging knowledge in diagnosis and management. Circulation. 2015;131:1608-39.

Q9. Answer d

Left-sided heart disease (LHD) is the most common cause of pulmonary hypertension (PH). In patients with LHD, elevated left atrial pressure causes a passive increase in pulmonary vascular pressure by hydrostatic transmission. In some patients, an active component caused by pulmonary arterial vasoconstriction and/or vascular remodelling superimposed on left-sided pressure elevation is observed. This "reactive" or "out-of-proportion" PH, defined as PH due to LHD with a transpulmonary gradient (TPG) > 12 mm Hg, confers a worse prognosis. However, TPG is sensitive to changes in cardiac output and left atrial pressure. The prognostic value of diastolic pulmonary vascular pressure gradient (DPG) (i.e., the difference between invasive diastolic pulmonary artery pressure and mean pulmonary capillary wedge pressure) is better to prognosticate death in "out-of-proportion" PH. DPG identifies patients with "out-of-proportion" PH who have significant pulmonary vascular disease and increased mortality.

Gerges C, Gerges M, Lang MB, et al. Diastolic pulmonary vascular pressure gradient: a predictor of prognosis in "out-of-proportion" pulmonary hypertension. Chest. 2013;143(3):758-66. doi: 10.1378/chest.12-1653.

Q10. Answer c

The circulatory and biochemical variables are managed by the general principle of the "Rule of 100" suggesting targets of SBP ≥100 mmHg, urine output ≥100 mL/h, hemoglobin of ≥100 g/L, PaO_2 ≥100 mm Hg and blood sugar targeted at 100% normal. Other elements of donor management are listed below: (i) Temperature: The aim is to keep the core temperature >35°C prior to organ donation. Circulating hot air blankets, warmed intravenous fluids and adjustments of ambient temperature may be needed to achieve this goal. (ii) Fluid management: These patients are often polyuric and dehydrated which is worsened by a vasoplegic state resulting in central volume depletion. (iii) Inotropes and cardiovascular system: Dopamine is the first choice of inotrope in hypotension unresponsive to volume and has beneficial effects on the renal graft. Though it has no renal protective effect and may predispose to arrhythmias, the benefits are probably related to moderation of preservation injury and inflammation, donor cardiovascular effects, or recipient treatment. Nor-adrenaline in doses >0.05 mcg/kg/min resulted in impaired cardiac contractility in transplanted hearts and in particular impairment of right ventricular performance. (iv) Ventilatory management: The principles are along the lines of management of acute lung injury (ALI), i.e. low tidal volume 6–8 mL/kg, minimum plateau pressure, lung recruitment. The lowest FiO_2 needed should be used, and optimal PEEP with a restrictive fluid strategy improves graft harvesting for lung transplants. (v) Replacement of hormones after brain death: Standardization of hormone therapy after brain death in combination with a central venous pressure <10 mmHg significantly improved utilization of the heart and lungs for transplant without affecting other organ systems. The recommended replacements are: Vasopressin, Methylprednisolone, Insulin, Thyroxine (T4) etc.

Kumar L. Brain death and care of the organ donor. J Anaesthesiol Clin Pharmacol. 2016;32(2):146-52.

K Type Answers

Q1. Answer TTTFT

Heart transplant is a treatment option for patients with advanced heart failure who continue to be symptomatic despite the use of recommended optimal medical therapy and cardiac resynchronization therapy as per ACC/AHA guideline. However in view of the scarcity of the organ any surgically amenable cardiac condition should be treated first before transplantation is considered. As per the ACC/AHA guidelines the indications for cardiac transplant are: (i) Refractory cardiogenic shock requiring intra-aortic balloon pump counterpulsation or left ventricular assist device (LVAD), (ii) Cardiogenic shock requiring continuous intravenous inotropic therapy (i.e., dobutamine, milrinone, etc.), (iii) Peak VO_2 (VO_2 max) less than 10 mL/kg per min, (iv) NYHA class of III or IV despite maximized medical and resynchronization therapy, (v) Recurrent life-threatening left ventricular arrhythmias despite an implantable cardiac defibrillator, antiarrhythmic therapy, or catheter-based ablation, (vi) End-stage congenital HF with no evidence of pulmonary hypertension, (vii) Refractory angina without potential medical or surgical therapeutic options.

Jessup M, Abraham WT, Casey DE, et al. 2009 focused update: ACCF/AHA guidelines for the diagnosis and management of heart failure in adults: A report of the American college of cardiology foundation/American Heart Association task force on practice guidelines: Developed in collaboration with the international society for heart and lung transplantation. Circulation. 2009;119:1977-2016.

Q2. Answer TFTTT

VO_2max is an indicator of exercise capacity and assesses cardiac reserve and peripheral adaptations to a reduced cardiac output much more accurately than NYHA classification. Currently it is the gold standard for assessing the severity of cardiac impairment. Patients who have impaired resting hemodynamics but with preserved exercise capacity (peak exercise VO_2 of more than 14 mL/min/kg), have survival and functional capacity equal to those afforded by cardiac transplantation. Contrarily, patients with compensated CHF and a peak oxygen consumption of less than 14 mL/kg/min or <50% predicted have poor long-term survival and must be considered for transplantation. This approach suggests that cardiac transplantation can be safely deferred in ambulatory patients with severe left ventricular dysfunction and a peak oxygen consumption of greater than 14 mL/kg/min. Beta blocker therapy has improved survival rates in patients with systolic HF including patients with very low VO_2max to as low as 10 mL/kg per min. With the use of current evidence-based HF therapy including beta-blockers, spironolactone, angiotensin converting enzyme inhibitors and devices (i.e., implantable cardioverter-defibrillator and cardiac resynchronization therapy), a VO_2max ≤10 mL/kg/min rather than the traditional cut-off value ≤14 mL/min/kg may be more useful for risk stratification.

Alraies MC, Eckman P. Adult heart transplant: indications and outcomes. J Thorac Dis. 2014;6(8):1120-8.

Q3. Answer TTTTF

According to ACC/AHA guidelines the absolute contraindications for heart transplant include: (i) Advanced irreversible renal failure with Cr >2 or creatinine clearance <30–50 mL/min without plans for concurrent renal transplant; (ii) Advanced irreversible liver disease; (iii) Advanced irreversible pulmonary parenchymal disease or (FEV_1 <1 L/min); (iv) Advanced irreversible pulmonary artery hypertension (pulmonary artery systolic pressure >60 mm Hg, pulmonary vascular resistance >4–5 wood units despite vasodilators) due to risk of acute right ventricular failure soon after transplant from insufficient accommodation of the donor heart to high pulmonary vascular resistance pressures; (v) History of solid organ or hematologic malignancy within the last 5 years due to probability of recurrence.

The following are generally considered relative contraindications for heart transplant: (i) Severe peripheral vascular disease; (ii) Severe cerebrovascular disease; (iii) Severe osteoporosis; (iv) Severe obesity (BMI >35 kg/m^2) or cachexia; (v) Acute pulmonary embolism (vi) Active infection (excluding LVAD-related infections); (v) Advanced age (>70 years old); (vi) Psychological instability (e.g., PTSD); (vii) Active or recent (within 6 months) substance abuse (alcohol, cocaine, opioids, tobacco products, etc.); (viii) Diabetes mellitus with end organ damage; (ix) Lack of social support or sufficient resources to permit ongoing access to immunosuppressive medication and frequent medical follow-up.

Yancy CW, Jessup M, Bozkurt B, et al. 2013 ACCF/AHA guideline for the management of heart failure: A report of the american college of cardiology foundation/american heart association task force on practice guidelines. J Am Coll Cardiol. 2013;62:e147-239.

Mancini D, Lietz K. Selection of cardiac transplantation candidates in 2010. Circulation. 2010;122:173-83.

Q4. Answer FTTTF

In the days when cardiac transplantation was started the upper limits of acceptable organs was 35 years of age. This has been gradually increased over the past several decades, with most centers now using donor age <55 years as a cut off. However, there are centres where donors up to age 65 or even greater are accepted. Most of the donor hearts which have undergone cardiopulmonary resuscitation, a neurologic insult, thoracic trauma or are on vasoactive/inotropic drugs display non-specific ST changes on electrocardiogram and can have elevated cardiac enzyme levels. It has been observed that modestly elevated donor cardiac troponin I levels do not have a negative influence in post-transplant mortality or need for mechanical circulatory support it is important to correlate the findings with echocardiographic examination. All potential donors should undergo a detailed echocardiographic examination and it is the single most important tool for examination of donor heart function. Special attention is paid to the presence of left ventricular hypertrophy (LVH), significant physiologic valvular dysfunction, and depressed ventricular function.

Coronary angiography is indicated in donor hearts >40 years of age or with significant risk factors (hypertension, diabetes mellitus, hyperlipidemia, family history, smoking or concerning findings on echocardiogram). Blood group matching is done prior to heart transplantation. HLA matching is not employed in cardiac transplant.

Kilic A, Emani S, Chittoor B. et al. Donor selection in heart transplantation. J Thorac Dis. 2014;6(8):1097-1104. doi: 10.3978/j.issn.2072-1439.2014.03.23.

Q5. Answer TTTTF

Cardiac transplant rejection manifests in 1 or more of the following 3 ways: acute cell-mediated rejection, antibody-mediated rejection (AMR), and allograft vasculopathy. Acute cell-mediated rejection is primarily a host T-lymphocyte-mediated response mounted against the allograft tissue.

AMR refers to allograft injury resulting from activation of the complement system, typically by recipient-generated antibodies directed against the allograft tissue. AMR most commonly occurs months to years following transplantation, a rare subtype, hyperacute rejection, can occur within minutes to hours after transplantation. Cardiac allograft vasculopathy (CAV) also called accelerated graft arteriosclerosis refers to concentric luminal narrowing of the epicardial and intramural coronary arteries. This process generally occurs months to years following transplantation and is currently the limiting factor in long-term allograft survival. This also is thought to represent a manifestation of an antibody-mediated response.

Patel JK, Kobashigawa JA. Improving survival during heart transplantation: diagnosis of antibody-mediated rejection and techniques for the prevention of graft injury. Future Cardiol. 2012;8(4):623-35.

Tan CD, Baldwin WM, Rodriguez ER. Update on cardiac transplantation pathology. Arch Pathol Lab Med. 2007;131(8):1169-91.

Q6. Answer TTFTT

Despite significant improvements in exercise tolerance compared with the end-stages of heart failure, patients still show a reduction in maximum achievable exertion when compared with normal individuals of the same age. This is accounted for by the chronotropic incompetence of the denervated heart as well as peripheral factors. The normal heart will show a rapid acceleration in heart rate in response to exercise that peaks during exercise and rapidly recovers. The transplanted heart shows a delayed chronotropic response to exercise due to a reliance on circulating catecholamines. Norepinephrine and epinephrine levels are either normal or elevated in the transplant recipient. The lack of nervous supply and reliance on humoral mechanisms causes a shift from predominately type-1 to type-2 beta adrenergic receptors on cardiac myocytes. Secondary to lack of parasympathetic tone the heart transplant recipients have a higher average resting heart rate of 95 beats per minute (bpm) compared with 66 bpm for non-transplant cardiac patients.

Fallen EL, Kamath MV, Ghista DN, Fitchett D. Spectral analysis of heart rate variability following human heart transplantation: evidence for functional reinnervation. J Auton Nerv Syst. 1988; 23(3):199-206.

Nytrøen K, Gullestad L. Exercise after heart transplantation: an overview. World J Transplant. 2013;3(4):78.

Q7. Answer TTTTT

CAV is an accelerated form of coronary artery disease (CAD) that is characterized by concentric fibrous intimal hyperplasia along the length of coronary vessels. Both immunologic and nonimmunologic risk factors contribute to the development of CAV by causing endothelial dysfunction and injury eventually leading to progressive intimal thickening. The diagnosis of CAV remains a challenge as angiography, the standard method for detecting focal plaques, lacks sensitivity in detecting CAV, and intravascular ultrasonography, a more sensitive method, lacks the ability to evaluate the entire coronary tree. The disease is difficult to treat and results in significant morbidity and mortality. Since treatment of CAV is limited and usually involves repeat transplantation, prevention or mitigation of immunologic and nonimmunologic risk factors is critically important. CAV prevention may involve therapy that provides protection against endothelial injury implemented just before transplantation, during storage and transplantation as well as after transplantation.

Before transplantation, preventing endothelial injury at brain death, reducing cold ischemic time and subsequent tissue damage, and improving myocardial preservation during storage and transportation of the graft all aid in post-transplant cardiac function and longevity. In a study on prolonged cold storage, the longer cold ischemic times produced greater endothelial dysfunction in cardiac allografts and that the composition of the storage medium affected the extent of allograft tissue damage.

Ramzy D, Rao V, Brahm J, et al. Ross cardiac allograft vasculopathy: a review. Can J Surg. 2005;48(4):319-27.

Q8. Answer FTFTT

Management of post-transplant persistent pulmonary arterial hypertension is a challenge. The diagnosis and surveillance of the pulmonary hypertension and right ventricular dysfunction is done by means of a pulmonary artery catheter (CVP, MPAP, PCWP, CO, SvO_2) and transesophageal echocardiography. The basic concepts involved in management include – avoidance of potentially PVR raising substances – ketamine, histamine-releasing muscle relaxants (mivacurium, atracurium) – ensuring sufficient oxygenation (paO_2 100 mm Hg) by raising the FiO_2 – careful recruitment of non-ventilated lung areas, use of a moderate PEEP level (< 10 mbar), avoidance of high peak pressure during artificial respiration – avoidance of respiratory acidosis, moderate hyperventilation (pCO_2 30–35 mm Hg) – neutralization of existing metabolic acidosis/ alkalization with sodium bicarbonate – careful volume therapy under strict monitoring of the preload parameters/optimization of the cardiac filling pressures (CVP 10–12 mm Hg, PCWP 12–15 mm Hg) – administration of systemic intravenous vasodilatators (nitroglycerin, sodium nitroprusside, the prostacyclin (PGI2) analogon iloprost (Ilomedin).

Simsch O, Gromann T, Knosalla C, et al. The intensive care management of patients following heart transplantation. Applied Cardiopulmonary Pathophysiology. 2011;15:230-40.

Q9. Answer TFFTT

Left ventricular dysfunction is managed by epinephrine infusion > 0.1 µg/kg/min. If the peripheral vascular resistance is > 1000 dyn* sec *cm, the administration of phosphodiesterase inhibitors might help. In addition, a heart rate of 100–120 bpm should be aimed at by means of atrial stimulation under monitoring of the cardiac output. With low MAP (< 65 mm Hg), persistent oliguria and acidosis refractory to therapy in spite of high-dose catecholamine support, the implantation of an intra-aortic balloon pump is indicated. Mechanical circulatory support remains the final option.

Simsch O, Gromann T, Knosalla C, et al. The intensive care management of patients following heart transplantation. Applied Cardiopulmonary Pathophysiology. 2011;15:230-40.

Q10. Answer TFTTT

Tacrolimus is one of the most nephrotoxic agents currently in use. It can cause hyperkalemia and acute kidney injury. Nephrotoxicity is reversible if tacrolimus is stopped early in the course of toxicity.

Corticosteroids cause diabetes mellitus, hypertension, peptic ulcer disease and leukocytosis. Mycophenolate is known to cause pancytopenia.

Azole group of antifungals inhibit the metabolism of tacrolimus and therefore increase plasma levels of tacrolimus.

Lehmkuhl H, Dandel M, Hiemann N, et al. Induction therapy in heart transplantation. Applied Cardiopulmonary Pathophysiology. 2011;15:241-4.

TRANSPLANTATION: LIVER

Ankit Sharma, Shrikanth Srinivasan, Deepak Govil

A Type Questions
(One best answer)

1. Surgical intervention will be most commonly required in which of the following complications of portal hypertension, in a patient with End Stage Liver Disease:
   a. Hypersplenism
   b. Variceal hemorrhage
   c. Ascites
   d. Encephalopathy
   e. Hepatic hydrothorax

2. "Achilles' heel" of liver transplantation refers to:
   a. Bile duct complications
   b. Neurologic complications
   c. Vascular thrombosis
   d. Primary non-function
   e. Hepatorenal syndrome

3. Most common cause of renal failure in cirrhosis is:
   a. Hepatorenal syndrome
   b. Spontaneous bacterial peritonitis
   c. Hypovolemia due to hematemesis
   d. Intrinsic renal pathology
   e. Massive ascites

4. In a cirrhotic patient, which one of the following conditions is considered as an indication for urgent referral for liver transplantation?
   a. Portal vein thrombosis
   b. Hepatic encephalopathy Grade 4
   c. Type 1 hepatorenal syndrome
   d. HCC with common bile duct obstruction
   e. Upper GI bleeding

5. Time of maximum instability during liver transplant is during which of the following phases?
   a. Pre-anhepatic
   b. Anhepatic
   c. Reperfusion
   d. Neohepatic
   e. Both a. and b.

6. Cut-off scores for MELD and Child Turcotte Pugh (CTP), for referring a patient for transplant evaluation are:
   a. MELD score of at least 10 or a CTP score of at least 7
   b. MELD score of at least 20 or a CTP score of at least 10
   c. MELD score of at least 20 or a CTP score of at least 15
   d. MELD score of at least 15 or a CTP score of at least 10
   e. MELD score of at least 5 or a CTP score of at least 2

7. Which one of the following statements about primary nonfunction (PNF), post liver transplant is not TRUE?
   a. PNF is the most severe manifestation of graft dysfunction
   b. It is described as liver function inconsistent with recipient survival, either progressing to patient death or requiring retransplantation within 7 days of surgery
   c. Clinical manifestations include persistent encephalopathy and metabolic acidosis, marked hypoglycemia, coagulopathy and reduced or absent bile production associated with progressive increase in serum AST levels
   d. PNF is characterized by laboratory changes (one or more of the following variables were present: serum bilirubin levels ≥10mg/dL; INR ≥1.6 on postoperative day 7; and serum AST or ALT levels >2,000IU/L within the first 7 days of surgery) and has full graft recovery
   e. PNF after liver transplantation is life threatening

8. Magnesium replacement post- liver transplant (LTx) is of paramount importance for all of these reasons except:
   a. Hypomagnesemia is associated with decreased effects of immunosuppressants
   b. Hypomagnesemia can cause severe arrhythmias
   c. Prolonged hypomagnesemia occurs regardless of the pre transplant Mg level due to using immunosuppressants like Tacrolimus
   d. During surgery, a huge amount of citrate in blood products is administered chelating Mg and Ca, further aggravating the hypomagnesemia which already exists in variable degrees because of underlying malnutrition

e. Hypermagnesemia (>3 mg/dL) can exert an anti-calcium effect on the cardiovascular system

9. **Cytomegalovirus in transplant recipients, all of the following statements are TRUE except:**
   a. It can cause pneumonitis, retinitis, CNS disease, diarrhea and carditis
   b. It can also have an immunomodulatory effect in liver recipients, further enhancing the immunosuppression and predisposition to opportunistic infections with bacteria, fungi or other viruses
   c. Serology to demonstrate CMV IgG in the blood of transplant recipients is recommended for the diagnosis of acute CMV infection after transplantation
   d. Treatment of choice is IV ganciclovir, at 5 mg/kg twice daily, or valganciclovir, at 900-mg orally twice daily
   e. CMV is the most common and single most important viral infection in solid organ transplant recipients

10. **Tacrolimus related toxicity in a liver transplant recipient can manifest as all of the following except:**
    a. Hyperkalemia and hypertension
    b. Hypoglycemia
    c. Seizures
    d. Nephrotoxicity
    e. Hypomagnesemia

K Type Questions
[Marked True (T)/False (F)]

1. **Regarding ascites in a cirrhotic patient the Grade I, class I recommendations are:**
   a. If patients undergo paracentesis and have no clinically evident fibrinolysis or disseminated intravascular coagulation, then they should not receive fresh frozen plasma or platelet replacement before paracentesis unless the international normalized ratio ≥2.5 and platelet count ≤100,000/cu mm
   b. If patients have clinically apparent (i.e., moderate to severe) ascites and normal renal function, then they should be managed with both salt restriction and diuretics (including a combination of spironolactone and loop diuretics)
   c. If hospitalized patients with ascites have an ascitic fluid polymorphonuclear count of >250 cells/mm^3, then they should receive empiric antibiotics within 6 hours of the test result
   d. If patients have a documented episode of spontaneous bacterial peritonitis (SBP), then they should receive long-term outpatient antibiotics with first prescription within 1 week of hospital discharge
   e. If patients with ascites have serum sodium of 110 mEq/L or less, then they should be managed with discontinuation of diuretics and fluid restriction

2. **Regarding variceal bleeding in a cirrhotic patient, following statements are TRUE:**
   a. If patients without prior variceal bleeding are found to have no varices on esophagogastroduodenoscopy (EGD), then they should not receive nonselective beta-blockers to prevent bleeding
   b. If patients have cirrhosis, no documented history of previous GI bleeding, and have medium/large varices on endoscopy, then they should receive either nonselective beta-blockers or endoscopic variceal ligation (EVL) within 1 month of varices diagnosis
   c. If patients with cirrhosis are admitted with or develop suspected variceal bleeding, then they should receive somatostatin or analogues (somatostatin, octreotide, terlipressin) within 12 hours of presentation
   d. If patients with cirrhosis present with hematemesis, then they should receive upper endoscopy within 72 hours of presentation
   e. If patients with cirrhosis are found to have bleeding esophageal varices, then they should receive EVL or sclerotherapy at the time of index endoscopy

3. **Recommendations for the management of hepatic encephalopathy are the following:**
   a. Oral disaccharides or Rifaximin
   b. Somnolence to semi-stupor, but responsive to verbal stimuli: refers to Grade 2 of West Haven grading hepatic encephalopathy
   c. Protein restriction has no beneficial effect in cirrhotic patients with hepatic encephalopathy
   d. Intubation and sedation are recommended in grade III encephalopathy because of the

attendant risks to airway and possibilities of raised intracranial pressure
e. Liver transplant remains the only effective therapy

4. **Regarding fulminant hepatic failure (FHF), consider the following statements:**
   a. FHF can only occur in the setting of pre-existing chronic liver disease
   b. Coagulopathy and coma are important findings in patients with FHF
   c. Liver transplant should not be attempted in patients with FHF because of the high mortality rate, regardless of the treatment used
   d. The main cause of death in these patients is cerebral edema
   e. One of the most important factors in prognosis of FHF is the cause of liver disease

5. **Which of the following statements about hepatic artery thrombosis following liver transplantation is/are correct?**
   a. Thrombosis of the hepatic artery following liver transplantation is more common in children than in adult patients
   b. Thrombosis of the hepatic artery usually occurs several weeks after transplant as a result of arteriosclerosis
   c. Thrombosis of the hepatic artery in the early days following transplantation is a serious complication leading to death unless retransplantation can be performed within 36 to 72 hours
   d. Late thrombosis of the hepatic artery may present as biliary complication or intrahepatic abscesses
   e. Thrombosis of the portal vein is more frequent than hepatic artery thrombosis following liver transplantation

6. **Regarding hepatorenal syndrome (HRS), consider the following statements:**
   a. Vasodilatation in splanchnic circulation due to NO release
   b. Insufficient cardiac output leading to effective hypovolemia
   c. Type-2 HRS is characterized by rapid progressive renal failure defined by doubling of the initial serum creatinine concentrations to a level greater than 226 mmol/L in less than 2 weeks
   d. Presence of shock is must for the diagnosis of HRS
   e. Liver transplantation is the treatment of choice for both type-1 and type-2 HRS

7. **King's College criteria for liver transplantation in AHF, for overdose of Acetaminophen (APAP) include the following:**
   a. INR > 6.5
   b. pH <7.3
   c. Duration of jaundice before encephalopathy/7 days
   d. Serum bilirubin >17.5 mg/dL
   e. INR>6.5, serum creatinine >3.4 mg/dL, and grade III/IV encephalopathy

8. **Post reperfusion syndrome (PRS), the following statements are TRUE:**
   a. Mild PRS, defined by a decrease of MAP and/or heart rate (HR) not reaching 30% of baseline value, lasting for less than 5 min, and responsive to an intravenous bolus dose of calcium chloride (1 g) and/or epinephrine (≤ 100 mcg) without the need to start a continuous infusion of vasopressors
   b. Can lead to sudden drop in SVRI, MAP, PVRI, PAP
   c. After reperfusion, an increase in serum potassium and a reduction in serum calcium are usually observed
   d. Significant PRS, defined by greater hemodynamic instability, a drop in MAP/HR exceeding 30% of baseline
   e. Preservation solutions, the transplantation technique and the washout technique used before reperfusion have no effect on the incidence of PRS

9. **Risk factors associated with bacterial infections after orthotopic liver transplantation are:**
   a. Increased length of preoperative stay
   b. Duct to duct anastomosis
   c. Higher volume of transfused blood products
   d. Preoperative higher MELD and CTP scores
   e. CMV status of the donor and the recipient

10. **Small-for-size syndrome in living donor liver transplantation has following features:**
    a. Is defined as a < 0.8% Graft-to-recipient body weight ratio (GRWR)
    b. Associated with excessive bile production
    c. Delayed synthetic functions of liver
    d. Intractable ascites
    e. Higher incidence of Graft vs Host disease and rejection

ANSWERS

A Type Answers

Q1. Answer b

Surgery has no role in primary prophylaxis. Its role in acute variceal bleeding is exceedingly limited, because therapy with endoscopic treatment controls bleeding in 90% of patients. A transjugular intrahepatic portosystemic shunt (TIPS) is a viable option and is less invasive for patients whose bleeding is not controlled. However, if TIPS is not available, then staple transection of the esophagus is an option when endoscopic treatment and pharmacologic therapy have failed. Surgical intervention is considered for the prevention of rebleeding when pharmacologic and/or endoscopic therapies have failed. As per the Baveno II consensus conference on portal hypertension, failure is defined as a single episode of clinically significant rebleeding (transfusion requirement of 2 U of blood or more within 24 hours, a systolic blood pressure < 100 mm Hg or a postural change of >20 mm Hg, and/or a pulse rate greater than 100 bpm).

Surgical interventions include the following:
- Portosystemic shunts
- Devascularization procedures
- Orthotopic liver transplantation (OLT) - Treatment of choice in patients with advanced liver disease.

De Franchis R. Updating consensus in portal hypertension: report of the Baveno III Consensus Workshop on definitions, methodology and therapeutic strategies in portal hypertension. J Hepatol. 2000;33(5):846-52.

Q2. Answer a

Biliary complications are regarded as the Achilles' heel of liver transplantation, especially for living donor liver transplantation (LDLT) due to smaller, multiple ducts and difficult ductal anatomy.

Vij V, Makki K, et al. Targeting the Achilles' heel of adult living donor liver transplant: Corner-sparing sutures with mucosal eversion technique of biliary anastomosis. Liver Transpl. 2016;22(1):14-23.

Q3. Answer b

Bacterial infections are the most common cause of renal failure in cirrhosis. The pathogenesis is related to an exacerbation of the systemic arterial vasodilation already present in patients with cirrhosis because of bacterial products, cytokines, or vasoactive mediators that appear in relation with the infection. This hemodynamic effect occurs mainly in patients who develop spontaneous bacterial peritonitis and spontaneous bacteremia, but it may occur with any bacterial infection. Therefore, the possibility of a bacterial infection should be meticulously examined in any patient with cirrhosis and renal failure.

Isabel G. Diagnostic approach to renal failure in cirrhosis. Clin Liver dis. 2013;2(3):128-31.

Q4. Answer c

Patients with cirrhosis and type 1 hepatorenal syndrome have a median survival of less than 2 weeks and should be urgently referred to a transplant center for an expedited transplant evaluation. In addition, patients diagnosed with hepatopulmonary syndrome or portopulmonary hypertension, attributed to cirrhosis, should be referred for consideration of transplantation. In addition, patients with acute liver failure also should have urgent referral and transfer to a liver transplantation centre.

O'Leary JG, Lepe R, Davis GL. Indications for liver transplantation. Gastroenterology. 2008;134(6):1764-76.

Q5. Answer c

Table 1: Phases of the liver transplant procedure with associated features

Phase	Pre-anhepatic	Anhepatic	Reperfusion	Neohepatic
Timing	From incision to isolation of native liver from circulation	From isolation of native liver from circulation to reperfusion	A brief event at which the new liver is introduced into the patients circulation	From reperfusion to the end of the procedure

Contd...

Contd...

Phase	Pre-anhepatic	Anhepatic	Reperfusion	Neohepatic
Features	• Anesthesia induction • Line placement, skin incision • Dissection to allow removal of diseased liver • Obvious and insidious blood losses • Fluid shifts • Poterntial compression of native vessels during dissection	• Isolation of native liver from circulation • Removal of diseased liver • Implantation of new liver	• Introduction of new liver into the circulation • Time of most instability • Postassium load, cytokine load, emboli, cold fluid	• From reperfusion to end of precedure • Reconstruction of hepatic artery • Construction of biliary anastomoses • New liver begins to function • Hemostasis
	• Worsening of preexisting coagulopathy	• Decrease in venous return (degree dependent on technique; modern "piggyback technique" affects venous return less than complete inferior vena cava occlusion technique) • Progressive coagulopathy • Progressive metabolic acidosis • Hypocalcemia	• Hypotension common • Intracranial pressure may rise • Pulmonary hypertension may worsen • Arrhythmias • Coagulopathy may worsen	• Continuing correction of coagulopathy, metabolic and acid base disorders • Optimization of cardiovascular parameters • Preparation for emergence

Keegan MT, David J. Perioperative care of the liver transplant patient. Crit Care Clin. 2016;32:453-73.

Q6. Answer a

The Model for End-Stage Liver Disease (MELD) score consists of serum bilirubin and creatinine levels, International Normalized Ratio (INR) for prothrombin time. It is a reliable measure of mortality risk in patients with end-stage liver disease and is suitable for use as a disease severity index to determine organ allocation priorities.

Kamath PS, et al. A model to predict survival in patients with end-stage liver disease, Hepatology. 2001;33(2):464-70.

Q7. Answer d

According to the strict criteria established by the United Network for Organ Sharing (UNOS; American transplantation regulatory body), PNF is defined as serum AST levels ≥3,000 associated with at least one of the following: INR ≥ 2.5, acidosis corresponding to arterial pH ≤7.30 or venous pH ≤7.25 and/or serum lactate levels ≥4mMol/L. Researchers supporting definitions based on objective criteria argue this would simplify PNF diagnosis and promote fast reinclusion in organ transplant waiting lists, the only alternative to prevent patient death.

Douglas BN, et al. Primary graft dysfunction of the liver: definitions, diagnostic criteria and risk factors. Einstein (São Paulo). 2016;14(4):24.

Q8. Answer a

Hypomagnesaemia induced morbidity during and after LTx are described in many studies, intraoperatively during orthotropic liver transplantation, associated with ventricular extrasystoles, and Torsades de Pointes developed during the anhepatic phase in a previous report of our group. It was associated with neurological complications in pediatrics and central pontine myelinolysis after LTx. Pretransplant hypomagnesaemia was considered as a predictor for new onset diabetes after both renal and LTx.

Hamed ME. Pretransplant serum magnesium level predicts outcome after pediatric living donor liver transplantation. Ann Transplant. 2012;17(2):29-37.

Q9. Answer c

CMV remains the single most devastating viral infection causing morbidity and mortality in liver transplant patients. It is known that contributions from both the innate and adaptive immune system are necessary for a complete immune response to CMV. Ganciclovir (and valganciclovir) is the most commonly used antiviral drug. High-risk D+/R- liver transplant patients require a more aggressive form of prevention, which in many centers have translated to longer duration of antiviral prophylaxis. Gold standard for diagnosis of tissue invasive CMV disease remains the demonstration of CMV pathology in a biopsy specimen from the involved organ.

Jasmine RM, Beam E, Razonable RR. Cytomegalovirus infection in liver transplant recipients: Updates on clinical management, World J Gastroenterol. 2014;20(31):10658-67.

Q10. Answer b

Features of tacrolimus toxicity include the following nephrotoxicity, neurotoxicity, hyperglycemia (require insulin), GI disturbances, hperkalemia, hypomagnesemia, hypertension and anaphylaxis, etc.

Ghufran A, Lucey MR (Eds.). A Textbook of Liver Disease, 7th edn. Elsevier. 2018; chapter 52.

K Type Answers

Q1. Answer FTTTF

Cirrhosis is a prevalent and expensive condition. Explicit quality indicators (QIs) for their treatment was established by 11-member, multidisciplinary expert panel and followed modified Delphi methods to systematically identify a set of QIs for cirrhosis. These provide physicians and institutions with a tool to identify processes amenable to quality improvement. This tool is intended to be applicable in any setting where care for patients with cirrhosis is provided.

Kanwal F, Kramer J, Asch SM, et al. An explicit quality indicator set for measurement of quality of care in patients with cirrhosis. Clinical gastroenterology and hepatology. 2010;8:709-17.

Q2. Answer TTTFT

Final set of Explicit quality indicators (QIs) for their treatment was established by 11-member, multidisciplinary expert panel and followed modified Delphi methods to systematically identify a set of QIs for cirrhosis. These provide physicians and institutions with a tool to identify processes amenable to quality improvement. This tool is intended to be applicable in any setting where care for patients with cirrhosis is provided.

Kanwal F, Kramer J, Asch SM, et al. An Explicit Quality Indicator Set for Measurement of Quality of Care in Patients With Cirrhosis. Clin gastroenterology and hepatology. 2010;8:709-717.

Q3. Answer TFTTT

Final set of explicit quality indicators (QIs) for their treatment was established by 11-member, multidisciplinary expert panel and followed modified Delphi methods to systematically identify a set of QIs for cirrhosis. These provide physicians and institutions with a tool to identify processes amenable to quality improvement. This tool is intended to be applicable in any setting where care for patients with cirrhosis is provided.

Kanwal F, Kramer J, Asch SM, et al. An Explicit Quality Indicator Set for Measurement of Quality of Care in Patients With Cirrhosis. Clinical Gastroenterol Hepatol. 2010;8:709-17.

Q4. Answer FTFTT

FHF corresponds to the rapid loss of hepatic function in the absence of pre-existing liver disease, causing jaundice, coagulopathy, and coma. One of the major prognostic factors is the cause of the liver disease. Early admission to an intensive care unit and management by physicians experienced in liver transplantation are mandatory. The major cause of death in these patients is cerebral edema. In patients who rapidly develop coma, subdural intracerebral pressure monitoring is mandatory for optimal management as well as for identification of patients who can benefit from liver transplantation. The survival rate for patients with FHF who undergo liver transplantation is currently above 65%. This is the only cure in most patients with FHF.

Lee WM, Larson AM, Stravitz RT. AASLD Position Paper: The Management of Acute Liver Failure: Update 2011. Available from: https://www.aasld.org/sites/default/files/guideline_documents/alfenhanced.pdf (Accessed 17th August, 2017).

Q5. Answer TFTTF

Hepatic artery thrombosis (HAT) is the most serious vascular complication after LTx with an overall incidence that varies from 2% to 9%. The exact mechanism of HAT development remains unclear and is likely multifactorial. Many risk factors, both operative and nonoperative, have been implicated. Close postoperative monitoring of these patients and clinical judgment are mandatory.

Bile ducts are exclusively dependent on the blood supply from the hepatic artery (HA). HAT usually presents with biliary ischemic lesions such as necrosis with biliary leakage, ischemic stricture(s), cholangitis, and ultimately multiorgan failure and graft dysfunction. Routine surveillance of HA anastomoses with Doppler ultrasonography (US) facilitates the early detection and treatment of these complications before irreversible graft dysfunction.

Early thrombosis of the hepatic artery leads to rapid liver failure with a fatal outcome unless a transplant can be performed within 36 to 72 hours. Although thrombolytic therapy through percutaneous or surgical access can be successful, most of these patients require retransplantation. Stenosis of the hepatic artery or late thrombosis of the hepatic artery can lead to multiple intrahepatic strictures of the bile duct and/or hepatic abscesses. This complication also often requires retransplantation. Portal vein thrombosis is a rarer complication. It is a devastating condition when it occurs early, but can be tolerated well if it develops after several months. Portal hypertension due to late portal vein thrombosis can often be treated successfully by a shunt procedure.

Mourand MM, Liosis C, Gunson BK, et al. Etiology and management of hepatic artery thrombosis after adult liver transplantation. Liver Transpl. 2014;20(6):713-23.

Q6. Answer TTFFT

HRS is a life-threatening complication arising in patients with liver cirrhosis and triggered by a series of complex hemodynamic and neurohormonal changes linked to the liver disease. The condition carries a very poor prognosis and high morbidity and mortality rates.

Type I HRS is characterized by acute onset and rapidly progressing kidney failure with a doubling of serum creatinine to > 2.5 mg/dL (corresponding to a 50% reduction in the creatinine clearance rate) in less than 2 weeks, usually associated with multiorgan damage. The prognosis is poor with only 10% of patients surviving longer than 90 days.

Type II HRS represents the final kidney response to hemodynamic impairments in cirrhosis. This type presents as a less severe and more gradual decline in renal function associated with refractory ascites. The increase in creatinine is gradual with mean values of 1.5-2.0 mg/dL. Type II HRS predisposes patients to the development of type I HRS after a precipitating event. The average survival rate is six to eight months after onset.

The current therapeutic armamentarium includes drugs with specific vasoconstrictive effects on the splanchnic circulation in addition to renal and liver replacement therapies which can be artificial or natural (liver transplantation). Liver transplant remains the only truly effective treatment but is limited by the high mortality rate in HRS patients and the shortage of available organs.

Baraldi O, Valentini C, Donati G, et al. Hepatorenal syndrome: Update on diagnosis and treatment. World J Nephrol. 2015;4(5):511-20.

Q7. Answer FTFFT

King's College criteria for liver transplantation in AHF.

APAP-associated AHF	All other causes of AHF
pH < 7.3 or INR > 6.5, serum creatinine > 3.4 mg/dL, and grade III-IV encephalopathy	INR > 6.5 or Three of the following variables: 1. Age <10 or >40 years 2. Cause is nonA, nonB, hepatitis or idiosyncratic drug reaction 3. Duration of jaundice before encephalopathy > 7 days 4. INR > 3.5 5. Serum bilirubin > 17.5 mg/dL

APAP: Acetaminophen; INR: International normalized ratio.

Castaldo ET, Chari RS. Liver transplantation for acute hepatic failure. HPB. 2006;8:29-34.

Q8. Answer TFTTF

Mild PRS, defined by a decrease of MAP and/or heart rate (HR) not reaching 30% of baseline value, lasting for less than 5 min, and responsive to an intravenous bolus dose of calcium chloride (1 g) and/or epinephrine ($\leq$ 100 mcg) without the need to start a continuous infusion of vasopressors; and significant PRS, defined by greater hemodynamic instability, a drop in MAP/HR exceeding 30% of baseline, asystole or hemodynamically significant arrhythmias; or the need to start the infusion of vasopressors during the intraoperative period and to continue throughout the postoperative period. Other presentations of significant PRS include a prolonged (defined as lasting more than 30 min) or recurrent (defined as reappearing within 30 min after resolution) fibrinolysis that requires treatment with antifibrinolytic agents. PRS is frequently characterized by a rapid fall of ABP, a reduction of HR and SVRI associated to an increase or, sometimes, a reduction in cardiac index (CI). Pulmonary capillary wedge pressure (PCWP) can decrease or increase, stroke volume index decreases (SVI) while there is usually an increase of both pulmonary vascular resistance index (PVRI) and pulmonary arterial pressure (PAP).

> Siniscalchi A, Gamberini L, et al. Post reperfusion syndrome during liver transplantation: From pathophysiology to therapy and preventive strategies, World J Gastroenterol. 2016;22(4):1551-69.

Q9. Answer TFTTF

Bacterial organisms are the leading cause of infection post-OLT, with an incidence that ranges from 53% to 70%. The risk factors associated with increased risk of bacterial infections are described in the following table:

- Older age
- Length of preoperative stay
- CMV infection
- Duration of surgery
- Retransplanation
- Volume of transfused blood products
- Preoperative MELD and CTP scores
- Bilioenteric anastomosis
- Technical complications (e.g. biliary leak, HAT)
- Renal replacement therapy
- Hyperglycemia

CMV: Cytomegalovirus; CTP: Child-Turcotte-Phgh; HAT: Hepatic artery thrombosis; MELD: Model for end-stage liver disease.

> Hernandez MDP, Martin P, et al. Infectious complications after liver transplantation. Gastroenterol Hepatol. 2015;11(11):741-53.

Q10. Answer TFTTF

SFSG (small for size graft) is defined as a <0.8% graft-to-recipient body weight ratio (GRWR). It is reported that the use of SFSG leads to SFSS, including poor bile production, delayed synthetic function, prolonged cholestasis and intractable ascites, with subsequent septic complications and higher mortality.

> Yagi S, Uemoto S. Small-for-size syndrome in living donor liver transplantation. Hepatobiliary Pancreat Dis Int. 2012;11(6):570-76.

CHAPTER 16

Infectious Diseases

Om Srivastava, Indraneel Raut

A Type Questions
(One best answer)

1. A 37-year-old male with immunodeficiency due to retroviral disease presents with chest infection diagnosed as *Pneumocystis jirovecii*. He is responsive to treatment but on tenth day in hospital he has massive hemoptysis and required intubation. His total leukocytes counts are 7800/mm^3 with 630 CD4 cells. Chest X-ray shows multiple cystic lesions. Most likely diagnosis is:
   a. P. jirovecii disseminated disease
   b. Vasculitis and angiopathy of HIV
   c. Disseminated tuberculosis
   d. Angioinvasive aspergillosis

2. A 23-year-old man with history of childhood asthma presents with a 3 day history of shortness of breath and wheezing. His parameters are otherwise normal other than eosinophil count of 31%. His CXR shows bilateral infiltrative shadows. An Aspergillus precipitin test is negative and a Galactomannan assay is unremarkable. Next investigation to prove your diagnosis would be:
   a. Pulmonary function tests to show reversible airways disease
   b. CT Chest in sitting and supine position to exclude aspergilloma
   c. Total serum IgE to establish Allergic Bronchopulmonary Aspergillosis (ABPA)
   d. Bronchoscopy to exclude mechanical obstruction

3. Regarding treatment of invasive aspergillosis:
   a. Surgical excision of fibrotic lung is gold standard
   b. Reduction of tacrolimus dose on Voriconazole therapy
   c. Posaconazole and Amphotericin are mainstay in initial treatment
   d. Immunosuppression in transplant patients should be withdrawn immediately

4. The most common commensal site of *Candida albicans* is:
   a. Female genitourinary tract
   b. Central nervous system
   c. Pluripotent stem cells
   d. Macrophages and glial cells

5. The most likely cause of endogenous candidemia in endophthalmitis is:
   a. Immunosuppression
   b. Total parenteral nutrition
   c. GI surgery
   d. Diabetes mellitus

6. A 44-year-old jute farm worker presents with a friable, painless papular lesion on his forearm, unproductive cough for ten days associated with non-migratory joint pains. A chest X-ray reveals moderate right pleural effusion. Patients CD4 count is 170 cells/mm^3. Biopsy of the skin lesion shows areas of necrosis in epithelial cells with minimal inflammation. Most likely diagnosis is:
   a. Cutaneous nocardiosis
   b. Disseminated cryptococcosis
   c. Systemic histoplasmosis
   d. Atypical mycobacterial infection

7. The biggest indicator of adverse clinical event in retroviral infection is:
   a. CD4 counts
   b. CD4 percentage of total leukocyte count
   c. CD4:CD 8 ratio
   d. Viral load of HIV

8. A 21-year-old girl with a three month history of diarrhea presents with painful peripheral neuritis and headache with blurred vision of recent onset. In the initial workup her western blot for HIV is positive and her CD4 count is 27 cells/mm³. Most likely diagnosis is:
   a. CMV colitis and retinitis
   b. HIV neuropathy
   c. Isospora Belli infection
   d. Salmonellosis

9. A family of three members all diagnosed positive for H1N1 and was started on treatment. A fourth member in contact with this family is post renal transplant on immunosuppression is asymptomatic. The recommended treatment is:
   a. Isolation, oseltamivir after throat swab
   b. Prophylactic oseltamivir at half dose
   c. Hospitalization for Oseltamivir and Zanamivir dual therapy
   d. Close observation for seven days

10. An elderly farmer presents with a fracture of right forearm and index finger non-resolving abscess. Investigations reveal pathological fracture of radius and ulna, right carpal tunnel syndrome. Drainage of abscess and microscopy reveals gray brown smooth conidia. He has failed treatment with Caspofungin and Amphotericin B. He has:
    a. Mycobacterium abscessus infection
    b. Streptococcus milleri infection
    c. Scedosporium infection
    d. Lujo hemorrhagic fever

11. A middle aged man with flu like symptoms has undergone a workup. Platelet count is 30,000/mm³. In further workup his ELISA for HIV is positive and his Western blot is indeterminate. He needs:
    a. Single donor platelet transfusion
    b. No therapy is indicated
    c. Bone marrow aspirate and biopsy
    d. Bone marrow transplant

12. Fetal ultrasound in a pregnant patient with Parvovirus B19 infection reveals fetal distress with a heart rate of 180 beats per minute. Best therapeutic option is:
    a. Medical termination of pregnancy
    b. IV Immunoglobulins to mother for 5 days
    c. IV acyclovir for 5 days
    d. IV amiodarone and beta blockers

13. In pregnant patients undergoing treatment for active tuberculosis, when a diagnosis of retroviral disease is established:
    a. Antiretroviral therapy should be initiated immediately
    b. ART is ideal only in third trimester
    c. ART is indicated after completion of antitubercular therapy
    d. ART is indicated after patient has delivered.

14. In Toxoplasmosis and pregnancy:
    a. Asymptomatic patients need not be evaluated or treated
    b. Intrauterine growth retardation is not a feature
    c. Lymphadenopathy should be evaluated vigorously to initiate potential treatment
    d. Termination of pregnancy is always indicated

15. A 54-year-male presents with a fourth event of salmonella bacteremia in one calendar year associated with 7 kg weight loss. He has now got oral thrush and signs of cerebral irritation. Most likely reason for his recurrent salmonellosis is:
    a. Incorrect treatment
    b. Drug resistanat infection
    c. Patient is a carrier state for salmonella
    d. AIDS defining illness

16. A 56-year-old professional pet trainer presents to emergency Department with abdominal bloating, vomiting and fever. Her initial blood show transaminitis and an initial USG abdomen is labeled Peliosis hepatis. Her likeliest diagnosis is.
    a. Bartonella henselae infection
    b. Hepatitis B
    c. Hepatitis C
    d. Chronic granulomatous disease

17. A 77-year-old man has undergone a seven day history of a febrile illness 3 weeks ago for which he took no treatment. Now he presents

with altered sensorium, pain abdomen and orthopnea. A CT scan of the chest shows pulmonary hemorrhages and in the workup a real time PCR is positive for leptospirosis. The treatment of choice is:
   a. Doxycycline
   b. Crystalline Penicillin
   c. Clarithromycin
   d. Levofloxacin

18. The most likely surgical emergency in Infectious Mononeuclosis is:
   a. Suppurative tonsillitis
   b. Spinal abscess and cord compression
   c. Catastrophic gastrointestinal bleeding
   d. Spontaneous rupture of spleen

19. A 20-year-old female presents with seizures, arthralgias and palpitations for 3 days. There is a history of travel to rain forests of countries in southeast Asia 2 months ago, longest duration in Vietnam. Family also describes a rash that appears to be migratory in nature. Once samples are collected for routine tests, cultures and serology, the next best step is:
   a. Lumbar puncture and MRI brain
   b. EEG
   c. Commence treatment with Ceftriaxone and Crystalline Penicillin
   d. Await serology for Lyme disease

20. A 55-year-old male with a clinical diagnosis of filariasis presents to emergency with hemodynamic collapse and shock. He has taken a single dose of Diethylcarbamazine (DEC) 2 hours before this event. This event is:
   a. Septecemia and shock
   b. Myocarditis and complete heart block
   c. Encephalitis due to microfilariae
   d. Mazzotti reaction

21. A post cerebral malaria and ARDS affected patient recovering in ICU goes into pancytopenia, and is comatose with a GCS of 3 within two hours. There is no obvious cause of bleeding and a peripheral smear shows fragmented and dyskaryotic cell lines which is confirmed by bone marrow. The likeliest diagnosis is:
   a. Myelodysplastic syndrome
   b. Acute myeloid leukemia
   c. Bone marrow suppression secondary to malaria
   d. Hemophagocytoic syndrome

22. In the same patient, the treatment of choice is:
   a. IVIG
   b. Quinine plus sulfadiazine/pyrimethamine
   c. Dexamethasone and Etoposide
   d. Bone marrow transplant

23. A 17-year-old boy is being discharged from hospital after recovering from bronchopneumonia and ARDS. This was his ninth chest infection in the previous 2 years and on 6 occasions. *S. pneumoniae* has been isolated from sputum and blood cultures. The most likely reason is:
   a. A hyper IgM syndrome
   b. Lack of Pneumococcal neutralizing antibodies
   c. Hypereosinophilia
   d. Complement deficiency

24. A 54-year-old male with a history of recurrent gut infections has grown *shigella* and *campylobacter* repeatedly in a background of dermatomyositis on azathioprine maintenance. Best investigation would be to establish:
   a. Muscle biopsy and myonecrosis
   b. Bone marrow for aplastic anemia
   c. Colonoscopy for colon cancer
   d. HLA – DR link association for muscle atrophy

25. A 47-year-old male on azathioprine for rheumatoid arthritis presents with urosepsis and septic shock. A lymphocyte enumeration panel shows T and B cell population to be below 5%. The duration of antibiotic cover based on T cell population recovery will be:
   a. Seven days
   b. Forty-eight hours
   c. Four months
   d. Three weeks

26. A 33-year-old male post renal transplant presents with an acute myocardial infarction. In his workup, he has pancytopenia, a creatinine of 7.3 mg/dL, and a nine fold normal transaminitis. A CT coronary angiogram while on CVVHD shoes diffuse atherosclerotic changes of coronary arteries, renal arteries and aorta. His most likely diagnosis is:
   a. Cytomegalovirus (CMV) infection
   b. Polyangiitis overlap syndrome
   c. Vaso-occlusive disease
   d. Drug induced bone marrow depression

27. A 23-year-old female with retroviral infection has a three week history of painful dysphasia and altered bowel movements. Her last CD4 counts 5 days ago were 54 cells/mm^3. Three stool

cultures are negative for microorganisms. She now has hematemesis and undergoes upper and lower gastrointestinal endoscopy showing multiple varied sized ulcers throughout the GI tract. She is likeliest to have:
   a. Helicobacter pylori disseminated disease
   b. B cell lymphoma of HIV
   c. Cytomegalovirus infection
   d. Ulcerative oesophagitis and inflammatory bowel disease

28. A 57-year-old female diagnosed with Dengue both on NS1 antigen and IgM for dengue is hospitalized with fever. Her platelet count on admission was 46,000/mm^3 which was reduced to 31,000/mm^3 within 24 hours.
   She is given six units of random donor platelets. On the fourth day she develops a left hemiparesis and a non-contrast CT shows a large intracerebral bleed. In the absence of other hematological evaluation, the most likely reason for the bleed is:
   a. Hypertensive stroke
   b. Auto antibodies and anti-platelet antibodies
   c. DIC
   d. Dengue induced encephalopathy

29. A 56-year-old female with chronic hepatitis C has a flare with transaminitis x 10 fold after she has discontinued her medications four months ago. She now has a wet gangrene involving her right foot and a lobar pneumonia. Her Coombs test in her workup is positive. Her last viral load is 3, 83,790 copies/mm^3. She has:
   a. Thrombo embolic disease
   b. Cold agglutinin disease associated with mycoplasma
   c. Varicose veins of Hepatitis C
   d. Primary vasculitis

30. The biggest risk factor for systemic complications of Hepatitis E infection is:
   a. Hepatorenal syndrome
   b. IVDU
   c. Paracetamol ingestion
   d. Pregnancy

31. A 38-year-old bone marrow transplant recipient presents with fever, generalized weakness and dyspnea of 5 days duration. On clinical examination she has hepatosplenomegaly, palpable lymph nodes in her neck, axilla and groin. Her post-transplant immunosuppression has been altered after a recent pancytopenia. She has a childhood history of infectious mononucleosis that resolved completely. Her likeliest diagnosis is:
   a. Epstein-Barr virus (EBV) associated Post-transplant Lymphoproliferative Disorder (PTLD)
   b. Disseminated Cytomegalovirus (CMV)
   c. Drug induced pancytopenia
   d. Burkitt's Lymphoma

32. A 27-year-old male presents with acute dyspnea of 3 days duration. He has immunodeficiency of retroviral illness and is stable on HAART with a CD4 count of 210 cells/mm^3. He works on a shop that feeds pigeons daily. In his evaluation his CT chest and PFT show restrictive airways disease with fine reticular shadows. He is likely to have:
   a. HIV associated lymphocytic pneumonia
   b. Allergic bronchopulmonary aspergillosis
   c. Bird Fancier's lung –hypersensitivity alveolitis
   d. Pneumocystis Jiroveci pneumonia

33. In treatment of pneumocystis jiroveci in immunocompromised patients with Trimethoprim/Sulfamethoxazole:
   a. Duration of treatment is 5 days
   b. Prophylaxis is lifelong
   c. Patients are best monitored as outpatients
   d. Patients will need steroid cover to prepare for initial worsening

34. A 36-year-old female is brought to emergency in a comatose condition. Her examination reveals multiple crusting skin lesions on trunk and arms, and her left breast has a crimson red appearance. On further evaluation her CSF shows evidence of meningitis, a left shoulder and right hip osteomyelitis and multiple pockets of abscess in her chest and abdomen. Her only significant medical history is a left breast implant surgery 6 weeks ago. She has:
   a. Bacteroides septicemia
   b. Collagen vascular disease with suppuration
   c. Gram positive bacteremia
   d. Mycobacterium fortuitum

35. A 27-year-old girl presents with a degloving injury of her face after being in contact with an undomesticated cat. She has presented ten hours after injury. In her treatment, the most effective regimen is:
   a. Tetanus toxoid and surgical opinion
   b. TT, rabies immunoglobulin, anti-rabies vaccine and surgery of cheek
   c. Only anti rabies vaccine
   d. Surgical repair and observation for ten days. Cats do not transmit rabies.

ANSWERS

A Type Answers

Q1. Answer d

Aspergillosis- The most common sites of infection are the respiratory tract (lungs, sinuses) and these infections can be:
1. Invasive
2. Non-invasive (e.g. Allergic Bronchopulmonary Aspergillosis - ABPA)
3. Chronic pulmonary and aspergilloma (e.g. chronic cavitary, semi-invasive)
4. Severe asthma with fungal sensitization (SAFS)

Chronic pulmonary aspergillosis (CPA) is a long-term aspergillus infection of the lung and Aspergillus fumigatus is almost always the species responsible for this illness. Patients fall into several groups as listed as follows:
1. Aspergillus nodule
2. Chronic cavitary pulmonary aspergillosis (CCPA) where cavities are present in the lungs, but not necessarily with a fungal ball (aspergilloma)
3. Chronic fibrosing pulmonary aspergillosis this may develop where pulmonary aspergillosis remains untreated and chronic scarring of the lungs occurs. Unfortunately scarring of the lungs does not improve.

In the presence of angioinvasive disease, *Aspergillus* spp can disseminate beyond the respiratory tract to multiple different organs, including the skin, brain, eyes, liver, and kidneys. Disseminated infection is associated with a very poor prognosis.

> Denning DW, Riniotis K, Dobrashian R, Sambatakou H. Chronic cavitary and fibrosing pulmonary and pleural aspergillosis: case series, proposed nomenclature change, and review. Clinical Infectious Diseases. 2003;37(3):S265-80.

Q2. Answer b

Chest radiography is an initial examination of choice in patients with respiratory symptoms or suspected pulmonary disease. However, many different causes of bronchiectasis including ABPA cannot be accurately diagnosed on chest radiographs. Also, radiographic features of pulmonary aspergillosis are generally nonspecific. Although the computed tomography (CT) scan features of ABPA are not specific, the demonstration of bronchial dilatation, wall thickening, and centrilobular nodules in an asthmatic patient should suggest the diagnosis. The demonstration of a mobile mass within a cavity on supine and prone scans is virtually diagnostic of mycetoma.

The CT scan appearances of chronic necrotizing aspergillosis are also nonspecific, but CT does provide useful information regarding the extent of pulmonary disease and any associated pleural thickening. CT scan findings in angioinvasive aspergillosis are more specific, and the presence of nodules with a halo of ground-glass attenuation in the appropriate clinical setting allows confident diagnosis.

> Agarwal R. Allergic bronchopulmonary aspergillosis. *Chest.* 2009;135(3):805-826.

Q3. Answer b

Aspergillus infection occurs frequently in the organ transplant recipients during the post-transplant period because of immunosuppression. The azole antifungals widely prescribed prophylactically are known to have many drug-drug interactions. Voriconazole treatment leads to a dramatic increase in tacrolimus concentration. The drug-drug interaction can be attributed to a strong inhibitory effect on cytochrome P450-3A4 activity by Voriconazole. When Voriconazole and tacrolimus are coadministered, close monitoring of tacrolimus blood levels is recommended. Reduction of tacrolimus dose by one-third may not be satisfactory.

> Kauffman CA. Treatment and prevention of invasive aspergillosis. Available at: https://www.uptodate.com/contents/treatment-and-prevention-of-invasive-aspergillosis (Accessed 23 August 2017).

Q4. Answer a

During the past several decades, the many published surveys of vaginal flora specimens obtained from asymptomatic women have clearly shown that *Candida albicans* may be present without the typical symptoms of vaginitis. Candida species may be present in stable association with the genital epithelium. Moreover, the majority of women who have vaginal yeast also carry the organism in the gut. The typical rate of yeast carriage varies among populations and increases both after puberty and during pregnancy which suggests an important role for host physiology in cases of vaginal candidiasis.

Weinstein L. The bacterial flora of the human vagina. Yale J Biol Med. 1938;10(3):247-60.

Q5. Answer a

Systemic risk factors for patients with endogenous fungal endophthalmitis caused by molds were iatrogenic immunosuppression and a history of solid organ transplantation. Shorter duration of symptoms before diagnosis and higher rates of hypopyon occurred in mold cases. While endogenous fungal endophthalmitis is generally associated with poor visual acuity outcomes, infection with mold species was associated with worse visual acuity on presentation and on final follow-up than infection with yeast species.

Sridhar J, Flynn HW, Kuriyan AE, Miller D, Albini T. Endogenous fungal endophthalmitis: risk factors, clinical features, and treatment outcomes in mold and yeast infections. J Ophthalmic Inflamm Infect. 2013;3:60.

Q6. Answer c

Most individuals with histoplasmosis are asymptomatic. Those who develop clinical manifestations are usually immunocompromised or are exposed to a high quantity of inoculum. Histoplasma species may remain latent in healed granulomas and recur resulting in impairment of cell-mediated immunity.

Clinical presentations include asymptomatic pulmonary histoplasmosis, symptomatic pulmonary histoplasmosis, acute diffuse pulmonary histoplasmosis, chronic pulmonary histoplasmosis, acute respiratory distress syndrome, disseminated histoplasmosis, broncholithiasis, mediastinal granuloma, fibrosing mediastinitis, endobronchial histoplasmosis, and lung nodules.

Fayyaz J, Lessnau KD. Histoplasmosis clinical presentation. Available at: http://emedicine.medscape.com/article/299054-clinical (Accessed 19 March 2017).

Q7. Answer c

The CD4:CD8 ratio acts as a surrogate marker of T cell compartment balance: CD4 T cell recovery and CD8 T cell expansion.

Long-term Anti-Retroviral Therapy (ART) has successfully restored CD4 T cell counts in a large proportion of HIV-positive patients. However, the majority of these patients still demonstrate a persistent elevation of CD8 T-cell count as well as dysfunction of CD8 T cell compartments. The balance between immune reconstitution and immune activation/inflammation may be involved in the trend towards the normalization of the CD4:CD8 ratio with ART.

Collectively, a persistently low CD4:CD8 ratio during long-term effective ART represents a marker of continuing immune dysfunction, 'inflammaging' and high-risk of non-AIDS morbidity and mortality. In long-term treated patients, the progressive correction of the CD4:CD8 ratio is solely a result of CD4 recovery, as CD8 T cell counts remains constant. Encouragingly, earlier ART initiation contributes to a more rapid CD4:CD8 ratio normalization when compared to late treatment initiation. However, when ART is initiated in chronic phase, a moderate increase in the CD4:CD8 ratio is observed.

Serrano-Villar S, Perez-Elias MJ, Dronda F, et. al. Increased risk of serious non-AIDS-related events in HIV-infected subjects on antiretroviral therapy associated with a low CD4/CD8 ratio. PLoS One. 2014;9(1):85798.

Q8. Answer a

In immunocompromised individuals, symptomatic disease usually manifests as a mononucleosis syndrome. Symptomatic CMV disease can affect almost every organ of the body resulting in fever of unknown origin, pneumonia, hepatitis, encephalitis, myelitis, colitis, uveitis, retinitis, and neuropathy. Rarer manifestations of CMV infections in immunocompetent individuals include Guillain-Barré syndrome, meningoencephalitis, pericarditis, myocarditis, thrombocytopenia, and hemolytic anemia. Cystoisospora belli previously known as Isospora belli is a parasite that causes an intestinal disease known as cystoisosporiasis.

In patients with HIV infection, CMV involves the entire GI tract. Retinitis is the most common manifestation of CMV disease in patients who are HIV positive.

Akhter K. Cytomegalovirus. Available at: https://emedicine.medscape.com/article/215702-overview (Accessed 14 October 2017).

Q9. Answer d

High-risk asymptomatic patients in close contact with infected ones are treated with home quarantine without antiviral therapy unless they begin to show symptoms of infection.

Avian influenza: guidelines. recommendations, descriptions. Available at: http://www.who.int/influenza/resources/documents/guidelinestopics/en/(Accessed 14 October 2017).

Q10. Answer c

Human disease Scedosporium prolificans has been recognized as an agent of opportunistic human disease since the 1990s. This species is primarily associated with subcutaneous lesions arising from injury following ciedosporidium (Disseminated) 'traumatic implantation' of the agent via contaminated splinters or plant thorns. The majority of S. prolificans infections in immunologically normal people remain localized, characteristically with bone or joint involvement. Disseminated infections from S. prolificans are largely limited to people with pre-existing immune impairment. Notably, S. prolificans exhibits varying tolerance to all currently available antifungal agents. This is particularly true of strains recovered from disseminated infections, and these infections carry a high mortality. Scedosporium prolificans has also been known to cause disseminated disease secondary to myeloblastic leukemia and following lung transplant. In otherwise healthy people, it was recorded as a cause of corneal infection following a lawn trimmer mishap, and bone infection following trauma.

Drug resistance Infections caused by S. prolificans are recognized to be difficult to treat due to the tendency of this species to exhibit resistance to many commonly used antifungal agents. Successful control of disseminated Scedosporium prolificans infection can be obtained with a combination of voriconazole and terbinafine, but some strains are resistant to this treatment. Drugs that might also be of help are posaconazole, miltefosine and albaconazole.

Cortez KJ, Roilides E, Quiroz-Telles F, et. al. Infections caused by Scedosporium spp. Clinical Microbiology Reviews. 2008; 21(1):157-97.

Q11. Answer b

Seroconversion from HIV negative status to HIV positive status is often characterized by flu like syndrome and western blot may require repeat samples at 3 month duration before it is clearly positive.

Thrombocytopenia is frequently associated with HIV infection. In the Multicenter AIDS Cohort Study, platelet counts were measured in over 1,500 HIV-seropositive participants who did not have CDC-defined AIDS; 6.7% of participants had platelet counts of less than 150,000 cells/mm^3 on at least one semiannual visit, and 2.6% of participants had platelet counts of less than 150,000 cells/mm^3 on two successive semiannual visits. In a Swiss study, platelet counts of less than 100,000 cells/mm3 were noted in 9% of 321 HIV-seropositive injection drug users and in 3% of 359 HIV-seropositive homosexual men. A smaller study from London reported platelet counts of less than 150,000 cells/mm^3 in 30% (6 of 20) of patients with advanced HIV disease and 8% (5 of 59) of patients with persistent generalized lymphadenopathy. Possible etiologies of thrombocytopenia in patients with HIV infection include immune-mediated destruction, thrombotic thrombocytopenic purpura, impaired hematopoiesis, and toxic effects of medications. In many instances, however, thrombocytopenia is a relatively isolated hematologic abnormality associated with a normal or increased number of megakaryocytes in the bone marrow and elevated levels of platelet-associated immunoglobulin. These patients have the clinical syndrome commonly referred to as immune thrombocytopenic purpura (ITP).

Zon LI, Groopman JE. Hematologic manifestations of the human immunodeficiency virus (HIV). SeminHematol. 1988;25:208-218.

Q12. Answer b

Fifth disease or erythema infectiosum is only one of several expressions of Parvovirus B19. The associated bright red rash of the cheeks gives it the nickname 'slapped cheek syndrome'. Any age may be affected, although it is the most common in children aged six to ten years. It is so named because it was the fifth most common cause of a pink-red infection associated rash to be described by physicians (many of the others such as measles and rubella are rare now). Once infected, patients usually develop the illness after an incubation period of four to fourteen days. The disease commences with high fever and malaise, when the virus is most abundant in the bloodstream, and patients are usually no longer infectious once the characteristic rash of this disease has appeared. The following symptoms are characteristic:

Generally, erythema infectiosum is self-limited and does not require treatment. Patients with arthralgia may require nonsteroidal anti-inflammatory drug treatment. Patients in transient aplastic crisis may require erythrocyte transfusions while the marrow recovers. Chronic red cell aplasia, if severe, may require intravenous immune globulin therapy. This treatment may improve anemia symptoms, but it may precipitate a rash or arthropathy. Intravenous immune globulin also has been used in several case reports of severe illness.

Servey JT, Reamy BV, Hodge J. Clinical presentations of parvovirus B19 infection. Am Fam Physician. 2007;75(3):373-6.

Q13. Answer a

All HIV-infected pregnant women with active TB should be started on ART as early as feasible, both for treatment of maternal HIV infection and to prevent perinatal transmission of HIV (AIII). The choice of ART should be based on efficacy and safety in pregnancy and should take into account potential drug-drug interactions between ARVs and rifamycins.

World Health Organization. Global Tuberculosis Report 2015. Available at: http://apps.who.int/iris/bitstream/10665/191102/1/9789241565059_eng.pdf.

Q14. Answer c

Congenital toxoplasmosis is the consequence of transplacental hematogenous fetal infection by T gondii during primary infection in pregnant women. Primary infection in an otherwise healthy pregnant woman is asymptomatic in 60% of cases. Symptoms during pregnancy are frequently mild. The most common manifestations are fatigue, malaise, a low-grade fever, lymphadenopathy and myalgias. Latent toxoplasma infection with reactivation during pregnancy may lead to congenital infection only in immunocompromised women (most commonly those with AIDS).

The classic triad of chorioretinitis, hydrocephalus, and intracranial calcifications cannot be used as a strict diagnostic criterion for congenital toxoplasmosis because a large number of cases would be missed. Congenital toxoplasmosis may occur in the following forms:
- Neonatal disease
- Disease occurring in the first months of life
- Sequelae or relapse of previously undiagnosed infection
- Subclinical infection

When clinically recognized in the neonate, congenital toxoplasmosis is very severe. Spontaneous abortions, prematurity, or stillbirth may result. Signs of generalized infection such as the following are usually present:
- Intrauterine growth restriction
- Fever
- Chorioretinitis (usually bilateral)
- Cerebral calcification
- Abnormal cerebrospinal fluid (xanthochromia and pleocytosis)
- Vomiting
- Eosinophilia
- Abnormal bleeding
- Jaundice
- Hepatomegaly
- Splenomegaly
- Rash

Paquet C, Yudin MH. Toxoplasmosis in Pregnancy: Prevention, Screening, and Treatment. J Obstet Gynaecol Can. 2013; 35(1):78-81.

Q15. Answer d

Salmonella septicemia is a condition wherein the presence of *Salmonella* bacteria in the blood triggers a potentially life-threatening, whole-body inflammatory response. Host risk factors for nontyphoidal (not involving gastrointestinal tract). Salmonella bacteremia include extremes of age and chronic or immunosuppressing conditions including malignancy, rheumatological disease, TNF blockade (e.g., agents such as etanercept or infliximab), transplantation, HIV infection, and congenital immune defects. Recurrent Salmonella septicemia is classified as an AIDS-defining condition by the US. Centers for Disease Control and Prevention (CDC). Other predisposing comorbidities include liver disease, hemoglobinopathies (especially sickle cell disease), schistosomiasis, and chronic granulomatous disease. Alteration of the GI tract also predisposes to progression from enteric to systemic salmonellosis (e.g., by suppression of gastric acid, malnutrition, recent antibiotic use, or rotavirus infection).

> Hohmann EL. Nontyphoidal Salmonella bacteremia. Available at: https://www.uptodate.com/contents/nontyphoidal-salmonella-bacteremia(Accessed 19 March 2017).

Q16. Answer a

Cat scratch disease (CSD), Bartonella henselae

People can get CSD from the scratches of domestic or feral cats, particularly kittens. The disease occurs most frequently in children under 15. Cats can harbor infected fleas that carry *Bartonella* bacteria. These bacteria can be transmitted from a cat to a person during a scratch. Some evidence suggests that CSD may be transmitted directly to humans by the bite of infected cat fleas, although this has not been proven.

CSD occurs worldwide and may be present wherever cats are found. Stray cats may be more likely than pets to carry *Bartonella*.

> Hansmann Y, DeMartino S, Piémont Y et al. Diagnosis of cat scratch disease with detection of Bartonella henselae by PCR: a study of patients with lymph node enlargement. J Clin Microbiol. 2005;43(8):3800-6.

Q17. Answer b

Treatment of leptospirosis should be started as soon as possible. Treatment is begun empirically in patients with a plausible exposure history, compatible symptoms, as culture times for Leptospira are long, and recovery rates are low. The criterion standard for serologic identification of leptospirosis, microscopic agglutination testing (MAT) is available only at reference laboratories. Paired acute and convalescent serum specimens can provide delayed confirmation of the diagnosis.

In uncomplicated infections that do not require hospitalization, oral Doxycycline has been shown to decrease the duration of fever and most symptoms. In hospitalized patients, intravenous penicillin G has been the treatment of choice. Patients with severe leptospirosis (Weil disease) require supportive therapy and careful management of renal, hepatic, hematologic, and central nervous system complications.

> Day N. Treatment and prevention of leptospirosis. Available at: https://www.uptodate.com/contents/treatment-and-prevention-of-leptospirosis?(Accessed 12 March 2017).

Q18. Answer d

Fatalities secondary to infectious mononucleosis (IM) most often are the result of splenic rupture. Other fatal occurrences have been attributed to secondary bacterial infection, hepatic failure, and myocarditis.

Airway obstruction can occur due to massive edema of the Waldeyer ring.

Serious nonfatal complications also are rare and may include involvement of the CNS or the hematologic system.

CNS complications can include meningitis, encephalitis, hemiplegia, psychosis, cranial nerve palsies, Guillain-Barré syndrome, transverse myelitis, and peripheral neuritis. Evidence also exists to suggest Epstein-Barr virus infection as an adult is a risk factor for the development of multiple sclerosis. Hematologic complications can include development of autoimmune hemolytic anemia, pancytopenia, red cell aplasia, severe thrombocytopenia, or agranulocytopenia.

> Andy CM Won, Ethell A. Spontaneous splenic rupture resulted from infectious mononucleosis. International Journal of Surgery Case Reports. 2012;3(3)97-99.

Q19. Answer c

In endemic areas, patients with probable erythema migrans and a recent source of tick exposure should be started on treatment without blood tests. In the absence of erythema migrans, serologic testing is used. CDC recommends a two-step testing procedure. The first step typically consists of a screening enzyme immunoassay (EIA) or enzyme-linked immunosorbent assay (ELISA); if results are positive or equivocal, a Western immunoblot test is performed to confirm the results. Other tests and procedures (e.g. electrocardiogram, cerebrospinal fluid analysis) depend on the presentation.

Antibiotic selection, route of administration, and duration of therapy for Lyme disease is guided by the patient's clinical manifestations and stage of disease, as well as the presence of any concomitant medical conditions or allergies. First-line agents include doxycycline, penicillins, cefuroxime, and ceftriaxone; however, doxycycline is contraindicated in patients younger than 8 years and in pregnant women.

Wright WF, Riedel DJ, Talwani R et al. Diagnosis and management of Lyme disease. Am. Fam. Physician. 2012;85(11):1086-93.

Q20. Answer d

Treatment of loiasis involves chemotherapy or, in some cases surgical removal of adult worms followed by systemic treatment. The current drug of choice for therapy is diethylcarbamazine (DEC), though ivermectin use is not unwarranted. The recommend dosage of DEC is 6 mg/kg/d taken three times daily for 12 days. The pediatric dose is the same. DEC is effective against microfilariae and somewhat effective against macrofilariae (adult worms).

In patients with high microfilaria load, however, treatment with DEC may be contraindicated, as the rapid microfilaricidal actions of the drug can provoke encephalopathy. In these cases, albendazole administration has proved helpful, and superior to ivermectin which can also be risky despite its slower-acting microfilaricidal effects.

The Mazzotti reaction, first described in 1948, is a symptom complex seen in patients after undergoing treatment of onchocerciasis with the medication diethylcarbamazine (DEC). Mazzotti reactions can be life-threatening, and are characterized by fever, urticaria, swollen and tender lymph nodes, tachycardia, hypotension, arthralgias, oedema, and abdominal pain that occur within seven days of treatment of microfilariasis. The Mazzotti reaction correlates with intensity of infection; however, there are probably multiple infection intensity-dependent mechanisms responsible for mediating this complex reaction. Patch test: The phenomenon is so common when DEC is used for the treatment of onchocerciasis that this drug is the basis of a skin patch test used to confirm that diagnosis.

Francis H, Awadzi K, Ottesen EA. The Mazzotti reaction following treatment of onchocerciasis with diethylcarbamazine: clinical severity as a function of infection intensity. Am J Trop Med Hyg. 1985;34(3):529-36.

Q21. Answer d

Hemophagocytic lymphohistiocytosis (HLH) is a rapidly progressive, life-threatening syndrome of excessive immune activation. Prompt initiation of treatment for HLH is essential for the survival of affected patients.

The treatment and prognosis of patients with HLH and the macrophage activation syndrome (MAS), a form of HLH in patients with juvenile idiopathic arthritis and other rheumatologic conditions, will be discussed here. The genetics, clinical features, and diagnosis of HLH are presented separately.

Overview and indications for treatment-HLH: It is a progressive syndrome of unchecked immune activation and tissue damage. If left untreated, patients with HLH survive for only a few months due to progressive multi-organ failure. In 1994, the Histiocyte Society organized the first treatment protocol for HLH (HLH-94), which dramatically increased this survival rate to 54% with a median follow-up of 6 years.

Often, the greatest barrier to treatment and a successful outcome for individuals with HLH is a delay in diagnosis. Several aspects of the clinical presentation of HLH contribute to this delay including the rarity of the syndrome, the variable clinical presentation, and the lack of specificity of the clinical and laboratory findings. Diagnostic criteria for HLH are based upon those used in the major HLH studies, and therefore may be too stringent to capture all patients with HLH. Thus, treatment is appropriate for some who do not meet the strict diagnostic criteria but for whom there is a high degree of clinical suspicion for HLH. Any patient with suspected HLH should be seen by a hematologist, and those who are acutely ill should be transferred emergently to a facility where they can receive HLH therapy.

The goal of the therapy for the patients with HLH is to suppress life-threatening inflammation by destroying immune cells. Induction therapy based on the HLH-94 protocol consists of a series of weekly treatments with dexamethasone and etoposide. Intrathecal methotrexate and hydrocortisone are given to those with central nervous system disease. After induction, patients who are recovering are weaned off therapy, while those who are not improving are continued on therapy as a bridge to allogeneic hematopoietic cell transplantation (HCT). HCT will be required in those with an HLH gene mutation, central nervous system disease, or disease relapse.

Q22. Answer c

Q23. Answer d

Deficiencies of complement proteins may be acquired or inherited. Acquired complement deficiencies are relatively common and may occur as a result of decreased synthesis, increased protein loss, or increased consumption. The liver is the most important organ for the synthesis of several complement proteins, and therefore, low complement levels are often seen in persons with advanced liver disease. Patients with alcoholic cirrhosis and low levels of C3, C4, and CH50 were reported to have an increased risk of infections, including pneumonia caused by *Streptococcus pneumoniae* and septicemia with Staphylococcus aureus and E. coli. Complement deficiencies may result from increased protein loss associated with nephritic syndrome or protein-losing enteropathies. Increased consumption of complement often accompanies immune complex disease, vasculitis, or development of autoantibodies against complement proteins.

Schwartz RA. Complement Deficiencies. Available at: https://emedicine.medscape.com/article/135478-overview (Accessed 14 October 2017).

Q24. Answer c

How long is cancer risk increased?
- Risk is highest within the first year of diagnosis
- In those with polymyositis, the risk fell to expected rates 5 years after diagnosis
- In those with dermatomyositis, the risk did not fall to expected rates
    - Ovarian, pancreatic, lung remained high up to 5 years
    - Pancreatic and colorectal cancer risks remained elevated past 5 years.

Hill CL, Zhang Y, Sigurgeirsson B, Pukkala E, Mellemkjaer L, Airio A, Evans SR, Felson DT. Frequency of specific cancer types in dermatomyositis and polymyositis: a population-based study. Lancet. 2001; Jan 13;357(9250):96-100.

Q25. Answer d

While the biological half-life of azathioprine is usually 8-10 hours after dosing, the presence of active metabolites in circulation may persist for upto 3 weeks after discontinuation of the last dose and impact on both T cell and B cell function.

Myelosuppression is known to occur with azathioprine. Physicians must remain sensitive to possibility of azathioprine induced severe bone marrow suppression. Frequent monitoring of blood counts is probably the best way to avoid this complication specially.

Hadda V, Pandey BD, Gupta R, Goel A. Azathioprine induced pancytopenia: a serious complication. J Postgrad Med. 2009;55(2):139-40.

Q26. Answer a

CMV infection may cause direct or indirect effects. Direct effects include bone marrow suppression, pneumonia, myocarditis, GI disease, hepatitis, pancreatitis, nephritis, retinitis, and encephalitis, among others. The main indirect effects include acute and chronic graft rejection, accelerated atherosclerosis (heart transplants), secondary bacterial or fungal infections, EBV-associated post transplant lymphoproliferative disease (PTLD), and decreased graft and patient survival.

CMV infection may predispose accelerated atherosclerosis. These observations by themselves do not demonstrate that viruses have a role in the pathogenesis of atherosclerosis, but they support a working hypothesis of the steps involved.

Melnick JL, Adam E, Debakey ME. Cytomegalovirus and atherosclerosis. Eur Heart J. 1993;14 Suppl K:30-8.

Q27. Answer c

In patients with HIV infection, CMV involves the entire GI tract. In the upper GI tract, CMV has been isolated from esophageal ulcers, gastric ulcers, and duodenal ulcers. Patients with upper GI tract, esophageal disease can present with painful dysphagia. Patients with CMV disease of the lower GI tract may present with diarrhea (colitis). CMV colitis frequently affects only the right colon, necessitating full colonoscopy and multiple biopsies for accurate diagnosis. Diagnosis of CMV, GI disease depends on a biopsy specimen demonstrating the typical CMV intranuclear inclusions.

Nasa M, Sharma Z, Sud R, Lipi L. Cytomegalovirus infection of gastrointestinal tract . Community Acquir Infect. 2016;3:4-9.

Q28. Answer b

The immune mechanisms that lead to dengue hemorrhagic fever are complex. Low avidity cross reactive T cells may produce an altered profile of cytokines leading to plasma leakage. Ongoing prospective studies that include epidemiological, virological and immunological risk factors are crucial. WHO guidelines do not recommend platelet transfusion for hemodynamically stable patients. In situation of severe bleeding and hemodynamic instability, transfusion of platelets is indicated. Other treatments considered for dengue-induced thrombocytopenia include immunoglobulin (IVIG). Viral infection may also cause abnormal immune responses that disrupt the balance of host immunity.

Sharone G, Alan R. Immunopathological mechanisms in dengue and dengue hemorrhagic fever. Current Opinion in Infectious Diseases. 2006;19(5):429-36.

Q29. Answer b

Cold antibody hemolytic anemia (CAHA) is classified as primary (idiopathic) or secondary. In most cases, CAHA is a primary disorder that typically becomes apparent at 50 to 60 years of age. Cold antibody hemolytic anemia may also occur as a secondary disorder in association with a number of different underlying disorders such as certain infectious diseases (e.g. mycoplasma infection and infectious mononucleosis) and lymphoproliferative diseases (e.g. non Hodgkin's lymphoma and chronic lymphocytic leukemia).

Extrapulmonary complications may present before, during, after, or in the absence of pulmonary signs. An increase in cold agglutinin titers is frequently observed during *M. pneumoniae* infection; it has been reported that 50%-60% of these patients had cold agglutinins in which appear 1 week after the onset of the illness and decline toward undetectable levels after 2 to 6 weeks. Cold agglutinins appear to be more specific for I antigen of the red blood cell surface and often result in mild, subclinical hemolysis and mild reticulocytosis. Severe hemolytic anemia is rare and is usually associated with marked pulmonary involvement. In 90% of such patients, cold agglutinin disease is mediated by an IgM molecule.

The induction of cold agglutinins may be triggered by the formation of mycoplasma-receptor complexes in which the lipid-rich mycoplasma surface plays the role of an adjuvant. The phagocytic and other destructive cells of the immune system do not have receptors for IgM as they do for IgG and IgA. Thus, since cold agglutinins are usually IgM, destruction of RBCs is primarily complement-mediated, occurring either by direct destruction of the membrane (direct lysis) or immunoadherence mediated by target-bound components (indirect lysis). Both of these processes are relatively inefficient in the absence of exposure to cold.

Typical laboratory features common to all forms of extravascular hemolysis include indirect hyperbilirubinemia and increased concentration of lactate dehydrogenase, whereas the hallmarks of intravascular hemolysis include a decrease in the serum level of haptoglobin and an increase in plasma-free hemoglobin. The existence of elevated serum levels of lactate dehydrogenase and bilirubin with low levels of haptoglobin is common in hemolytic anemia caused by cold agglutinins. Our patient showed both features of extra- and intravascular hemolysis.

Clues to the diagnosis of cold agglutinin disease include acrocyanosis and Raynaud's phenomenon. Moreover, auto agglutination on the peripheral blood film which disappears on warming the blood sample suggests a cold antibody.

Diagnosis of CAHA is based on a positive direct Coombs test in the presence of cold agglutinins.

Clyde WA Jr. Clinical overview of typical Mycoplasma pneumoniae infections. Clin Infect Dis. 1993;17(Suppl 1):S32-6.

Q30. Answer d

Hepatitis E infection with genotype 1 during the third trimester can lead to maternal mortality upto 15% to 25% of cases. Most of the studies showing high maternal mortality are from India, where infection occurs in epidemics. There is a very high-risk of vertical transmission of HEV from the mother to the fetus. During a Delhi epidemic, a hospital-based study revealed that HEV infection during pregnancy was associated with miscarriage, stillbirth, or neonatal death in 56% of infants. One recent study highlights that HEV infection might be responsible for 2400 to 3,000 stillbirths each year in developing countries with many additional fetal deaths linked to antenatal maternal deaths. There is a very high-risk of preterm delivery in pregnant women with HEV infection with poor neonatal survival rates. In two separate studies from India, 15% to 50% of live-born infants of mothers with HEV infection died within 1 week of birth. During an outbreak in Sudan in 2010 to 2011, among 39 pregnant women with HEV infection there were 14 intrauterine deaths and 9 premature deliveries.

Rein DB, Stevens GA, Theaker J, et al. The global burden of hepatitis E virus genotypes 1 and 2 in 2005. Hepatology. 2012; 55(4):988-97.

Q31. Answer a

Diseases caused by the EBV are of great significance among organ transplant recipients. PTLD is a major complication among organ transplant recipients. Management of this entity is problematic due to the difficulties with laboratory surveillance, diagnosis, prevention and treatment. The Epstein-Barr virus (EBV) is recognized primarily for its etiological role in infectious mononucleosis, a usually benign lymphoproliferative disorder most prevalent in adolescents and young adults. Under conditions of severe T cell immunosuppression, which prevail in patients with AIDS and transplant recipients, EBV-infected B cells may expand unchecked resulting in malignant lymphoproliferation. In this context, the virus is able to transform and immortalize B lymphocytes leading to their uncontrolled proliferation. This is particularly likely in settings where the host lacks adequate cytotoxic T lymphocyte surveillance. One such setting occurs when transplant recipients experience primary EBV infection.

Pope JH, Horne MK, Scott W. Transformation of foetal human leukocytes in vitro by filtrates of a human leukemic cell line containing herpes-like virus. Int J Cancer. 1968;3:857-66.

Q32. Answer c

Hypersensitivity pneumonitis (HP), also called extrinsic allergic alveolitis is a complex syndrome of varying intensity, clinical presentation, and natural history rather than a single, uniform disease. Numerous inciting agents have been described including but not limited to agricultural dusts, bio aerosols, microorganisms (fungal, bacterial, or protozoal), and certain reactive chemical species.

King TE. Diagnosis of hypersensitivity pneumonitis (extrinsic allergic alveolitis). Available at: https://www.uptodate.com/contents/diagnosis-of-hypersensitivity-pneumonitis-extrinsic-allergic-alveolitis?source=search_result&search=Bird%20Fancier%E2%80%99s%20lung&selectedTitle=2~8(Accessed 13 October 2017).

Q33. Answer d

Corticosteroids given in conjunction with anti-Pneumocystis therapy can decrease the incidence of mortality and respiratory failure associated with PCP. Without steroids, patients with PCP may worsen clinically after 2 to 3 days of therapy, presumably due to increased inflammation in response to dying organisms. Several randomized trials have demonstrated the benefits of administering corticosteroids to patients with PCP who have abnormalities in oxygen exchange at the time of presentation. These findings were illustrated in a Cochrane Database review of seven randomized controlled trials that evaluated the effects of adjunctive corticosteroids in HIV-infected patients with moderate to severe disease.

Sax PE. Treatment and prevention of Pneumocystis infection in HIV-infected patients. Available at: https://www.uptodate.com/contents/treatment-and-prevention-of-pneumocystis-infection-in-hiv-infected-patients?(Accessed 20 May 2017).

Q34. Answer d

Skin and soft tissue infections due to rapidly growing mycobacteria are associated with systemic comorbidities including the use of immunosuppressive medications. There are significant differences in the demographic and clinical features of patients who acquire specific organisms, including association with immunosuppression and surgical procedures.

Kothavade RJ, Dhurat RS, Mishra SN, Kothavade UR. Clinical and laboratory aspects of the diagnosis and management of cutaneous and subcutaneous infections caused by rapidly growing mycobacteria. European Journal of Clinical Microbiology and Infectious Diseases. 2013;32(2):161-88.

Q35. Answer b

Types of contact are:

Category I—touching or feeding animals, licks on the skin

Category II—nibbling of uncovered skin, minor scratches or abrasions without bleeding, licks on broken skin

Category III—single or multiple transdermal bites or scratches, contamination of mucous membrane with saliva from licks; exposure to bat bites or scratches.

For category I no treatment is required, whereas for category II immediate vaccination and for category III immediate vaccination and administration of rabies immune globulin are recommended in addition to immediate washing and flushing of all bite wounds and scratches. Depending on vaccine type, the post-exposure schedule prescribes intramuscular doses of 1 ml or 0.5 ml given as four to five doses over four weeks. For rabies-exposed patients who have previously undergone complete pre-exposure vaccination or post-exposure treatment with cell-derived rabies vaccines, two intramuscular doses of a cell-derived vaccine separated by three days are sufficient. Rabies immune globulin treatment is not necessary in such cases. The same rules apply to persons vaccinated against rabies who have demonstrated neutralizing antibody titers of at least 0.5 IU/ml.

WHO. Guide for post-exposure prophylaxis. Available at: http://www.who.int/rabies/human/postexp/en/.

CHAPTER 17

Biostatistics and Research Methodology

Manish Kumar Singh

A Type Questions
(One best answer)

1. **Which of the following represents data?**
   a. A single value
   b. Only two values
   c. A group of values in a data set
   d. Both a & b
   e. None of the above

2. **For normally distributed data:**
   a. Mean = Median = Mode
   b. Mean > Median > Mode
   c. Mean < Median < Mode
   d. Mean = Median < Mode
   e. Mean < Median = Mode

3. **Whether test is one sided or two sided depends on:**
   a. Null Hypothesis
   b. Alternative Hypothesis
   c. Composite Hypothesis
   d. Simple Hypothesis
   e. None of the above

4. **Level of significance is the probability of:**
   a. Type I error
   b. Type II error
   c. Both Type I and Type II error
   d. Other than above error
   e. Not committing error

5. **Power of a test is related to:**
   a. Type I error
   b. Type II error
   c. Type I error and Type II error both
   d. Other than above error
   e. Not committing error

6. **The inference of a statistical test with 5% level of significance will be interpreted as follows:**
   a. Null hypothesis is rejected if $p < 0.05$
   b. Null hypothesis is rejected if $p > 0.05$
   c. Null hypothesis is accepted if $p < 0.05$
   d. Null hypothesis is rejected if $p = 0.10$
   e. None of the above

7. **In a series of 21 values arranged in ascending order, the median is:**
   a. 11th value in the ordered series
   b. The mean of 10th and 12th value in the series
   c. 12th value in the series
   d. 10th value in the series
   e. None of the above

8. **For which type of data the mode is the most appropriate measure of central tendency?**
   a. Nominal
   b. Ordinal
   c. Continuous
   d. Grouped data
   e. Rate

9. **If the mean of a data series is 20 and variance as 16, the coefficient of variation is:**
   a. 40%
   b. 20%
   c. 80%
   d. 10%
   e. 100%

10. Following table presents the results of diagnostic test vis-à-vis gold standard.

Diagnostic test	Gold Standard		
	Positive	Negative	Total
Positive	90	60	150
Negative	10	40	50
Total	100	100	200

The sensitivity (Sn) and specificity (Sp) of the diagnostic test is a:
a. Sn: 90/100 × 100 = 90% & Sp: 40/100 × 100 = 40%
b. Sn: 90/150 × 100 = 60% & Sp: 130/200 × 100 = 65%
c. Sn: 90/200 × 100 = 45% & Sp: 40/50 × 100 = 80%
d. Sn: 150/200 × 100 = 75% & Sp: 100/200 × 100 = 50%
e. Sn: 100/200 × 100 = 50% & Sp: 50/200 × 100 = 25%

K Type Questions
[Marked True (T)/False (F)]

1. Characteristics of statistics are:
   a. Collection of data
   b. Presentation of data
   c. Analysis of data
   d. Interpretation of data
   e. None of the above

2. Features of a reliable data:
   a. Complete
   b. Accurate
   c. Consistent
   d. Heterogeneous
   e. Representing the population

3. Sample size estimation is based on:
   a. Primary aim of the study
   b. Secondary aim of the study
   c. Both primary and secondary aim of the study
   d. Neither primary nor secondary aim of the study
   e. Investigator choice

4. Choice of a graph depends on:
   a. The purpose of the display of data
   b. Types of data
   c. Number of attributes
   d. Duration of the study
   e. Readers/viewers

5. Measure of dispersion are:
   a. Range
   b. Mean deviation
   c. Quartile deviation
   d. Standard deviation
   e. Mean

6. Range of simple correlation coefficient is:
   a. < -1
   b. -1 to 0
   c. 0 to +1
   d. -1 to +1
   e. None of the above

7. Confounding variables can cause following problems:
   a. Introduce bias
   b. Influence outcome
   c. Influence exposure
   d. Neither outcome nor exposure
   e. Cause a spurious association

8. Qualitative variables are:
   a. Age
   b. Gender
   c. Disease severity
   d. Hemoglobin
   e. BMI

9. Measure of central location are:
   a. Mean
   b. Median
   c. Mode
   d. Variance
   e. Standard deviation

10. Which of the following statements are true?
    a. Categorical variables is also known as qualitative variables
    b. Categorical variables is also known as quantitative variables
    c. Quantitative variables can be continuous variables
    d. Quantitative variables can be categorical variables
    e. All above is correct

ANSWERS

A Type Answers

Q1. Answer c

Data is a collection of information on different characteristics for each of the individual subject. The data is collected on a sample of study subjects. The collection of information is either through observations or experimentation or mix of both methods. The data is any set of characters that has been gathered for the purpose of analysis. Since the collection of information is on group of subjects, the answer (c) is correct.

Park K. Parks textbook of preventive and social medicine. India: Bhanot Publishers; 2015.

Q2. Answer a

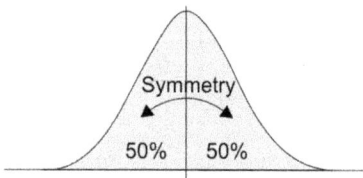

A normal distribution is a bell-shaped curve. In normally distributed data, the mean, median and mode are all equal.

Park K. Parks textbook of preventive and social medicine. India: Bhanot Publishers; 2015.

Q3. Answer b

Null Hypothesis: A null hypothesis is negation of difference and generally expressed in terms of no difference, no effect, no relation, no association and no correlation. Generally, Null Hypothesis indicates that the effect of interest is zero.

Common null hypothesis (H_0) is depicted below:

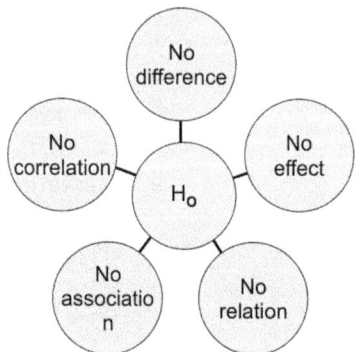

Alternative Hypothesis: The effect of interest is not zero. This includes both two directional or unidirectional situations. If one is testing the difference which is two directional – positive and negative, it is two tailed test. In one tailed test, possibility of test difference is only in one direction - either positive or negative.

H_0: P1 = P2
H_1: P1 # P2   Two tailed
    P1 > P2   One tailed
    P1 < P2   One tailed

There is another categorization of hypothesis into simple and composite hypothesis. A simple hypothesis completely specifies the distribution. A composite does not. Therefore, the correct answer is (b) - alternative hypothesis.

Park K. Parks textbook of preventive and social medicine. India: Bhanot Publishers; 2015.

Q4. Answer a

There are two types of statistical errors, namely Type I and Type II error depicted below:

Types of Error in Hypothesis Tests		
Statistical Inference	Actual/Real Situation	
	Null Hypothesis is True	Null Hypothesis is False
Null Hypothesis is rejected	Incorrect Decision Type I Error (α)	Correct Decision (Power = 1-β)
Null Hypothesis is not rejected	Correct Decision (Confidence level = 1- α)	Incorrect Decision Type II error (β)

Type I error occurs when one rejects the Null hypothesis which is actually true. For example, diagnosing a person wrongly as suffering from the disease, when he/she is not. Level of significance is the probability of type I error and denoted by α. Type II error occurs when one accepts the null hypothesis but it is actually false. For example, missing the diagnosis and person is declared as free from the disease when he/she is actually suffering from the disease. Power of a test is denoted by 1-β. Where β is the probability of Type II error.

Park K. Parks textbook of preventive and social medicine. India: Bhanot Publishers; 2015.

Q5. Answer b

The power of any test of statistical significance is defined as the probability that it will reject a false null hypothesis. Statistical power is inversely related to beta or the probability of making a Type II error. In short, power = 1 - β. Statistical power is the likelihood that a study will detect an effect when there is an effect there to be detected. If statistical power is high, the probability of making a Type II error, or concluding there is no effect when, in fact, there is one, goes down. Statistical power is affected chiefly by the size of the effect and the size of the sample used to detect it. Bigger effects are easier to detect than smaller effects, while large samples offer greater test sensitivity than small samples.

Park K. Parks textbook of preventive and social medicine. India: Bhanot Publishers; 2015.

Q6. Answer a

The level of significance is defined as probability of Type I error that is rejecting a null hypothesis which is true. The p-value is the probability of the computed test statistic based on the sample observations. If the calculated value of p is less than the level of significance, the null hypothesis is rejected. In the present case the level of significance is 5% and in alternative (a) the calculated value of p is less than 0.05 and hence null hypothesis rejected.

Zar JH. Biostatistical analysis. Upper Saddle River, NJ: Pearson; 2010.

Indrayan, A. and Holt, MP: Concise Encyclopedia of Biostatistics for Medical Professionals. CRC Press. 2016.

Q7. Answer a

Median value is the middle most value in the series after arranging in the ascending or descending order. In the present case the number of observation are 21 which is an odd number. The median value is the (n+1)/2th value in case of odd number of observation, where n is the total number of values in the series. Thus the median is (21+1)/2 = 11th value in the order series.

Bland M. An introduction to medical statistics. Oxford: Oxford University Press; 2015.

Q8. Answer a

There are three most commonly used measures of central location that is mean, median and mode.
- The mean is the sum of all observation divided by number of observations.
- Median value is the middle most value in the series.
- Mode is the number which appears most frequent in a set of observations.

The types of data/variables are defined as under:
- Nominal scale: A nominal variable is recorded as a word. Examples - gender (male or female), genotype (AA, Aa, or aa), Blood groups (A+, A-, B+, B-, AB+, AB -).
- Ordinal scale, are those for which the individual observations can be put in order from smallest to largest, even though the exact values are unknown. Thus, Ordinal Scale are qualitative which can be graded. Example - Severity of cancer: stage I, stage II, stage III and stage IV.
- Continuous variable can take any value within a given range. Examples - blood glucose, urinary creatinine excretion and bilirubin level.
- Grouped data are data formed by aggregating individual observations of a continuous variable into groups, so that a frequency distribution of these groups serves as a convenient means of summarizing or analyzing the data.
- Rate: Many a times some indicators such as mortality and morbidity are expressed in terms of rates. A rate is a ratio of the form a*/(a+b); where
  - a* = the frequency of events (death or disease) during a certain time period and
  - a+b = the number at risk of the event during that time period

The best measure of central tendency with respect to the different types of variable is summarized as under.

Type of variable	Best measure of central tendency
Nominal	Mode
Ordinal	Median
Continuous	Mean
Grouped Data	Mean
Rate	Ratio

Bland M. An introduction to medical statistics. Oxford: Oxford University Press; 2015.

Q9. Answer b

The coefficient of variation is the ratio of standard deviation and mean, expressed in percentage, where:
The mean is the sum of all observation divided by number of observations.
Standard deviation is the square root of variance.
The variance is defined as the mean of the squared deviations of individual values around their mean.
In this question standard deviation is 4, which is square root of variance and mean is 20.
Thus   CV = (SD/Mean) * 100% = (4/20)*100% = 20%

Bland M. An introduction to medical statistics. Oxford: Oxford University Press; 2015.

Q10. Answer a

| Diagnostic test | Gold Standard | | |
	Positive	Negative	Total
Positive	a (TP)	b (FP)	a + b
Negative	c (FN)	d (TN)	c + d
Total	a + c (Total diseased)	b + d (Total normal)	N = a + b + c + d

The sensitivity is defined as number detected as positive by the diagnostic test out of total positive by gold standard.

$$\text{Sensitivity} = a/(a+c)$$

In the present case out of 100 true positives the test detected only 90 as positive and hence the sensitivity as 90%.

The specificity is defined as number detected as negative by the diagnostic test out of total negative by gold standard.

$$\text{Specificity} = d/(b+d)$$

In the present case out of 100 true negatives the test detected only 40 as negative and hence the specificity as 40%.

Thus the true answer is (a).

Bland M. An introduction to medical statistics. Oxford: Oxford University Press; 2015.

K Type Answers

Q1. Answer TTTTF

Statistics is defined as the science of collection, presentation, analysis and interpretation of numerical data.

Sundaram KR, Dwivedi SN, Sreenivas V. Medical statistics: principles & methods. Tunbridge Wells: Anshan; 2010.

Q2. Answer TTTFT

A data set is reliable when data set is complete (free from missing values), accurate (measured with correct scales and free from outliers), observations are consistent and homogeneous (similar characteristics, satisfying inclusion and exclusion criteria) representing the population.

Sundaram KR, Dwivedi SN, Sreenivas V. Medical statistics: principles & methods. Tunbridge Wells: Anshan; 2010.

Q3. Answer TFFFF

An essential part of any medical research is to decide how many subjects needs to be studied. The sample size is the number of patients or subjects included in the study. The main aim of the sample size is capable of answering the primary aim.

Sundaram KR, Dwivedi SN, Sreenivas V. Medical statistics: principles & methods. Tunbridge Wells: Anshan; 2010.

Q4. Answer TTTFT

The main factors play role for selection of graph are objective of the study, types of data, number of factors or variables and most importantly readers/viewers for whom graph is prepared.

Sundaram KR, Dwivedi SN, Sreenivas V. Medical statistics: principles & methods. Tunbridge Wells: Anshan; 2010.

Q5. Answer TTTTF

Dispersion tells us the scatteredness of the observation from the central value. The range is the difference between the minimum and maximum values in a set of observations. Mean deviation is the deviation of each observation from the mean value of the same set of observation.

The quartiles are the values which divide the whole distribution into four equal parts. Quartile deviation is calculated as, $Q.D. = (Q_3 - Q_1)/2$, where Q_1 and Q_3 are first and third quartile respectively.

The standard deviation is defined as the square root of the mean of the squared deviations of individual values around their mean.

The mean is the average of the numbers: a calculated "central" value of a set of observation and calculated as the sum of all observation divided by number of observations.

Zar JH. Biostatistical analysis. Upper Saddle River, NJ: Pearson; 2010.

Indrayan, A. and Holt, MP: Concise Encyclopedia of Biostatistics for Medical Professionals. CRC Press. 2016.

Q6. Answer FFFTF

Correlation measures the strength of association between two variables and the direction of the relationship. The range of correlation coefficient is -1 to +1. The correlation coefficient is zero when there is no correlation between the two variables. When the correlation is complete or perfect the correlation coefficient will be either +1 or -1.

Zar JH. Biostatistical analysis. Upper Saddle River, NJ: Pearson; 2010. Indrayan, A. and Holt, MP: Concise Encyclopedia of Biostatistics for Medical Professionals. CRC Press. 2016.

Q7. Answer TTTFT

A confounder (also confounding variable or confounding factor) is a variable that influences both the dependent variable (outcome) and independent variable causing a spurious association.

> Zar JH. Biostatistical analysis. Upper Saddle River, NJ: Pearson; 2010. Indrayan, A. and Holt, MP: Concise Encyclopedia of Biostatistics for Medical Professionals. CRC Press. 2016.

Q8. Answer FTTFF

Qualitative variable can take values that are names or labels.

> Zar JH. Biostatistical analysis. Upper Saddle River, NJ: Pearson; 2010. Indrayan, A. and Holt, MP: Concise Encyclopedia of Biostatistics for Medical Professionals. CRC Press. 2016.

Q9. Answer TTTFF

Measure of central location indicates the concentration of observation in the central part of distribution.

Variance is a measurement of the spread between numbers in a data set. The variance measures how far each number in the set is from the mean.

> Zar JH. Biostatistical analysis. Upper Saddle River, NJ: Pearson; 2010. Indrayan, A. and Holt, MP: Concise Encyclopedia of Biostatistics for Medical Professionals. CRC Press. 2016.

Q10. Answer TFTFF

Variables can be classified in two parts, as qualitative or quantitative. Qualitative variables also known as categorical variable take on values that are names or labels. Quantitative variables are numeric values.

> Sokal RR, Rohlf JF. Biometry: The principles and practice of statistics in biological research. New York: W.H. Freeman and Company; 2007.

CHAPTER 18

Transfusions in Critical Care

Aseem Kumar Tiwari, Qurat Ul Ain Makhdoomi

A Type Questions
(One best answer)

1. There is a need of emergency transfusion in a Road-Traffic-Accident (RTA) case of 30 years old male. The blood group of patient is not known. Which of the following statements regarding emergency transfusion is NOT TRUE?
   a. Group 'O' Rh-negative packed red cells without cross-match can be transfused
   b. An Rh-negative male patient or an older female patient can be transfused Rh-positive RBCs
   c. Delaying blood transfusion in emergency situations may be more dangerous than the small risk of transfusing incompatible blood before the antibody screen and cross match are completed
   d. After transfusion of O blood, there is no use of blood grouping and antibody screening
   e. Ensure a pre-transfusion sample is taken for subsequent testing

2. You are consulted regarding Red Blood Cell (RBC) transfusion in a 45 years old male patient admitted in ICU with diagnosis of pneumonia, and having hemoglobin (Hb) of 7.5 g/dL; well compensated. There is no signs of active bleeding, petechiae or ecchymosis. The correct advice would be:
   a. Transfuse RBC to maintain Hb between 9 and 10 g/dL
   b. Transfuse RBC, FFP and platelets in ratio of 1:1:1
   c. No need for red blood cell transfusion at present
   d. Patient should be regularly transfused red blood cells over next few days, so that his Hb is maintained above 10 g/dL
   e. Fresh whole blood should be transfused

3. You receive a call from emergency department for a case of 23-year-old female patient having gastrointestinal bleeding from varices. You decided to activate massive transfusion protocol. Which of the following is NOT TRUE for massive transfusion protocol (MTP)?
   a. It can be defined as administration of 10 RBC units or more to an adult patient in less than 24 hours or replacement of one or more blood volume(s) within 24 hours
   b. The maximum citrate infusion rate should be 0.02 mmol/kg per minute
   c. 10% calcium gluconate, 10 to 20 mL should be given intravenously (into another vein) for each 500 mL of blood infused
   d. Protocol follows the ratio of transfusion of red cells, FFP and platelets in the ratio of 1:1:1
   e. Calcium gluconate may be preferable to calcium chloride in the presence of abnormal liver function

4. Regarding transfusion reaction all of the following are true except:
   a. Acute hemolytic transfusion reaction (AHTR) is a life-threatening reaction caused by acute intravascular hemolysis of transfused red blood cells

b. Anaphylactic transfusion reaction is allergic reaction including angioedema, wheezing or hypotension
c. Febrile non-hemolytic transfusion reaction (FNHTR) is release of cytokines from white blood cells in a product that has not been leukoreduced
d. Primary hypotensive reactions have been reported most commonly with platelet transfusion
e. Urticarial transfusion reaction (UTR) is a contraindication to continuing the transfusion

5. **A 35-year-old female with multiple myeloma is undergoing transfusion. You are asked by the nursing staff for the suggested guidelines for the flow rate of administration of RBC transfusion. You will suggest to:**
   a. Start for the first 15 minutes at the rate of 1-2 mL/min (i.e. 60-120 mL/hr), then if the patient is stable after 15 minutes approximately at 4 mL/min or 240 ml/hr; infusion duration should not exceed 4 hours
   b. Start for the first 15 minutes with the rate of 2-5 ml/min (i.e. 120-300 mL/hr), then if the patient is stable after 15 minutes approximately at 240 mL/hr; infusion can be given over 2 hours
   c. Start for the first 15 minutes with the rate of 1 mL/min (i.e. 60 mL/hr), then if the patient is stable after 15 minutes continue approximately at 60-120 mL/hr; infusion can be given over 6 hours
   d. Start for the first 15 minutes with the rate of 2-5 mL/hr (i.e. 120-300 mL/hr), then if patient is stable, it can be given as rapidly as possible
   e. Slowly transfuse over 8-12 hours

6. **In clinical practice major exceptions to the use of a threshold of 7 to 8 g/dl, where evidence is insufficient to guide therapy, include all of the following except:**
   a. Case of a 25-year-old female case of swine flu, pneumonia complicated by ARDS on high ventilator support
   b. Case of a 43-year-old man who presented with an anterior wall ST elevation myocardial infarction and was thrombolysed
   c. A 32-year-male after hit by car sustaining polytrauama on massive transfusion protocol
   d. Severe thrombocytopenia in case of myelodysplastic syndrome patients at risk of bleeding
   e. Symptomatic chronic transfusion-dependent anemia

7. **A 45 years old male was scheduled for elective orthopedic surgery after 3 months. He opted for autologous blood donation and preserving (freezing RBCs) his red cells. His blood group was O negative and was k negative (cellano negative). Which of the following is FALSE regarding deglycerolized RBC:**
   a. Expires after 24 hours of thawing
   b. Inexpensive process
   c. Cryopreservation is usually used for rare antigen type donor blood
   d. The expected hematocrit increase for deglycerolized RBCs is the same that for regular red blood cells units
   e. Compared with refrigerated RBC, frozen deglycerolized cells were non-inferior with respect to increasing hematocrit and clinical outcomes

8. **A 20-years-old female patient with blood group as O positive received RBC transfusion as her Hb was 6 gm/dL. After receiving approximately 20 ml of RBC, patient started complaining of fever with chills and rigors. She was hypotensive, dyspneic and also had pain in abdomen and over the flanks. Transfusion was immediately stopped. The duty doctor noticed that on the blood bag the group was 'A' positive. All of the following steps should be followed next regarding patient management and to prevent such occurrences except:**
   a. Immediately stop the transfusion
   b. Infusion of saline should be started and continued to maintain venous access, treat hypotension, and maintain renal blood flow
   c. The unit of blood should be returned to the blood bank, along with post-transfusion sample and urine sample of the patient
   d. Institutional policies and procedures should be in the place to minimize the likelihood of such errors
   e. Pre-transfusion administration of antipyretics or anti-histamines should be commonly ordered

9. **Regarding red blood cell transfusion in a 28 years old patient with IgA deficiency. All of the following are true except:**

a. Washed RBC are indicated in IgA deficiency
b. The red blood cells administered to the patient should be washed with normal saline
c. Irradiated red blood cells are indicated
d. Washed RBCs have lifespan of 24 hours
e. Appropriate staff and medication should be available to treat anaphylaxis

10. A 21-year-old lady presents with pallor and bruising. Her Complete Blood Count (CBC) reveals pancytopenia (Hb 3.4 g/dL, WBC $1.2 \times 10^3/mm^3$, platelets 9,000/mm^3) and reticulocytosis. Leukoreduced blood products should be advised for her as:
    a. Leukoreduction eliminates the risk of bacterial contamination
    b. Leukoreduction reduces the risk of HLA-sensitization
    c. Leukoreduction completely prevents allergic transfusion reaction
    d. It eliminates the risk of transfusion-associated graft-versus-host disease (ta-GVHD)
    e. Diminish the risk of postoperative infections

11. Most suitable patient for cryoprecipitate transfusion is:
    a. Cardiac patient with intracranial hemorrhage requiring immediate neurosurgery but has developed Warfarin toxicity
    b. Five-year-old child with Factor IX deficiency planned for adenoidectomy
    c. Newborn with suspected Hemophilia B in a setting where no Factor IX is available
    d. Trauma victim who has received 3 times the total blood volume red cells, 3 units of Single Donor Platelets (SDP) with fibrinogen levels of 60 mg/dL
    e. Postoperative patient with overt sepsis complicated by DIC

12. An adult male patient with uncontrolled bleeding after minor trauma was tested for Hemophilia after his wife gave a positive family history of Hemophilia from his mother's family. Investigations revealed a PTT – 75 seconds, Factor VIII - <1%, Factor IX – 62%. What is the transfusion product of choice?
    a. FFP
    b. Cryoprecipitate
    c. Whole blood
    d. Recombinant factor VIII concentrate
    e. Plasma cryoprecipitate reduced

13. Compared to one unit of FFP, one unit of cryoprecipitate has:
    a. More Factor VIII and in higher concentration
    b. Less Factor VIII and in higher concentration
    c. More fibrinogen and in higher concentration
    d. Less Factor XIII and in lower concentration

14. The first line of therapy in the rapidly bleeding patient should be:
    a. Whole blood transfusion
    b. Packed red blood cell transfusion
    c. Transfusion of packed red blood cells and fresh frozen plasma
    d. Infusion of crystalloid solution
    e. Infusion of colloid solution

15. A 40-year-old patient with liver disease receives FFP transfusion. Patient develops urticarial and dyspnea after one unit is transfused. On questioning, patient informs about two such similar episodes in the past. All of the following actions are appropriate for the Physician except:
    a. Discontinue transfusion
    b. Assess the patient
    c. Repeat FFP transfusion without any investigations
    d. Send IgA level
    e. X-ray Chest PA view

16. A patient develops Cytomegalovirus (CMV) infection after hospital admission. During his hospital stay, the patient had received transfusions of red cells, platelet concentrates and plasma products. Which of the following carries the least risk of CMV transmission?
    a. Red cells
    b. Random Donor Platelet Concentrate (RDPC)
    c. Single Donor Platelet Concentrate (SDPC)
    d. Fresh Frozen Plasma (FFP)
    e. Whole blood

17. A European suffering from severe Hemophilia, traveling to India, runs out of factor concentrate and develops a knee bleed. He visits a local hospital where plasma derived factor concentrate is available. The concentrate is solvent detergent treated. Pathogen most likely to be transmitted is:
    a. HIV
    b. HBV

c. HCV
d. CMV
e. Parvovirus B19

18. Five patients are admitted in a ward with the following diagnosis:
    1. Severe Hemophilia A
    2. Mild Hemophilia B
    3. von Willebrand Disease
    4. Hypoprothrombinemia
    5. Hypofibrinogenemia
    Cryoprecipitate is a good choice of treatment for patients with:
    a. 1,2,5
    b. 1,3,5
    c. 1,4,5
    d. 3,4,5
    e. 2,4,5

19. A 32-year-old female falls from the roof of her house and is rushed to the emergency of the nearest hospital with massive bleeding. Initially she received six units of red cells followed by four units over next 6 hours. Patient lands into a state of dilutional coagulopathy. Immediate next step is:
    a. Transfuse three doses each of platelets (10 mL/kg) and FFP (15 mL/kg)
    b. Transfuse platelets only
    c. Perform PT/aPTT/platelet count stat and then decide
    d. PT/aPTT/platelet count/Fibrinogen stat and then transfuse FFP (15 mL/kg), platelets (10 mL/kg) and cryoprecipitate (I bag/10 kg) appropriately.
    e. Cryoprecipitate alone is sufficient

20. A patient is undergoing liver transplant for ethanol related chronic liver disease. As a part of preoperative preparation, cryoprecipitate is requested. Cryoprecipitate would be:
    a. Irradiated
    b. Rich in factor IX
    c. Rich in fibrinogen and factor VIII
    d. Stored for 48 hours at room temperature after thawing
    e. Carrying viable lymphocytes

21. All are true regarding platelet count thresholds that are used for following procedures except:
    a. Central line placement – 50,000/mm^3
    b. Endoscopic procedures – 50,000/mm^3 for therapeutic procedures
    c. Bronchoscopy with bronchoalveolar lavage (BAL) – 20,000 to 30,000/mm^3
    d. Lumbar puncture –greater than 40,000 to 50,000
    e. Bone marrow aspiration/biopsy – 20,000/mm^3

22. Regarding platelets transfusion all are true except:
    a. Adults dose is approximately one random donor unit per 10 kg of body weight
    b. Apheresis platelets have the advantages of limiting the recipient exposure to a single donor
    c. Leukoreduction removes most of the contaminating white blood cells (WBC) from the platelet transfusion
    d. Platelets express ABO as well as Rh antigens on their surface
    e. Platelet irradiation is used to prevent transfusion associated -Graft Versus Host Disease (GVHD)

23. A 44-year-old female with Acute Lymphoblastic Leukemia (ALL) is admitted for pancytopenia and fever. Her platelet count is less than 10,000/mm^3. The patient blood type is 'A' positive. The blood bank is low on platelet inventory and can only dispense 'O' positive platelets. Which of the following platelet product choice is best to prepare and transfuse to patient?
    a. Transfuse 10 mL/kg 'O' positive SDPC that are leukoreduced and irradiated
    b. Transfuse 10 mL/kg 'O' positive SDPC that are volume reduced pre-storage leukoreduced and irradiated
    c. Wait to transfuse despite active bleeding because it is unsafe to transfuse 'O' positive leukoreduced, irradiated SDPC to 'A' positive patient
    d. Transfuse 10 mL/kg 'O' positive SDPC that are irradiated only
    e. Transfuse 10 mL/kg 'O' positive SDPC without any special preparation

24. Regarding spontaneous bleeding in thrombocytopenia all statements are true except:
    a. There are no ideal tests for predicting who will bleed spontaneously
    b. Bleeding is much more likely at platelet counts less than 5,000/mm^3
    c. Mucosal bleeding and epistaxis are generally not thought to be predictive of serious bleeding
    d. Coexisting inflammation, infection, and fever also increase bleeding risk

e. Tests for platelet-dependent hemostasis are generally not used to predict bleeding in thrombocytopenic patients

25. **Regarding the treatment of immune thrombocytopenia (ITP) all of the following are true except:**
    a. Immediate platelet transfusion for patients with severe bleeding and a platelet count <30,000/µL
    b. ITP is a contraindication to the use of myelosuppressive chemotherapy
    c. The usual dose of anti-D is 50 to 75 mcg/kg intravenously
    d. IVIG dose is 400 mg/kg daily for five days
    e. Dose of dexamethasone 40 mg orally per day for 4 days with no taper

26. **Regarding platelet irradiation, all are true except:**
    a. Useful in Immunosuppression from hematopoietic or solid organ transplant
    b. Irradiation can be substituted for leukoreduction
    c. Irradiation is inadequate to kill pathogens such as bacteria and viruses
    d. Indicated in Hodgkin lymphoma and other hematologic malignancies
    e. Indicated in Congenital immunodeficiency

27. **Leukoreduction can be adequately used for following indications except:**
    a. Reduction of HLA alloimmunization
    b. Reduction of CMV transmission
    c. Reduction of transfusion-associated immunomodulation
    d. Reduction of lung injury during and after cardiopulmonary bypass
    e. Prevent ta-GVHD

28. **A patient receiving a transfusion of 6 units FFP started having shortness of breath. On examination, he was dyspneic, temperature 36.4°C, HR:90/min, BP:95/40 mm Hg, RR:35/min and SpO$_2$ was 88%. On auscultation, there was bilateral scattered crepts with no bronchospasm. His oxygen requirement has increased. His chest radiograph was suggestive of homogenous bilateral alveolar opacities. His NT-ProBNP was found to be elevated. The patient may be experiencing which of the following?**
    a. Transfusion-related-acute lung injury (TRALI)
    b. Transfusion associated circulatory overload (TACO)
    c. Allergic transfusion reaction
    d. Transfusion associated dyspnea
    e. ARDS

29. **An adult male postoperative patient for perforated appendicitis on mechanical ventilation in ICU received 6 units RDPC for sepsis induced thrombocytopenia and surgical intervention. His oxygen requirement suddenly increased 2 hours after completing transfusion. On examination his temperature was 36.4°C, HR:110/min, BP:110/60 mm Hg, and SpO$_2$ was 86% on FiO$_2$ of 1.0. Chest X-ray was showing bilateral homogenous alveolar opacities. ET secretion was clear. His CVP was 10 cm H$_2$O. Which of the following is most likely diagnosis?**
    a. Transfusion-related-acute lung injury (TRALI)
    b. TRALI with other ALI risk factors
    c. Transfusion associated circulatory overload
    d. ARDS
    e. Fluid overload

30. **One unit of random donor platelet usually increases the platelet count in an adult by:**
    a. 5000
    b. 10000
    c. 15000
    d. 20000
    e. 30000

K Type Questions
[Marked True (T)/False (F)]

1. **A 13-year-old boy from Tamil Nadu is posted for knee surgery, which was injured. His medical history is suggestive of sickle cell anemia. The following guidelines seem to be appropriate for this patient undergoing surgery:**
    a. Preoperative RBC transfusions are warranted when prolonged general anesthesia is indicated
    b. A desirable preoperative HbS is 15% to 20%
    c. No special measures need to be taken in sickle cell trait
    d. It is not necessary to obtain a full red cell antigen profile before transfusion therapy

2. **Intravenous (IV) fluids compatible with red blood cells infusion are:**
    a. 0.9% sodium chloride injection
    b. 5% dextrose
    c. Ringer lactate
    d. 5% Albumin

3. A 25 years old road traffic accident patient got transfused with 11 units of red blood cells in the last 24 hours. Complications that can occur in this patient in context to RBC transfusion are:
   a. Hypercalcemia
   b. Hyperkalemia
   c. Hypothermia
   d. Hemostatic abnormalities

4. Cryoprecipitate:
   a. Is prepared from FFP
   b. Must be transfused within 6 hours of thawing
   c. Contains 150–250 mg of fibrinogen
   d. Shelf life of frozen cryoprecipitate is 30 days

5. Regarding fresh frozen plasma:
   a. FFP is plasma prepared from whole blood through the primary centrifugation of whole blood
   b. The most labile coagulation factors are preserved for a year if FFP is kept at 0-4°C
   c. Should be transfused as soon as possible after thawing
   d. Dose is 5 mL/kg

6. Cryoprecipitate poor plasma:
   a. Is a by-product of FFP preparation
   b. Lacks labile clotting factors V and VIII and fibrinogen
   c. Cryoprecipitate poor plasma deplete the vitamin K-dependent clotting factors
   d. Cryoprecipitate-poor plasma contains 50% of the amount of Factor V in FFP and cannot be used as an alternative to FFP

7. Fresh frozen plasma can be indicated in:
   a. Disseminated Intravascular Coagulation (DIC)
   b. Anti-thrombin III deficiency
   c. Volume expansion
   d. Deficiency of Factors II, VII, IX and X

8. Regarding Prothrombin Complex Concentrate (PCC):
   a. Contains Factors II, IX and X and to varying degree of factor VII
   b. Also known as Anti-inhibitor coagulation complex (AICC)
   c. Used for the treatment of patients with high titers of antibodies to factor VIII
   d. Used to treat Hemophilia A

9. Platelet products are contaminated commonly:
   a. By entry of skin plug into collection plug
   b. By environmental contamination during processing
   c. By storing platelet at 20°- 24°C for 5 days
   d. By storing platelet with continuous agitation

10. A 22-year-old woman presents with easy bruising and fatigue. A complete blood count reveals hemoglobin 9.0 g/dL, haematocrit: 27%, WBC: 15,000/µL, and platelet count 15,000/µL. The hematologist plans to perform a bone marrow biopsy and aspiration, which of the following is correct?
    a. Platelet transfusion not indicated
    b. Platelet transfusion should be initiated
    c. One unit of RDPC is enough, which contain at least $5.5 *10^{10}$ platelet
    d. Platelet should be preferably leucodepleted if transfused

11. Mark true or false about Single Donor Platelet Concentrate (SDPC) and Random Donor Platelet Concentrate (RDPC):
    a. SDPC must be constantly agitated and stored at 4°C, while RDPC can be stored at room temperature
    b. SDPC platelets and RDPC contain a similar number of thrombocytes
    c. Both platelet types decrease the possibility of multiple donor exposures and bacterial contamination
    d. Both platelet types can be stored for 5 days and are suspended in donor plasma

12. The following are true about current storage time and storage temperature for platelet concentrates and apheresis platelet components:
    a. It can be stored for 5 days at 24°-27°C
    b. It can be stored for 5 days at 20°-24°C
    c. It can be stored for 7 days at 24°-27°C
    d. It can be stored for 7 days at 20°-24°C

13. About Corrected Count Increment (CCI) in platelet refractoriness:
    a. Platelet refractoriness is suspected when CCI is less than 20% at 10 minute and one hour post platelet transfusion
    b. Platelet refractoriness is suspected when CCI is less than 30% at 10 minute and one hour post platelet transfusion
    c. Platelet refractoriness is suspected when CCI is less than 40% at 10 minute and one hour post platelet transfusion
    d. Platelet refractoriness is suspected when CCI is less than 50% at 10 minute and one hour post platelet transfusion

ANSWERS

A Type Answers

Q1. Answer d

In case of urgency, uncross-matched group 'O' RBCs can be transfused if the patient's ABO group is unknown. It is preferable to give D-negative blood if the recipient's D type is unknown especially if the patient is a female of childbearing potential. It should be documented that compatibility testing was not completed before transfusion and benefit outweighs risk of transfusion reaction. After 'O' blood transfusion in emergency situations (without cross match), compatibility testing should be continued and completed promptly by blood bank.

> Grossman B, Hillyer C. Pre-transfusion Testing. In: Downes K, Shulman I, Fung M (eds.). Technical manual. 18th edition. 2014. Bethesda, United States: AABB; p.385-386.
>
> Lynne U, Arthur JS, Jennifer ST (eds.). Pretransfusion testing for red blood cell transfusion. Available from: https://www.uptodate.com/contents/pretransfusion-testing-for-red-blood-cell-transfusion (Accessed 14th Oct 2017).

Q2. Answer c

At the end of TRICC Trial, the authors concluded that 'the use of a threshold for red-cell transfusion as low as 7.0 g of hemoglobin per deciliter, combined with the maintenance of hemoglobin concentrations in the range of 7.0 to 9.0 g per deciliter (restrictive transfusion strategy), was at least as effective as and possibly superior to a liberal transfusion strategy (threshold, 10.0 g per deciliter; maintenance range 10.0 to 12.0) in critically ill patients with normovolemia. There was a trend toward decreased 30 day mortality among patients who were treated according to the restrictive transfusion strategy. The significant differences in mortality rates during hospitalization, rates of cardiac complications, and rates of organ dysfunction all favored the restrictive strategy.'

> Hébert PC, Wells G, Blajchman MA, et. al. A multicenter, randomized, controlled clinical trial of transfusion requirements in critical care. Transfusion requirements in clinical care investigators, Canadian critical care trials group. N Engl J Med. 1999;340:409-17.

Q3. Answer e

Massive transfusion, historically defined as the replacement by transfusion of 10 units of red cells in 24 hours is a response to massive and uncontrolled hemorrhage. With more rapid and effective therapy, alternative definitions such as 3 units over 1 hour are more sensitive in identifying patients needing rapid issue of blood products for serious injuries because of uncontrolled hemorrhage. MTP is designed to interrupt the lethal triad of acidosis, hypothermia and coagulopathy that develops with massive transfusion thereby improving outcome. MTP describes the process of management of blood transfusion requirements in major bleeding episodes, assisting the interactions of the treating clinicians and the blood bank and ensuring judicious use of blood and blood components. By developing locally agreed and specific guidelines that include clinical, laboratory, blood bank and logistic responses, clinicians can ensure effective management of massive blood loss and improve outcome.

MTP have a predefined ratio of RBCs, FFP/cryoprecipitate and platelets units (random donor platelets) in each pack (e.g. 1:1:1 or 2:1:1 ratio) for transfusion. The physiology supporting the 1:1:1 (FFP:platelets:RBCs) approach derives from the existence of the acute coagulopathy of trauma and the dilute nature of conventional blood products. Resuscitation with FFP, platelets, and RBCs at 1:1:1 unit ratios means that the actual blood being given has a coagulation factor concentration of 65 percent of normal, a platelet count of 88×10^9/L, and a hematocrit of 29 percent. The maximum citrate infusion rate should be 0.02 mmol/kg per minute (since this represents the maximum rate of citrate metabolism) and the citrate concentration in whole blood is 15 mmol/L (0.015 mmol/mL). If 10 percent calcium gluconate is used, 10 to 20 mL should be given intravenously (into another vein) for each 500 mL of blood infused. If 10 percent calcium chloride is used; only 2 to 5 mL per 500 mL of blood should be given. Calcium chloride may be preferable to calcium gluconate in the presence of abnormal liver function.

> Patil V, Shetmahajan M. Massive transfusion and massive transfusion protocol. Indian J Anaesth. 2014;58:590-5.
>
> John R, Arthur J (ed), Jennifer S (ed). Massive blood transfusion. Available from: https://www.uptodate.com/contents/massive-blood-transfusion (Accessed 14th Oct 2017).

Q4. Answer e

AHTR is a life-threatening reaction caused by acute intravascular hemolysis of transfused red blood cells (RBCs). Presenting symptoms include fever, chills, flank pain, and oozing from intravenous sites. Treatment involves aggressive hydration and diuresis. Febrile non-hemolytic transfusion reaction (FNHTR) is characterized by fever, usually accompanied by chills in the absence of other systemic symptoms. The most common cause of FNHTR is release of cytokines from white blood cells (WBCs) in a product that has not been leukoreduced. In the case of platelet transfusion, a similar reaction characterized by chills and/or rigors can occur in the absence of a temperature change. Management is symptomatic. Primary hypotensive transfusion reactions are rare transfusion reactions in which there is a drop in blood pressure without other causes of hypotension. Blood pressure (systolic, diastolic, or both) decreases by 30 mm Hg or more within minutes of onset of transfusion and returns to baseline once the transfusion is stopped. The mechanism is thought to involve vasoactive kinins (e.g. bradykinin). The reactions are rapidly reversible and generally do not require specific treatment or prevention except for possible avoidance of ACE inhibitors prior to planned transfusion or apheresis. Urticarial reactions are associated with hives but no other allergic findings (i.e. no wheezing, angioedema, hypotension). UTR is not a contraindication to continuing the transfusion as long as it is clear there are no other allergic symptoms.

> Arthur J, Steven K (ed), Jennifer S (ed). Massive blood transfusion. Available from: https://www.uptodate.com/contents/approach-to-the-patient-with-a-suspected-acute-transfusion-reaction (Accessed 14th Oct 2017).

Q5. Answer a

The infusion should start slowly at approximately 2 mL per minute, for the first 15 minutes while the transfusionist remains near the patient. Severe reactions may occur after as little as 10 mL has been transfused. Potentially life-threatening reactions most commonly occur within 10 to 15 minutes of the start of a transfusion. The rate of transfusion should be increased after 15 minutes to ensure the unit is administered within the 4 hour window. The advantages of using relatively rapid transfusion rates (e.g. 240 mL/hour) include correction of deficiency as rapidly as possible as well as reduced patient and nursing time dedicated to transfusion.

> Maynard K, Fung M, Administration of Blood Components. Technical manual. 18th edition. Bethesda, United States: AABB; 2014. p.553-554.
>
> Jun T, Donald H Carrie A (eds.). Red blood cell transfusion in infants and children: Administration and complications. Available from: https://www.uptodate.com/contents/approach-to-the-patient-with-a-suspected-acute-transfusion-reaction (Accessed 14th Oct 2017).

Q6. Answer a

Major exceptions to the use of a threshold of 7 to 8 g/dL, where evidence is insufficient to guide therapy include the following:
  i. Symptomatic patients may be transfused at higher hemoglobin levels to treat symptoms.
  ii. Patients with acute coronary syndromes have not been adequately evaluated in clinical trials and may require higher thresholds for transfusion. Threshold-based transfusion is not appropriate for patients requiring massive transfusion such as in the setting of trauma because it requires waiting for hemoglobin levels to be reported.
  iii. Severe thrombocytopenia in hematology/oncology patients at risk of bleeding.
  iv. Chronic transfusion-dependent anemia.

> Jeffrey L. Indications and hemoglobin thresholds for red blood cell transfusion in the adult. Available from: https://www.uptodate.com/contents/indications-and-hemoglobin-thresholds-for-red-blood-cell-transfusion-in-the-adult (Accessed 14th Oct 2017).

Q7. Answer b

Predeposit autologous donation is usually reserved for patients anticipating a need for transfusion such as for a scheduled major surgery. Predeposit autologous transfusion is expensive because about half of the donated units are not used.

In addition, patients present for surgery with lower hematocrits which increases transfusion of homologous units in addition to autologous units. However, patients with multiple RBC antibodies or antibodies to high-incidence antigens may store frozen units for use by themselves or others.

Compared with refrigerated RBC, frozen deglycerolized cells were non-inferior with respect to increasing hematocrit, effects on thromboelastography parameters, and clinical outcomes.

Kennedy M, Harmening D (eds.). Transfusion Therapy. Modern blood banking & transfusion practices. Sixth edition. Philadelphia, PA: FA Davis Company; 2012.p.360.

Q8. Answer e

Although antipyretics (e.g. acetaminophen) were commonly ordered in the past to reduce the risk of febrile nonhemolytic transfusion reaction, indications for their use are controversial. Prophylactic use of antipyretics may mask the elevated temperature and other symptoms and signs that result from a transfusion reaction. In the absence of definitive evidence-based studies, pre-transfusion medication to prevent transfusion reactions should not be encouraged. In a Cochrane review of studies on premedication to prevent allergic reactions and febrile non-hemolytic transfusion reactions (FNHTRs), the authors stated that current evidence from three randomized controlled trials (RCTs) involving 462 patients indicate that no pre-transfusion medication regimen reduces the risk of allergic reaction or FNHTR. They further state that no evidence shows that pre-transfusion medications prevent NHTR.

Maynard K, Fung M (eds). Administration of Blood Components. Technical manual. 18th edition. Bethesda, United States: AABB; 2014. p.547.

Q9. Answer c

Washed RBC are indicated for IgA deficient patients to avoid severe allergic/anaphylactic reactions. RBC are washed with 2-3 liters of normal saline. Since the procedure is an 'open' procedure, the shelf-life reduces to 24 hours.

There is no indication for irradiated RBC for IgA deficient patients. Indications for transfusion of irradiated blood components are as follows:

- Bone marrow transplant or Peripheral blood stem cells recipients
- Neonates/intrauterine transfusion recipients
- Neonatal exchange transfusion recipients
- Premature newborns (less than 1200 g)
- Immunocompromised or immunosuppressed recipients
- Recipients of first-degree relative donors blood

Saran RK (ed). Transfusion Medicine: Technical Manual. Directorate General of Health Services. Second edition. New Delhi:Mehta Offset Pvt. Ltd. 2003. p. 213, 258.

Q10. Answer b

Donor leukocytes present in cellular blood components have been linked to a wide range of complications in transfusion recipients. Both acute and long-term complications can result directly from exposure to donor leukocytes, prompting the adoption of leukocyte reduction as a highly effective and widely practiced prevention strategy.

Current high-performance leukocyte removal filters can reduce the residual white cell (WBC) content at least 3 logs and typically achieve 4 log or greater removal. As a result, the proportion of filtered units with less than 10^6 residual leukocytes has steadily increased to 99% or greater.

Established indications for leukoreduction are the following:

- Reduce frequency of recurrent febrile non-hemolytic transfusion reactions to Red Blood Cells (RBCs)
- Reduce rate of alloimmunisation to leukocyte antigens for patients (especially in patients with hematologic malignant disease)
- Reduce the risk of transmission of cytomegalovirus (CMV) among persons at risk of infection by transfusion.

Triulzi D, Dzik W, Simon T, Snyder E, Solheim B. Leukocyte-Reduced Blood Components: Laboratory and Clinical Aspects. In: Rossi's Principles of Transfusion Medicine. Stowell C, Strauss (eds.). Fourth Edition. West Sussex, UK: Blackwell Publishing Ltd; 2009.p. 233.

Q11. Answer d

Cryoprecipitate is indicated in fibrinogen deficiency and in massive transfusion with dilutional coagulopathy. In option a, administration of vitamin K is preferred over Fresh Frozen Plasma (FFP) or cryoprecipitate in order to correct vitamin K deficiency (or coumarin over dose). In severe cases where volume overload and time is concerned prothrombin complex concentrate (PCC) may be administered. However, FFP may be required to act immediately; before vitamin K starts its action. In option b, and c, cryoprecipitate is not preferred for use in factor IX deficiency/Hemophilia B because it is a not a rich source of factor IX. FFP may be used in factor IX deficiency when the individual factor IX concentrate is not available. Option d is correct because cryoprecipitate is indicated in massive transfusion and fibrinogen deficiency. There is no definite indication of cryoprecipitate in DIC without evidence of hypofibrinogenemia.

Management strategy for massive transfusion are as follows:
- Restore blood volume to maintain tissue perfusion and blood pressure
- Maintain Oxygen-carrying capacity
- Treat any surgical source of bleeding
- Correct coagulopathy by the judicious use of
  - FFP
  - Platelet transfusion
  - Cryoprecipitate (if fibrinogen is low)
- Prevent hypothermia

Saran R (ed). Transfusion Medicine Technical Manual. Directorate General of Health Services. Second edition. Mehta Offset Pvt. Ltd. New Delhi. 2003. p. 219-221, 253.

Q12. Answer d

Although, earlier effective treatment for Hemophilia A used to be cryoprecipitate transfusion, purified plasma-derived factor or recombinant factors are preferred because of no risk of transfusion transmissible infections (TTI). Patients with moderate (1%-5% Factor VIII activity) or severe (<1% activity) disease are now treated exclusively with a recombinant or purified plasma-derived concentrate. Similar treatment has evolved for patients deficient in Factor IX.

Factor VIII Concentrate preparations that are available:
1. Factor VIII prepared from large pools of plasma (plasma-derived factors)
   - Vials of freeze-dried protein labelled with content usually 250 IU of factor VIII.
   - It is reconstituted aseptically with the diluents provided with the vial.
   - One IU is the factor activity present in 1 mL of normal pooled plasma less than 1 hour old.
   - It is inactivated for viruses by heat treatment, solvent/detergents or purified with monoclonal antibodies.
2. Recombinant DNA technology is currently used to manufacture of factor VIII concentrate which is commercially available. It is clinically equivalent to factor VIII derived from plasma.

Saran R (ed). Plasma Derivatives & Plasma Substitutes. Transfusion Medicine Technical Manual. Directorate General of Health Services. Second edition. Mehta Offset Pvt. Ltd. New Delhi; 2003. p. 377.

Q13. Answer b

Each unit of cryoprecipitate has approximately:
  Plasma 10-15 mL
  Factor VIII 80-100 IU
  Fibrinogen 150-250 mg
  von-Willebrand Factor 40-70%
  Fibronectin 55 mg
  Factor XIII 20-30% of the original
Contents of 1 unit of FFP prepared from 450 mL of whole blood:
  Plasma 175-230 mL
  All coagulation Factors 1 IU/mL of each factor
  (Including Factors V and VIII)

Fibrinogen 200–400 mg/dL

Therefore, compared to one unit of FFP, one unit of cryoprecipitate has less Factor VIII but in higher concentration.

<small>Saran R (ed). Blood Components Preparation and Their Uses. Transfusion Medicine Technical Manual. Directorate General of Health Services. Second edition. Mehta Offset Pvt. Ltd. New Delhi; 2003. p. 219-221.</small>

Q14. Answer d

In patients with active bleeding, the hemodynamic status and need for emergency intervention must be determined and weighed before start of any therapy. Crystalloids are administered to maintain the intravascular volume. Red cell transfusions are administered rapidly to maintain adequate oxygen-carrying capacity. Clinical judgment and hemoglobin measurements at regular intervals is needed to estimate how much more bleeding may occur and how much lower the hemoglobin level would decrease, and then perform transfusion. Vital signs are examined for a decrease in blood pressure and tachycardia. Vigil is maintained for symptoms and signs that can result from anemia like fatigue, dizziness, weakness, and orthostatic hypotension unresponsive to intravenous fluids, cardiac ischemia (chest pain), congestive heart failure (dyspnea, paroxysmal nocturnal dyspnea and edema).

Restoration of circulating volume is initially achieved by rapid infusion of crystalloids or colloids through a large-bore (14 gauge or larger) peripheral cannula. The use of albumin and non-albumin colloids versus crystalloids for volume replacement have long been the subject of debate. Ringer's Lactate solution or normal saline is recommended as initial therapy.

Crystalloid is infused at 3:1 ratio for every unit of volume lost. Therapy is monitored by hemodynamic response and return of tissue perfusion (measured by mental status, urine output, capillary refill and absence of acidosis).

<small>Jeffrey LC, Hébert P. Anaemia and red blood cell transfusion. In: Toby LS, Jeffrey McCullough, Edward LS, Bjarte GS, Ronald GS. (eds.) Rossi's principles of Transfusion Medicine. 5th edition. West Sussex UK: John Wiley and Sons, Ltd. 2016. p. 123-124.

Transfusion Practice in Clinical Medicine. In: Saran RK. (ed.) Directorate General of Health Services Ministry of Health & Family Welfare Government of India. 2nd ed. New Delhi: Mehta Offset Pvt. Ltd.; 2003. p. 254.</small>

Q15. Answer c

Patients with a suspected transfusion reaction should undergo a thorough workup before transfusion of another unit. It is advised to discontinue the transfusion immediately in case of any type of transfusion reaction. Vital signs should be taken at once if there is a suspected transfusion reaction.

A three tier laboratory investigations of any such suspected adverse event with respect to transfusion must be done to provide safe transfusion to the recipient as follows:

First-Tier Investigations
- Post transfusion serum hemoglobin (qualitative)
- Post transfusion Direct Antiglobulin Test (DAT)
- Confirmation of post-transfusion ABO and Rh D

Second-Tier Investigations
- Repeat pre-transfusion ABO and Rh D
- Pre and post-transfusion antibody screen
- Repeat special antigen typing, if needed
- Crossmatch with pre and post-reaction specimens

Third-Tier Investigations
- Antibody identification panels on pre and post-reaction samples
- Enhanced antibody screening method: Polyethylene glycol (PEG), extended incubation, gel, enzymes
- Red cell eluate on pre and post-reaction samples
- Investigation of transfusion technique and blood storage conditions
- Check of the blood bag, tubing, and segments for haemolysis
- Enhanced crossmatches: PEG, enzymes
- Minor crossmatches of implicated units
- Antibody detection tests on donor units

- Quantitative serum hemoglobin
- Serum bilirubin (conjugated and unconjugated)
- Urine hemoglobin and hemosiderin
- Bacterial culture and Gram stain of blood bags
- Blood urea and serum creatinine
- Peripheral blood smear
- Serial hemoglobin, hematocrit and platelet count
- Blood coagulation studies (PT, fibrinogen, FDP)
- DAT on donor units

Always, rule out hemolysis (DAT, inspect for hemoglobinuria, repeat patient ABO), rule out cardiogenic pulmonary edema by a chest X-ray. Patients with two or more severe allergic reactions can undergo testing for IgA deficiency to rule out a relative deficiency of IgA because it is a known cause of both a severe allergic and anaphylactic reactions.

Therefore, option c is incorrect. Any patient with signs of transfusion reaction should not receive any further transfusions until the present reaction is investigated for the cause of reaction.

Robertson DD, Martin HB, Toby L, McCullough, Edward L, Bjarte G (eds). Hemolytic transfusion reactions. Fourth Edition. West Sussex, UK: Blackwell Publishing Ltd. 2009. p. 643-646.

Q16. Answer d

CMV is known to be transmitted through red blood cells and leukocytes. Therefore, blood components containing white blood cells are more likely to transmit CMV infection. Plasma-derived components and derivatives are not likely infectious for CMV as they do not have any cellular component.

Immunosuppressed patients are at greater risk of CMV infection transmitted by blood transfusion. This can be avoided or reduced by transfusing blood that is tested and contains no CMV antibodies or by the use of leukocytes-depleted blood components. Finding a unit which is CMV negative is very difficult; leucodepletion seems to be the best option to avoid CMV transmission.

Hence, option d is correct; FFP is least likely to be associated with the risk of CMV transmission.

Saran RK (ed.). Blood Transfusion Transmitted Diseases. Transfusion Medicine Technical Manual. Directorate General of Health Services. Second edition. Mehta Offset Pvt. Ltd. New Delhi; 2003. p. 144,169.

Q17. Answer e

Solvent detergent plasma is treated with the solvent tri n-butyl phosphate (TBP) and the detergent Triton X-100. Solvent detergent techniques destroy the viral envelope in lipid - enveloped viruses such as hepatitis B, hepatitis C and HIV. The solvent – detergent treatment has no effect on non-lipid enveloped viruses such as hepatitis A and Parvovirus B19. The coagulation factors of solvent/detergent plasma are comparable to FFP. Indications for its use are the same as that of FFP. Hence, option e Parvovirus B19 is likely to be transmitted by transfusion of SD plasma.

Saran RK. Blood Components Preparation and their uses. Transfusion Medicine Technical Manual. Directorate General of Health Services. Second edition. Mehta Offset Pvt. Ltd. New Delhi. 2003. p. 221.

Q18. Answer b

Indications of cryoprecipitate:
- Hemophilia A
- von Willebrand disease
- Congenital or acquired fibrinogen deficiency
- Acquired Factor VIII deficiency (e.g. DIC, massive transfusion)
- Factor XIII deficiency
- Source of fibrin glue used as topical hemostatic agent in surgical procedures.

Therefore, option is b is correct. Severe Hemophilia A, vWD and hypo-fibrinogenemia are indications for cryoprecipitate transfusion.

Saran RK (ed.). Blood Components Preparation and their uses. Transfusion Medicine Technical Manual. Directorate General of Health Services. Second edition. Mehta Offset Pvt. Ltd. New Delhi; 2003. p. 218-220.

Q19. Answer d

Coagulation factor deficiency is the primary cause of coagulopathy in patients with massive transfusion.
- Massive or large volume transfusion can result in disorders of coagulation due to dilution of clotting factors and platelets.
- Prolongation of activated partial thromboplastin time (aPTT) and prothrombin time (PT) to 1.5 to 1.8 times of the control values is correlated with an increased risk of clinical coagulopathy and requires correction. Fresh frozen plasma (15 mL/kg body weight) is given to correct coagulation abnormalities.
- Continued bleeding together with severely disturbed coagulation needs more aggressive therapy. Platelet concentrates, FFP or cryoprecipitate are given particularly when there is an evidence of disseminated intravascular coagulopathy (DIC). Cryoprecipitate will replace fibrinogen and factor VIII. Infusion of FFP should be considered after one blood volume has been lost. FFP alone, if given in sufficient quality will correct fibrinogen and most coagulation factor deficiencies, but large volume may be required if fibrinogen remains critically low (<10 g/L), and therefore cryoprecipitate therapy should be considered for providing fibrinogen. If fibrinogen is low (< 80 mg/dL), cryoprecipitate (10 units/ kg body weight.) can be given.
- If the platelet is count is less than 50×10^9/L, and the patient is bleeding, give platelet concentrates 4-6 units or one unit of apheresis platelets.

   Saran RK (ed.). Blood Components Preparation and their uses. Transfusion Medicine Technical Manual. Directorate General of Health Services. Second edition. Mehta Offset Pvt. Ltd. New Delhi; 2003. p. 254-257

Q20. Answer c

Cryoprecipitate is rich in factor VIII, von willebrand factor, fibrinogen (Factor XIII) and fibronectin; not factor IX.

Gamma irradiation inactivates lymphocytes in blood. Routinely either Cesium-137 (^{137}Cs) or Cobalt-60 (^{60}Co) is used as the source of gamma rays. The usual dose is 25 Gray (Gy) at the center of the bag. (1 Gray=100 rads). This dose inactivates 85 to 95% of lymphocytes in the blood components without any major adverse effect on other cellular components (red cells, platelets and granulocytes) of blood. Products such as FFP and cryoprecipitate do not require irradiation because they do not carry viable lymphocytes. Thawed Cryoprecipitate can be stored for 6 hours at 2-6°C. Therefore, option c is correct.

   Saran RK (ed.). Blood Components Preparation and their uses. Transfusion Medicine Technical Manual. Directorate General of Health Services. Second edition. Mehta Offset Pvt. Ltd. New Delhi; 2003. p. 257-260.

Q21. Answer a

Platelets are transfused in preparation for an invasive procedure if the thrombocytopenia is severe and the risks of bleeding are deemed high. Most of the data is used to determine bleeding risk come from retrospective studies of patients who are afebrile and have thrombocytopenia but not coagulopathy. Typical platelet count thresholds that are used for some common procedures are as follows:
- Neurosurgery or ocular surgery – 100,000/mm³
- Most other major surgery – 50,000/mm³
- Endoscopic procedures – 50,000/mm³ for therapeutic procedures; 20,000/μL for low risk diagnostic procedures
- Bronchoscopy with bronchoalveolar lavage (BAL) – 20,000 to 30,000/mm³
- Central line placement – 20,000/mm³
- Lumbar puncture – 10,000 to 20,000/μL in patients with hematologic malignancies and greater than 40,000 to 50,000 in patients without hematologic malignancies, but lower in patients with immune thrombocytopenia (ITP)
- Epidural anesthesia – 80,000/mm³
- Bone marrow aspiration/biopsy – 20,000/mm³

   Shan Y, Dennis G, Arthur J (eds.). Clinical and laboratory aspects of platelet transfusion therapy. Available from: https://www.uptodate.com/contents/clinical-and-laboratory-aspects-of-platelet-transfusion-therapy (Accessed 14th Oct 2017).

Q22. Answer d

A standard dose of platelets for prophylactic therapy in adults is approximately one RDPC per 10 kg of body weight, which translates to 4 to 6 units of pooled platelets or 1 apheresis unit (SDPC), both providing approximately 3 to 4×10^{11} platelets. Apheresis platelets have the advantages of limiting the recipient exposure to a single donor which potentially reduces the possibility of infection and alloimmunization; some centers use apheresis platelets exclusively. Leukoreduction removes most of the contaminating white WBC from the platelet transfusion. Platelet irradiation is used to prevent ta-GVHD in which contaminating WBCs attack host tissues and cause serious, even fatal, outcomes in both immunosuppressed and some immunocompetent individuals. Irradiation damages the nuclei of donor lymphocytes in the transfusion so that they cannot proliferate and mount an immune response against the recipient. Platelets are anucleate so their functions are unaffected by irradiation. Platelets express ABO antigens on their surface, as well as HLA class I antigens. They do not express Rh or HLA class II antigens.

Shan Y, Dennis G, Arthur J, Jennifer S (eds.). Clinical and laboratory aspects of platelet transfusion therapy. Available from: https://www.uptodate.com/contents/clinical-and-laboratory-aspects-of-platelet-transfusion-therapy (Accessed 14th Oct 2017).

Q23. Answer b

This patient requires platelet transfusion. However, administrating 'O' platelet to 'A' group patient without knowing titre of anti-A is unacceptable. The titers of anti-A and anti-B is not routinely performed in India.

The plasma 'O' platelet contains both anti-A and anti-B and can result in hemolysis of RBC in the recipient. Thus in any patient volume reduction of plasma or washing of platelet can be performed.

Melanie S, Garratty G (eds.). Transfusion Therapy. Modern blood banking and transfusion practices, Harmening. 6th edition. New Delhi, India: Jaypee Brothers Medical Publishers (P) Ltd.; 2012. p.354-356.

Q24. Answer c

There are no ideal tests for predicting who will bleed spontaneously. Studies of patients with thrombocytopenia suggest that patients can bleed even with platelet counts greater than 50,000/µL. However, bleeding is much more likely at platelet counts less than 5000/µL. The platelet count at which a patient bleed previously can be a good predictor of future bleeding. Petechial bleeding and ecchymoses are generally not thought to be predictive of serious bleeding, whereas mucosal bleeding and epistaxis (so-called 'wet' bleeding) are thought to be predictive. Coexisting inflammation, infection, and fever also increase bleeding risk. The underlying condition responsible for a patient's thrombocytopenia also may help in estimating the bleeding risk. Tests for platelet-dependent hemostasis (i.e. bleeding time, thromboelastography, and other point of care tests) are generally not used to predict bleeding in thrombocytopenic patients.

Shan Y, Dennis G, Arthur J, Jennifer S (eds.). Clinical and laboratory aspects of platelet transfusion therapy. Available from: https://www.uptodate.com/contents/clinical-and-laboratory-aspects-of-platelet-transfusion-therapy (Accessed 14th Oct 2017).

Q25. Answer b

Immediate platelet transfusion is indicated for patients with severe bleeding (e.g. intracranial, gastrointestinal) and a platelet count <30,000/µL. The most common treatment regimens are high-dose dexamethasone, typically administered as 40 mg orally per day for 4 days with no taper, or oral prednisone at 1 mg/kg daily for one to two weeks followed by a gradual taper. Doses for IVIG is 1 g/kg daily for one or two days though 1 g/kg for one day is often sufficient. Alternative dosing can also be used (e.g. 400 mg/kg daily for five days). The usual dose of anti-D is 50 to 75 mcg/kg intravenously. ITP is not a contraindication to the use of myelosuppressive chemotherapy.

James N, Donald M, Lawrence L, Jennifer S (eds.). Immune thrombocytopenia (ITP) in adults: Initial treatment and prognosis. Available from: https://www.uptodate.com/contents/immune-thrombocytopenia-itp-in-adults-initial-treatment-and-prognosis (Accessed 14th Oct 2017).

Q26. Answer b

Platelet irradiation is used to prevent transfusion associated GVHD in which contaminating WBCs attack host tissues and cause serious, even fatal, outcomes in both immunosuppressed and some immunocompetent individuals. Irradiation damages the nuclei of donor lymphocytes in the transfusion, so that they cannot proliferate and mount an immune response against the recipient. Platelets are anucleate, so their functions are unaffected by irradiation, although there may be a slight effect on platelet survival due to membrane damage. Irradiation is not a substitute for leukoreduction because lymphocytes inactivated by irradiation still express human leukocyte antigens (HLA) on their surfaces and can elicit an anti-HLA antibody response from the host. Irradiation is also inadequate to kill pathogens such as bacteria and viruses. Irradiation is used for all Immunosuppressed states secondary to transplant, cytotoxic chemotherapy, congenital immunodeficiency, hematologic malignancies etc.

Shan Y, Dennis G, Arthur J, Jennifer S (eds.). Clinical and laboratory aspects of platelet transfusion therapy. Available from: https://www.uptodate.com/contents/clinical-and-laboratory-aspects-of-platelet-transfusion-therapy (Accessed 14th Oct 2017).

Q27. Answer e

Leukoreduction removes most of the contaminating WBC from platelet transfusion. In some centers leukoreduction is standard practice. In other centers, leukoreduction is used for the following indications:
- Reduction of HLA alloimmunization
- Reduction of CMV transmission
- Reduction of transfusion-associated immunomodulation
- Reduction of lung injury during and after cardiopulmonary bypass
- Reduction of febrile nonhemolytic transfusion reactions (FNHTR)

Leukoreduction is done by passing platelets through a filter that blocks passage of most white blood cells. Apheresis platelets can be leukoreduced during collection, and pooled platelets can be leukoreduced shortly after collection or at bedside before transfusion.

Leukoreduction can reduce the risks of several potential complications of contaminating WBC, but it is not adequate to prevent ta-GVHD because some WBC can pass through the leukoreduction filter. Therefore, irradiation must be used to prevent ta-GVHD.

Arthur J, Steven K, Jennifer S (eds.). Leukoreduction to prevent complications of blood transfusion. Available from: https://www.uptodate.com/contents/leukoreduction-to-prevent-complications-of-blood-transfusion (Accessed 14th Oct 2017).

Q28. Answer b

This patient is having the signs and symptoms of volume overload, pulmonary edema most likely secondary to transfusion. Over and above his raised NT-proBNP is suggestive of TACO, and help differentiating from TRALI. Differentiation from TRALI is very important as diuretics are helpful in this rather than in TRALI. Allergic reaction cannot be ruled out completely but absence of wheezing, erythema, pruritus along with feature of volume overload is favouring TACO. Transfusion-associated dyspnea is a transfusion reaction with acute respiratory distress occurring within 24 hours of cessation of transfusion and/or that do not meet the criteria for other transfusion reactions.

Melanie S, Garratty G, Denise M (eds.). Transfusion Therapy. Modern blood banking and transfusion practices, Harmening. 6th edition. Jaypee Brothers Medical Publishers (P) Ltd. New Delhi, India; 2012;378-380.

Steven K, Daryl J, Arthur J, Scott M, (eds.). Transfusion-related acute lung injury (TRALI). Available from: https://www.uptodate.com/contents/transfusion-related-acute-lung-injury (Accessed 14th Oct 2017).

Q29. Answer b

This patient's respiratory deterioration is showing temporal relationship with transfusion. Transfusion related acute lung injury is a presence of new acute respiratory distress occurring during or within 6 hours after blood product administration, documented by hypoxemia and an abnormal chest radiograph. Though TRALI has been associated with virtually all blood products, high-plasma-volume components such as plasma, apheresis platelet concentrates, and whole blood have been consistently shown to carry the greatest risk per component or per transfusion episode. When a clear temporal relationship to an alternative risk factor for ARDS coexists like here it is sepsis a formal diagnosis of TRALI cannot be made. In these circumstances, 'possible TRALI' or Transfusion-related acute lung injury with other ALI risk factors or more recently endorsed 'transfused ARDS' is the more appropriate diagnosis. Normal CVP is unlikely in volume overload.

Steven K, Daryl J, Arthur J (eds.). Transfusion-related acute lung injury (TRALI). Available from: https://www.uptodate.com/contents/transfusion-related-acute-lung-injury (Accessed 14th Oct 2017).

Q30. Answer a

The increment in platelet count depends on many factors but if all other factors are absent then one unit of whole blood derived random platelets usually increases the platelet count by 5,000/mm³ per square metre.

   Melanie S, Garratty G, Denise M (eds.). Transfusion Therapy. Modern blood banking and transfusion practices, Harmening. Jaypee Brothers Medical Publishers (P) Ltd. New Delhi. 2012. p. 378-380.

K Type Answers

Q1. Answer TFTF

Preoperative RBC transfusions are warranted when prolonged general anesthesia is used or anticipated. For uncomplicated minor procedures in which brief inhalation anesthetic is used (e.g. some dental procedures), transfusion is seldom necessary. The specific method of transfusion, i.e. regular or partial exchange is not as important as the hematologic endpoint. A preoperative HbS of 30% to 40% and hemoglobin concentration in an intermediate range (10 to 12 g/dL) are desirable. Patients with sickle cell trait probably do not even require transfusion before cardiopulmonary bypass. However, prophylactic transfusion may well be appropriate for patients with sickle cell trait who will be undergoing orthopedic surgery requiring prolonged tourniquet application. Whenever there is a prolonged or repeated requirement for transfusion, it is prudent to obtain a full red cell antigen profile (including, e.g. C, E, K, Fya, and Jkb phenotypes) of the recipient before transfusion therapy is initiated. This information will be very useful later if alloimmunization is suspected.

   Sharon B, Simon T, Snyder E, Solheim B, Stowell CP, Strauss R (eds.). Management of Congenital Hemolytic Anemias. Rossi's Principles of Transfusion Medicine. Fourth Edition. West Sussex, UK: Blackwell Publishing Ltd. 2009. p. 459-460.

Q2. Answer TFFT

No medications or solutions other than 0.9% sodium chloride injection, USP, or albumin should be administered with blood components through the same tubing. Solutions containing dextrose alone may cause red cells to swell and lyse. Lactated Ringer's solution or other solutions containing high levels of calcium may overcome the buffering capacity of the citrate anticoagulant in the blood preservative solution and cause clotting of the component.

   Maynard K, Fung M (eds.). Administration of Blood Components. Technical manual.18th ed. Bethesda, United States: AABB; 2014. p.552.

Q3. Answer FTTT

The potential complications of massive transfusion usually defined as the receipt of more than 10 RBC units within 24 hours include metabolic and hemostatic abnormalities, immune hemolysis, and air embolism. Metabolic abnormalities can depress ventricular function. Hypothermia from refrigerated blood, citrate toxicity, and lactic acidosis from under perfusion and tissue ischemia which are often complicated by hyperkalaemia, can contribute to this effect.

   Mazzei C, Popovsky M, KopkoP, Fung M(eds.). Non-infectious Complications of Blood Transfusion. Technical manual.18th ed. Bethesda, United States: AABB. 2014. p. 684-6.

Q4. Answer TTTF

Cryoprecipitate are precipitated proteins of plasma, rich in factor VIII and fibrinogen, obtained from a single unit of fresh frozen plasma. It is rich in factor VIII, von Willebrand factor, fibrinogen (Factor XIII) and fibronectin. Cryoprecipitate contains at least 80 units of anti-hemophilic factor and 150-250 mg of fibrinogen; this product is indicated for hemophilia A, factor XIII deficiency and hypofibrinogenemia. Shelf life at –25°C or colder is for up to 1 year. Must be transfused within 6 hours of thawing.

   Saran RK (ed). Blood Components Preparation and Their Uses. Directorate General of Health Services Ministry of Health & Family Welfare Government of India. 2nd ed. New Delhi: Mehta Offset Pvt. Ltd.; 2003. p. 205-207.

   Clinical Transfusion Practice Guidelines for Medical Interns. Available from http://www.who.int/bloodsafety/transfusion_services/ClinicalTransfusionPracticeGuidelinesforMedicalInternsBangladesh.pdf (Accessed 15th Oct 2017).

Q5. Answer TFTF

FFP is plasma obtained from a single donor either by normal donation or by plasmapheresis and rapidly frozen within 6-8 hours of being collected.
Collection of blood for FFP should follow the following standards:
- Blood should be collected by a clean, single venipuncture.
- Draw of blood should be rapid and constant.
- Total time taken to collect 450 mL of blood should not be more than 8 minutes. It has been shown that the most labile coagulation factors are preserved for 1 year if FFP is kept at -30°C or below. If FFP is not used within one year, it is redesignated as single donor plasma which can be kept further for 4 years at -30°C or below. The FFP should be administered as soon as possible after thawing, and in any event within 24 hours if kept at 2-6°C.

   Saran RK. (ed). Blood Components Preparation and Their Uses. Directorate General of Health Services Ministry of Health & Family Welfare Government of India. 2nd ed. New Delhi: Mehta Offset Pvt. Ltd.; 2003. p. 205-207.

   Clinical Transfusion Practice Guidelines for Medical Interns. Available from: http://www.who.int/bloodsafety/transfusion_services/ClinicalTransfusionPracticeGuidelinesforMedicalInternsBangladesh.pdf (Accessed 15th Oct 2017).

Q6. Answer FTFF

Cryoprecipitate poor plasma is a by-product of cryoprecipitate preparation. It lacks labile clotting factors V and VIII and fibrinogen. It contains adequate levels of the stable clotting factors II, VII, IX and X. It is frozen and stored at -30°C or lower temperature for 5 years. Cryoprecipitate-poor plasma contains 80% of the amount of factor V in FFP and can be used as an alternative to FFP. Indications include:
- In deficiency of stable clotting factors (e.g. coagulopathies due to warfarin drugs)
- Burns
- Therapeutic plasma exchange (especially in patients with Thrombotic Thrombocytopenic Purpura and Hemolytic Uremic Syndrome).

Dose is same as that of FFP.

   Saran RK. (ed). Blood Components Preparation and Their Uses. Directorate General of Health Services Ministry of Health & Family Welfare Government of India. 2nd ed. Mehta Offset Pvt. Ltd. New Delhi; 2003. p. 205-207, 221.

   Arthur J, Steven K, Jennifer S (eds.). Clinical use of plasma components. Available from: https://www.uptodate.com/contents/clinical-use-of-plasma-components (Accessed 14th Oct 2017).

Q7. Answer TTFT

Indications of Fresh Frozen Plasma:
- Active bleeding and multiple coagulation factor deficiencies such as liver diseases, Disseminated Intravascular Coagulation (DIC), coagulopathy in massive transfusion, Thrombotic Thrombocytopenic Purpura or when specific disorder cannot be or has not yet been identified.
- Familial factor V deficiency if concentrated factor V is not available
- Deficiency of factors II, VII, IX and X
- Anti-thrombin III deficiency
- Congenital or acquired coagulation factor deficiency when individual purified factor is not available

Transfusion of FFP is not indicated in:
- Blood volume expansion
- Hypoproteinemia
- Source of immunoglobulins
- When the prothrombin time is < 18 seconds.

   Saran RK. (ed). Blood Components Preparation and Their Uses. Directorate General of Health Services Ministry of Health & Family Welfare Government of India. 2nd ed. New Delhi: Mehta Offset Pvt. Ltd.; 2003. p. 219-221.

Q8. Answer TTTF

Procoagulants that require vitamin K for appropriate carboxylation and normal activity Factors II (prothrombin), VII, IX and X—are called the 'vitamin K-dependent factors.' They have long been known to be separable from plasma by simple chemical means and are known as factor IX complex concentrate or PCC. PCC contains factors II, IX and X and to a varying degree factor VII. Also known as Anti-inhibitor coagulation complex. It is used for the treatment of patients with high titers of antibodies to factor VIII.

Indications:
- Treatment of hemophilia B (Christmas disease)
- To treat prolonged prothrombin time (PT) and patients with high titer of antibodies to factor VIII.
- can be used to rapidly correct the effects of warfarin

   Saran RK. (ed.) Blood Components Preparation and Their Uses. Directorate General of Health Services Ministry of Health & Family Welfare Government of India. 2nd ed. Mehta Offset Pvt. Ltd. New Delhi; 2003. p. 375-378.

   Nester T. Jain S. Poisson J, Fung M (ed.), Grossman B (ed), Hillyer C (ed.) et al. Hemotherapy Decisions and Their Outcomes. Technical Manual. 18th ed. United States; AABB. p. 527.

Q9. Answer TFFF

Platelet can be contaminated either because of inadequate cleaning of venepuncture site or entry of skin plug into collection bag. To prevent this venepuncture site has to be cleaned adequately preferably with methylated spirit/alcohol, 10% povidone-iodine solution (betadine). Collecting initial 5 mL of blood in diversion pouch also reduces the risk of contamination. Platelet product is processed in a closed circuit so, there are lesser chances of contamination because of environmental contamination. Continuous agitation of platelet ensures enough oxygen delivery which helps maintain pH.

   Melanie S, Garratty G (eds.). Transfusion Therapy. Modern blood banking and transfusion practices. 6th edition. Jaypee Brothers Medical Publishers (P) Ltd. New Delhi; 2012. p.15-17.

   Shan Y, Dennis G, Arthur J, Jennifer S (eds.). Clinical and laboratory aspects of platelet transfusion therapy. Available from: https://www.uptodate.com/contents/clinical-and-laboratory-aspects-of-platelet-transfusion-therapy (14th Oct 2017).

Q10. Answer FTTT

The platelet count is below 15,000/μL with bruising; therefore, a platelet transfusion is indicated. Without the platelet transfusion, she would be at increased risk of bleeding from the site of the bone marrow biopsy. Dose of platelet concentrate is, 1 unit of platelet concentrate/10 kg; for an adult of 60-70 kg, 4-6 single donor units containing at least 240 × 109 platelets should raise the platelet count by 20–40 × 109 /L. Increment will be less if there is splenomegaly, disseminated intravascular coagulation or septicemia. Platelet should be preferably leucodepleted to reduce the occurrence of febrile haemolytic transfusion reaction. Typical platelet count thresholds that are used for some common procedures are as follows:
- Neurosurgery or ocular surgery – 100,000/μL
- Most other major surgery – 50,000/μL
- Endoscopic procedures – 50,000/μL for therapeutic procedures; 20,000/μL for low risk diagnostic procedures
- Bronchoscopy with bronchoalveolar lavage (BAL) – 20,000 to 30,000/μL
- Central line placement – 20,000/μL
- Lumbar puncture – 10,000 to 20,000/μL in patients with hematologic malignancies and greater than 40,000 to 50,000 in patients without hematologic malignancies, but lower in patients with immune thrombocytopenia (ITP)
- Epidural anesthesia – 80,000/μL
- Bone marrow aspiration/biopsy – 20,000/μL.

   Melanie S, Garratty G (ed.). Transfusion Therapy. Modern blood banking and transfusion practices. 6th edition. New Delhi, India: Jaypee Brothers Medical Publishers (P) Ltd.; 2012. p.378-380, 354-355.

   Clinical Transfusion Practice Guidelines for Medical Interns. Available from: http://www.who.int/bloodsafety/transfusion_services/ClinicalTransfusionPracticeGuidelinesforMedicalInternsBangladesh.pdf (Accessed 15th Oct 2017).

   Shan Y, Dennis G, Arthur J, Jennifer S(eds.). Clinical and laboratory aspects of platelet transfusion therapy. Available from: https://www.uptodate.com/contents/clinical-and-laboratory-aspects-of-platelet-transfusion-therapy (14th Oct 2017).

Q11. Answer FFFT

Both platelets are stored for 5 days and are suspended in donor plasma. Both products need constant agitation, are stored at room temperature (20-24° C). SDPC has 6 times more platelets. There is multiple blood donor exposure for patient with RDPC since six RDPCs makes one adult dose; while single SDPC is an adult dose.

Melanie S, Garratty G (eds.). Transfusion Therapy. Modern blood banking and transfusion practices. 6th edition. New Delhi, India: Jaypee Brothers Medical Publishers (P) Ltd.; 2012. p.12-17.

Q12. Answer FTFF

Storing platelet at 1°-6°C results in marked reduction in platelet in vivo viability, manifested as reduction in vivo life span, after 18 hours of storage. In 1986, when platelets were stored for 7 days and transfused to patients, reports of septic transfusion reaction were reported due to 50% increase in bacterial contamination. When platelets were stored for 5 days at 24°-27°C, pH of platelet fell below 6.2 and platelet changed their shape from disk to sphere which was irreversible. So, platelet should be stored at 20°-24°C to maintain Ph of 6.2, hence maintain shape and viability.

Melanie S, Garratty G, Denise M (eds.). Transfusion Therapy. Modern blood banking and transfusion practices, Harmening. 6th edition. Jaypee Brothers Medical Publishers (P) Ltd. New Delhi; 2012.p.12-17.

Clinical Transfusion Practice Guidelines for Medical Interns. p 13. Available from http://www.who.int/bloodsafety/transfusion_services/ClinicalTransfusionPracticeGuidelinesforMedicalInternsBangladesh.pdf (Accessed 15th Oct 2017).

Q13. Answer FFFT

Refractoriness to platelet transfusion is defined as a platelet count response significantly less than expected to two or more platelet transfusions. Platelet refractoriness can be diagnosed by CCI. CCI using a 10-minute to 1-hour post-transfusion platelet count can be calculated by formula:

CCI = [PPI × BSA (m^2)] × 10^{11}/ number of platelets transfused

[PPI - post-transfusion platelet increment, BSA- body surface area, CCI- corrected count increment].

Melanie S, Garratty G (eds.). Transfusion Therapy. Modern blood banking and transfusion practices. 6th edition. Jaypee Brothers Medical Publishers (P) Ltd. New Delhi. 2012. p.378-380, 354-355.

Dennis G, Arthur J, Jennifer S (eds). Refractoriness to platelet transfusion therapy. Available from: https://www.uptodate.com/contents/refractoriness-to-platelet-transfusion-therapy (14th Oct 2017).

CHAPTER 19

Medical Law and Ethics

Srinivas Samavedam, Kamal Lashkari

A Type Questions
(One best answer)

1. **A claim of medical negligence is valid only if the claimant can conclusively prove that:**
   a. There was a breach of duty
   b. The doctor had an obligation to the patient to treat him
   c. There was an injury to the patient
   d. All of the above
   e. None of the above

2. **While giving consent, all of the following are ascertained except:**
   a. The person is competent to give consent
   b. He is above 18 years of age
   c. He is capable of paying the bills
   d. He understands the spoken language
   e. He has no impediments to communication

3. **The Bolam test establishes the relationship between:**
   a. Patient and caregiver
   b. Caregiver and Institution
   c. Caregiver and Law
   d. Patient and Institution
   e. Patient and Law

4. **The branch of medicine which brings the medical professional into relationship with Law is:**
   a. IPC
   b. Criminal Procedure Code
   c. Code of Civil Conduct
   d. Medical Jurisprudence
   e. Medical Council Act

5. **An advance decision on not opting for life sustaining therapies is valid even if it is not written and witnessed:**
   a. True
   b. False
   c. There is no validity for advance decision in India
   d. Advance Will is now legal in India
   e. None of the above

6. **In cases of alleged medical negligence, a medical professional is expected to provide:**
   a. Standard of care considered as acceptable by experts in the field
   b. Standard of care considered appropriate by majority of doctors
   c. Standard of care considered as reasonable standard
   d. Standard of care expected by patient or his/her family
   e. Standard of care expected by accreditation agencies

7. **When a patient walks into an outpatient clinic of a physician, his consent is:**
   a. Implicit
   b. Implied
   c. Imposed
   d. Insisted
   e. Incorporated

8. **In the case of 'GOOD SAMARITAN' situation.**
   a. Duty of care concept cannot be invoked
   b. Duty of care concept will apply mandatorily
   c. Duty of care applies only if valid consent is taken

d. Good Samaritan act will protect against subsequent disputes
e. Negligence cannot be alleged if there is a 'GOOD SAMARITAN' situation

9. Vicarious liability applies only if:
   a. The employee is currently employed
   b. The employee is paid for his service
   c. The employee has worked for at least 1 year
   d. Employer employee relationship is established
   e. Employee discontinues his service to the employer

10. Which of the following qualifies for criminal negligence?
    a. Facial nerve injury during parotid surgery
    b. Limb ischemia after IABP insertion
    c. Pneumothorax after Central Line
    d. Skin infection after Burns
    e. Surgery on wrong side

11. Law of confidentiality is:
    a. Arbitrary
    b. Absolute
    c. Ambiguous
    d. Anecdotal
    e. Avoidable

12. As per MCI norms, case records of all patients should be maintained for at least:
    a. 2 years
    b. 7 years
    c. 3 years
    d. Till the death of the patient

13. Record of investigations done on a patient are the property of:
    a. Individual
    b. Institution
    c. Third party payer
    d. All of the above
    e. Government

14. Prescription of drugs has to be written as:
    a. Generics only in BOLD
    b. Generics and Brands in BOLD
    c. Brands in BOLD which the patient is expected to buy to avoid confusion
    d. Generics in BOLD is mandatory; Brands is optional
    e. Brands in BOLD, Generics is optional

15. Fees for a medical professional service should be announced to the patient:
    a. After rendering service
    b. Anytime during the interaction
    c. Should not be announced
    d. Within one day
    e. Prior to rendering service

16. The law binds a physician to treat every patient who seeks his/her service:
    a. True
    b. False
    c. The law does not but MCI rules do
    d. Law does but MCI does not
    e. None of the above

17. A medical practitioner is allowed to advertise all of the following except:
    a. Change of practice address
    b. Starting practice
    c. Felicitation by NGOs
    d. Temporary absence from duty
    e. Additional qualifications

18. Article 21 of the Indian Constitution refers to obligation to:
    a. Provide Legal support
    b. Provide Medical advice
    c. Protect Life
    d. Prevent Medical Negligence
    e. Prevent Malpractice

19. Which of the following acts/laws does not pertain to sale and storage of drugs and safe medication?
    a. Drugs and Cosmetics Rules
    b. Narcotics and Psychotropic Drugs Act
    c. Pharmacy Act
    d. Drugs and Magic Remedies advertisement Act
    e. None of the above

20. Which of the following acts protects the safety of patients, staff and public in a hospital?
    a. Maternity benefits Act
    b. Equal remuneration Act
    c. AERB Safety code 2001
    d. Industrial dispute Act
    e. None of the above

21. All the following statements regarding CLABSI are true *except*:
    a. It is expressed as per 1,000 central line days
    b. If a patient has two central lines on the given day it is taken as two central line days
    c. CLABSI is considered only if 48 hours have elapsed since CVC insertion

d. It is not synonymous with CRBSI
   e. CLABSI criteria is different for HD catheters

22. **Which of the following is NOT an indicator for quality of structure of an ICU?**
   a. Beds per 1,000 population
   b. Intensivist availability
   c. Length of stay in the ICU
   d. Patient nurse ratio
   e. Availability of handwash facility

23. **All of the following are indicators for the quality of processes in an ICU *except*:**
   a. SMR
   b. Bed occupancy rates
   c. Compliance with care bundles
   d. Blood sugar values in target range
   e. Reintubation rates

24. **Hang hygiene compliance is a measure of quality of:**
   a. Structure
   b. Process
   c. Outcome
   d. All of the above
   e. None of the above

25. **Rates of infection acquired in an ICU are a measure of quality in:**
   a. Structure
   b. Process
   c. Outcome
   d. None of the above
   e. All of the above

26. **Presence of an End of Life Pathway is a measure of quality in:**
   a. Structure
   b. Process
   c. Outcome
   d. None of the above
   e. All of the above

27. **SMR is defined as:**
   a. Observed mortality/predicted mortality
   b. Predicted mortality/observed mortality
   c. Observed mortality – predicted mortality/ crude mortality
   d. Observed mortality – predicted mortality/ predicted mortality
   e. None of the above

28. **Ideal SMR should be:**
   a. < 1
   b. 1
   c. 1

   d. None of the above
   e. Depends on national average

29. **Quality of nutritional support is calculated and based on percentage of eligible patients initiated on enteral nutrition within:**
   a. 6 hours of ICU admission
   b. 12 hours of ICU admission
   c. 24 hours of ICU admission
   d. 48 hours of ICU admission
   e. During course of hospitalization

30. **Having a daily goal sheet for documentation of nutrition is a measure of quality in:**
   a. Structure
   b. Process
   c. Both
   d. None
   e. It is not a measure of quality

31. **Readmission within 48 hours of ICU discharge is a measure of quality in:**
   a. Process
   b. Outcome
   c. Both
   d. None

32. **Which of the following is a fundamental marker of quality in cardiac care?**
   a. Door-to-balloon time
   b. Therapeutic hypothermia after cardiac arrest
   c. Door-to-angioplasty time
   d. Beta blocker administration in ACS
   e. ECG interpretation by qualified cardiologist

33. **Which of the following is not a fundamental marker of infection control/surveillance in ICU?**
   a. Early antibiotic therapy in sepsis
   b. CLABSI rate
   c. CAUTI rate
   d. VAP rate
   e. SSI rate

34. **Survival of patients is:**
   a. Overestimated by physicians
   b. Underestimated by physicians
   c. Accurately estimated by physicians
   d. Cannot be done by physicians
   e. Is not in the Physicians domain

35. **Which of the following is not a reason for varied EOL policies in different countries?**
   a. Differences in religion
   b. Differences in legislation

c. Differences in organization of ICU
d. None of the above
e. All of the above

36. In ABCD of 'dying with dignity' D stands for:
   a. Disability
   b. De-escalation
   c. Dialogue
   d. Dementia
   e. Dispute

37. The right to life and personal liberty is guaranteed under Article -- of the Constitution:
   a. 34
   b. 21
   c. 370
   d. 56
   e. 24

38. Administration of a lethal drug by a physician as an act of mercy is called:
   a. Euthanasia
   b. Terminal treatment
   c. Palliative care
   d. None of the above
   e. Allowing natural death

39. Fiduciary obligation to always act in the best interests of the patient relates to:
   a. Beneficence
   b. Non-malfeasance
   c. Social justice
   d. None of the above
   e. All of the above

40. The principal of Primum non nocere relates to:
   a. Beneficence
   b. Non-malfeasance
   c. Social justice
   d. Patient rights
   e. None of the above

41. The situation when adequate analgesia and sedation which unintentionally shortens the dying process relates:
   a. Doctrine of non-malfeasance
   b. Doctrine of double effect
   c. Doctrine of beneficence
   d. All of the above
   e. None of the above

42. Allocating resources appropriate to the condition of the patient relates to:
   a. Principle of non-malfeasance
   b. Principle of beneficence
   c. Principle of double effect
   d. Principle of social justice
   e. Principle of equality

43. Which of the following is not a goal of communication?
   a. Establishing consensus among caregivers
   b. Providing accurate information to the family
   c. Keeping the administration and management satisfied
   d. Ensuring transparency and accountability
   e. Addressing concerns about the EOL process that may arise

44. In the SOLER acronym for nonverbal communication, R stands for:
   a. Rational thinking
   b. Relaxed posture
   c. Reconciliation
   d. Return queries
   e. Rapid decision

45. During communication with family, a professional who conveys information fast and with no warning and understanding is labeled as:
   a. The inexperienced messenger
   b. The emotionally burdened expert
   c. The rough and ready expert
   d. The empathic professional
   e. The experienced counselor

46. A doctor who comes across as not too involved in the discussion of EOL issues is labeled as:
   a. The inexperienced messenger
   b. The emotionally burdened expert
   c. The rough and ready expert
   d. The experienced counselor
   e. The empathic professional

47. Which of the following is NOT a virtue of a Rough and Ready medical professional?
   a. Delivers message quick and fast
   b. Message is clear
   c. Body language is terse
   d. Wants to finish quickly
   e. Listens long enough

48. A professional who is unable to pick up the verbal and nonverbal cues of the family is labeled:
   a. Rough and ready
   b. Inexperienced messenger

c. Benevolent tactless
   d. Distanced
   e. Philosophical

49. **Which of the following statements regarding a distanced expert is FALSE?**
   a. Gives precise information
   b. Appears calm
   c. Is emotionally involved
   d. Perceived by family as disinterested
   e. All of the above

50. **A medical professional who can deliver the message with right mix of balance and competence is labeled:**
   a. Empathic professional
   b. Efficient professional
   c. Emotional professional
   d. Effective professional
   e. Educated professional

51. **In the SPIKES approach to patient centred communication, 'I' stands for Invitation. This means:**
   a. Invitation to patient to be part of the discussion
   b. Invitation to family members to visit the patient
   c. Invitation to patient and family to attend other similar counseling
   d. Confirming whether patient wishes to receive information regarding diagnosis and prognosis
   e. Invitation to seek second opinion

52. **Which of the following is NOT a patient/family factor during conflict at EOLD?**
   a. Level of medical education
   b. Socioeconomic status
   c. Ethnicity and religion
   d. Emotional stress
   e. Acceptance of the disease

53. **Which of the following is NOT a physician factor during conflict at EOLD?**
   a. Communication skills
   b. ICU culture
   c. Grounding in medical ethics
   d. Type of hospital
   e. Medical knowledge

54. **Treatment that has less than 1% chance of succeeding is labeled:**
   a. Quantitative futility
   b. Lethal condition futility
   c. Qualitative futility
   d. Imminent demise futility
   e. Economic futility

55. **An intervention that will not change the probability of dying of a patient is:**
   a. Quantitative futility
   b. Lethal condition futility
   c. Qualitative futility
   d. Imminent demise futility
   e. Clinical futility

K Type Questions
[Marked True (T)/False (F)]

1. **The following Acts governs medico-legal aspects:**
   a. Consumer Protection Act
   b. NBE rules for PG training
   c. Law of Torts
   d. Ethical guidelines for Biomedical research on Human Subjects
   e. Fundamental principles of state policy

2. **The following are the statements regarding reporting obligations of a hospital:**
   a. The MTP reports have to be filed daily
   b. Communicable diseases have to be reported monthly
   c. Needle stick injuries have to be reported monthly
   d. Radiation Exposure badges (TLD) have to be renewed quarterly
   e. SMR has to be reported monthly

3. **Following statements regarding diagnosis of death are true:**
   a. CPR is synonymous with death
   b. No cardiac activity with intact brain activity is synonymous with death
   c. Brainstem death is synonymous with death
   d. No brain activity with brainstem activity is synonymous with death
   e. Cardiac death is definition of death

4. **The following can give consent for organ donation:**
   a. The donor prior to death
   b. The next of kin prior to death
   c. The next of kin after death
   d. The treating physician after death
   e. Hospital Panel after death

5. Regarding live related organ donation:
   a. It is legal in India
   b. It is directed at a specific individual
   c. The blood relative can take money for the organ donated
   d. It need not be directed at a specific individual
   e. It has to be ratified by a state appointed panel

6. Regarding direct liability of a hospital:
   a. Cleanliness of the hospital is a direct liability
   b. Providing equipped ambulance is a direct liability
   c. Providing safe equipment is a direct liability
   d. Employing competent professionals is a direct liability
   e. Providing adequate lab facilities is a direct liability

7. State True or False for the following statements:
   a. Head end elevation is a fundamental marker of quality of respiratory care
   b. Initiation of DVT prophylaxis is a fundamental marker of quality of respiratory care
   c. HME filter change every 48 hours is a fundamental marker of quality of respiratory care
   d. Chlorhexidine mouthwash everyday is a fundamental marker of quality of respiratory care
   e. Initiation of Stress Ulcer Prophylaxis is a fundamental marker of quality of respiratory care

8. Regarding Aspirin usage in ACS:
   a. Its usage is considered as a marker of quality
   b. Time limit for initiation of therapy is 24 hours
   c. Denominator is no of patients dying of ACS
   d. It is a marker of outcomes
   e. It is a marker of process

9. Urgent invasive strategy for NSTEMI is:
   a. Not a quality indicator
   b. It is applied only if complications occur
   c. It is an outcome indicator
   d. It is a process indicator
   e. Expected compliance is 100%

10. Door to Needle time:
    a. Applies only to patients admitted in ER
    b. Applies to percutaneous interventions also
    c. Denominator is hospital discharge
    d. Denominator is number of ACS admissions
    e. It is a marker of process quality

11. Regarding quality indicators among patients undergoing heart surgery:
    a. Number of re-explorations is a marker
    b. Prolonged mechanical ventilation is a marker
    c. Postoperative renal failure is not a marker
    d. Perioperative MI is not a marker
    e. Perioperative transfusion is a marker

12. Quality of mechanical ventilation for respiratory failure includes:
    a. Incidence of barotrauma is an indicator
    b. Minimum duration of ventilation needed is 48 hours
    c. Includes line related pneumothorax
    d. Accepted standard is < 3%
    e. Includes post-extubation stridor

13. Quality of Prone ventilation for ARDS is:
    a. Is a quality indicator
    b. Accidental extubation is a marker
    c. ET tube block is a marker
    d. Decubitus ulcers are markers
    e. Deterioration is a marker

14. Regarding unplanned extubation:
    a. Self extubation is not included
    b. Denominator is the number of intubated patients
    c. Standard is 20 per 1,000 ventilator days
    d. It is a marker of processes
    e. It is a marker of outcomes

15. Examination of all severe trauma patients by intensivists:
    a. Is a quality marker
    b. Denominator is the total number of patients with severe trauma in hospital
    c. It is a process marker
    d. Applies only to trauma centers
    e. Accepted standard is 95%

16. Critical illness polyneuropathy incidence is considered as a marker of quality in ICU:
    a. It reflects the safety environment in the ICU
    b. Duration of ICU stay is atleast 72 hours
    c. It is an outcome parameter
    d. It has diagnosis based rates
    e. Accepted standard is < 70%

17. Incidence of VAP is an indicator of quality in ICU:
    a. Applied to Non-Invasive Ventilation also
    b. Duration cut-off is atleast 48 hours

c. It is a process indicator
d. Accepted standard is 20 per 1000 ventilator days
e. Applies to outpatient care also

18. **Antimicrobial therapy usage is an marker of quality:**
    a. Empirical antibiotic therapy is accepted for 48 hours
    b. Incorrect dose is one of the markers
    c. Penetration of antibiotics into the probable source is a factor
    d. Accepted default rate is 10%
    e. Defined daily dosage is one of the markers

19. **Quality markers for parenteral nutrition in ICU:**
    a. Blood glucose for hyperglycemia random value cut-off is 110 mg/dL
    b. Bilirubin is not a marker
    c. Hyperglycemia rate should be < 10%
    d. Liver dysfunction rate should be < 25%
    e. Nutrition is not part of quality assessment

20. **Quality of enteral nutrition delivery is monitored with:**
    a. Feeding tube position
    b. Patient position
    c. Daily electrolytes
    d. Monitoring feed tolerance
    e. Achieving nutritional targets in defined time

21. **Regarding analgesia and sedation:**
    a. At least 80% of patients should have interruption of sedation
    b. At least 80% of nonventilated patients should have pain assessment
    c. At least 80% of ventilated patients should have pain assessment
    d. Neuromuscular blockade should be justified in at least 80% patients
    e. Analgesia and sedation monitoring are optional parameters

22. **Regarding Defined Daily Dosage:**
    a. It is the assumed average maintenance dose per day
    b. It is used for non-antibiotics also
    c. The concept is based on monotherapy
    d. It applies to topical agents also
    e. It is the same as duration of therapy

23. **Consider the following:**
    a. As soon as a decision is taken on inappropriateness of therapy, each member of the team counsels the family individually
    b. Pulse oximetry is an essential monitoring during EOL process
    c. Pain relief is an essential part of EOL process
    d. Allow natural death is an accepted concept in India
    e. Involvement of a palliative care team is considered as a failure on part of the treating team

24. **Consider the following:**
    a. Number of unplanned extubations per 100 ventilator days is a quality indicator for outcome
    b. Ventilator circuit change at 7 days is a fundamental indicator of quality
    c. Inappropriate transfusion of packed red cells is a fundamental marker of quality
    d. Survey about perceived quality of care at ICU discharge is a fundamental measure of quality
    e. Scientific publications from the department of critical care is a quality marker for the ICU

25. **Consider the following:**
    a. Absence of a clear EOL policy leads to increased incidence of burnout among clinicians
    b. The difference between palliative care and EOL care is that palliative care extends to the family beyond the death of the patient
    c. The ideal process of End of Life Care is a single step process
    d. It is unlawful to document discussions involving personal issues
    e. There is no guidelines to address futile care in India

ANSWERS

A Type Answers

Q1. Answer d

A claim of medical negligence should have some basic strength. The first is whether the doctor had an obligation to treat the patient by virtue of an implied consent. This would mean a patient seeks an appointment for or walks in for a consultation. Once this obligation is satisfied the doctor is expected to fulfil it without a breach. If this breach of obligation results in an injury to the patient, a claim of medical negligence will be valid. This claim of medical negligence can be filed either with the consumer forum or as a criminal negligence.

Joga Rao SV. Medical Negligence liability under the Consumer Protection Act: A review of Judicial Perspective. Indian journal of Urology. 2009;25(3):361-71.

Q2. Answer c

When consent is sought, it has to be ensured that the procedure, its implications and complications are understood by the patient or by his surrogate representative in totality. Therefore, the person giving consent has to be mentally capable and mature to understand and consent for a procedure. It implies that a child younger than 18 years of age cannot consent for himself or for his kin. It is also essential that the details which are discussed are understood by the person consenting. Therefore, such discussions and documentation should be in the spoken language of the person who is giving the consent. The person who is consenting should also have no impediments to listening, comprehending and reacting to the information provided. Financial obligations and abilities are not the part of the consent process.

Joga Rao SV. Medical Negligence liability under the Consumer Protection Act: A review of Judicial Perspective. Indian journal of Urology. 2009;25(3)361-71.

Q3. Answer a

The Bolam test is based a landmark judgement with reference to medical negligence. It is based on a judgement passed in 1957 in a dispute between Bolam vs. Frien Hospital Management. The Bolam principle is that 'the test is the standard of the ordinary skilled man exercising and professing to have those specials skills. A man need not possess the highest expert skill, it is well established law that it is sufficient if he exercises the ordinary skill of an ordinary competent man exercising' that particular art (a healthcare professional) is not guilty of negligence if he has 'acted in accordance with a practice accepted as proper by a responsible body of medical man skilled in the particular act'. Whenever a claim of negligence is made against a medical professional, the Bolam test is applied. The question that has to be answered is 'Did the professional show minimum expected skills related to the speciality which he claims to specialize in?' Claim of negligence is strong if the professional fails the Bolam test.

Brazier M. Medicine, Patients and the Law. Third Edition, Harmondsworth: Penguin Books. 2003.

Q4. Answer d

Medical Jurisprudence is the branch of medicine which brings the profession into relationship with Law. It is sometimes referred as Forensic Medicine, but Jurisprudence has a wider cover. IPC and CPC are statutes which decide the method of investigation and the quantum of punishment for a crime irrespective of who commits it. Code of civil conduct also applies to all members of the civil society. The Medical Council Act is a set of rules and regulations for the behavior and conduct of the medical professionals. Breach of this act also comes under the purview of Medical Jurisprudence

Q5. Answer b

An advanced directive for not opting life sustaining therapies is valid in India only if it is written down and witnessed by at least two individuals who are not next of kin nor beneficiaries of the demise of the person executing the directive. But an advance will although proposed is yet to become legal in India.

Bhat A practitioner guide to contemporary issues. Reflections on Medical Law and Ethics in India. 2016.

Q6. Answer c

When an allegation of Medical Negligence is investigated, the Bolam principle is applied. Accordingly a medical professional is expected to show a reasonable standard of skill and expertise that appears reasonable for the speciality being practised by the professional. A professional is not expected to possess extraordinary skills or exercise care which is the best in the speciality show. Similarly, the care shown by majority of doctors is also not a factor used to judge allegations of negligence. Family expectations, although expected are not criteria to judge the genuineness of a negligence claim.

> THE CONSUMER PROTECTION ACT,1986 & RULES, 1987.

Q7. Answer b

Consent in the context of Medical Law is governed by the Law of Torts and the Article 21 of the Indian Constitution. When a patient walks into the outpatient clinic of a physician, having taken an appointment, his consent for being examined and evaluated by the physician is implied in the act of taking an appointment. However, this consent does not extend to any invasive examinations or procedures which the physician may need to do. A new consent has to be sought (verbal or written) and properly documented for carrying out the invasive tests. Failure to seek a new consent for invasive examinations and procedures amounts to breach of privacy of the patient.

> Nurenberg code, Law of Torts,

Q8. Answer b

A medical professional is considered to behaved as a 'good samaritan' if he attends to a victim of medical emergency with an intention of doing good, even though there was no implied consent. However, in doing so, the professional is expected to show reasonable skill and knowledge and follow the principle of 'primum non nocere'. Duty of care will be invoked and no consent is needed for acting as a good samaritan. Acting as a good samaritan cannot be used as an excuse for acts of negligence.

> Law of Torts.

Q9. Answer d

Vicarious liability refers to the responsibility of the mentor to the acts of commission and omission of the mentoree. It also refers to the responsibility of the employer to the actions of the employee. For this liability to be established, the relationship between the employer and employee has to be formally established in the form of a contract, agreement or job description.

> Pandit MS, Pandit S. Medical negligence: Coverage of the profession, duties, ethics, case law, and enlightened defense - A legal perspective. Indian J Urol. 2009;25(3):372-78.

Q10. Answer e

The law pertaining to criminal negligence warrants the demonstration of harm and an intention to do harm. Procedural complications like facial nerve injury and Limb ischemia are expected complications. Pneumothorax after a central line is also a known complication. However, operating on the wrong side reflects a sense of complacency and inattention to the patient's actual problem. It is liable to be treated as criminal negligence.

> Naveen S, Kumar PM. Doctor and Criminal Negligence. J Indian Med Assoc. 2011;109(11):823-5.

Q11. Answer b

The law of confidentiality in medicine applies to the disclosure of information about the patients disease and its implications to parties other than the patient himself or herself. Irrespective of how grave the situation is, the patient should be the first to receive information about his disease, if he is capable of comprehending the information. All others are expected to be informed after the consent of the patient. In this regard the Law of confidentiality is deemed to be absolute.

> Watwe JM. Disclosure of confidential medical information. Issues Med Ethics. 2016;6(2):56.

Q12. Answer c

Maintenance of medical records is also governed by the law. Specific situations warrant maintenance of the records for specific periods of time. For all records, the minimum duration of preservation is 3 years. However, for medico-legal cases which are not under litigation for 7 years preservation period is recommended. Records of those cases which are under investigation and sub judice will be preserved until cleared by the court of Law.

Singh H, Vij K, et al. Maintenance of records....... how vital? J Punjab Acad Forensic Med Toxicol. 2012;12(2).

Q13. Answer a

The law pertaining to the maintenance of records clearly states that all documents pertaining to the investigation and treatment of a patient, remain the property of the patient and patient alone. However, in certain situations like insurance claims and medico legal problems, relevant agencies can request the hospital or health care facility to provide a separate set of records for the purpose of investigation or claim settlement. At no point, however, the patient or his kin can be denied to have the possession of the original records.

Singh H, Vij K, et al. Maintenance of records....... how vital? J Punjab Acad Forensic Med Toxicol. 2012;12(2).

Q14. Answer d

The Drugs and Cosmetics Act as well as the Medical Council Act describe the principles of writing a medical prescription. Writing the generic name of drugs (pharmacological name) is mandatory. The same has to be transcribed in Bold using an indelible ink with dose, frequency and special instructions. Commonly expected side effects are also expected to be written. The MCI act allows a prescription to include a brand name as an optional item. All the prescriptions have to be signed by the prescribing professional along with the registration number with the medical council.

Q15. Answer a

According to the drugs and cosmetics rules, fees for rendering service are secondary to delivery of the service. Although the hospital can announce and display tariffs and fees for common procedures, the professional should disclose the fees after ensuring the patient has been attended to and his concerns addressed.

The drug and cosmetics rules (Amendment 2005) 1945.

Q16. Answer b

The Medical Council Act defines ethical conduct. Once a doctor agrees to see a patient and starts interaction, the law of Torts is active, and the professional is bound to deliver safe and prompt service. However, the doctor is not bound by law to offer his service to every person who approached him for help. The professional is entitled to refuse to see a patient for the first time. However, this does not apply to review visits, postoperative visits, complications arising from previous interactions or in emergency situations.

Indian medical council (professional conduct, etiquette and ethics) regulations, 2002.

Q17. Answer c

The Medical Council Act describes the flexibility of spreading word about the availability and skills of a medical professional. When a professional starts a practice or facility, he is entitled to let the community know about his location and availability. Similarly, if the professional changes the address of his practice, he is entitled to let his clients as well as public know. When a medical professional acquires additional qualifications or acquires new competencies, he is entitled to let the community know of this progress. Similarly, the professional can also use media of communication to advice his patients and the community about non-availability. However, displaying information about being felicitated or honored by agencies and groups is deemed to be advertisement and is not permitted under the MCI act.

Indian medical council (professional conduct, etiquette and ethics) regulations, 2002.

Q18. Answer d

Article 21 of the constitution defines the right to life for every citizen. With reference to medical law, every patient has a right to live and it is the duty of every medical professional to uphold that right. In addition, the implications of Article 21 extend to the realm of EOL discussions and withdrawal of support. Right to dignified living is an integral part of Article 21 and needs to be respected when dealing with futility of care.

Article 21 of the Constitution of India – Right to Life and Personal Liberty.

Q19. Answer d

Regulation of sale and storage of drugs and administering medications safely is governed by several laws. The drugs and cosmetics rules act deals with the licensing of pharmacies and dispensing of drugs. The narcotics and psychotropic drugs act defines drug, scheduled drugs and the precautions to be followed in dispensing and storage of such drugs. These acts are in corollary to the Pharmacy Act. The Drugs and Magic remedies advertisement act does not deal with the sale and storage or safe medication of drugs.

The Drugs and Magic Remedies (Objectionable Advertisements) Act, 1954.

Q20. Answer b

Safety of patients, employees, visitors and professionals working in a hospital are addressed in several laws. One of the important codes is related to the exposure to radiation in a hospital. This is covered in the AERB Safety code, 2001. The rest of the acts mentioned deal with the privileges and work benefits of employees and professionals working in the hospital.

AERB safety code no. AERB/SC/Med -2 (REV), 2001.

Q21. Answer b

Infections acquired by patients who have a central venous cannula are measured by either Central Line-Associated Bloodstream Infections (CLABSI) rated or Catheter-Related Bloodstream Infection (CRBSI) rates. Although numerator and denominator in both the definitions are essentially the same, the method of capturing infection is different between the two. While CLABSI uses a clinical correlation of fever in a patient with a central line that resolves on line removal, CRBSI depends on differential time to positivity (DTTP) to identify infections. Both are expressed in terms of 1000 catheter days. Generally a catheter has to be in situ for at least 48 hours for the definitions to be applied. Criteria are the same for all central venous catheters. However, if a patient has two central lines on a given day, the number of central line days is still taken as one.

Ray B, Samaddar P, et al. Quality indicators for ICU: ISCCM guidelines for ICUs in India; Indian J Crit Care Med. 2009;13(4): 173-206.

Quality Indicators in Critically Ill Patients – Update 2011. http://www.semicyuc.org/temas/calidad/indicadores-de-calidad

Q22. Answer c

Structure of an ICU has a lot of influence on the outcome of critically ill patients. Availability of ICU beds for a fixed number of population is a broad indicator of quality. Similarly, staffing of the designated units and the ratio of nurses to patients are also markers of structure of an ICU. The results of structure and processes influence the outcome of patients. Length of stay is one of the simplest and commonly used marker of outcomes in an ICU.

Ray B, Samaddar DP, et al. Quality indicators for ICU: ISCCM guidelines for ICUs in India; Indian J Crit Care Med. 2009; 13(4):173-206.

Quality Indicators in Critically Ill Patients – Update 2011 http://www.semicyuc.org/temas/calidad/indicadores-de-calidad

Q23. Answer a

Quality indicators are directed at measuring the effect of structure, process and outcomes. Bed occupancy rates are related to the process of admission and adherence to admission criteria. Similarly, compliance with the care bundle, glycemic control policies and assessment for extubation, all are related to processes being followed in the ICU. However, SMR is a marker of outcome that is obtained by comparison of observed with predicted mortality and is a marker of outcomes in the ICU.

Ray B, Samaddar DP, et al. Quality indicators for ICU: ISCCM guidelines for ICUs in India; Indian J Crit Care Med. 2009; 13(4):173-206.

Quality Indicators in Critically Ill Patients – Update 2011. http://www.semicyuc.org/temas/calidad/indicadores-de-calidad

Q24. Answer b

Hand hygiene is an essential component of most Infection control programs. Education and training related to hand hygiene and compliance rates are the markers of the infection control processes in the hospital in general and ICU in particular.

> Ray B, Samaddar DP, et al. Quality indicators for ICU: ISCCM guidelines for ICUs in India; Indian J Crit Care Med. 2009; 13(4):173-206.
>
> Quality Indicators in Critically Ill Patients – Update 2011. http://www.semicyuc.org/temas/calidad/indicadores-de-calidad

Q25. Answer c

Infections acquired by patients while being hospitalized occur due to breach of certain practices in the delivery of health care. This has an association with both clinical outcomes like morbidity and administrative outcomes like length of stay in the hospital. All rates of infection therefore represent markers of quality of outcomes among hospitalized patients.

> Ray B, Samaddar DP, et al. Quality indicators for ICU: ISCCM guidelines for ICUs in India; Indian J Crit Care Med. 2009; 13(4):173-206.
>
> Quality Indicators in Critically Ill Patients – Update 2011. http://www.semicyuc.org/temas/calidad/indicadores-de-calidad

Q26. Answer b

Most patients are admitted to the hospital in anticipation of definitive treatment. However, in certain situations and conditions, the gravity of situation might necessitate invoking discussion on End Of Life (EOL) Issues. All hospitals should have a process in place to initiate, analyse, communicate, execute and document EOL discussions.

> Ray B, Samaddar DP, et al. Quality indicators for ICU: ISCCM guidelines for ICUs in India; Indian J Crit Care Med. 2009;13(4): 173-206.
>
> Quality Indicators in Critically Ill Patients – Update 2011. http://www.semicyuc.org/temas/calidad/indicadores-de-calidad

Q27. Answer a

Standardized mortality ratio is a marker of quality of ICU and represents the difference which the care delivered has made to the severity of the underlying disease. In effective intensive care units, the observed mortality tends to be lower than the predicted mortality. The predicted mortality is derived from various scoring systems which take into account the disease severity with / without chronic problems. SMR is obtained as a ration of observed mortality to predicted mortality. Good units tend to have an SMR of < 1

> Ray B, Samaddar B P et al Quality indicators for ICU: ISCCM guidelines for ICUs in India; Indian J Crit Care Med. 2009 Oct-Dec; 13(4):173-206.
>
> Quality Indicators in Critically Ill Patients – Update 2011 http://www.semicyuc.org/temas/calidad/indicadores-de-calidad

Q28. Answer a

Ref to explanation of Q27.

Q29. Answer d

Enteral nutrition is the mainstay of achieving nutritional targets in the ICU. Immediate initiation and establishment of target nutrition may not be possible soon after ICU admission. It is expected that atleast 24 hours may be needed to stabilize the hemodynamic and metabolic status of an ICU patient. However, initiation of enteral feed later than 48 hours of ICU admission reflects on a suboptimal quality of intensive care.

> Ray B, Samaddar DP, et al Quality indicators for ICU: ISCCM guidelines for ICUs in India; Indian J Crit Care Med. 2009;13(4): 173-206.
>
> Quality Indicators in Critically Ill Patients – Update 2011. http://www.semicyuc.org/temas/calidad/indicadores-de-calidad

Q30. Answer c

Nutrition in the ICU is a specialized therapeutic intervention, which has a bearing on the length of stay of the patient in the ICU as well as in the hospital. Proper planning and execution of nutrition strategy needs a daily assessment of issues and setting of goals and targets. Having a daily goal sheet for documentation of the targets and the means to achieve the targets reflects the processes in place and impacts the outcome of patients in the ICU.

> Ray B, Samaddar DP, et al Quality indicators for ICU: ISCCM guidelines for ICUs in India; Indian J Crit Care Med. 2009;13(4): 173-206.
>
> Quality Indicators in Critically Ill Patients – Update 2011. http://www.semicyuc.org/temas/calidad/indicadores-de-calidad

Q31. Answer c

ICU discharge is an activity which is linked to the assessment of the patient as well as to the care that is provided outside the ICU. Inappropriate discharge from ICU resulting in readmission is associated with significant morbidity and sometimes mortality. Therefore, readmission to the ICU within 48 hours of discharge for the same indication as what necessitated the ICU admission in the first instance reflects both the processes and outcomes associated with ICU discharge.

> Ray B, Samaddar DP, et al Quality indicators for ICU: ISCCM guidelines for ICUs in India; Indian J Crit Care Med. 2009;13(4): 173-206.
>
> Quality Indicators in Critically Ill Patients – Update 2011. http://www.semicyuc.org/temas/calidad/indicadores-de-calidad

Q32. Answer b

Quality assessment for patients admitted for cardiac care includes attention to safety, diagnosis and appropriate therapy. For patients admitted to the ICU with ACS, door to needle time is an essential aspect of care irrespective of the modality of revascularization. ECG interpretation should be done by a professional trained in its interpretation, but not necessarily a cardiologist. Beta blocker is not a mandatory prescription and has to be tailored to patient's clinical condition. Some of these markers may be optional markers of quality but not fundamental markers. However, initiation of targeted temperature management is an essential and fundamental marker to be captured for all patients being managed after a cardiac arrest.

> Quality Indicators in Critically Ill Patients – Update 2011. http://www.semicyuc.org/temas/calidad/indicadores-de-calidad

Q33. Answer c

Most infections acquired in the ICU need to be captured, analyzed and compared with local and international benchmarks. Infections related to the process of ventilation, venous cannulation and surgery are essential components of most of the quality assurance programs. Initiation of antibiotics during the golden period is increasingly being seen as a marker of quality. CAUTI rates are not easy to obtain because of the ambiguity in the diagnosis and criteria for reporting.

> Quality Indicators in Critically Ill Patients – Update 2011. http://www.semicyuc.org/temas/calidad/indicadores-de-calidad.

Q34. Answer a

Patients requiring hospitalization need to be triaged and assessed for the severity of the disease and the effectiveness of the therapy. This is increasingly relevant for patients admitted to the High Intensity care areas. Several scoring systems and predictors are in use which help the physicians to assess the severity of the patients' disease and their survival. None of them is absolute and can predict survival with near perfection. A combination of clinical judgement and scoring systems comes closest to determining the survival of patients. However, despite all this the ability of Physicians in estimating the survival of patients tends to lean towards overestimation in a large number of situations.

> Myatra SN, Salins N, et al End-of-life care policy: An integrated care plan for the dying; A Joint Position Statement of the Indian Society of Critical Care Medicine (ISCCM) and the Indian Association of Palliative Care (IAPC): Indian Journal of Critical Care Medicine. 2014;18(9).
>
> Mani RK. Constitutional and legal protection for life support limitation in India. Indian J Palliat Care. 2015;21(3):258-61.

Q35. Answer e

EOL policies are increasingly being seen as essential aspects of quality of intensive care. In addition, awareness about the methods involved in EOL discussions are incorporated in most curricula of ICU training. The level of educational qualification of the individual and his/her personalities determine the varied policies of EOL in different countries.

> Karnik S, Karnekar A; Ethical issues surrounding end of life care – a narrative review. Healthcare (Basel). 2016;(2)4Pii. 24.

Q36. Answer c

Dying with dignity is the fundamental right of an individual. Medical professionals dealing with death have to ensure that this right is preserved and protected. Attitude, Behavior, Compassion and Dialogue are the ABCDs of ensuring dignified death. Dialogue is all about enquiring the values which are very important for the patient. Getting to know the stakeholders in the EOL decision is also a part of the Dialogue.

> Myatra SN, Salins N, et al. End-of-life care policy: An integrated care plan for the dying; A Joint Position Statement of the Indian Society of Critical Care Medicine (ISCCM) and the Indian Association of Palliative Care (IAPC). Indian Journal of Critical Care Medicine. 2014;18(9):615-35.
>
> Rocker G, Cook D. Dying with dignity in the intensive care unit. N Engl J Med. 2014;370(26):2506-14.

Q37. Answer b

Article 21 deals with the right to life and privacy of every individual in the country. Its implications for the medical profession are many. No patient should be denied access to treatment for a condition that can endanger his life. Any information shared between the patient and the caregiver has to be treated as confidential. The right to accept or refuse the treatment offered is also protected under this article of the constitution.

Q38. Answer a

Euthanasia - literally means good death. Two types of Euthanasia are recognized. Passive and Active. Administration of drugs or therapy directly resulting the termination of life is active euthanasia. This does not have legal sanctity in India. The withdrawal of certain modalities of life sustaining treatment in patients in persistent vegetative state is passive euthanasia. This process has some legal validity in India dealt with in the 196TH report of the Law Commission of India.

> Mani RK. Constitutional and legal protection for life support limitation in India. Indian J Palliat Care. 2015;21(3):258-61.

Q39. Answer a

The principle of Non-malfeasance comes from the doctrine of 'first of all do no harm'. This stems from the principle of Primum non nocere – first do no harm. This has different implications while dealing with an EOL situation. The principle of Beneficence represents the fiduciary obligation to act always in patient's best interests. The doctrine (or principle) of double effect explains a situation of an action taken in the best interest of the patient but results in harm to the patient.

> Myatra SN, Salins N et al. End-of-life care policy: An integrated care plan for the dying; A Joint Position Statement of the Indian Society of Critical Care Medicine (ISCCM) and the Indian Association of Palliative Care (IAPC) Indian Journal of Critical Care Medicine September 2014 Vol 18 Issue 9.

Q40. Answer b

Ref to Explanation of Q39.

Q41. Answer b

Ref to Explanation of Q39.

Q42. Answer d

Ref to Explanation of Q39.

Q43. Answer c

Communication in a healthcare setting is an important tool for providing quality patient care and improving patient satisfaction. Medical professionals should be able to convey their thought process to satisfy the patients' and families' queries. Effective communication is targeted to patients and their loved ones satisfaction, establishing consensus among caregivers, providing accurate information to the family, ensuring transparency and accountability and addressing concerns about the EOL process that may arise etc. Keeping the administration and management satisfied is not the primary goal in this process.

> Myatra SN, Salins N et al. End-of-life care policy: An integrated care plan for the dying; A Joint Position Statement of the Indian Society of Critical Care Medicine (ISCCM) and the Indian Association of Palliative Care (IAPC). Indian Journal of Critical Care Medicine. 2014;18(9).

Q44. Answer b

The SOLER pneumonic is a useful tool for adopting good body language for better communication. S stands for face of the patient/family squarely at eye level to indicate your interest and involvement. O stands for Adopt an Open body posture (do not cross your arms, do not sit across the table). L implies Lean toward the patient/family. E recommends Use Eye contact to show that you are paying careful attention. R warrants maintaining a Relaxed body posture.

> Myatra SN , Salins N, et al End-of-life care policy: An integrated care plan for the dying; A Joint Position Statement of the Indian Society of Critical Care Medicine (ISCCM) and the Indian Association of Palliative Care (IAPC). Indian Journal of Critical Care Medicine. 2014;18(9):615-35.

Q45. Answer a

The inexperienced messenger delivers information fast with no warning and with no understanding of the specific medical, psychosocial, spiritual, or emotional issues involved in EOLD. Patients or family will perceive this as a junior inexperienced doctor without empathy.

> Myatra SN, Salins N, et al. End-of-life care policy: An integrated care plan for the dying; A Joint Position Statement of the Indian Society of Critical Care Medicine (ISCCM) and the Indian Association of Palliative Care (IAPC) Indian Journal of Critical Care Medicine. 2014;18(9):615-35.

Q46. Answer b

Communication by an emotionally burdened expert is careful and good but doctor comes across as someone who is too involved and under emotional strain.

> Myatra SN, Salins N, et al End-of-life care policy: An integrated care plan forthe dying; A Joint Position Statement of the Indian Society of Critical Care Medicine (ISCCM) and the Indian Association of Palliative Care (IAPC). Indian Journal of Critical Care Medicine. 2014;18(9):615-35.

Q47. Answer e

Delivery of information is quick, clear, and delivered in terse sentences with closed body language. Listening is minimal and patient/family emotions are not acknowledged. Doctor is perceived by the patient/ family as unemotional, uncaring, and lacking respect.

> Myatra SN , Salins N, et al End-of-life care policy: An integrated care plan for the dying; A Joint Position Statement of the Indian Society of Critical Care Medicine (ISCCM) and the Indian Association of Palliative Care (IAPC). Indian Journal of Critical Care Medicine. 2014;18(9):615-35.

Q48. Answer c

A Benevolent tactless expert delivers information competently with a sympathetic attitude but there is a lack of ability to pick up emotional verbal and nonverbal cues from the family. The doctor comes across as someone who is well-meaning but without an understanding of the family or patient situation.

> Myatra SN , Salins N, et al End-of-life care policy: An integrated care plan forthe dying; A Joint Position Statement of the Indian Society of Critical Care Medicine (ISCCM) and the Indian Association of Palliative Care (IAPC). Indian Journal of Critical Care Medicine. 2014;18(9):615-35.

Q49. Answer c

Information given is to the point, precise, and is delivered calmly in an objective manner. There is a lack of emotional involvement and the expert tends to avoid emotional and psychosocial issues. Patient/family perceives the expert as someone who was disinterested and did not really care about the patient as a person with hopes and feelings.

> Myatra SN, Salins N, et al. End-of-life care policy: An integrated care plan for the dying; A Joint Position Statement of the Indian Society of Critical Care Medicine (ISCCM) and the Indian Association of Palliative Care (IAPC). Indian Journal of Critical Care Medicine. 2014;18(9):615-35.

Q50. Answer a

Various categories of professionals are identified with reference to the ability to communicate with patients and their families. A professional who can balance the gravity of the situation with due understanding of the ensuing reactions is called an empathic professional.

Myatra SN, Salins N, et al End-of-life care policy: An integrated care plan for the dying; A Joint Position Statement of the Indian Society of Critical Care Medicine (ISCCM) and the Indian Association of Palliative Care (IAPC). Indian Journal of Critical Care Medicine. 2014;18(9):615-35.

Q51. Answer d

The SPIKES approach is one of the recommended methods of overcoming barriers to communication. S stands for setting up. This involves a mental plan on how to communicate the news to the patient or the family. An idea about how to answer any queries that maybe asked forms part of setting up. P stands for perception. This implies the process of understanding what the patient or the family already know about the disease and its outcome. I stands for invitation. This involves knowing how the patient would like the information regarding the disease to be given. K stands for knowledge. This is the process of the medical professional educating the stakeholders regarding the disease, its outcome and the options available. E stands for empathy and emotions. The medical professional should be prepared to let the patient express his emotions and should exhibit enough empathy. S stands for strategy and summary. This includes the planned course of action and the pathway being followed and finally a gist of the discussion and conclusion.

Baile WF, Buckman R, Lenzi R, et al. SPIKES- A six step protocol for delivering bad news: application to the patient with cancer. Oncologist. 2000;5(4):302-11.

Q52. Answer a

Patient/family factors are as important as professional and organizational factors in successful EOL discussions. Acceptance of the disease and treatment implications are very essential to convey the concept of futility. Ethnic and religious factors sometimes hinder the discussions regarding the EOL situation. Families who are emotionally stressed may not be able to take a meaningful part in EOL discussions. Level of medical knowledge is however a professional factor that acts as a barrier during EOL discussions.

Myatra SN, Salins N, et al End-of-life care policy: An integrated care plan for the dying; A Joint Position Statement of the Indian Society of Critical Care Medicine (ISCCM) and the Indian Association of Palliative Care (IAPC). Indian Journal of Critical Care Medicine. 2014;18(9):615-35.

Q53. Answer d

Several barriers have been identified with regards to ineffective communication during EOL discussions. Physician related factors are most often implicated in failed EOL discussions. Basic skills of communication, the culture of discussion between team members, the kind of grounding they have in medical ethics and etiquette coupled with their core medical knowledge are important attributes. The type of hospital is an organizational factor.

Myatra SN, Salins N, et al. End-of-life care policy: An integrated care plan for the dying; A Joint Position Statement of the Indian Society of Critical Care Medicine (ISCCM) and the Indian Association of Palliative Care (IAPC). Indian Journal of Critical Care Medicine. 2014;18(9):615-35.

Q54. Answer c

Quantitative futility represents the likelihood that an intervention will benefit the patient is exceedingly poor. Lethal condition futility implies that the patient has an underlying disease that is not compatible with long-term survival, regardless of the intervention, even if he she could survive to be discharged from the current hospitalization. Qualitative futility implies that the quality of benefit an intervention will produce is exceedingly poor. Imminent demise futility means that the patient will die before discharge regardless of the intervention. EOL discussions are usually evoked in situations of Imminent demise futility.

Myatra SN, Salins N, et al. End-of-life care policy: An integrated care plan for the dying; A Joint Position Statement of the Indian Society of Critical Care Medicine (ISCCM) and the Indian Association of Palliative Care (IAPC). Indian Journal of Critical Care Medicine. 2014;18(9):615-35.

Mohindra RK; Medical futility – a conceptual model; J Med Ethics. 2007;33(2):71-7586.

Q55. Answer d

Ref to explanation of Q54.

K Type Answers

Q1. Answer TFTFF

Medico-Legal aspects of health care are based on the relationship between the doctor and the patient. While the interaction between the two is governed by the law of Torts, the privileges and safety of the patient are protected by the consumer protection act. The patient and doctor association is similar to a contract. NBE rules do not apply to patient doctor interactions nor do the guidelines for research. Fundamentals principles of state policy define the right to health for all citizens but do not cover patient doctor relationships.

  Consumer Protection Act 1986,
  ETHICAL GUIDELINES FOR BIOMEDICAL RESEARCH ON HUMAN PARTICIPANTS – ICMR 2006

Q2. Answer FFFTT

The epidemic diseases act specify the reporting schedule of communicable diseases. All communicable diseases have to be reported to the designated health authorities as soon as they are diagnosed in the hospital. Needle stick injuries have to be reported on a quarterly basis and MTPs on a monthly basis. SMR has to be reported monthly.

  Rakesh PS. The Epidemic Diseases Act of 1897. Indian Journal of Medical Ethics. 2016;1(3)
  The Medical Termination Of Pregnancy Act, 1971 (Act No. 34 of 1971)
  AERB safety code no. AERB/SC/Med -2 (REV) 2001.

Q3. Answer FFTFF

Certification of brain death is also mentioned in the THOA act of 1994. India follows the british convention of accepting brainstem death as brain death. A person is considered dead, once he is certified as 'Brain Dead'. Presence of any signs of brainstem activity makes declaration of death untenable.

  THE TRANSPLANTATION OF HUMAN ORGANS ACT, 1994 No.42 OF 1994
  Transplantation of Human Organs and Tissues Rules, 2014
  Management of Potential Organ Donor: Indian Society of Critical Care Medicine (ISCCM) - Position Statement

Q4. Answer FFTFF

Consent for organ donation is clearly defined in the THOA 1994. Next of kin of the deceased are the only parties entitled to agree of refuse for organ donation. The treating physician is not part of the team that certifies the death of the patient. A hospital designated panel only carries out the tests to confirm death but does not have the privilege of sanctioning an organ harvest.

  THE TRANSPLANTATION OF HUMAN ORGANS ACT, 1994 No.42 OF 1994
  Transplantation of Human Organs and Tissues Rules, 2014
  Management of Potential Organ Donor: Indian Society of Critical Care Medicine (ISCCM) - Position Statement

Q5. Answer TTFFT

Organ donation is increasingly being encountered in hospitals. In India unrelated live organ donation is not accepted unless it is verified and ratified by a panel constituted by the respective state governments. Live related organ donation is directed at a specific individual and cannot be commercialised under any circumstance.

  THE TRANSPLANTATION OF HUMAN ORGANS ACT, 1994 No.42 OF 1994
  Transplantation of Human Organs and Tissues Rules, 2014.
  Pandit RA, Zirpek G, et al. Management of potential organ donor: Indian society of critical care medicine (ISCCM) - position statement. 2017;21(5):303-16.

Q6. Answer TTTTT

According to the Medical Council and the Consumer Protection Acts, every hospital has a responsibility of making the facility safe for all users. This responsibility of the organization extends to making the safest equipment available to medical professionals. The competence and skills of the professionals hired by a hospital is also a direct liability. Similarly, the lab facilities and their reliability are also the scope of a hospital's responsibility.

Consumer Protection Act 1986.

Medical Council Act; 2002.

Q7. Answer TTFFT

Respiratory care gets lot of attention in the number of markers of quality which are recorded. Head end elevation is considered as a fundamental aspect of care. Prevention of VTE with use of appropriate prophylaxis is an important aspect of care. It is however, not restricted to pharmaco-prophylaxis alone. Similarly, initiation of stress ulcer prophylaxis is a component of the care bundle. Oral hygiene is an essential aspect but use of chlorhexidine is not an essential marker. Time lines for change of HME filter are not rigid and may vary based on the clinical situation.

Ray B, Samaddar DP, et al. Quality indicators for ICU: ISCCM guidelines for ICUs in India; Indian J Crit Care Med. 2009;13(4): 173-206.

Quality Indicators in Critically Ill Patients – Update 2011. http://www.semicyuc.org/temas/calidad/indicadores-de-calidad

Q8. Answer TTFFT

Aspirin is one of the mainstay for the management of ACS. Initiation of Aspirin therapy after a diagnosis of ACS is a marker of quality of the processes being followed in the ICU. Initiation is expected within 24 hours after a diagnosis of ACS is made, irrespective of what treatment modality has been used for the ACS. The denominator is the number of patients diagnosed with ACS, while the number of patients receiving aspirin occupies the numerator.

Quality Indicators in Critically Ill Patients – Update 2011. http://www.semicyuc.org/temas/calidad/indicadores-de-calidad

Q9. Answer FFFTF

NSTEMI management is one of the quality indicators for all ICUs. It applies to all aspects of NSTEMI management from diagnosis to discharge. It applies to all patients irrespective of their outcome from therapy. It is an indicator of process and is expected to be followed in atleast 90% of patients.

Quality Indicators in Critically Ill Patients – Update 2011. http://www.semicyuc.org/temas/calidad/indicadores-de-calidad

Q10. Answer FFFTT

Quality of care for patients admitted to the hospital for management of AMI rests on the time taken for appropriate measures taken for achieving revascularization. This applies to both patients admitted for management of AMI or have developed AMI during hospitalization. The methods taken for revascularization could be pharmacological or interventional. The denominator is the number of ACS admissions and reflects the process in place for management of ACS.

Quality Indicators in Critically Ill Patients – Update 2011. http://www.semicyuc.org/temas/calidad/indicadores-de-calidad

Q11. Answer TTFFF

Patients undergoing cardiac surgery are a specific subset of patients with specific targets of therapy and thresholds for intervention. Majority of these patients are expected to be liberated from mechanical ventilation on day 1. However, the incidence of postoperative renal failure reflects the standards of perioperative monitoring and optimization. The occurrence of MI in the perioperative period is a statement on the patency and adequacy of the grafts and prostheses. As with most other surgical processes, perioperative transfusion in reasonable limits is not a marker of quality of surgery.

Quality Indicators in Critically Ill Patients – Update 2011. http://www.semicyuc.org/temas/calidad/indicadores-de-calidad

Q12. Answer TFFTT

Mechanical ventilation is a common intervention in ICU. Complications occur in a proportion of patients. This proportion is not expected to exceed 3%. The duration of ventilation taken as a cut off for assessing safety is 24 hours. Post-extubation stridor is a marker of safety pertaining to the process of intubation and maintenance of the tube. Line related pneumothoraces, although seem often in ventilated patients are to be seen as quality markers of the process of venous cannulation and not of mechanical ventilation.

Quality Indicators in Critically Ill Patients – Update 2011. http://www.semicyuc.org/temas/calidad/indicadores-de-calidad

Q13. Answer TTTTF

Prone ventilation is an important rescue measure for management of refractory hypoxemia. However, attention to safety during prone ventilation is an essential precaution and is deemed as a quality issue. Dislodgement of tubes during the process of prone ventilation is an obvious safety and therefore a quality issue. Mobilization of secretions is a normal accompaniment of prone ventilation. The treating team is expected to anticipate this and monitor and prevent tube blocks. In the prone position new pressure areas like malleolar prominences, iliac crests, malar eminences etc. are involved. These areas should be actively protected and development of pressure ulcers on these areas is a marker of quality. A proportion of patients deteriorate after being turned prone independent of the attention being paid to the process. Deterioration is not therefore a marker of quality.

Ray B, Samaddar DP, et al Quality indicators for ICU: ISCCM guidelines for ICUs in India; Indian J Crit Care Med. 2009;13(4): 173-206.

Quality Indicators in Critically Ill Patients – Update 2011. http://www.semicyuc.org/temas/calidad/indicadores-de-calidad

Q14. Answer FFFFT

Extubation success is a prime marker of quality for the outcomes of mechanical ventilation in ICU. Planned extubations are the norm. Unplanned extubations include self extubations and accidental dislodgement of tubes. Both are associated with significant morbidity and adverse outcomes. It is generally expressed as the number of unplanned extubations per 1000 extubations. It is a marker of outcomes and has an acceptable rate of 5-10 per 1000 extubations.

Ray B, Samaddar DP, et al Quality indicators for ICU: ISCCM guidelines for ICUs in India; Indian J Crit Care Med. 2009;13(4): 173-206.

Quality Indicators in Critically Ill Patients – Update 2011. http://www.semicyuc.org/temas/calidad/indicadores-de-calidad

Q15. Answer TTTFT

Management of trauma is an essential aspect of hospital care and therefore for assessment of quality. Examination of all trauma victims by an ICU team member is considered as an essential aspect of quality. It is a marker of quality for both trauma and non-trauma centers. Atleast 95% of trauma victims arriving to the ED are expected to be seen by an intensivist.

Quality Indicators in Critically Ill Patients – Update 2011. http://www.semicyuc.org/temas/calidad/indicadores-de-calidad

Q16. Answer TTTFF

Critical Illness Polyneuropathy is a marker of quality in ICU. It reflects the awareness of the team about the triggering factors and precipitating events. The LOS cutoff for making a diagnosis of CIP is atleast 72 hours. It is therefore considered as a marker of outcome of critical illness. The underlying diagnosis has no bearing on the accepted prevalence of CIP which is currently < 40%.

Ray B, Samaddar DP, et al. Quality indicators for ICU: ISCCM guidelines for ICUs in India; Indian J Crit Care Med. 2009;13(4): 173-206.

Quality Indicators in Critically Ill Patients – Update 2011. http://www.semicyuc.org/temas/calidad/indicadores-de-calidad

Q17. Answer FFFFF

The definition of Ventilator Associated Pneumonia is constantly being revised to incorporate the knowledge regarding the etiopathogenesis of this common condition in the ICU. At this stage, the term VAP is being reserved for episodes of pneumonia occurring among patients being ventilated invasively. The cutoff has been revised to atleast 24 hours of invasive ventilation. It does not apply to patients who are under outpatient care and follow-up. Such patients might be included in Health Care-Associated Pneumonia. It is an indicator of outcomes of invasive ventilation. Accepted standards are 12-14 episodes per 1000 ventilator days.

Ray B, Samaddar DP, et al. Quality indicators for ICU: ISCCM guidelines for ICUs in India; Indian J Crit Care Med. 2009;13(4): 173-206.

Quality Indicators in Critically Ill Patients – Update 2011. http://www.semicyuc.org/temas/calidad/indicadores-de-calidad

Q18. Answer FTTTT

Antimicrobial therapy and its monitoring are integral parts of quality assessment programs. Empirical antibiotic therapy is accepted for 24-36 hours after which is a definitive microbiological diagnosis and therapy are

Medical Law and Ethics 437

expected to be in place. Appropriate antimicrobial therapy implies the use of the right drug in the right dose for the appropriate duration. Choice of antibiotic is guided by the tissue which the drug has to penetrate. One of the indices to measure appropriate use of antibiotics is Defined Daily Dosage. A default rate of 10% is accepted for compliance to antimicrobial discipline.

> Ray B, Samaddar DP, et al. Quality indicators for ICU: ISCCM guidelines for ICUs in India; Indian J Crit Care Med. 2009;13(4): 173-206.
>
> Quality Indicators in Critically Ill Patients – Update 2011. http://www.semicyuc.org/temas/calidad/indicadores-de-calidad

Q19. Answer FFTTF

Parenteral nutrition is increasingly being viewed as a bride to achieve nutritional targets in ICU. Monitoring of patients who are on parenteral nutrition is a quality marker in ICU. Patients in ICU who receive parenteral nutrition need to have a plan to monitor its adequacy as well as adverse effects. Some of the well documented adverse effects include hyperglycemia (target 130 mg/dL), hyperbilirubinemia and hepatic dysfunction. Hyperglycemia is an important predictor of morbidity in ICU and is supposed to occur in < 10% of patients on PN. Similarly, liver dysfunction is not expected to occur in more than 25% of patients receiving PN. All these parameters imply that nutrition is an essential aspect of quality assessment in ICU.

> Quality Indicators in Critically Ill Patients – Update 2011. http://www.semicyuc.org/temas/calidad/indicadores-de-calidad

Q20. Answer TTTTT

Monitoring of nutrition prescription and delivery is a mandatory parameter for quality assessment in ICU. It is expected that the medical and nutrition teams ascertain the position of the feeding tube atleast once a day before finalising the feeding plan. It is the responsibility of the medical and nursing teams to ensure that the head end of the bed is elevated during the initiation and execution of the feeding plan. Electrolytes like sodium, potassium and magnesium need to be monitored for ensuring proper nutrition planning as well as to anticipate intolerance. Tolerance to feeds and their components is also an essential aspect of nutrition planning. All these markers of quality are built in to ensure that the targets for nutrition are clearly defined and achieved within defined time lines.

> Ref: Ray B, Samaddar DP, et al. Quality indicators for ICU: ISCCM guidelines for ICUs in India; Indian J Crit Care Med. 2009;13(4):173-206.
>
> Quality Indicators in Critically Ill Patients – Update 2011. http://www.semicyuc.org/temas/calidad/indicadores-de-calidad

Q21. Answer TFFFF

Monitoring and Implementation of analgesia and sedation is an essential tool for the quality assessment in Intensive Care. A definitive plan for assessment for sedation and analgesia needs to be documented. Similarly, a plan for interruption of sedation also needs to be implemented and documented. It is expected that atleast 80% of the patients should have sedation interruption assuming that 20% might not be eligible for the interruption. Pain assessment is expected to be a universal phenomenon among ICU patients. Therefore, pain assessment plans and documentation is expected to be accomplished in 100% of ICU patients. Neuromuscular blockade use is also expected to be justified in nearly all patients. Compliance of 100% is expected for justification of use of neuromuscular blockade in the ICU. This essentially means that analgesia and sedation are the parameters which are essential parameters to be monitored for quality assessment in ICU

> Quality Indicators in Critically Ill Patients – Update 2011. http://www.semicyuc.org/temas/calidad/indicadores-de-calidad

Q22. Answer TTTFF

Defined Daily Dosage is a term used to describe the utilization of a particular antimicrobial agent. It is essentially a tool for antimicrobial stewardship which has been used as a quality indicator for antimicrobial drug use in ICU. For example, if a patient is prescribed Meropenem 1g 8 hrly for 5 days, the DDD of Meropenem becomes 3g. It can be used for other antimicrobials also. It is based on monotherapy, i.e. a single drug. Combinations like Ampicillin-Sulbactam or Amoxycillin. Clavulanate can be monitored using DDD. Topical agents cannot be included in the list for DDD monitoring. Duration of therapy is the total number of days a particular antibiotic is used. It is another method of monitoring drug usage but is not synonymous with DDD.

Q23. Answer FFTFF

Inappropriateness of therapy is a decision which is taken by the teams taking care of a critically ill patient. Any difference of opinion on the appropriateness of aggressive therapy has to be mutually discussed and a consensus arrived at. Once a consensus is reached, the teams dealing with the clinical care conveys a joint decision to the family. During the family counseling leading members of all teams involved should be available for clarifications. All members are expected to voice their unanimity of agreement on the inappropriateness of intensive care for the given patient. Individual counseling sessions are likely to give a fractured view and confuse the stakeholders.

Monitoring of patients for whom EOL discussions have been done and concluded involves comfort care and painless process of dying. Aggressive therapies such as fluid boluses, noninvasive ventilation etc. are not generally included in this process. As a result monitoring of hemodynamics and respiratory parameters is generally toned down once an EOL decision has been taken.

End of Life policy decisions depend on making the process of dying painless both to the patient as well as the family. Initiation of therapies such as renal replacement or high end antibiotics do not fit into the scope of EOL discussions. However, all forms of analgesia are core inclusions in EOL processes.

End of Life Care and Decisions and Limitation of therapy are still grey areas in India. However, the concept of Allow Natural Death which is prevalent in some European countries is a concept that does not have a legal or legislative sanction in India.

Palliative care is considered as a separate discipline in health care. Primary disciplines involved in the care of hospitalized patients are expected to involve palliative care teams for a structures approach and decision making. Involving such teams is considered as an effective quality initiative and should not be seen as a failure of any of the primary care giving teams.

Myatra SN, Salins N, et al. End-of-life care policy: An integrated care plan for the dying; A Joint Position Statement of the Indian Society of Critical Care Medicine (ISCCM) and the Indian Association of Palliative Care (IAPC) Indian Journal of Critical Care Medicine. 2014;18(9):615-35.

Mani RK. Constitutional and legal protection for life support limitation in India. Indian J Palliat Care. 2015;21(3):258-61.

Q24. Answer TFTTF

Extubation in the ICU is always a planned procedure. Parameters which are likely to compromise the patient's ability to sustain extubation should be corrected prior to the process. However, unplanned extubations - self and accidental - are important events which reflect the processes in the ICU and impact the outcomes of patients being ventilated.

Monitoring of the hardware associated with delivery of mechanical ventilation is an essential aspect of quality assessment. Integrity of ventilator circuits, HME filters, suction systems and ET tube holders need to be monitored. However, no definite time lines can be set for changing these components which has to be done on a need based process rather than on a fixed time based process.

Transfusion triggers in the ICU have been well established. Aims and purposes of such transfusions have to be documented and audited. Appropriate transfusion strategy should include the indication, threshold, quantum and effects of the intervention. Any deviation from accepted norms is considered as a quality default in the ICU.

Quality of care delivered to the patient reflects on the clinical and psychological state of the patient and his family at the time of ICU discharge. All aspects of ICU structure, process and outcomes will have an impact on the perceived quality of care at ICU discharge. The stake holders will be the patient and his family who have interacted with the ICU team during the ICU stay.

Scientific Publications are an integral part of the documentation and validation of the work done in academic training units. It may be an essential requirement for accreditation by training and validation agencies. But, to date, publications do not find mention in the assessment of quality of the ICU.

Ray B, Samaddar DP, et al. Quality indicators for ICU: ISCCM guidelines for ICUs in India. Indian J Crit Care Med. 2009;13(4): 173-206.

Q25. Answer TTFFF

Dealing with a difficult situation of EOL issue is a cause of stress and anxiety for specialists working in the ICU. A clear policy will help the professionals to streamline and execute the EOL discussions effectively. Absence of a policy will lead to unexpected situations and hostilities which may not be handled well by the professionals. This is one of the reasons for a burnout among clinicians.

Palliative care and EOL situations are two aspects of health care where definitive therapy is not likely to contribute to improve the quality of life or treat the underlying disease. Both aspects deal with a situation where death is inevitable. However, palliative care takes into account the steps and processes involved in the acceptance of death by the family and helping them in coming to terms with the demise of a family member

EOL process is a multiple step process starting from identification of the right clinical situation. This is followed by an agreement between the various teams regarding futility of care. Communicating and documenting the decision is followed by execution and an audit of such processes over a period of time.

Mani RK. Constitutional and legal protection for life support limitation in India. Indian J Palliat Care. 2015;21(3):258-61.

Myatra SN, Salins N, et al. End-of-life care policy: An integrated care plan for the dying; A Joint Position Statement of the Indian Society of Critical Care Medicine (ISCCM) and the Indian Association of Palliative Care (IAPC). Indian Journal of Critical Care Medicine. 2014;18(9):615-35.

Karnik S, Karnekar A; Ethical issues surrounding end of life care – a narrative review. Healthcare. 2016;4;24.

CHAPTER 20

Infection Control in Critical Care

Monika Rajani, Yash Javeri

A Type Questions
(One best answer)

1. Which one of the following is NOT a key component of Institute of Healthcare Improvement (IHI) Central Line Bundle?
   a. Hand washing
   b. Dressing when soiled/damp
   c. Aseptic handling
   d. Early removal
   e. Line listing

2. You have been looking after H1N1 patient admissions at your hospital amidst an outbreak. What is considered a safe distance for avoiding droplet infections?
   a. 2 feet
   b. 3 feet
   c. 4.5 feet
   d. 6 feet
   e. 12 feet

3. You finished securing a central line in ICU. The correct order to remove personal protective equipment (PPE) is:
   a. Apron first, eye protection second, mask and finally gloves
   b. Eye protection, then mask if worn, then apron and finally gloves
   c. Gloves first and after that any sequence
   d. Gloves first, face shield next, gown and finally mask
   e. It does not matter in what order they are removed

4. When using alcohol based hand rub, you should:
   a. Apply the hand rub and wave hands until dry
   b. Apply a sufficient quantity of hand rub and rub hands for 20–30 seconds, being sure to cover all areas: front, back, between fingers, nail beds and thumbs
   c. Apply the hand rub and rub palms together for 10 seconds
   d. Apply hand rub when you see an infected patient
   e. You should rub for at least 60 seconds in all directions

5. Identify the device and grade the level of recommendation from Center of Disease Control (CDC) for infection prevention.

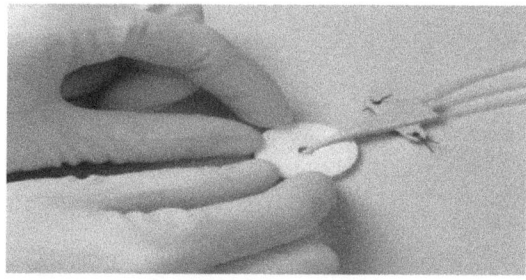

   a. Alcohol impregnated sponge dressing -Category 1B
   b. Impermeable dressing -Category 1A
   c. Chlorhexidine-impregnated sponge dressing -Category 1A

Infection Control in Critical Care — 441

d. Chlorhexidine-impregnated sponge dressing-Category 1B
e. None of the above

6. You are a visiting ICU consultant for a nursing home facility. Several of the patients have developed influenza like symptoms and the community is in the midst of influenza A outbreak. None of the nursing home residents have received the influenza vaccine. What course of action is most appropriate?
    a. Give the influenza vaccine to all residents who do not have a contraindication to the vaccine (i.e. allergy to eggs)
    b. Give the influenza vaccine to all residents who do not have a contraindication to the vaccine plus also give amantadine for 2 weeks
    c. Give amantadine alone to all residents
    d. Do not give any prophylactic regimen
    e. Quarantine alone

7. You are asked to calculate attack rate for *Klebsiella pneumoniae* nosocomial infections for your neonatal intensive care unit (NICU). Which of the following formula correctly defines attack rate?
    a. (Number of new nosocomial infections acquired in a period/number of patients observed in the same period) × 100
    b. (Number of new nosocomial infections acquired in a period/number of patients observed in the same period) × 1000
    c. Number of new nosocomial infections acquired in a period/number of patients observed in the same period
    d. Number of new nosocomial infections acquired in a period/total patient days for the same period) × 1000
    e. None of the above

8. Which of the following is false regarding Coagulase negative staphylococci (CoNS) implicated bacteremia?
    a. CoNS usually represent the contamination of blood culture bottles when blood cultures are obtained
    b. CoNS continue to be frequently isolated in blood cultures and represent the most common cause of pseudobacteremia
    c. Patients with CoNS bloodstream contaminants had longer hospital LOS and infection-related LOS
    d. Coagulase-negative staphylococci (CoNS) are part of the normal flora of human skin
    e. All of the above

9. For prevention of CLABSI one of the following is true:
    a. Infusion tubing should be used for no longer than 96 hours
    b. Tubing used to administer blood products or lipid emulsions should be changed every 48 hours
    c. In-line filters should be used as they decrease the rate of infection
    d. Central intravascular catheters should be routinely changed
    e. Use CVC with maximum number of ports so that each port is used less frequently

10. While designing an ICU, following are the measures to be taken to prevent hospital acquired infections except:
    a. The unit should be away from the ward areas
    b. Air should be filtered to 99% efficiency down to 5 μm
    c. ICU is planned with 15 air changes per hour (5 fresh + 10 re-circulation)
    d. Each bed should ideally have 8 sqm floor space
    e. Provision for separate area for medication preparation

11. What is true about selective oropharyngeal decontamination (SOD) and selective digestive decontamination of digestive tract (SDD)?
    a. Reduces mortality
    b. Is recommended in ICU's with high anti-microbial resistance
    c. Reduces mortality in ICU's with low anti-microbial resistance
    d. SDD is part of VAP bundle
    e. SDD reduces the risk of VAP but not HAP

12. You as an ICU Director are requested by Infection Control team to draft a cleaning policy for your unit. Which of the following will not be included by you in your policy?
    a. High-quality cleaning and disinfection of all patient-care areas is important, especially surfaces close to the patient (e.g. bedrails, bedside tables, doorknobs, and equipment)
    b. EPA-registered disinfectants or detergents that best meet the overall needs of the ICU should be used

c. Routine surface cleaning only with alcohol
d. Frequency of cleaning: surface cleaning (walls) twice weekly, floor cleaning two to three times per day
e. Terminal cleaning (patient bed area) after discharge or death

13. **Modes of transmission are numbered below as 1 to 5:**
    1. **Contact - fecal oral route**
    2. **Contact - droplet transmission**
    3. **Common vehicle - via fomites in the hospital**
    4. **Sharp's injury**
    5. **Airborne**

    Which of the following methods is correct means by which rotavirus is commonly transmitted?
    a. 1 and 2 only
    b. 1 and 3 only
    c. 2 and 3 only
    d. 4 and 5 only
    e. 1 only

14. In the Six Sigma DMAIC format, the D represents:
    a. Document
    b. Develop
    c. Define
    d. Demonstrate
    e. Denominator

15. When a patient is on contact precautions for Methicillin-resistant *Staphylococcus aureus* (MRSA) cellulitis on hand, which of the following is correct?
    a. Wear gown and gloves whenever entering the room
    b. Enter the room without PPE if no patient contact planned
    c. Wear gloves only if anticipating patient contact
    d. Wear gown, gloves, and faceguard whenever entering the room
    e. Any one of the above

16. You as ICU Director approach infection control committee and recommend an educational campaign aimed at all ICU staff and attending physicians who insert and maintain catheters aimed at prevention bundles to reduce the HAI risk. Which of the following is correct?
    a. Infection control education and implementation of prevention bundles; Re: Catheter insertion and maintenance cannot reduce the incidence of CRBSI
    b. Infection control education and implementation of prevention bundles; Re: Catheter insertion and maintenance can reduce the incidence of CRBSI, however CRBSI do not independently lead to increased ICU length of stay so such a program is unwarranted
    c. Infection control education and implementation of prevention bundles; Re: Catheter insertion and maintenance can reduce the incidence of CRBSI, since CRBSI do independently lead to increased ICU length of stay so such a program is warranted
    d. Infection control education is required only for dedicated vascular access teams
    e. None of the above

17. Your Human Resources Department wants to have a policy for influenza prophylaxis for ICU staff. Which of the following statements is NOT TRUE?
    a. Annual influenza vaccination is the best way to prevent influenza
    b. Vaccine is recommended for Healthcare Provider (HCP) to protect not only themselves, but also their patients and vulnerable colleagues
    c. WHO guidelines state that individuals at high risk of severe disease who have been exposed to a patient with influenza may benefit from presumptive treatment with a full twice-daily 5-day course of antivirals, even if they do not show signs and symptoms of infection
    d. Stay at home until symptoms have resolved (at least 7 days after fever has defervesced)
    e. The best time to vaccinate is before the influenza season starts, but getting it later will still protect during the rest of the season

18. Which of the following is NOT TRUE regarding infection control policies for bronchoscopy suite?
    a. Store bronchoscope in a hanging position to prevent moisture accumulation
    b. Rinse with filtered tap water followed by 70% ethyl alcohol or sterile water after disinfection
    c. The bronchoscopy area should have engineering controls that will allow for negative air pressure, at least 6 air changes per hour

d. N95 particulate respirator is a minimally acceptable alternative during bronchoscopy of a TB patient
e. All of the above

19. **A child is admitted to the PICU with a diagnosis of suspected meningococcal meningitis. Which of the following infection control measures should be instituted?**
   a. Isolation of patients is recommended for at least 96 hours after adequate antibiotic treatment
   b. No isolation required
   c. Standard (universal) precautions alone be observed
   d. Respiratory droplet precautions (used in addition to standard precautions)
   e. None of the above

20. **The ICU fellow gets needle stick exposure from an HIV infected patient in trauma bay. Which of the following is NOT TRUE regarding steps to be taken after exposure to HIV infected blood?**
   a. Needle stick injuries should be washed with soap and water
   b. Splashes to the nose, mouth or skin should be flushed with water
   c. Postexposure prophylaxis (PEP) should be started after 96 hr of exposure
   d. Follow-up HIV testing is typically concluded 6 months after an HIV exposure
   e. PEP is recommended when occupational exposures to HIV occur

K Type Questions
[Marked True (T)/False (F)]

1. **You are the champion for your ICU infection control program. There are other measures you must take to ensure hand hygiene is effective in minimising the spread of infection:**
   a. Cover all cuts and abrasions with a waterproof plaster
   b. Bare your arms below the elbow and remove watches and bracelets
   c. Keep nails short and clean
   d. Do not wear nail varnish or nail extensions
   e. Wear no rings other than a plain band

2. **Regarding body fluids which can cause contamination:**
   a. Urine
   b. Vomit
   c. Feces
   d. Saliva
   e. Tears

3. **Concerning prevention of CRBSI in your ICU:**
   a. The use of the subclavian route carries the lowest risk of CRBSI
   b. CVC should be changed at 4 days before a threshold load of organisms is reached
   c. Current evidence suggests the universal use of antibiotic-coated catheters to reduce CRBSI
   d. A dry gauze dressing is acceptable over the CVC site
   e. Povidone iodine antiseptic ointment at the hemodialysis catheter exit site after catheter insertion and at the end of each dialysis session

4. **Proper disposal technique as per Biomedical Waste Management Rules 2016 in India:**
   a. Human tissues, organs, body parts—red colored non-chlorinated plastic bags
   b. Expired or discarded medicines—yellow colored non-chlorinated plastic bags or containers
   c. Broken or discarded and contaminated glass including medicine vials—Cardboard boxes with blue colored marking
   d. Wastes generated from disposable items such as tubing, bottles, intravenous tubes and sets, catheters, urine bags, syringes—red colored non-chlorinated plastic bags or containers
   e. Metallic body implants—cardboard boxes with red colored marking

5. **Regarding ventilator-associated event (VAE):**
   a. Groups all the conditions that result in a significant and sustained deterioration in oxygenation
   b. Only infectious conditions (such as tracheitis, tracheobronchitis, and pneumonia) are included
   c. Tier 1: ventilator-associated condition (VAC) —the patient develops hypoxemia (as defined above) for a sustained period of more than 2 days. The etiology of the hypoxemia is not infective
   d. Tier 2: infection-related ventilator-associated complication (IVAC)—hypoxemia develops in the setting of generalized infection or inflammation, and antibiotics are instituted for a minimum of 4 days

e. Tier 3: probable or possible ventilator-associated pneumonia (VAP)—additional laboratory evidence of white blood cells on Gram stain of material from a respiratory secretion specimen of acceptable quality, or (=possible)/and (=probable) presence of respiratory pathogens on quantitative cultures, in patients with IVAC

6. **Immunosuppressed transplant recipients should not have the following:**
   a. BCG vaccine
   b. Raw salads
   c. Varicella immune globulin
   d. Influenza vaccine
   e. Malaria prophylaxis

7. **Preventing opportunistic infections in patients undergoing bone marrow transplantation (BMT):**
   a. Appropriately designed facilities that have rooms with more than 12 air exchanges per hour and point-of-use high-efficiency particulate air (HEPA) filtration
   b. Laminar airflow rooms, in which air moves in one direction, have been shown to protect patients from *Aspergillus* infections during outbreaks
   c. Rooms should have positive air pressure compared to the hallway unless it is housing a patient who has active disease with a pathogen that has airborne transmission; in that case, a negative pressure room is recommended
   d. Granulocyte transfusion appears to be beneficial, in the presence of profound neutropenia
   e. The advent of ganciclovir for prophylaxis has profoundly decreased severe CMV disease

8. **Isolation facilities include the following types:**
   a. Neutral or standard room air pressure, e.g. standard air conditioning, also known as Class S
   b. Positive room air pressure where an immune-compromised patient is protected from airborne transmission of any infection, Class P
   c. Negative room air pressure, where others are protected from any airborne transmission from a patient who may be an infection risk, Class N
   d. Class Q is type of positive room with anteroom
   e. A negative pressure Isolation Room requires at least 80% outside air ventilation (i.e. no return air permitted), with low level exhaust ducts

9. **The following are recognised strategies in the prevention of VAP:**
   a. Daily sedation holds
   b. Head-up positioning of 30° to 45°
   c. Prone positioning
   d. Chlorhexidine mouth care
   e. Daily ventilator tubing changes

10. **Concerning CRBSI:**
    a. Any positive culture from a CVC should be interpreted as likely CRBSI
    b. The "Matching Michigan" project showed a post implementation mean rate of CRBSI/1000 catheter days
    c. *Staphylococcus aureus* CRBSI should prompt a search for metastatic infection, including endocarditis.
    d. CoNS CRBSI may get better without antibiotics
    e. Guidewire exchange is encouraged as a routine at 14 days in ICU patients

11. **Regarding CAUTI bundle implementation in your unit:**
    a. Maintain an open drainage system
    b. Maintain unobstructed urine flow
    c. Urinary catheter should be placed and taped below the thigh
    d. Urinary bag should hang below the level of the bladder
    e. The urinary bag should never have floor contact

12. **According the National Nosocomial Infections Surveillance System (NNIS), an infection of a prosthetic hip requiring prosthesis removal can be reported as a surgical-site infection (SSI) if it occurs within:**
    a. 7 days of surgery
    b. 30 days of surgery
    c. 60 days of surgery
    d. 90 days of surgery
    e. 1 year of surgery

13. **Postoperative CNS infection (PCNSI):**
    a. Staphylococcus species is rare cause
    b. CSF leak is independent risk factor

c. No antibiotic prophylaxis
d. Shunt procedure is not a risk factor
e. Duration of surgery is a risk factor

14. **Which of the following is a risk factor for Vancomycin Intermediate *Staphylococcus aureus* (VISA)/Vancomycin Resistant Enterococci (VRE) acquired in ICU?**
    a. Hemato-oncology patients
    b. Immunosuppressed patients
    c. Gut breach- GI surgery
    d. Mucosal barrier injury
    e. Liver transplant recipients

15. **Regarding healthcare-associated aspergillosis:**
    a. Do not perform routine, periodic cultures of the nasopharynx of asymptomatic patients at high-risk healthcare-associated aspergillosis
    b. Healthcare-associated aspergillosis is most commonly acquired via inhalation of airborne spores resulting in pulmonary aspergillosis
    c. Only few outbreaks have occurred as a result of airborne spores from non-water environmental sources
    d. Internal construction or renovation with failure to control spread of contaminated dust or debris can cause outbreaks
    e. Use seamless carpeting in hallways and rooms occupied by severely immunocompromised patients

16. **You have a confirm patient with H1N1 pneumonia admitted under your care. Regarding the infection control practices:**
    a. Articles like swabs/gauges, etc. are to be discarded in the yellow colored autoclavable biosafety bags after use, the bags are to be autoclaved followed by incineration of the contents of the bag
    b. Use phenolic disinfectants, quaternary ammonia compounds, alcohol or sodium hypochlorite
    c. Use N-95 masks during aerosol-generating procedures
    d. To avoid possible aerosolization of virus, sweeping should be performed
    e. Remove mask by pulling front side of mask

17. **Concerning Ventilator Associated Tracheobronchitis (VAT) and VAP:**
    a. Patients with VAT should receive antibiotic
    b. Noninvasive respiratory sampling refers to endotracheal aspiration
    c. Suspected VAP, we recommend including coverage for *S. aureus*, *Pseudomonas aeruginosa*, and other gram-negative bacilli in all empiric treatment
    d. All patients with VAP should receive at least 15 days of antibiotic therapy
    e. Discontinuation of antibiotic therapy be based on CPIS

18. **Regarding infection control practices for a burns unit:**
    a. Quantitative cultures of burn wound tissue biopsy with concomitant histological analysis are not preferred infection surveillance approach for burn areas that have not been or cannot be excised
    b. Strict infection control practices and appropriate empirical antimicrobial therapy are essential
    c. Invasive burn wound infections due to *Candida* spp., *Aspergillus* spp., and other opportunistic fungi are important emerging causes of early onset morbidity and mortality
    d. Herpesvirus group, particularly HSV and varicella-zoster virus but less commonly CMV, are rarely reported but increasingly recognized causes of wound infections in burns
    e. Laboratory surveillance as well as routine microbial surveillance cultures of the burn wound and other sources should be monitored to rapidly identify epidemic pathogens and/or antibiotic-resistant strains

19. **Regarding to the results of HBV blood test in cases of needle stick injuries:**
    a. Immediately following any exposure, whether or not the source is known to pose a risk of infection, the wound should be washed immediately and thoroughly with soap and water
    b. If HBV blood test of the patient is positive and the intensivist is non-vaccinated, intensivist must receive HB hyperimmune globulins and start an HB vaccine series
    c. Postexposure treatment should begin after 7 days
    d. If HBV blood test of the patient is negative and the intensivist is vaccinated, no further action can be done

e. For a susceptible person, the risk from a single needle stick to HBV-infected blood ranges from 1–3%

20. **Regarding CAUTI prevention interventions:**
   a. Hand hygiene does not need to be performed if you are wearing gloves
   b. The periurethral area should be cleaned vigorously and with a special antimicrobial solution
   c. Data are insufficient to make a recommendation as to whether use of antibiotic coated catheters reduces CA-bacteriuria or CA-UTI in patients with long-term catheterization
   d. A 3-day antimicrobial regimen may be considered for women aged ⩽65 years who develop CA-UTI without upper urinary tract symptoms after an indwelling catheter has been removed
   e. Daily meatal cleansing with povidone-iodine solution, silver sulfadiazine, polyantibiotic ointment or cream, or green soap and water is not recommended for routine use in men or women with indwelling urethral catheters to reduce CA-bacteriuria

Infection Control in Critical Care 447

ANSWERS
A Type Answers

Q1. Answer e

Line listing is a table in which critical information from an outbreak is listed.

Each column represents an important variable (e.g. identifier, age, sex) and each row represents a different case. A line listing is produced by epidemiologists in outbreak investigations. A line listing allows information about time, person, and place to be organized and reviewed quickly. It is also a good way to keep track of different categories of cases.

<small>How-to Guide: Prevent Central Line-Associated Bloodstream Infections (CLABSI). Cambridge, MA: Institute for Healthcare Improvement; 2012. Available from: www.ihi.org (Accessed 13 February 2018).</small>

Q2. Answer b

During periods of increased prevalence of respiratory infections in the community, offer masks to coughing patients and other symptomatic persons (e.g. persons who accompany ill patients) upon entry into the facility and encourage separation, ideally by a distance of at least 3 feet, from others in common areas.

<small>Siegel JD, Rhinehart E, Jackson M, et al. Guideline for Isolation Precautions: Preventing Transmission of Infectious Agents in Healthcare Settings. Available from: https://www.cdc.gov/infectioncontrol/guidelines/isolation/index.html (Accessed 13 February 2018).</small>

Q3. Answer d

The sequence for removing PPE is intended to limit opportunities for self contamination. The gloves are considered the most contaminated pieces of PPE and are therefore removed first. The face shield or goggles are next because they are more cumbersome and would interfere with removal of other PPE. The gown is third in the sequence, followed by the mask or respirator.

<small>Sequence for putting on personal protective equipment (PPE). Available From: https://www.cdc.gov/hai/pdfs/ppe/ppe-sequence.pdf (Accessed 8 December 2017).</small>

Q4. Answer b

When using an alcohol-based hand rub, apply a coin sized amount of product into the palm of one hand and rub hands together, covering all surfaces of hands and fingers, until hands are dry. This complete procedure takes 20–30 seconds.

<small>Pittet D, Allegranzi B, Boyce J. et al. The WHO guidelines on hand hygiene in health care and their consensus recommendations. Infection Control and Hospital Epidemiology. 2009;30:611-22.</small>

Q5. Answer c

For patients aged 18 years and older: Chlorhexidine-impregnated dressings with an FDA-cleared label that specifies a clinical indication for reducing catheter-related bloodstream infection (CRBSI) or catheter-associated bloodstream infection (CABSI) are recommended to protect the insertion site of short-term, non-tunneled central venous catheters (Category I A recommendation).

<small>Updated Recommendations on the Use of Chlorhexidine-Impregnated Dressings for Prevention of Intravascular Catheter-Related Infections. (https://www.cdc.gov/infectioncontrol/guidelines/bsi/c-i-dressings/index.html).</small>

Q6. Answer b

Influenza A is a potentially lethal disease in the elderly and chronically ill patients. This calls for prophylaxis in this setting. All residents should receive the vaccine unless they have known egg allergy. Since protective antibodies to the vaccine will not develop for 2 weeks, amantadine can be used for protection against influenza A during the interim 2-week period.

<small>Interim Guidance for Influenza Outbreak Management in Long-term Care Facilities. Available from: https://www.cdc.gov/flu/pdf/professionals/interim-guidance-outbreak-management.pdf (Accessed 13 February 2018).</small>

Q7. Answer a

Attack rate is another type of incidence rate expressed as cases per 100 populations (or a percentage). It is used to describe the new and recurrent cases of disease that have been observed in a particular group during a limited time period in special circumstances, such as during an outbreak.

> Richards C, Alonso-Echanove J, Caicedo Y, Jarvis W. *Klebsiella pneumoniae* Bloodstream Infections Among Neonates in a High-Risk Nursery in Cali, Colombia. Infection Control & Hospital Epidemiology. 2004;25(3):221-5.

Q8. Answer c

CONS isolated from blood culture are usually contaminants but are also a significant cause of bacteremia. False positive blood culture leads to additional laboratory tests, unnecessary antibiotic use and longer hospitalization of patients that increases the patients care costs.

> Becker K, Heilmann C, Peters G. Coagulase-negative staphylococci. Clin Microbiol Rev. 2014;27:870.

Q9. Answer a

In patients not receiving blood, blood products or fat emulsions, replace administration sets that are continuously used, including secondary sets and add-on devices, no more frequently than at 96-hour intervals, but at least every 7 days (Category IA).

Replace tubing used to administer blood, blood products, or fat emulsions within 24 hours of initiating the infusion (Category IB).

For reducing the risk for CRBSI, no strong recommendation can be made in favor of using in-line filters.

> Guidelines for the Prevention of Intravascular Catheter-Related Infection. Available from: https://www.cdc.gov/infectioncontrol/guidelines/bsi/index.html (Accessed 13 February 2018).

Q10. Answer d

Each bed should ideally have 14 sqm of floor space. Separation of critical areas like OT, ICU from general traffic and avoidance of air movement from areas like laboratories and infectious diseases wards towards ICU.

> Recommendations for the prevention of hospital acquired infection. Am J Infect Control. 1996;22:267-92.

Q11. Answer c

SOD or SDD is not a new concept. Recent studies demonstrated that SDD and, to some extent, SOD suppress the load of antibiotic resistant bacteria in the gut, reduce mortality and reduce transmission.

> Muskiet ERR. Development of antibiotic resistance related to selective decontamination of the digestive tract. Neth J Crit Care. 2014;1:4-9.

Q12. Answer c

Select EPA-registered disinfectants use them in accordance with the manufacturer's instructions. Do not use high-level disinfectants/liquid chemical sterilants for disinfection of either noncritical instruments or devices or any environmental surfaces. Clean noncritical medical equipment surfaces with a detergent/disinfectant followed by application of EPA-registered hospital disinfectant. Do not use alcohol to disinfect large environmental surfaces.

> Favero MS, Bond WW. Chemical disinfection of medical and surgical materials. In: Block SS (ed). Disinfection, Sterilization, and Preservation, 5th edition. Philadelphia, PA: Lippincott Williams and Wilkins, 2001.

Q13. Answer b

Rotavirus is highly infectious and shed in the feces of infected individuals. These infective particles can spread onto contaminated surfaces by infectious excreta and can then infect multiple patients from a single contaminated source.

Q14. Answer c

The Six Sigma DMAIC (Define, Measure, Analyze, Improve, and Control) methodology can be thought of as a roadmap for problem solving and product/process improvement. Six Sigma "DMAIC" approach is effective in reducing the HAI rate.

> Eldridge NE, Woods SS, Bonello RS, et al. Using the Six Sigma process to implement the centers for disease control and prevention guideline for hand hygiene in 4 Intensive Care Units. J Gen Intern. 2006;21 Suppl 2:S35-42.

Q15. Answer a

Modes of spread of MRSA- Patients "colonized" with MRSA may carry the bacteria on skin or in nose. MRSA may spread from person to person by: touching the skin or contaminated surface (such as a countertop, door handle, or phone). Other patients admitted in the ICU may have risk factors for MRSA infection such as a surgical wound and/or intravenous (IV) line, being hospitalized for a prolonged period of time, recent use of antibiotics, having a weakened immune system due to a medical condition or its treatment, being in close proximity to other patients, family members, etc.

In addition to Standard Precautions, Contact Precautions are needed for specified patients known or suspected to be infected or colonized with epidemiologically important microorganisms that can be transmitted by direct contact with the patient (hand or skin-to-skin contact that occurs when performing patient-care activities that require touching the patient's dry skin) or indirect contact (touching) with environmental surfaces or patient-care items in the patient's environment (Category IB).

Precautions to Prevent Spread of MRSA. Available from: https://www.cdc.gov/mrsa/healthcare/clinicians/precautions.html (Accessed 13 February 2018).

Q16. Answer c

The problem of CLABSI has gained increasing attention in recent years. They cause a great deal of morbidity and deaths, and increase healthcare costs. Central venous catheters (CVCs) are increasingly used in hospitals to manage critically ill patients. CRBSIs occurring in the intensive care unit (ICU) are common, costly and potentially lethal. CRBSIs are considered among the first and most "preventable" classes of nosocomial infections. Patients with CVCs are at risk of developing local as well as systemic infectious complications like local insertion-site infection, CRBSI, septic thrombophlebitis, endocarditis and other metastatic infections. The most serious complications are bacteremia, sepsis and death. The definitive diagnosis of catheter infection can be made by using a combination of clinical signs and symptoms together with the quantitative culture techniques. CVC catheterization is often associated with serious infectious complications, mostly CRBSI, resulting in significant morbidity, increased duration of hospitalization and additional medical costs. The majority of CRBSIs are associated with CVCs, and the relative risk for CRBSI is significantly greater with CVCs than with peripheral venous catheters. CRBSI is associated with high rates of morbidity and mortality in critically ill patients.

Pronovost PJ, Berenholtz SM, Goeschel CA. Improving the quality of measurement and evaluation in quality improvement efforts. Am J Med Qual. 2008;23:143-6.

Q17. Answer d

Annual flu vaccine is the first and best way to protect against influenza. This recommendation is same even during years when the vaccine composition remains unchanged from the previous season. Vaccination of HCP reduces the risk that HCP will become infected with influenza, thus reducing the risk of transmission to susceptible patients and co-workers. HCP excluded from work until at least 24 hours after they no longer have a fever or respiratory symptoms.

WHO Guidelines for Pharmacological Management of Pandemic Influenza A(H1N1) 2009 and other Influenza Viruses. Available from: http://www.who.int/csr/resources/publications/swineflu/h1n1_guidelines_pharmaceutical_mngt.pdf?ua=1 (13 February 2018).

Q18. Answer c

The bronchoscopy area should have engineering controls that will allow for negative air pressure, at least 14 air changes per hour.

Infection Control in the Bronchoscopy Suite. American Journal of Respiratory and Critical Care Medicine. 2003;167(8):1050-56.

Q19. Answer d

Isolation of patients is recommended for at least 24–48 hours after adequate antibiotic treatment (for elimination of carriage) and patients should not be admitted into an overcrowded ward. Respiratory droplet precautions (used in addition to standard precautions).

Guidelines for the management, prevention and control of Meningococcal Disease in south Africa. Available from: www.doh.gov.za 2011 (Accessed 13 February 2018).

Q20. Answer c

PEP is recommended when occupational exposures to HIV occur and the HIV status of the exposure source patient should be determined, if possible, to guide need for HIV PEP. PEP medication regimens should be started as soon as possible after occupational exposure to HIV, and they should be continued for 4 week duration. Follow-up HIV testing is typically concluded 6 months after an HIV exposure. Patients with an occupational exposure should seek treatment as soon as possible, as studies have shown the efficacy of postexposure HIV prophylaxis is highest when initiated within the first 72 hours of exposure.

> Kuhar DT, Henderson DK, Struble KA, et al. Updated US Public Health Service guidelines for the management of occupational exposures to human immunodeficiency virus and recommendations for postexposure prophylaxis. Infect Control Hosp Epidemiol. 2013;(9):875-92.

K Type Answers

Q1. Answer TTTTT

Nails should be short and clean and no nail polish or extensions. Wrist watches must not be worn. No other jewellery should be worn around the wrist. No rings with stones should be worn however one plain band is permitted. Sleeves must be short or rolled securely up to the elbow.

> 'Bare Below the Elbow' Supplementary Policy for Hand Hygiene 2.0
> 'Bare Below the Elbow' Supplementary Policy for Hand Hygiene. Available from: http://www.tamesidehospital.nhs.uk/documents/barebelowtheelbowsupplementpolicy.pdf (Accessed13 February 2018).

Q2. Answer FFFTF

Blood and body fluids, such as saliva, semen and vaginal fluid, can contain viruses that can be passed on to other people. Body fluids, like sweat, tears, vomit or urine have very low risk.

Semen and vaginal secretions should also be considered potentially contagious. Similarly, CSF, amniotic fluid, pleural fluid, synovial fluid, peritoneal and pericardial fluids carry a significant risk.

> Lohiya GS, Tan-Figueroa L, Lohiya S, Lohiya S. Human bites: bloodborne pathogen risk and postexposure follow-up algorithm. J Natl Med Assoc. 2013;105(1):92-5.

Q3. Answer TFFTT

Use a subclavian site, rather than a jugular or a femoral site, in adult patients to minimize infection risk for nontunneled CVC placement (Category IB).

There is no need to replace peripheral catheters more frequently than every 72–96 hours to reduce risk of infection and phlebitis in adults (Category IB).

Use a chlorhexidine/silver sulfadiazine or minocycline/rifampicin -impregnated CVC in patients whose catheter is expected to remain in place >5 days if, after successful implementation of a comprehensive strategy to reduce rates of CLABSI, the CLABSI rate is not decreasing (Category IA).

Use either sterile gauze or sterile, transparent, semipermeable dressing to cover the catheter site (Category IA).

Use povidone iodine antiseptic ointment or bacitracin/ gramicidin/polymyxin B ointment at the hemodialysis catheter exit site after catheter insertion and at the end of each dialysis session (Category IB).

> Guidelines for the Prevention of Intravascular Catheter-Related Infections. Available from: ww.cdc.gov/infectioncontrol/guidelines/bsi/recommendations.html (Accessed 13 February 2018).

Q4. Answer FTTTF

(1) Human tissues, organs, body parts—Yellow colored non-chlorinated plastic bags (2) Metallic body implants—Cardboard boxes with blue colored marking.

> Biosafety manual for public health laboratories Edition: July 2016
> National Centre for Disease Control Directorate General of Health Services Ministry of Health and Family Welfare.

Q5. Answer TFFTT

VAE includes all the conditions that result in a significant and sustained lowering of oxygenation, including both infectious and non-infectious etiology.

Tier 1: Ventilator-associated condition (VAC)—the patient develops hypoxemia for a sustained period of more than 2 days. The etiology of the hypoxemia is not considered.

Tier 2: Infection-related ventilator-associated complication (IVAC) —hypoxemia develops in background of generalized infection or inflammation, and antibiotics are given for a minimum of 4 days.

Tier 3: Probable or possible VAP —additional laboratory evidence of WBC or Gram stain of a respiratory specimen of acceptable quality, or (=possible)/and (=probable) presence of pathogens on quantitative cultures, in patients with IVAC.

>Lilly CM, Ellison RT 3rd. Quality measures for critically ill patients: where does ventilator-associated condition fit in? Chest. 2013;144(5):1429-30.

Q6. Answer TTFFF

Immunosuppressed patients in general should not receive live vaccines like BCG, MMR, oral polio, oral typhoid or rubella vaccine. Inactivated vaccines, such as influenza, hepatitis A or B, pneumococcal and adsorbed tetanus vaccine are permitted. Varicella immune globulin is used in immunosuppressed patients who have come into contact with chicken pox. Patients are advised to avoid eating foods likely to be contaminated like salads.

>Walter EA, Bowden RA. Infection in the bone marrow transplant recipient. Infect Dis Clin North Am. 1995;9:823-47.

>Rhame FS, Streifel AJ, Kersey JH, McGlave PB. Extrinsic risk factors for pneumonia in the patient at high risk of infection. Am J Med. 1984;76(Suppl 5A):42-52.

Q7. Answer TTTFT

Granulocyte transfusion does not appear to be beneficial, even in the presence of profound neutropenia.

>Rhame FS, Streifel AJ, Kersey JH, McGlave PB. Extrinsic risk factors for pneumonia in the patient at high risk of infection. Am J Med. 1984;76(Suppl 5A):42-52.

>Hassan IA, Chopra R, Swindell R, Mutton KJ. Respiratory viral infections after bone marrow/peripheral stem-cell transplantation: the Christie hospital experience. Bone Marrow Transplantation. 2003;32:73-77.

Q8. Answer TTTFF

Negative room air pressure with additional barriers including an anteroom (also known as Class Q) for quarantine isolation.
  A negative pressure Isolation Room requires 100% outside air ventilation (i.e. no return air permitted), with low level exhaust ducts.
Isolation Rooms.

>Available from: http://healthfacilityguidelines.com/Guidelines/ViewPDF/iHFG/iHFG_part_d_isolation_rooms (Accessed 13 February 2018).

Q9. Answer TTFTF

Daily sedation holds helps reduce patient time spent on the ventilator, and thus reduce the incidence of VAP. Head-up positioning of 30 to 45° reduces micro-aspiration, and thus VAP. Prone positioning impact on VAP rates per se is as yet unclear. Daily changes of ventilator tubing may increase the VAP risk due to cross-contamination from excess handling of equipment.

>Hunter JD. Ventilator-associated pneumonia. Br Med J. 2012;344:e3325.

>Guerin C, Reignier J, Richard JC, et al. Prone positioning in severe acute respiratory distress syndrome. Now Engl J Med. 2013:368(2):159-68.

Q10. Answer FFTTF

Positive culture from CVP could represent contamination, luminal colonization or CRBSI. The "Matching Michigan" project showed a post implementation mean rate of 1.4 CRBSI/1000 catheter days. Wire exchange not recommended for CRBSI.

>Bion J, Richardson A, Hibbert P, et al. 'Matching Michigan': a 2-year stepped interventional programme to minimise central venous catheter-blood stream infections in intensive care units in England. BMJ. 2012.

Q11. Answer FTFTT

For CAUTI prevention maintain closed drainage system. Urinary catheter should be placed and taped above the thigh.

> Lo E, Nicolle LE, Coffin SE, et al. Strategies to prevent catheter-associated urinary tract infections in acute care hospitals: 2014 update. Infect Control Hosp Epidemiol. 2014;35:464-79.

Q12. Answer e

A deep incisional infection is diagnosed if the deep tissues around an implant are infected within one year.

> **Protocol for surveillance of surgical site infection.** Health Protection Agency. Available from: http://www.hpa.org.uk/web/HPAwebFile/HPAweb_C/1194947388966 (Accessed 13 February 2018).

Q13. Answer FTTFT

PCNSI *Staphylococcus aureus* is a common etiology.

Shunt is an independent risk factor.

In a case of a shunt infection the early appropriate antibiotics and the removal of the shunt should be contemplated.

> McClelland S, Hall WA. Postoperative central nervous system infection: incidence and associated factors in 2111 neurosurgical procedures. Clin Infect Dis. 2007;45:55-59.

Q14. Answer TTTTT

> Moore ZC, Eden S, et al. Factors associated with acquisition of vancomycin-resistant enterococci (VRE) in roommate contacts of patients colonized or infected with VRE in a tertiary care hospital. Infection Control and Hospital Epidemiology. 2008;29(5):398-403.

Q15. Answer TTFTF

Establish and maintain surveillance for airborne environmental disease (e.g. aspergillosis) as appropriate during construction, renovation, repair, to ensure safety of immunocompromised patients. *Aspergillus* spp has been isolated from hospital water supply and implicated in outbreaks.

> Thio CL, Smith D, Merz WG. et al. Refinements of environmental assessment during an outbreak investigation of invasive aspergillosis in a leukemia and bone marrow transplant unit. Infect Control Hosp Epidemiol. 2000;21:18-23.

Q16. Answer TTTFF

Damp sweeping is done to avoid possible aerosolization of virus Mask is removed by grasping elastic behind ears and front portion of mask should not be touched.

> World Health Organization. Seasonal influenza. In. WHO website 2016, Available from: http://www.who.int/mediacentre/factsheets/fs211/en/ (Accessed 13 February 2018).

Q17. Answer FTTFF

Patients with VAT, we suggest not providing antibiotic therapy (*weak recommendation, low-quality evidence*).

For patients with VAP, we recommend a 7-day course of antimicrobial therapy rather than a longer duration (*strong recommendation, moderate-quality evidence*).

For patients with suspected HAP/VAP, we suggest not using the CPIS to guide the discontinuation of antibiotic therapy *(weak recommendation, low-quality evidence)*.

> Management of Adults With Hospital-acquired and Ventilator-associated Pneumonia: 2016 Clinical Practice Guidelines by the Infectious Diseases Society of America and the American Thoracic Society. Available at: www.idsociety.org/Guidelines/Patient_Care/IDSA_Practice_Guidelines/Infections_by_Organ_System/Lower/Upper_Respiratory/Hospital-Acquired___Ventilator_-_Associated_Pneumonia_(HAP/VAP)/#recommendations (Accessed 13 February 2018).

Q18. Answer FTFTT

Invasive burn wound infections due to *Candida* spp., *Aspergillus* spp., and other opportunistic fungi (including *Alternaria* spp., *Fusarium* spp., *Rhizopus* spp., and *Mucor* spp.) are important emerging causes of late onset morbidity and mortality in patients with major burns.

> Weber JM. Epidemiology of Infections and Strategies for Control. In: Carrougher GJ (Ed). Burn Care and Therapy. St. Louis, MO: Mosby, Inc; 1998: pp. 185-211.

Q19. Answer TTFTF

HCP who have received hepatitis B vaccine and developed immunity to the virus are at virtually no risk for infection. For a susceptible person, the risk from a single needle stick or cut exposure to HBV-infected blood ranges from 6–30% and depends on the hepatitis B antigen (HBeAg) status of the source individual. HBsAg positive individuals who are HBeAg positive are more likely to transmit HBV than those who are HBeAg negative. While there is a risk for HBV infection from exposures of mucous membranes or non-intact skin, there is no known risk for HBV infection from exposure to intact skin.

Hepatitis B immune globulin (HBIG) alone or in combination with vaccine (if not previously vaccinated) is effective in preventing HBV infection after an exposure. The decision to begin treatment is based on several factors.

Postexposure treatment should begin as soon as possible after exposure, preferably within 24 hours, and no later than 7 days.

Exposure to Blood What Healthcare Personnel Need to Know

Information from the Centers for Disease Control and Prevention National Center for Infectious Diseases Divison of Healthcare Quality Promotion and Division of Viral Hepatitis. Available from: www.cdc.gov/hai/pdfs/bbp/exp_to_blood.pdf (Accessed 13 February 2018).

Q20. Answer FFTTT

Gloves play a key role in preventing hand contamination, but glove use does not replace proper hand hygiene. Hand hygiene should always be performed both before and after any contact with patient, handling an indwelling catheter or the drainage system. Periurethral care should be gently performed using only soap and water.

Tambyah PA. Catheter-associated urinary tract infections: diagnosis and prophylaxis. Int J Antimicrob Agents. 2004;24 (Suppl 1):S44-S8.

CHAPTER 21

Model Question Papers

MODEL QUESTION PAPER I
Jaya Susan Jacob, Nita George

A Type Questions
(One best answer)

A1. **Cardiogenic shock due to RV failure can be treated by all of the following EXCEPT:**
   a. Adequate FiO_2
   b. Volume expansion
   c. Inhaled nitric oxide
   d. IV Nitroglycerine
   e. Levosimendan

A2. **Treatment of C. difficile infection includes all the following EXCEPT:**
   a. Stopping all antibiotics
   b. IV vancomycin
   c. Subtotal colectomy
   d. Oral fidaxomicin
   e. Fecal transplantation

A3. **Scorpion envenomation:**
   a. Causes coagulopathy
   b. Results in tetany
   c. Causes hypophosphatemia
   d. Results in 'adrenergic storm'
   e. Should be treated primarily with corticosteroids

A4. **Which of the following is true in acute respiratory distress syndrome (ARDS)?**
   a. Permissive hypercapnia is permitted in all patients with ARDS
   b. Recruitment maneuvers (RMs) have been shown to decrease mortality
   c. Higher Positive End-Expiratory Pressures (PEEP) is associated with improved survival
   d. Driving pressure was most strongly associated with survival
   e. Pressure control modes are better than volume control modes

A5. **Most common vascular injury reported with central venous cannulation is:**
   a. Right atrial perforation
   b. Vena Caval injury
   c. Arterial puncture
   d. Mediastinal perforation
   e. Pericardial tamponade

A6. **The role of damage control surgery in blast injuries is:**
   a. Early recognition of patients likely to benefit from surgery
   b. Relies on resuscitation first and subsequent surgery
   c. Emphasizes the importance of early correction of the altered anatomy
   d. Is ineffective in preventing development of the 'lethal triad'
   e. Indicated in less severe or non life-threatening injuries only

A7. **The medication that is ineffective in preventing delirium in the critically ill patients is:**
   a. Risperidone
   b. Haloperidol

c. Rivastigmine
d. Dexmedetomidine
e. Low dose ketamine

A8. **Most likely cause of persistent abdominal pain in a patient with organophosphorus poisoning and low pseudocholinesterase level is:**
a. Intestinal obstruction
b. Mesenteric ischemia
c. Acute pancreatitis
d. Hepatitis
e. Gallbladder calculi

A9. **Medication errors in critically ill patients:**
a. Lead to more harm to patients outside of the ICU than in the ICU
b. Is the single most common type of error in healthcare
c. Are more commonly prescription errors than administration errors
d. Transdermal drug delivery is an effective and safe alternative to subcutaneous route
e. Are more likely to be reported than those occurring in patients admitted in wards

A10. **Acute kidney injury (AKI) occurring as a consequence of snake bite is commonly caused by all of the following EXCEPT:**
a. Severe persistent hypotension leading to acute tubular necrosis
b. Rhabdomyolysis and subsequent myoglobinuria
c. Vasculitis
d. Volume overload from transfusions
e. Acute extracapillary proliferative glomerulonephritis

A11. **With regard to the use of N-acetyl cysteine (NAC) for the treatment of paracetamol poisoning:**
a. Oral route of administration of NAC is currently recommended in patients with early liver failure
b. Oral route of administration of NAC is recommended in pregnant patients
c. Standard oral regimen is for 21 hours as compared to intravenous regimen for 72 hours
d. Timely use of NAC improves prognosis of paracetamol poisoning
e. NAC should be continued until INR and ALT normalize

A12. **Cardiac output measurement by thoracic electrical bioimpedance (TEB) is reliable in the following conditions EXCEPT:**
a. Early cardiac failure
b. Severe septic shock
c. Rejection after heart transplantation
d. Drug resistant hypertension
e. Early recognition of shock in high risk trauma

A13. **Besides Oseltamivir treatment options for H1N1 infection includes:**
a. Ribavarin
b. Zanamivir
c. Ganciclovir
d. Amantadine
e. Valganciclovir

A14. **Rabies infection:**
a. Has an incubation period of 2-5 days
b. Is caused by Lyssa virus
c. Can be transmitted to humans from birds and reptiles as well
d. May result in Guillain Barre syndrome
e. Is more commonly transmitted through non-bite exposures

A15. **Acute viral encephalitis:**
a. Is a self-limiting disease in most cases
b. Is most commonly caused by adenovirus
c. Is confirmed by polymerase chain reaction (PCR) test for the virus in the cerebrospinal fluid (CSF)
d. Responds to steroid therapy
e. Is best diagnosed by CT imaging of the brain

A16. **Methicillin resistant Staphylococcus aureus (MRSA) infections can be treated with all of the following EXCEPT:**
a. Ticarcillin
b. Vancomycin
c. Linezolid
d. Daptomycin
e. Ceftobiprole

A17. **The trigger for developing posterior reversible encephalopathy syndrome (PRES) is commonly:**
a. Severe hypotension
b. Acute hypertension
c. Drug intoxication
d. Acute psychotic illness
e. Seizures

A18. New onset refractory status epilepticus (NORSE) is usually caused by:
a. Severe hyponatremia
b. Drug intoxication
c. Traumatic brain injury
d. Autoimmune encephalitis
e. Intracranial space occupying lesion

A19. Refeeding syndrome:
a. Is seen in patients who have had little or no nutritional intake for at least > 10 days
b. Is precipitated by high lipid load
c. Can be associated with respiratory and neuromuscular complications
d. Maybe prevented with a diet supplying around 2000 kcal
e. Can be minimized with antacid and proton pump inhibitor therapy

A20. Ventilator Associated Pneumonia (VAP) prevention may include all EXCEPT:
a. Selective digestive decontamination (SDD)
b. Use of silver coated endotracheal tubes
c. Use of subglottic suction endotracheal tube
d. Chlorhexidine oral care
e. Avoiding re-intubation

A21. Basic practices recommended to prevent MRSA infection includes all EXCEPT:
a. Implementation of MRSA monitoring program
b. Promotion of hand hygiene
c. Contact precautions while handling MRSA colonized patients
d. Decolonization of close healthy contacts of MRSA colonized patients
e. MRSA risk assessment

A22. Side effects of chronic inhaled anticholinergics in elderly patients include all EXCEPT:
a. Osteoporosis
b. Supraventricular tachycardias
c. Paradoxical bronchoconstriction
d. Blurred vision
e. Acute glaucoma

A23. Antibiotic dosing in a patient on extracorporeal membrane oxygenation (ECMO) is affected by all of the following EXCEPT:
a. Drug sequestration in circuit
b. Increased Vd
c. Increased drug clearance
d. Capillary leakage
e. Vasodilation and capillary leak

A24. In patients with severe pulmonary artery hypertension (PAH), medication recommended as first-line therapy is:
a. Iloprost
b. Sildenafil
c. Treprostinil
d. Epoprostenol
e. Bosentan

A25. Full resuscitation of the severely injured patient results in:
a. Producing the 'no-reflow' phenomenon
b. Restoring 'fluid creep'
c. Hemostatic resuscitation
d. End organ homeostasis
e. Activation of noradrenergic axis

A26. The salient source of strain among family members of critically ill patients in the ICU is:
a. Finance
b. Depression
c. Decision-making burden
d. Treatment preferences
e. Treatment withdrawal

A27. The osmotic demyelization syndrome is seen as a result of:
a. Rapid correction of hyponatremia
b. Seen more in acute hyponatremia
c. Risk of developing this syndrome is much less alcoholics
d. It is less often seen in malnourished patients.
e. ADH therapy is the antidote to this therapy

A28. Regarding viral hemorrhagic fever with renal syndrome (HFRS):
a. Is autoimmune in origin
b. Affects young adults maximally
c. Is self-limiting
d. Most serious type is caused by Hantaan virus infection
e. Rarely requires dialysis

A29. The cornerstone of medical management in the treatment of acute aortic dissection is:
a. Control of heart rate by beta blockers
b. Control of blood pressure by nitrates
c. Analgesia by opioids
d. Rhythm control by antiarrhythmics
e. Maintaining urine output by adequate fluids

A30. **Vagal maneuvers used to terminate SVT:**
   a. Valsalva maneuver is more effective than carotid sinus massage
   b. Carotid sinus massage can be performed in all age groups
   c. May be repeated multiple times
   d. Should be attempted only when medical management fails
   e. May be performed in patients with hemodynamically stable and unstable SVT

A31. **A clinical sign often overlooked in a patient with abdominal sepsis is:**
   a. Stool consistency
   b. Hypothermia
   c. Skin color
   d. Altered mental state
   e. Gastric residuals

A32. **All of the following are accepted treatment modalities for the management of severe ovarian hyperstimulation syndrome (OHSS) EXCEPT:**
   a. Subcutaneous heparin
   b. Hyperosmolar intravenous therapy with 25% albumin
   c. Saline infusions
   d. Abdominal paracentesis
   e. Surgical aspiration of cysts

A33. **The primary cause of death in severe pulmonary embolism is:**
   a. PE induced myocarditis
   b. Right ventricular (RV) failure
   c. Ventricular desynchronization
   d. Acute RBBB
   e. Resultant catecholamine storm

A34. **Noninvasive positive pressure ventilation (BPAP) may be considered in all the following conditions EXCEPT:**
   a. Hypercapnic respiratory failure
   b. Acute hypoxemic respiratory failure
   c. Cardiogenic pulmonary edema
   d. Respiratory arrest
   e. Weaning from mechanical ventilation in COPD

A35. **All of the following drugs can cause lactic acidosis in a critically ill patient EXCEPT:**
   a. Acetaminophen
   b. Highly active antiretroviral therapy (HAART)
   c. Linezolid
   d. Isoniazid
   e. Propofol

A36. **Heparin induced thrombocytopenia (HIT):**
   a. Can occur spontaneously without previous heparin exposure
   b. Causes severe thrombocytopenia
   c. Causes a bleeding tendency
   d. Unfractionated Heparin should be replaced by low molecular weight heparin (LMWH) for the treatment of HIT
   e. HIT can be treated with platelet transfusions

A37. **Invasive mechanical ventilation (IMV) for the treatment of acute respiratory failure may be indicated in the following clinical situations in critically ill cancer patients:**
   a. When no further life-extending anticancer therapies are available
   b. Patients undergoing 'ICU trial'
   c. Uncontrolled or refractory acute graft-versus-host disease after allogeneic stem cell transplant
   d. With lifespan of <1 year under ongoing anticancer therapy
   e. Those with poor performance status/bedridden over the past months

A38. **Clinically relevant severe hypothyroidism that is reversible upon withdrawal of the offending medication is seen with the use of:**
   a. Nitroglycerine
   b. Norepinephrine
   c. Phenylephrine
   d. Dopamine
   e. Epinephrine

A39. **The following statement is incorrect with regard to heparin induced thrombocytopenia (HIT):**
   a. Pathological antibodies to heparin-platelet factor 4 complex are formed
   b. Unfractionated heparin (UFH) is more immunogenic than low molecular weight heparin (LMWH)
   c. The resultant thrombocytopenia commonly causes severe bleeding
   d. Once the antibody titers are low, heparin can be given again
   e. Classical onset HIT occurs between 5-10 days after exposure to heparin

A40. **Idiopathic chronic pericardial effusion:**
   a. Exhibit features of distress early in the course of the disease

b. Has good prognosis
   c. Is treated with a course of corticosteroids
   d. May present with tamponade in the presence of hypovolemia
   e. Wide anterior pericardiectomy is the surgical treatment of overt tamponade

A41. **Bedside tools to facilitate weaning in ventilated patients with cervical spinal cord injuries include:**
   a. Pulse oximetry
   b. Diaphragmatic fluoroscopy
   c. Phrenic nerve conduction studies
   d. Spirometry
   e. Diaphragm needle electromyography

A42. **Leukoreduction (LR) of blood components has been proven to reduce the incidence of all of the following EXCEPT:**
   a. Febrile non-hemolytic transfusion reactions (FNHTR)
   b. Transfusion related acute lung injury (TRALI)
   c. HLA alloimmunization
   d. CMV transmission
   e. Platelet refractoriness

A43. **In normal cells, the largest intracellular source of reactive oxygen species (ROS) is:**
   a. Ribosomes
   b. Cytoplasm
   c. Golgi apparatus
   d. Mitochondria
   e. Peroxisomes

A44. **Endovascular treatment of intracranial atherosclerotic disease:**
   a. Is the current recommended primary treatment modality
   b. Aggressive blood pressure, diabetes, and dyslipidemia management per stroke guidelines are secondary considerations
   c. Perforator stroke may arise as a result of the 'snow plow' effect
   d. Bare metal stents and drug eluting stents are equally effective
   e. Acute stent thrombosis is the most life threatening peri procedure complication observed

A45. **In patients with traumatic brain injury decompressive craniectomy is advised for:**
   a. Elderly patients with head injury
   b. Prevention of development of intracranial hypertension
   c. When systemic disease does not allow implementation of aggressive ICH lowering measures
   d. In patients who are otherwise unlikely to survive > 24 hours
   e. As second-tier therapeutic arsenal in patients with refractory ICH to first-tier therapeutic measures

A46. **Immunonutrition in a surgical patient undergoing elective surgery:**
   a. Is beneficial only when administered in preoperative period
   b. Is beneficial in patients with severe sepsis
   c. Should be considered along with carbohydrate loading in preoperative period
   d. Is recommended through parenteral route
   e. Has shown good outcomes only in patients undergoing major abdominal surgery

A47. **Temporary manual occlusion of the aorta at the diaphragmatic hiatus during damage control surgery has all the following advantages EXCEPT:**
   a. Augmentation of cerebral perfusion
   b. Reduction of myocardial ischemia
   c. Quick control of abdominal exsanguination
   d. Prevention of visceral ischemia
   e. Facilitating volume replacement

A48. **Early interventional management of STEMI incorporates all of the following EXCEPT:**
   a. Primary PCI
   b. Intravenous fibrinolytic therapy
   c. Drug eluting stents
   d. Thrombus aspiration during PCI
   e. Radial artery access

A49. **ICU acquired hypernatremia may be caused by all of the following EXCEPT:**
   a. Fluid restriction
   b. Furosemide
   c. Dopamine
   d. Hydrocortisone
   e. 0.9% NaCl diluent for drug administration

A50. **In a parturient, disseminated intravascular coagulation (DIC) may complicate all the following conditions EXCEPT:**
   a. Abruption
   b. Amniotic fluid embolism
   c. Uterine atony
   d. Severe pre eclampsia
   e. Uterine sepsis

K Type Questions
[Marked True (T)/False (F)]

K1. '20 Minute Whole Blood Clotting Test' is performed during diagnostic phase of snake bite. Mark the following statements true/false in this regard:
   a. The reliability is inconsistent
   b. Fresh venous blood is drawn to perform the test
   c. Accuracy is improved when the test samples are maintained at body temperature
   d. Plastic tubes and syringes may give false readings

K2. Latest surviving sepsis guidelines recommend:
   a. Protocolized fluid resuscitation in patients with evidence of tissue hypoperfusion
   b. Target a CVP of 8-12 mm Hg
   c. Target a MAP of ≥ 65 mm Hg
   d. Target a central venous oxygen saturation of > 70%

K3. Mortality in acute iron overdose is a result of:
   a. GI bleeding
   b. Mitochondrial failure
   c. Hepatotoxicity
   d. Myocardial failure

K4. Etiology of rhabdomyolysis in acute alcohol intoxication includes:
   a. Coma
   b. Acid base disturbances
   c. Disruption of adenosine triphosphatase pump
   d. Direct toxic effect on skeletal muscles

K5. Successful resuscitation of established local anesthetic systemic toxicity (LAST) requires:
   a. Lipid emulsion therapy as first priority
   b. High quality basic life support
   c. Low dose epinephrine
   d. Vasopressin

K6. In a suspected case of corrosive poisoning treatment modalities include:
   a. Dilution of gastric contents
   b. Proton pump inhibitors
   c. Systemic steroids
   d. Prophylactic antibiotics

K7. Domestic cat and dog bite wounds cause infections from:
   a. Pasteurella
   b. Fusobacterium
   c. Capnocytophaga
   d. Methicillin resistant staphylococcus aureus

K8. Management of crush syndrome utilizes:
   a. Isotonic saline
   b. Mannitol
   c. Sodium bicarbonate
   d. Restrictive fluid resuscitation

K9. The following drugs in excess may cause hyperthermia:
   a. Cocaine
   b. Alcohol
   c. Lithium
   d. Monoamine oxidase inhibitors

K10. Type 3 cardiorenal syndrome occurs when:
   a. Acute kidney injury (AKI) precipitates development of acute cardiac injury
   b. Secondary to cirrhosis of the liver
   c. May be triggered by AKI related volume overload
   d. As a consequence of acute left ventricular dysfunction and accelerated fibrosis associated with AKI

K11. Monoclonal antibody therapy targeting B lymphocytes increases risk of reactivation of:
   a. Hepatitis B virus
   b. Cytomegalovirus
   c. Pneumocystis jiroveci
   d. Herpes simplex

K12. The treatment of acute onset severe hypertension during labor in a pregnant woman is with intravenous:
   a. Labetolol
   b. Enalaprilat
   c. Nicardipine
   d. Hydralazine

K13. Possible pathogenesis of Amniotic fluid embolism (AFE):
   a. Mechanical obstruction of pulmonary vessels by fetal squames
   b. Immune response to fetal antigens
   c. Complement system activation
   d. Coagulation system activation

K14. Nasotracheal intubation is absolutely contraindicated in:
   a. Epiglottitis

b. Midface instability
c. Patients with prosthetic heart valves
d. Apnea

K15. Infectious diseases transmitted by Aedes mosquito include:
a. Zika fever
b. Dengue
c. Japanese encephalitis
d. Chikungunya

K16. MDR-TB treatment regimens utilize:
a. Kanamycin
b. Amikacin
c. Ciprofloxacin
d. Capreomycin

K17. Management of posterior reversible encephalopathy syndrome (PRES) includes:
a. Corticosteroids
b. Ultrafiltration
c. Aggressive blood pressure management
d. Delivery in eclampsia

K18. Refractory status epilepticus is treated with anesthetics such as:
a. Propofol
b. Ketamine
c. Inhaled anesthetics
d. Barbiturates

K19. Trace elements that have been implicated in long-term toxicity of TPN solutions include:
a. Aluminum
b. Selenium
c. Chromium
d. Manganese

K20. Central line associated blood stream infections (CLABSI) can be prevented by:
a. Antimicrobial impregnated CVCs in adult patients
b. Alcohol containing dressings for CVCs
c. Antimicrobial locks for CVCs
d. Silver zeolite impregnated umbilical catheters in preterm infants

K21. The following statements are true about Retapamulin:
a. It is a pleuromutilin topical antibiotic
b. The spectrum of activity includes S. pyogenes and S. aureus
c. It is moderately active against gram negative and anaerobic bacteria
d. The most common adverse effect is local pruritus

K22. Major obstetric hemorrhage may be managed with the following techniques to avoid hysterectomy:
a. Uterine compression sutures
b. Intrauterine balloon tamponade
c. Intra-arterial balloon occlusion
d. IR arterial embolization

K23. Pharmacological therapy for ARDS to reduce mortality include:
a. Glucocorticoids
b. Nitric oxide
c. Surfactant
d. Statins

K24. The benefits of permissive hypercapnia in the management of severe ARDS are:
a. Increase in cardiac output
b. Leftward shift of oxygen dissociation curve
c. Anti-inflammatory effect
d. Potentiation of hypoxic pulmonary vasoconstriction

K25. Disadvantages of combination antimicrobial therapy includes:
a. Antibacterial synergy
b. Increased drug toxicity
c. Risk of superinfection
d. Possible antagonism

K26. Delivery of nebulized medications can be improved by:
a. Increasing the I:E ratio
b. Increasing inspiratory flow
c. Aerosol particle size 1-3 μm
d. Removing the heat/moisture exchanger

K27. Aggressive fluid resuscitation in a critically injured patient is necessary to:
a. Minimize secondary central nervous system (CNS) injury
b. Resolve critical acid–base and electrolyte disorders
c. Restore normothermia
d. Treat occult injuries

K28. "ABCDs" of dignity-conserving care in the dying patient deal with:
a. Attitudes
b. Behavior
c. Compassion
d. Drugs

K29. Viral hemorrhagic fevers are caused mainly by:
a. Filoviruses

    b. Arenaviruses
    c. Bunyaviruses
    d. Reoviruses
K30. **Main causes of fatigue in a patient with end stage cardiac failure are:**
    a. Anorexia
    b. Overdiuresis
    c. Beta blocker therapy
    d. Paroxysmal nocturnal dyspnea
K31. **Signs of acute aortic dissection seen on chest X-ray are:**
    a. Mediastinal widening
    b. Cardiac apical displacement
    c. Tracheal deviation to right
    d. Calcium sign
K32. **The role of magnesium in the treatment of acute asthma:**
    a. Is hampered by the side effects of inhaled magnesium in children
    b. Should be offered as first line in management of severe asthma
    c. Both intravenous and nebulization therapy should be employed in patients with life-threatening exacerbation
    d. Is superior to other treatment modalities
K33. **The recommended pharmacological treatment for termination of paroxysmal supraventricular tachycardia is:**
    a. Metoprolol
    b. Adenosine
    c. Verapamil
    d. Diltiazem
K34. **Consequences of paralytic ileus include:**
    a. Bacterial translocation
    b. Intra-abdominal hypertension
    c. Fluid sequestration with volume overload
    d. Abdominal compartment syndrome
K35. **Regarding specialty nutrition formulations:**
    a. Omega 3 fatty acids are recommended in ARDS
    b. Branched chain amino acids are to be given in hepatic encephalopathy
    c. High fat formulations are useful to wean off patients from the ventilator
    d. Immune-modulating enteral formulations with arginine may be useful in postoperative patients and patients with severe trauma

K36. **Important aspects to be considered in the management of asymptomatic bacteriuria are:**
    a. Prior treatment with antibiotics is the most important determinant
    b. Patients with chronic indwelling catheters maybe having continuous bacteriuria
    c. Acquisition of bacteriuria with an indwelling catheter is less common in adult male patients
    d. In acute care facilities, outbreaks of resistant organisms may be sourced to bacteria colonizing drainage bags
K37. **Risk factors for microaspiration in an intubated and mechanically ventilated patient are:**
    a. Underinflation of tracheal cuff
    b. Application of PEEP
    c. Tracheal suctioning
    d. Longitudinal folds in high-volume low-pressure cuffs
K38. **Respiratory failure in patients with pulmonary embolism results from:**
    a. Ventilation-perfusion mismatch
    b. Right to left shunting
    c. Hemodynamic instability
    d. Pulmonary artery occlusion
K39. **Investigative modalities for suspected pulmonary embolism in a pregnant patient are:**
    a. D-dimer testing
    b. Pulmonary angiography
    c. Lung scintigraphy
    d. CT angiography
K40. **Drugs recommended in the treatment of severe chemotherapy induced diarrhea (CID) are:**
    a. Budesonide
    b. Tincture of opium
    c. Octreotide
    d. Loperamide
K41. **Resuscitation failure is commonly seen following cardiac arrest in cancer patients with:**
    a. Acute renal failure
    b. Refractory shock
    c. On mechanical ventilation
    d. Sudden unexpected cardiac arrest

K42. **Hypothyroidism in a critically ill patient with prolonged ICU stay is related to:**
   a. Reduced hypothalamic stimulation of thyrotropes
   b. Increased pulsatility of TSH secretion
   c. Low plasma T3
   d. Low plasma T4

K43. **Established coagulopathy in a critically ill patient typically manifests with:**
   a. Immediate posttraumatic bleeding in coagulation abnormalities
   b. Delayed posttraumatic bleeding in severe thrombocytopenia
   c. Petechia in presence of thrombocytopathia
   d. Ecchymoses in patients with significant impairment of coagulation

K44. **Tools to differentiate persistent vegetative state from minimally conscious state include:**
   a. Glasgow Coma Scale
   b. Coma Remission Scale
   c. Aldrete's Scoring system
   d. Revised Coma Recovery Scale

K45. **In AKI, renal replacement therapy (RRT):**
   a. High dose CRRT (35 or 45 ml/kg/hour) is associated with lower mortality
   b. Positive fluid balance is associated with higher mortality in AKI
   c. CVVH improves mortality compared to IHD
   d. Removal of endotoxin by polymyxin B hemoperfusion improves mortality in sepsis

K46. **In critical illness survivors, posttraumatic stress disorder:**
   a. Is more prevalent in patients with comorbid psychopathology
   b. Maybe reduced with use of ICU diaries
   c. Is preventable with use of benzodiazepines for ICU sedation
   d. Occurs infrequently

K47. **Acute graft versus host disease mainly affects:**
   a. Skin
   b. Bone marrow
   c. Liver
   d. Gastrointestinal tract

K48. **'Rapid response teams' in health care settings:**
   a. Are aimed at replacing 'code teams'
   b. Comprise primarily of physicians, surgeons and intensivists
   c. Are intended to prevent deaths outside the ICU
   d. May increase hospital stay

K49. **In an unstable patient with blunt abdominal trauma and severe head injury:**
   a. Priority is given to the management of head injury
   b. Titrated fluid administration should be employed
   c. Simultaneous laparotomy and craniotomy may be indicated
   d. ICP monitoring may be beneficial

K50. **In the treatment of calcium channel blocker (CCB) poisoned patients, first-line therapy includes:**
   a. Monotherapy with high dose insulin
   b. Vasopressin monotherapy
   c. IV lipid emulsion therapy
   d. Dobutamine in presence of cardiogenic shock

ANSWERS

A Type Answers

QA1. Answer d

Definitive therapy for acutely decompensated RV failure requires primary treatment of the underlying condition in addition to hemodynamic support. Patients with RV failure are preload dependent. The initial treatment is volume expansion. In general, nitrates, morphine, diuretics, and other vasodilators should be avoided. However diuretics can be used judiciously when appropriate to decrease volume load on the distended RV. Hemodynamic support of the patient with decompensated RV failure may require combinations of vasopressors and inotropes such as dobutamine and norepinephrine. Milrinone and Amrinone (phosphodiesterase 3 inhibitor) increase contractility via a non-beta-adrenergic mechanism, do not increase myocardial oxygen demand, can be nebulized like prostaglandin, decreases pulmonary vascular resistance (PVR), i.e. afterload of the right ventricle but may cause hypotension. Levosimendan is calcium sensitizer with additional pulmonary vasodilatory effects.

Yucel E et al. Evidence based practice of critical care. 2nd Edn. Ch 54. 370-9.

QA2. Answer b

Metronidazole and oral vancomycin have been the mainstays of treatment for C. difficile infection. Fidaxomicin (200 mg twice a day for 10 days) a poorly absorbed, bactericidal, macrocyclic antibiotic with activity against specific anaerobic gram-positive bacteria, was approved by the Food and Drug Administration (FDA) in 2011. Options are limited for patients with severe colitis in whom vancomycin and fidaxomicin are ineffective. Emergency colectomy for fulminant C. difficile infection is associated with mortality as high as 80%. Other antibiotics that have activity against C. difficile are rifaximin, nitazoxanide, ramoplanin, teicoplanin, and tigecycline. However, because of limited data, high cost, unfavorable adverse-event profile, and resistance to C. difficile (associated with rifaximin in particular), the use of these agents is not recommended except in cases of unacceptable adverse effects associated with standard therapy, the need for salvage therapy for fulminant disease when surgery is not possible, and intractable recurrent infection. Fecal microbial transplantation, a procedure that was first reported in 1958, has recently emerged as an accepted, safe, and effective treatment for recurrent C. difficile infection.

Leffler DA et al. Clostridium difficile infection. N Engl J Med. 2015;372:1539-48.

QA3. Answer d

Overstimulation of the sympathetic system increases blood levels of catecholamines, resulting in a characteristic "adrenergic (autonomic) storm" which consists of cardiac (tachycardia, peripheral vasoconstriction, hypertension, diaphoresis), metabolic (hyperthermia, hyperglycemia), urogenital (bladder dilatation, urinary retention, ejaculation in males), respiratory (bronchial dilation, tachypnea), and neuromuscular (mydriasis, tremor, agitation, convulsions) complications.

It is indeed easy to treat pain with analgesics having an anti-inflammatory effect, such as salicylates.

Chippaux JP. Emerging options for the management of scorpion stings. Drug Des Devel Ther. 2012;6:165-73.

QA4. Answer d

The consequence of pressure and volume limited ventilation is permissive hypercapnia. There has been some suggestion that hypercapnic acidosis in ARDS may have an intrinsic protective effect beyond its associated ventilation strategies. However, surgical patient populations with concomitant cardiovascular disease or traumatic brain injury may suffer from the negative inotropic effects or increased intracranial pressure associated with hypercapnia, and should be avoided in these groups. The rationale for the use of RMs in ARDS is to promote alveolar recruitment, leading to an increased end-expiratory lung volume and thus decreased ventilator-induced lung injury (VILI). Not all patients respond to RMs and has not been shown to decrease mortality. At least two trials are ongoing to address whether RMs change the outcomes of ARDS patients. In an randomized control trial (RCT) of higher versus lower PEEP in patients with ARDS, a study of 549 patients showed no significant differences in mortality rates or the numbers of ventilator-free days, ICU-free days, or organ-failure- free days between the lower- and higher-PEEP study groups. As per a Cochrane review in 2015, currently available data from RCTs are insufficient to confirm or refute whether pressure-controlled or volume-controlled ventilation offers any advantage for people with ARDS. Driving pressure (ΔP) can be calculated at the bedside as plateau pressure minus positive end-expiratory pressure (Pplat − PEEP).

> Greer S. E et al. Acute respiratory distress syndrome and lung protective Ventilation. Principles of Adult Surgical Critical Care. 115-25.
>
> ARDSNET. Higher versus lower positive end-expiratory pressures in patients with the acute respiratory distress syndrome. N Engl J Med. 2004;351:327-36.

QA5. Answer c

While arterial injuries are more common, lacerations of the vena cava, mediastinal vessels, and right atrium have been reported. The proposed mechanism of these injuries is that the guidewire becomes trapped against a vessel wall, and subsequent insertion of dilator or catheter causes injury.

> Kornbau C, Lee KC, Hughes GD, et al. Central line complications. International Journal of Critical Illness and Injury Science. 2015;5(3):170-8.

QA6. Answer a

Damage control surgery is indicated when a person sustains an injury of such severity that it impairs their ability to maintain homeostasis. Severe hemorrhage then leads to triad of metabolic acidosis, hypothermia, and increased coagulopathy. This form of surgery puts more emphasis on preventing the above-mentioned trauma triad of death, rather than correcting the anatomy. A major component of the surgery is early recognition of a person who could benefit from it and thus patients are transported to the operating room upon arrival, and resuscitation ensues concurrently with surgery. Goals of damage control surgery to stop the bleeding remove contaminants and leave the wound open to avoid abdominal compartment syndrome.

> Samra T, Pawar M, Kaur J. Challenges in management of blast injuries in Intensive Care Unit: Case series and review. Indian J Crit Care Med. 2014;18(12):814-8.

QA7. Answer c

There is some evidence that delirium can be prevented. Outside the ICU, repeated reorientation, noise reduction, cognitive stimulation, vision and hearing aids, adequate hydration, and early mobilization can reduce the incidence of delirium in hospitalized patients. Haloperidol prophylaxis in patients undergoing hip surgery reduced the severity and duration of delirium. Four placebo-controlled trials have evaluated pharmacologic prophylaxis of delirium; low-dose haloperidol, low-dose risperidone and single low dose of ketamine during the induction of anesthesia reduced the incidence of delirium. Cholinesterase inhibitor rivastigmine was ineffective in preventing delirium. Sedation with dexmedetomidine rather than benzodiazepines appears to reduce the incidence of delirium in the ICU.

> Reade MC, Finfer S. Sedation and Delirium in the Intensive Care Unit . N Engl J Med. 2014;370:444-54.

QA8. Answer c

Organophosphate insecticides are the potent inhibitors of the acetylcholinesterase enzyme which lead to an increased acetylcholine activity, responsible for symptoms such as abdominal pain, diarrhea, vomiting and hypersalivation. Acute pancreatitis (toxic pancreatitis) is a rare complication of organophosphorus poisoning. It is mainly caused by acetylcholine release from the pancreatic nerves and the prolonged hyper stimulation of the acinar cells.

> L V, Rao VD, Rao MS, YM. Toxic pancreatitis with an intra-abdominal Abscess which was caused by organophosphate poisoning (OP). J Clin Diagn Res. 2013;7(2):366-8.

QA9. Answer b

Medication errors are estimated to account for 78% of all medical errors in ICUs, with an average of 1.75 medication errors per patient per day. Large volume resuscitations, positive pressure ventilation, surgical procedures, systemic inflammatory response, and changes in protein binding, all common in ICU patients, affect the pharmacokinetics of many drugs. Administration is vulnerable to error because it is the last step in the process before the patient receives the medication. Transdermal drug delivery is erratic in critically ill patients. Because perfusion to epidermal and subcutaneous tissue is often lower than normal, it can cause unpredictable and often less-than-optimal absorption. The transdermal route should not be a target for novel drug delivery in the critically ill patient population. Fear of negative consequences can be a major barrier to accurate reporting of errors, with as many as 50% to 96% going unreported.

    Kruer RM, Jarrell AS, Latif A. Reducing medication errors in critical care: a multimodal approach. Clinical Pharmacology: Advances and Applications. 2014;6:117-26.

QA10. Answer d

The pathogenesis of AKI due to snake bite may be multifactorial as follows: (1) Severe and persistent hypotension leading to acute tubular necrosis; (2) Myoglobin and rhabdomyolysis; (3) Part of DIC; (4) Vasculitis; (5) Acute diffuse interstitial nephritis; (6) Extracapillary proliferative glomerulonephritis etc.

    Ghosh S, Mukhopadhyay P, Chatterjee T. Management of snake bite in India. JAPI. 2016;64:11-14.

QA11. Answer d

NAC is used for the treatment of paracetamol (acetaminophen) overdose, mucolytic and dietary supplement, etc. Route of administration can be both intravenous and oral. Vomiting or altered mental status may preclude oral therapy. Patients who are treated for hepatic failure should receive intravenous therapy. Although these standard protocols are based on a prespecified duration of therapy, many toxicologists believe that the defined oral course (72 hours) is often too long and that the defined intravenous course (20 hours) may be too short for patients in whom hepatic injury develops or for those who have ingested massive amounts of acetaminophen. Treatment with intravenous NAC is preferred in pregnancy. Acetaminophen poisoning can have two situations: (1) Toxic acetaminophen concentration without liver injury and (2) Liver injury. NAC improves outcome in both of the two categories.

    Heard KJ. Acetylcysteine for Acetaminophen Poisoning. The New England journal of medicine. 2008;359(3):285-92.

QA12. Answer b

TEB is one of several noninvasive techniques that have been investigated to measure cardiac output and other hemodynamic parameters. TEB can be used for hemodynamic evaluation in circumstances such as: (1) Fluid management for heart failure; (2) Differentiation of cardiogenic from pulmonary causes of acute dyspnea (3) Optimization of atrioventricular interval in cardiac pacemakers; (4) Monitoring of patients for early diagnosis of rejection after heart transplantation; (5) Management of drug-resistant hypertension; (6) Evaluation of hemodynamic response in dehydrated patients; (7) Management of patients with severe cardiac illness during surgery; (8) Management of patients during intensive care; (9) Management of patients in the Emergency Department; (10) Noninvasive monitoring for early recognition; (11) Shock in high-risk trauma and surgical patients etc. TEB has been shown to have acceptable accuracy with lower cost per patient in those circumstances in which intracardiac pressures and mixed venous blood samples are not required.

    Stevanović P, Sćepanović R, Radovanović D, et al. Thoracic electrical bioimpedance theory and clinical possibilities in perioperative medicine. Signa vitae. 2008;3(1):S22-27.

QA13. Answer b

Presently government of India recommends Oseltamivir as a drug of choice which is available at all government health bodies. Human influenza A is susceptible to both oseltamivir and zanamivir, two antiviral medications approved for the prevention and treatment of influenza. Two classes of antiviral medication are available for the treatment of seasonal human influenza: (1) Neuraminidase inhibitors (oseltamivir and zanamivir) and (2) Adamantanes (rimantadine and amantadine). During the 2008-2009 influenza seasons, almost all circulating human influenza A (H1N1) viruses in the United States were resistant to oseltamivir. However, genetic and phenotypic analyses indicate that swine influenza is susceptible to oseltamivir and zanamivir but resistant to the adamantanes.

    Dandagi GL, Byahatti SM. An insight into the swine-influenza A (H1N1) virus infection in humans. Answer Lung India : Official Organ of Indian Chest Society. 2011;28(1):34-38.

QA14. Answer b

The genus Lyssa virus includes rabies virus and the antigenically and genetically related rabies like viruses: Lagos bat, Mokola, and Duvenhage viruses, and two suggested subtypes of European bat Lyssa viruses. Rabies virus is most commonly transmitted through the bite of an infected mammal, all of which may be susceptible, but to greatly varying degrees. In the United States, non-bite exposures were reported as the source of infection for only 5 (3 %) of the 154 cases reported from 1950 through 1980. Guillain-Barre syndrome may be mistaken for the paralytic form of rabies, and vice versa. The incubation period for rabies is typically 1-3 months but may vary from 1 week to 1 year, dependent upon factors such as the location of virus entry and viral load. Rabies is mostly transmitted to humans, and between animals, through the saliva of infected animals. Transmission is generally through a bite from any infected animal.

> Rupprecht CE. Rhabdoviruses: Rabies Virus. In: Baron S, editor. Medical Microbiology. 4th edition. Galveston (TX): University of Texas Medical Branch at Galveston; 1996. Chapter 61.

QA15. Answer c

Acute encephalitis constitutes a medical emergency. In most cases, the presence of focal neurological signs and focal seizures will distinguish encephalitis from encephalopathy. Acute disseminated encephalomyelitis is a non-infective inflammatory encephalitis that may require to be treated with steroids. The role of steroids in the treatment of acute viral encephalitis remains uncertain. Herpes simplex encephalitis (HSE) is the commonest sporadic acute viral encephalitis. Magnetic resonance imaging (MRI) of brain is the investigation of choice in HSE and the diagnosis may be confirmed by the PCR test for the virus in the CSF. With few exceptions (for example, acyclovir for HSE), no specific therapy is available for most forms of viral encephalitis. Mortality and morbidity may be high and long term sequelae are known among survivors. The emergence of unusual forms of zoonotic encephalitis has posed an important public health problem. Vaccination and vector control measures are useful preventive strategies in certain arboviral and zoonotic encephalitis.

> Chaudhuri A, Kennedy PGE. Diagnosis and treatment of viral encephalitis. Postgraduate Medical Journal. 2002;78:575-83.

QA16. Answer a

MRSA is resistant to penicillin-like beta-lactam antibiotics. However, a number of drugs still retain activity against MRSA, including glycopeptides (e.g., vancomycin and teicoplanin), linezolid, tigecycline, daptomycin, and even some new beta-lactams, such as ceftaroline and ceftobiprole.

> Ventola CL. The Antibiotic Resistance Crisis: Part 1: Causes and Threats. Pharmacy and Therapeutics. 2015;40(4):277-83.

QA17. Answer b

Hypertension is usually identifiable as most common trigger, but patients often have other comorbidities that may predispose them to developing PRES. Peak systolic blood pressure is usually between 170 mm Hg and 190 mm Hg, but 10-30% of patients have normal or only mildly elevated blood pressure.

> Hobson EV, Craven I, Blank SC. Posterior Reversible Encephalopathy Syndrome: A Truly Treatable Neurologic Illness. Peritoneal Dialysis International : Journal of the International Society for Peritoneal Dialysis. 2012; 32(6):590-4.

QA18. Answer d

NORSE is a rare condition characterized by the occurrence of a prolonged period of refractory seizures with no readily identifiable cause in otherwise healthy individuals. It is one of the causes of refractory status epilepticus (RSE) and super refractory status epilepticus (SRSE). Initially, the absence of a proven etiology was considered mandatory for the diagnosis of NORSE; however, recent reports have suggested autoimmune encephalitis as a common cause. Unidentified viral infections can also cause NORSE. As per a recent report, autoimmune encephalitis (paraneoplastic or non- paraneoplastic) is the most commonly identified cause of NORSE; however, half of these patients remain cryptogenic. Outcome of NORSE patients is generally poor but improves during the follow-up, and epilepsy develops in most patients.

> Dubey D, Kalita J, Misra UK. Status epilepticus: Refractory and super-refractory. Neurol India. 2017;65(Suppl S1):12-7.

QA19. Answer c

All patients who have had no or very little nutritional intake for >5 days are at risk of refeeding syndrome, which is associated with severe electrolyte abnormalities including hypokalemia, hypomagnesemia, and hypophosphatemia, caused by movement of phosphate, fluids, and other electrolytes intracellularly after a sudden carbohydrate load. A history of alcohol abuse or being on drugs such as insulin, chemotherapy, antacids, or diuretics are risk factors for developing refeeding syndrome. Refeeding syndrome can be associated with respiratory, cardiac, and neuromuscular complications. National Institute for Health and Care Excellence (NICE) guidelines advise commencing nutritional support at 50% of estimated energy requirements for 2 days in patients at risk of refeeding syndrome, thereafter increasing by 200–400 kcal every day. Nutrients and fluids should not be initiated without electrolytes and micronutrients. Close monitoring of serum potassium, magnesium, and phosphate levels is required once feeding has been initiated.

Macdonald K, Page K, Brown L. Parenteral nutrition in critical care. Contin Educ Anaesth Crit Care Pain. 2013;13:1-5.

QA20. Answer a

Some of the strategies to prevent VAP are: (1) Noninvasive positive pressure ventilation; (2) Daily weaning trials and sedation holidays; (3) Avoiding Reintubation; (4) Early tracheostomy when indicated; (5) Minimizing pooling of secretions above the endotracheal tube cuff by subglottic secretion endotracheal tube; (6) Oral hygiene that includes either chlorhexidine mouthwash or gel is associated with a 40% reduction in the odds of developing VAP. SDD is not practiced due to concerns about promoting the growth of resistant bacteria.

Yokoe DS, Anderson DJ, Berenholtz SM et al. A Compendium of Strategies to Prevent Healthcare-Associated Infections in Acute Care Hospitals: 2014 Updates. Infection control and hospital epidemiology : the official journal of the Society of Hospital Epidemiologists of America. 2014;35(8):967-77.

QA21. Answer d

Basic practices for preventing MRSA transmission and infection recommended for all acute care hospitals (1) Conducting MRSA risk assessment; (2) Implement an MRSA monitoring program; (3) Promote compliance with CDC or WHO hand hygiene recommendations; (4) Use contact precautions for MRSA-colonized and MRSA-infected patients; (5) Ensure cleaning and disinfection of equipment and the environment.

Yokoe DS, Anderson DJ, Berenholtz SM et al. A Compendium of Strategies to Prevent Healthcare-Associated Infections in Acute Care Hospitals: 2014 Updates. Infection control and hospital epidemiology : the official journal of the Society of Hospital Epidemiologists of America. 2014;35(8):967-77.

QA22. Answer a

Functional beta2-adrenoceptors are present in osteoblasts, and chronic use of beta-agonists has been implicated in osteoporosis. Inhaled anticholinergics are usually well-tolerated but may cause dry mouth, which can be troublesome in older people. Pupillary dilatation, blurred vision and acute glaucoma can occur from escape of droplets from loosely fitting nebulizer masks. Although ECG changes have not been seen in RCTs of long-acting inhaled anticholinergics, supraventricular tachycardias have been observed in a 5-year RCT of ipratropium bromide. Paradoxical bronchoconstriction can occur with inhaled anticholinergics as well as with beta-agonists, but tolerance has not been reported with anticholinergics. Anticholinergic drugs also cause central effects, most notably impairment of cognitive function, and these effects have been noted with inhaled agents.

Gupta P, O'Mahony MS. Potential adverse effects of bronchodilators in the treatment of airways obstruction in older people: recommendations for prescribing. Drugs Aging. 2008;25(5):415-43.

QA23. Answer c

Antibiotics are commonly required during ECMO; however, few data are available regarding antibiotic PK during ECMO. The major changes in ECMO are increased Vd and decreased drug clearance, although the extent of such changes remains poorly characterized. Antibiotic concentrations may be further altered during ECMO because of the circuit itself (with associated drug sequestration) and/or the associated systemic inflammation (with vasodilation and capillary leak).

Vincent JL, Bassetti M, François B, et al. Advances in antibiotic therapy in the critically ill. Crit Care. 2016;20:133.

QA24. Answer d

Epoprostenol is a synthetic analogue of prostacyclin, a naturally occurring substance in the body, which has effects on dilating blood vessels. Epoprostenol was approved for PAH by the United States FDA in 1995. Epoprostenol is an intravenous medication approved for the treatment of PAH in World Health Organization

(WHO). For patients with severe PAH, those patients who present with functional class IV disease or who progress and deteriorate while on therapy, the proceedings of the 5th World Symposium on Pulmonary Hypertension recommend first-line IV epoprostenol therapy, based on the highest level of evidence. Other PAH medications (ambrisentan, bosentan, iloprost, macitentan, riociguat, sildenafil, tadalafil and treprostinil) as monotherapy or initial combination therapy are recommended with lower evidence. Sequential combination therapy is advised for patients with severe PAH who do not adequately respond or deteriorate. Despite the evidence available for IV epoprostenol use in functional class IV patients, it has been shown that many patients die without having received epoprostenol therapy.

> Corris P, Degano B. Severe pulmonary arterial hypertension: treatment options and the bridge to transplantation. European Respiratory Review Dec. 2014;23(134):488-97.

QA25. Answer d

Once definitive hemostasis has been achieved, the patient may still be significantly hypo-perfused. Prolonged activation of the noradrenergic axis results in profound vasoconstriction, which may be aggravated by hypothermia. Hypoperfusion impairs cellular energetics and results in loss of endothelial integrity. Inflammatory cytokines and ischemia-reperfusion injury may result in cellular edema reducing the lumen of capillaries and producing the "no-reflow" phenomenon. Full resuscitation of the severely injured patient requires not only arrest of bleeding and restoring hemodynamic stability but also re-establishing micro-circulatory flow, restoring end-organ homeostasis, and repaying the "oxygen debt". Failure to do this may result in the development of subsequent organ dysfunction in the hemodynamically stable but still under-resuscitated patient. Therefore, assuring adequate completeness of resuscitation is the next critical challenge for the ICU physician after establishing hemostasis.

> Shere-Wolfe RF, Galvagno SM, Grissom TE. Critical care considerations in the management of the trauma patient following initial resuscitation. Scandinavian Journal of Trauma, Resuscitation and Emergency Medicine. 2012;20:68.

QA26. Answer c

Although preferences for decision-making roles vary among family members, physicians do not always clarify family preferences. Family members may lack confidence about their surrogate decision-maker role, regardless of the decision-making model, if they have had no experience as a surrogate or no prior dialogue with the patient about treatment preferences. Decision-making burden is postulated as a salient source of strain among family members of patients who are dying in the ICU; anxiety and depression are also prevalent.

> Cook D, Rocker G. Dying with Dignity in the Intensive Care Unit. N Engl J Med. 2014;370:2506-14.

QA27. Answer a

This syndrome is seen as a result of rapid correction of hyponatremia. It occurs due to sudden osmotic shrinkage of brain cells and is more commonly seen in correction of chronic hyponatremia since their brain volume has returned to near normal as a result of osmotic adaptive mechanisms. It is characterized by dysphasia, spastic quadriparesis, pseudobulbar palsy, mutism, delirium, coma, etc. The risk of osmotic demyelination syndrome (ODS) is high is alcoholics, malnutrition and hypokalemia. There is no specific treatment for this condition.

Sodium level in various infusate

Infusate	Sodium Level (mmol/L)
5% NaCl	855
3% NaCl	513
0.9% NaCl	154
Ringer Lactate	130
0.45% NaCl	77

> George GN. Osmotic demyelization syndrome. In: Kumar P (Ed). Renal replacement therapy – ICU Manual. 1st Edition. India: Jaypee Brothers Medical Publishers (P) Ltd, 2017.

QA28. Answer d

HFRS is caused by Hantaan virus (HTNV), Amur virus (AMV), Seoul virus (SEOV), Dobrava virus (DOBV), or Puumala virus (PUUV), each of which causes diseases with differing severity. HTNV or DOBV may cause the most severe form of HFRS and have the highest morbidity rates ranging from 5 to 10%. Kidney injury frequently occurs in HFRS and the most prominent pathological presentation is acute tubule interstitial nephritis following the infiltration of inflammatory cells. AKI often induces death in patients with HFRS, particularly in the oliguric phase. The elderly patients often develop severe AKI and are more likely to have shock, hematuria, thrombocytopenia and leukocytosis. The patients with severe AKI usually need dialysis or continuous blood purification and stay longer in hospital than non-AKI patients.

Jiang H, Du H, Wang LM, et al. Hemorrhagic Fever with Renal Syndrome: Pathogenesis and Clinical Picture. Frontiers in Cellular and Infection Microbiology. 2016;6:1.

QA29. Answer a

The cornerstone of medical management is beta blockade, titrated to a heart rate of 60 beats per minute. Widely available agents well suited to this purpose include metoprolol and esmolol, labetalol etc. When beta blockade has achieved its goal heart rate, blood pressure is the next therapeutic target. If systolic blood pressure is greater than 120 mm Hg, an additional agent should be added to lower blood pressure with a goal of less than 120 mm Hg, ideally titrated to as low a blood pressure as end organs allow.

Strayer RJ, Shearer PL, Hermann LK. Screening, Evaluation, and Early Management of Acute Aortic Dissection in the ED. Current Cardiology Reviews. 2012;8(2):152-7.

QA30. Answer a

Vagal maneuvers are an appropriate first treatment option in patients with hemodynamically stable SVT. Studies report an approximately 25% success rate, although reported rates vary widely in the literature (6–54%). The most commonly performed maneuvers are the Valsalva maneuver and carotid sinus massage. The increase in intrathoracic pressure resulting from the Valsalva maneuver stimulates aortic and carotid baroreceptors, causing an increase in vagal input into the atrioventricular node. Most recent studies advocate placing the patient in a supine position and attempting the maneuver for 15–20 seconds. The Valsalva maneuver has generally been shown to be most effective in adults, having a superior effect on SVT termination compared to carotid sinus massage. Caution is advised when considering whether to attempt carotid sinus massage in older patients, as there is a risk of carotid atheroembolism and stroke even in the absence of an audible bruit. No guidelines currently exist regarding the appropriate number of attempts prior to initiating other therapies, although most providers will try a maximum of 2 attempts. Several studies have suggested that vagal maneuvers are more effective in the termination of AVRT compared to AVNRT.

Sohinki D, Obel OA. Current trends in supraventricular tachycardia management. The Ochsner Journal. 2014;14(4):586-95.

QA31. Answer d

In a patient with abdominal sepsis, an often-overlooked clinical sign is altered mental status. This alteration initially may be so subtle that only close relatives can detect it. In ongoing sepsis, alterations in mental status can range from agitation, anxiety, somnolence, delirium, stupor, epileptic insult to coma. This is called septic or metabolic encephalopathy. Anorexia and nausea are frequent and may precede the emergence of abdominal pain by some time. Vomiting can be caused by hollow viscus obstruction or peritoneal inflammation. Other important elements are: the amount of gastric residuals, the aspect of gastric contents (feculent, bloody, bilious), and the presence of hematemesis. Diarrhea is another clinical sign and stool consistency can be changed (or mixed with blood) by alterations in gut mucosal flora or gut hypoperfusion. Fever is clearly the most common manifestation of abdominal sepsis, although it can be masked in immunocompromised patients with neutropenia or under corticosteroid therapy. A patient with severe sepsis can also present one with hypothermia. Some believe that the skin is the mirror of the "inner human being". If the skin is mottled the intestinal mucosa probably is too. One should look at the turgor of the skin and the presence or absence of sudor or sweating, and local or generalized signs of inflammation, the presence of central or peripheral cyanosis (livedo reticularis).

Blaser AR, Starkopf J, Malbrain MLNG. Abdominal signs and symptoms in intensive care patients. Anaesthesiol Intensive Ther. 2015;47(4):379-87.

QA32. Answer e

Severe OHSS is not common, but it is dangerous. Severe and critical forms of OHSS are potentially lethal disorders, and history taking and physical examination are paramount at the time of admission.

Medical treatment of severe OHSS is directed at maintaining intravascular blood volume. Simultaneous goals are correcting the disturbed fluid and electrolyte balance, relieving secondary complications of ascites and hydrothorax and preventing thromboembolic phenomena.

The main interventions are fluid management and correction of hypovolemia. These measures consist of initial fast intravenous administration of normal saline. Dextrose 5% in normal saline or normal saline is infused at a rate of 125–150 mL/hr with 4-hour tabulations of urine production. If urine production is restored or improved, a maintenance protocol is started. The patient should be closely monitored for clinical signs of overhydration. If urine output is unsatisfactory, hyperosmolar intravenous therapy is indicated with an infusion of 200 mL of 25% human albumin. The use of diuretics in patients with low urine production and hypovolemia is counterproductive and dangerous. To prevent thrombosis, subcutaneous heparin 5000–7500 U/d is begun on the first day of admission. It is stopped after adequate mobilization is achieved. To manage ascites, ultrasonographic-guided paracentesis is indicated if the patient has severe discomfort or pain or if she has pulmonary or renal compromise.

Kumar P, Sait SF, Sharma A, et al. Ovarian hyperstimulation syndrome. Journal of Human Reproductive Sciences. 2011;4(2):70-75.

QA33. Answer b

Acute PE interferes with both the circulation and gas exchange. RV failure due to pressure overload is considered the primary cause of death in severe PE.

2014 ESC Guidelines on the diagnosis and management of acute pulmonary embolism: The Task Force for the Diagnosis and Management of Acute Pulmonary Embolism of the European Society of Cardiology (ESC). European Heart Journal. 2014;35(43):3033-73.

QA34. Answer d

Multiple randomized, controlled trials have proven the benefits of BPAP in patients with hypercapnic respiratory failure resulting from an acute exacerbation of chronic obstructive pulmonary disease (COPD) and the benefits of both BPAP and CPAP in patients with cardiogenic pulmonary edema in the absence of shock or ischemia. BPAP has been shown to benefit patients with immune compromise, fever, and pulmonary infiltrates who have acute hypoxemic respiratory failure. It has also been shown to facilitate the transition from invasive ventilation to spontaneous breathing in patients with COPD. The only absolute contraindications to BPAP and CPAP are cardiac arrest and respiratory arrest.

Kelly CR, Higgins AR, Chandra S. Noninvasive Positive-Pressure Ventilation. N Engl J Med. 2015;372:e30.

QA35. Answer a

HAART has led to dramatic reductions in HIV-associated morbidity and mortality. However, lactic acidosis complicated this therapy, especially with the nucleoside and nucleotide reverse transcriptase inhibitor (NRTI)-based regimens: didanosine, stavudine, lamivudine, zidovudine, and abacavir. Combined use of these drugs further increases the risk of lactic acidosis. Linezolid is a long-term antibiotic against serious resistant Gram-positive organisms with adverse effects including bone marrow toxicity, optic/peripheral neuropathy, and lactic acidosis. Isoniazid is commonly used to treat tuberculosis. Dosing more than 300 mg/day can lead to refractory grand mal or localized seizure, coma, and lactic acidosis. Propofol is commonly used for induction and maintenance of anesthesia, sedation, and interventional procedures. Cases were reported on propofol-associated severe metabolic acidosis. Risk factors include severe head injury, critical illness, prolonged administration (>48 hours) of large doses (>4 mg/kg/hour, equivalent to 1.6 mmol/hour for a 70 kg person), and inborn errors of fatty acid oxidation.

Pham AQT, Xu LHR, Moe OW. Drug-Induced Metabolic Acidosis. F1000Research. 2015;4:F1000 Faculty Rev-1460.

QA36. Answer a

HIT is a potentially devastating immune mediated adverse drug reaction caused by the emergence of antibodies that activate platelets in the presence of heparin. Despite thrombocytopenia, bleeding is rare; rather, HIT is strongly associated with thromboembolic complications involving both the arterial and venous systems. Infection and surgical inflammation can also give rise to "spontaneous HIT" a clinical variant occurring without antecedent heparin exposure. Warfarin should not be used until the platelet count has recovered. The thrombocytopenia of HIT is typically of moderate severity, with median platelet counts ranging between 50–80×109/L. Severe thrombocytopenia (platelets < 15 × 10^9/L) is unusual. LMWH cannot be used in patients with HIT because of the strong cross reactivity of the HIT antibody with the LMWH-PF4 complex. Avoid prophylactic platelet transfusion because they may exacerbate the hypercoagulable state, leading to additional thrombosis.

<small>Ahmed I et al. Heparin induced thrombocytopenia: diagnosis and management update. Postgrad Med J. 2007;83:575-82.</small>

QA37. Answer b

The ICU trial is claimed as new admission policy for cancer patients requiring mechanical ventilation. Survival up to 40% in mechanically ventilated cancer patients who survived to day 5 and 21.8% overall can be expected. Reappraisal on day 6 in all nonbedridden cancer patients for whom lifespan extending cancer treatment is available. Such intensified intensive care measures of IMV or treatment of ARF may not be adequate for most patients in following situations: (1) no further life-extending anticancer therapies available; (2) uncontrolled or refractory acute graft-versus-host disease after allogeneic stem cell transplant; (3) lifespan of <1 year under ongoing anticancer therapy; (4) poor performance status/bedridden over the past months; (5) refusal of ICU admission by the patient.

<small>Schellongowski P, Sperr WR, Wohlfarth P et al. Critically ill patients with cancer: chances and limitations of intensive care medicine—a narrative review. ESMO Open. 2016;1(5):e000018.</small>

QA38. Answer d

Dopamine has been shown to induce clinically relevant and iatrogenic hypothyroidism in critically ill adults and children. Even in low doses, often used in ICU patients for a considerable amount of time, dopamine has shown to profoundly suppress TSH secretion, and to lower plasma T4 and T3 concentrations in adult and pediatric ICU patients, to levels that are compatible with severe iatrogenic hypothyroidism. Upon withdrawal of the dopamine infusion, the release of TSH was found to rebound, which brought about a substantial and sustained rise in T4 and T3. Treating pediatric ICU patients who are on a dopamine infusion with thyroid hormone was shown to improve intensive care outcome in a RCT.

<small>Van den Berghe G. Non-Thyroidal Illness in the ICU: A Syndrome with Different Faces. Thyroid. 2014;24(10):1456-65.</small>

QA39. Answer c

HIT is a rare, adverse drug reaction caused by heparin. It is an intensely prothrombotic disorder which can be fatal when there is a delay in diagnosis. High index of suspicion is to be maintained to facilitate diagnosis and treatment in this condition. The pathophysiology of HIT centers on the development of pathological antibodies to the combination of heparin and platelet factor 4 (PF4). These antibodies are able to activate platelets, triggering the release of their procoagulant substances and precipitating the development of pathological thrombus. Heparin binding causes a conformational change in the shape of the PF4 molecule, with loss of its negative charge. This facilitates coalescence of PF4 molecules and exposes new epitopes capable of generating an immune response. The activation and support of thrombin generation enables HIT to cause DIC. The probability of developing HIT is influenced by a patient's exposure to the different types of heparin. UFH is more immunogenic than LMWH. The antibody response is amnesiac and once the antibody has waned, usually after 100 days, the patient can be successfully re challenged with heparin. The timing of onset of the thrombocytopenia is of key importance; with classical onset HIT occurring between 5 and 10 days after exposure to heparin. A platelet count < 20 is uncommon and should prompt re-evaluation of the diagnosis. Bleeding, particularly mucocutaneous bleeding is unusual in HIT.

<small>Retter A, Barrett NA. The management of abnormal hemostasis in the ICU. Anesthesia. 2015;70:121-e41.</small>

QA40. Answer d

Most patients with a large (more than 20 mm), chronic (longer than 3 mo), idiopathic pericardial effusion are asymptomatic and may remain clinically stable for many years. However, this condition may entail a less than good prognosis, as unexpected overt tamponade can develop in up to 29% of such patients. The trigger of tamponade is unknown, but hypovolemia, paroxysmal tachyarrhythmias, and intercurrent acute pericarditis may precipitate tamponade; accordingly, these events should be vigorously managed. Medical therapy, particularly corticosteroids, colchicine or antituberculous therapy, is not useful. Pericardiocentesis is the first option in patients with overt tamponade. Elective pericardial drainage has to be performed as well in asymptomatic patients as a prophylactic measure to prevent unexpected tamponade.

Sagristà-Sauleda J, Mercé AS, Soler-Soler J. Diagnosis and management of pericardial effusion. World Journal of Cardiology. 2011;3(5):135-43.

QA41. Answer d

Exclusive monitoring by pulse oximetry is inadequate and requires arterial gasometry or capnography. The studies on phrenic nerve conduction, although essential for assessing the possibility of using diaphragmatic pacemakers, do not properly differentiate between patients who can be weaned and those who are ventilator dependent. Pathological studies do not distinguish between neuropraxia, atrophy, and axonotmesis. Similarly, normal results do not guarantee a sufficient diaphragmatic force. For similar reasons, diaphragmatic fluoroscopy does not predict the possibility of weaning from the respirator and should not be used as a prognostic marker.

As with monitoring the need for intubation, spirometry with measurement of the VC and the maximum negative inspiratory pressure are the best bedside markers for initiating weaning. More direct measures of diaphragmatic function such as transdiaphragmatic pressure and negative inspiration force diaphragm needle electromyography are invasive and of little use in clinical practice.

Vázquez RG, Sedes PR, Fariña MM, et al. Respiratory Management in the Patient with Spinal Cord Injury. BioMed Research International. 2013; ID 168757.

QA42. Answer b

LR can reduce following adverse reactions due to blood component transfusion: (1) FNHTR, (2) immunization against human leucocyte antigens (HLA) and human platelet antigens (HPA), which may cause refractoriness to platelet transfusion, (3) transmission of cytomegalovirus (CMV). Furthermore, LR improves the clinical outcome, in terms of reducing mortality and postoperative infections, in patients undergoing cardiac surgery. LR does not have an evidence-based role in the prevention of TRALI and TA-GVHD.

Bianchi M, Vaglio S, Pupella S et al. Leucoreduction of blood components: an effective way to increase blood safety? Blood Transfusion. 2016;14(3):214-27.

QA43. Answer d

In normal cells, mitochondria constitute the largest single intracellular source of O^{-2}. More than 90% of oxygen entering cells is reduced to water via the mitochondrial etc. under physiological conditions, about 1-2% of that oxygen is reduced to O^-_2, mainly due to "electron leak" at two sites in the chain: NADH ubiquinone oxidoreductase (Complex I) and ubiquinone/cytochrome C reductase (Complex III). Recent evidence indicates that non etc. sources of ROS may play a significant role in mitochondrial ROS production. Production of ROS by the mitochondria is significantly increased by I/R. A second mechanism contributing to I/R-induced increases in mitochondrial ROS is a decreased endogenous mitochondrial antioxidant capacity. Therefore, net ROS release from mitochondria likely reflects the balance between production versus disposal/scavenging.

Kalogeris T, Baines CP, Krenz M, et al. Cell Biology of Ischemia/Reperfusion Injury. International review of cell and molecular biology. 2012;298:229-317.

QA44. Answer c

When stenting is undertaken in perforator rich arteries there is a risk of the "snow plow" effect of pushing atheroma into the ostia of perforators and consequently causing a perforator stroke. Additionally a very important factor is that stenting should not be a substitute for aggressive risk factor control and continued attention to control all modifiable risk factors needs to be paid. This should include aggressive blood pressure, diabetes, and dyslipidemia management per stroke guidelines. Dangerous life threatening complications with severe morbidity and mortality are mainly from the risk of dissection and rupture of the parent vessel. Acute stent thrombosis can lead to occlusion of the stent and vessel predisposing to a malignant infarct and edema within the vessels vascular territory and usually occurs within a setting of suboptimal antiplatelet therapy.

Amongst the types of stents there is no randomized data comparing BMS to SEIS. The initial excitement with SEIS has been quelled by restenosis rates however on the other hand the trackability and deliverability of BMS seems to be inferior to that of SEIS.

Short JL, Majid A, Hussain SI. Endovascular treatment of symptomatic intracranial atherosclerotic disease. Frontiers in Neurology. 2010;1:160.

QA45. Answer e

According to the European Brain Injury Consortium and Brain Trauma Foundation guidelines for severe TBIs, DC should be incorporated to the second-tier therapeutic arsenal in patients with refractory ICH to first-tier therapeutic measures, i.e. when appropriate targeted surgery and medical treatment fails, DC is the option. Contraindications for DC (Lubillo et al., 2009)

- Patients with GCS 3 post-resuscitation, with dilated and fixed pupils
- Patient > 65 years old
- Devastating trauma that would not allow patient survive more than 24 hours.
- Irreversible systemic disease in the short term
- Uncontrollable ICH during more than 12hours besides all energetic therapeutic measures
- O_2 arterio-venous difference < 3, 2vol%, measured in the side of hemicraniectomy or a $PtiO_2$ < 10 mm Hg in the apparently health area since patient admission.

Alvis-Miranda H, Castellar-Leones SM, Moscote-Salazar LR. Decompressive Craniectomy and Traumatic Brain Injury: A Review. Bulletin of Emergency & Trauma. 2013;1(2):60-8.

QA46. Answer c

The American Society of Parenteral and Enteral Nutrition (ASPEN) recommends that patients who undergo major neck or abdominal cancer surgery, trauma, burns or are critically ill and on mechanical ventilation receive enteral formulations that are supplemented with arginine, glutamine, nucleic acid, omega-3 fatty acids and antioxidants. However, ASPEN does caution the use of these enteral formulations in patients with severe sepsis. The European Society of Parenteral and Enteral Nutrition (ESPEN) recommend the use of IMN formulas in malnourished patients undergoing major neck and abdominal cancer surgery. Additionally, ESPEN recommends that IMN should commence before surgery and continue for 5–7 days postoperatively. In 2012, the North American Surgical Nutrition Summit laid down consensus recommendations for the use of IMN in surgical patients. These included a greater emphasis on preoperative metabolic preparation and optimizing health status, performing preoperative nutritional risk assessments, perioperative IMN, considering carbohydrate loading preoperatively and the use of protocols to implement the appropriate surgical nutritional interventions.

Bharadwaj S, Trivax B, Tandon P, et al. Should perioperative immunonutrition for elective surgery be the current standard of care? Gastroenterology. 2016;4(2)87-95.

QA47. Answer d

In penetrating trauma, knowledge of the trajectory of the projectiles may aid in assessing potential sites of major bleeding or organ injury. Adequate packing should provide a good degree of hemorrhage control for most venous or solid organ bleeding. If the patient remains profoundly hypotensive after packing, a significant arterial source of hemorrhage is likely and control of aortic inflow should be obtained. Manual occlusion of the aorta at the diaphragmatic hiatus can be performed quickly to control abdominal exsanguination and give the anesthetic team sometime to catch up with volume replacement; this maneuver also has been shown to augment cerebral and myocardial perfusion. If prolonged occlusion is necessary, or if surgical hands need to be freed, a vascular clamp can be placed on the supraceliac aorta after minimal dissection in the abdomen or alternatively, the descending thoracic aorta if a thoracotomy is performed. Once clamped, the time should be noted as severe visceral ischemia will develop unless the clamp can be removed, or at least placed more distally, within a short period of time. In practice, it is desirable to move the clamp down the aorta sequentially as access and hemorrhage control is gained distally.

Lamb CM, MacGoey P, Navarro AP, Brooks AJ. Damage control surgery in the era of damage control resuscitation. BJA: British Journal of Anaesthesia. 2014;113(2):242-9.

QA48. Answer d

Emergency reperfusion of ischemic myocardium is the primary therapeutic goal. Coronary reperfusion is accomplished by means of primary PCI (angioplasty and stenting) or intravenous fibrinolytic therapy. Prompt PCI (with a performance goal of ≤90 minutes from the first medical contact) is the preferred approach at PCI-capable hospitals for STEMI with onset of symptoms within the previous 12 hours (ACC–AHA class I recommendation, evidence level A) and for STEMI with cardiogenic shock, regardless of the timing (ACC–AHA class I recommendation, evidence level B). Drug eluting stents has improved outcomes. The routine use of thrombus aspiration during PCI is not indicated since it does not improve clinical outcomes. In the high thrombus burden group, the trends toward reduced cardiovascular death and increased stroke or transient ischemic attack is a possibility. Radial artery access has been advocated for patients with STEMI, in whom bleeding at the access site is most common.

Anderson JL, Morrow DA. Acute Myocardial Infarction. N Engl J Med. 2017;376:2053-64.

QA49. Answer c

Two treatment-related factors that may have contributed to the shift from hyponatremia to hypernatremia are the less liberal use of intravenous fluids in combination with wider use of diuretic treatment and the increased use of steroids and in particular hydrocortisone. Fluid restriction may have contributed indirectly to the rising incidence of hypernatremia. More than one-third of the patients with ICU-acquired hypernatremia are actually still volume overloaded. This phenomenon is explained by the combination of large volumes of (approximately) isotonic fluids and a reduced urinary concentrating ability. In line with these observations, it was recently shown that NaCl 0.9% used to dilute drugs and keep catheters open contributes to the occurrence of ICU-acquired hypernatremia. In the group of patients with ICU-acquired hypernatremia, the plasma creatinine and dose of furosemide were also higher, again suggesting compromised urinary concentrating ability as an important contributor to hypernatremia. The widespread use of dopamine in past decades may have helped to avoid hypernatremia, since dopamine is a natriuretic agent.

Lansink-Hartgring AO, Hessels L, Weigel J et al. Long-term changes in dysnatremia incidence in the ICU: a shift from hyponatremia to hypernatremia. Annals of Intensive Care. 2016;6:22.

QA50. Answer c

The etiology of the coagulopathy of PPH relates to varying proportions of dilutional coagulopathy, localized consumption, disseminated consumption and/or increased fibrinolysis. Consumption localized to the placental bed and uterus may be marked in placental abruption and may also be a feature of uterine atony and retained or adherent placenta. DIC is uncommon during PPH but is associated with amniotic fluid embolus (AFE), infection and severe cases of abruption and pre eclampsia. It is unusual to develop an early coagulopathy when bleeding is caused by atony or trauma.

Collins P, Abdul-Kadir R, Thachil J. Management of coagulopathy associated with postpartum hemorrhage: guidance from the SSC of the ISTH. J Thromb Haemost. 2016;14:205-10.

K Type Answers
[Mark True (T)/False (F)]

QK1. Answer FTFT

20 Minute Whole Blood Clotting Test (20WBCT) is considered the most reliable test of coagulation and should be carried out at the bedside by treating physician. It can also be carried out in the most basic settings. A few milliliters of fresh venous blood is placed in a new, clean and dry, glass vessel and left at ambient temperature for 20 minutes. The vessel ideally should be a small glass test tube. The use of plastic bottles, tubes or syringes will give false, readings and should not be used. The test should be carried out every 30 minutes from admission for three hours and then hourly after that. If incoagulable blood is discovered, the 6 hourly cycles is then be adopted to test for the requirement for repeat doses of antisnake venom (ASV).

Ghosh S, Mukhopadhyay P, Chatterjee T. Management of snake bite in India. JAPI Aug. 2016;64:11-14.

QK2. Answer TFTF

Current guidelines recommend at least 30 mL/kg of IV crystalloid be given within the first 3 hours for sepsis-induced hypoperfusion. Additional fluids to be guided by frequent reassessment of hemodynamic status. Assessment of cardiac status with echocardiography and using dynamic over static variables to assess fluid responsiveness is recommended. CVP and $ScvO_2$ targets are no longer recommended.

> Rhodes A et al. Surviving Sepsis Campaign: International Guidelines for Management of Sepsis and Septic Shock: 2016. CCM. 2017; 45(3):486-552.
>
> Dellinger RP et al. Surviving Sepsis Campaign: International Guidelines for Management of Severe Sepsis and Septic Shock, 2012. Intensive Care Med. 2013; 39:165-228.

QK3. Answer FTTT

Acute iron overdose frequently leads to gastrointestinal disturbances. Intracellular iron exerts its toxic effect on mitochondria; this leads to anaerobic metabolism and thus metabolic acidosis. Myocardial failure, caused by ROS-induced myocardial damage results in profound shock observed in the later stages of illness. Once hepatotoxicity has developed the mortality rate can be 50% or more.

> Audimoolam VK, Wendon J, Bernal W, et al. Iron and acetaminophen a fatal combination? Transplant International. 2011; 24: e85-e88.

QK4. Answer TFTT

Although the pathophysiology of alcohol-induced rhabdomyolysis is not fully understood, it quite differs between short and long-term alcohol intoxication. In short-term alcohol intoxication, immobilization and coma are the main causative factors while in long-term alcohol abuse, acid–base and electrolyte disturbances (hypokalemia, hypophosphatemia, hypomagnesemia, and hypocalcemia) seem to be the main underlying causes of rhabdomyolysis. As a result, and according to basic research, we believe that the direct toxic effect of ethanol in skeletal muscles through disruption of adenosine triphosphatase pump function, breakdown of the muscle membrane, and alteration of the sarcoplasmic reticulum, or induction of cytochrome P450 may play a crucial role in the skeletal muscles' disintegration. Cases of alcohol-induced rhabdomyolysis without prolonged coma or seizures have rarely been described.

> Papadatos SS, Deligiannis G, Bazoukis G et al. Nontraumatic rhabdomyolysis with short-term alcohol intoxication – a case report. Clinical Case Reports. 2015;3(10):769-72.

QK5. Answer FTTF

Though minor differences exist among these versions, there is a generally accepted approach establishing airway management as the first priority in order to assure optimal oxygenation and ventilation; then seizure suppression, preferably with a benzodiazepine; then lipid emulsion infusion to reverse signs and symptoms of toxicity. Basic life support including chest compressions must be used when clinically indicated in order to assure tissue perfusion and circulation of resuscitation drugs including lipid.

The bolus injection is key to rapid clinical improvement since a large mass of lipid is apparently necessary to achieve the desired effect. Given that the lipid infusion must circulate to the coronary vascular bed, high quality basic life support is a necessary element of lipid resuscitation in the setting of a low output state. In toxic cardiomyopathy, raising peripheral vascular resistance with potent vasopressors can impair cardiac output and impede resuscitation. Therefore, vasopressin is not considered useful in this setting and epinephrine should be used in small doses (e.g., <1 μ/kg).

> Weinberg GL. Lipid Emulsion Infusion: Resuscitation for Local Anesthetic and other Drug Overdose. Anesthesiology. 2012; 117(1):180-187.

QK6. Answer FTFF

1. Dilution and neutralization: Dilution and neutralization of corrosive by nasogastric tube lavage generates heat and increases the risk of aspiration. Both have no proven benefit and hence are contraindicated.
2. Stabilized patient: Initial evaluation of a stabilized patient aims to identify the acute complications of corrosive ingestion and stratify the risk for acute and long-term complications mainly by endoscopic grading of corrosive lesions.

3. Corticosteroids: While there is no role of systemic steroids in the management of caustic ingestion, intralesional steroids can be given.
4. Antibiotics: Tissue destruction from caustic injury increases the risk of infection by enteric organisms. Antibiotics are not recommended prophylactically in corrosive poisoning. They are recommended in GI perforation.
5. Proton pump inhibitors (PPIs) and H_2-blockers: Gastroenterologists routinely recommend PPIs and H_2-blockers in caustic ingestion.

Ramulu Naik RR, Vadivelan M. Corrosive Poisoning. Indian Journal of Clinical Practice. 2012;23(3):131-4.

QK7. Answer TTTT

Bite infections can contain a mix of anaerobes and aerobes from the patient's skin and the animal's oral cavity, including species of *Pasteurella, Streptococcus, Fusobacterium,* and *Capnocytophaga*. Domestic cat and dog bite wounds can produce substantial morbidity and often require specialized care techniques and specific antibiotic therapy. Bite wounds can be complicated by sepsis. Disseminated infections, particularly those caused by *Capnocytophaga canimorsus* and *Pasteurella multocida,* can lead to septic shock, meningitis, endocarditis, and other severe sequelae. An emerging syndrome in veterinary and human medicine is methicillin-resistant Staphylococcus aureus (MRSA) infections shared between pets and human handlers, particularly community-acquired MRSA disease involving the USA300 clone. Skin, soft-tissue, and surgical infections are the most common. MRSA-associated infections in pets are typically acquired from their owners and can potentially cycle between pets and their human acquaintances.

Oehler RL, Velez AP, Mizrachi M, et al. Bite-related and septic syndromes caused by cats and dogs. Lancet Infect Dis. 2009; 9(7):439.

QK8. Answer TTTF

Crush syndrome is common in disaster-prone regions. Treatment of crush-related acute renal failure includes (1) Early fluid resuscitation (within the first six hours, preferably before the victim is extricated). The preferred fluid is isotonic saline, given at a rate of 1 L/hr (10 to 15 mL/kg of body weight per hour), while the victim is under the rubble, followed by hypotonic saline soon after rescue. (2) Sodium bicarbonate (50 mEq) to each second or third liter of hypotonic saline (usually a total of 200 to 300 mEq the first day) to maintain urinary pH above 6.5 and prevent intratubular deposition of myoglobin and uric acid. (3) Mannitol (20%) 50 mL- If urinary flow exceeds 20 mL/hr. 1 to 2 g per kilogram per day (total, 120 g), given at a rate of 5 g/hr, may be added to each liter of infusate.

Sever MS, Vanholder R, Lameire N. Management of Crush-Related Injuries after Disasters. N Engl J Med. 2006;354:1052-63.

QK9. Answer TFFT

Drugs, which have an anticholinergic or sympathomimetic effect, increase temperature. In contrast, organophosphates, opiates, barbiturates, β-blockers, benzodiazepines, alcohol, and clonidine cause hypothermia.

Mokhlesi B et al. Adult toxicology in critical care. Part I: General approach to the intoxicated person. Chest. 2003;123:577-92.

QK10. Answer TFTT

Type 3 cardiorenal syndrome, also defined as acute renocardiac syndrome, occurs when AKI contributes and/or precipitates development of acute cardiac injury. AKI may directly or indirectly produce an acute cardiac event; triggered by the inflammatory surge, oxidative stress and secretion of neurohormones following AKI. Other triggers for cardiac injury and dysfunction include AKI related volume overload, metabolic acidosis and electrolytes disorders such as hyperkalemia and hypocalcemia. Acute, left ventricular dysfunction and accelerated fibrosis have been also described in patients with AKI.

Di Lullo L, Barbera V, Russo L, et al. Pathophysiology of the cardio-renal syndromes types 1–5: An up to date. Indian Heart Journal. 2017;69(2):255-65.

QK11. Answer TTFT

Monoclonal antibodies that target B lymphocytes cause significant cellular immunosuppression predisposing to bacterial, fungal, and viral infections. Reactivation of hepatitis B virus (HBV) is more common compared to other viruses such as herpes simplex virus (HSV), varicella zoster virus (VZV), cytomegalovirus (CMV), and Epstein-Barr virus (EBV). These agents should not be administered to patients with active infection. Anti-CD20- directed monoclonal antibodies (rituximab, ofatumumab, and obinutuzumab) are used in the treatment of lymphoproliferative disorders. Their use is associated with HBV reactivation resulting in fulminant hepatitis, hepatic failure, and death.

Singh D, Bonomo RA. Infections in Cancer Patients. In: Oncology Critical Care Hoag JB (ed.). 2016.

QK12. Answer TFTT

In the rare circumstance that IV labetalol, hydralazine, or immediate release oral nifedipine fails to relieve acute onset severe hypertension and is given in successive appropriate doses, emergent consultation with an anesthesiologist, maternal-fetal medicine subspecialist or critical care subspecialist to discuss second line intervention is recommended. Second line alternatives to consider include nicardipine or esmolol by infusion pump.

El-Sayed YY, Borders AE. Emergent Therapy for Acute-Onset, Severe Hypertension During Pregnancy and the Postpartum Period. Available from: https://www.acog.org/Resources-And-Publications/Committee-Opinions/Committee-on-Obstetric-Practice/Emergent-Therapy-for-Acute-Onset-Severe-Hypertension-During-Pregnancy-and-the-Postpartum-Period (Accessed 13 February 2018).

QK13. Answer TTTT

Historically, AFE was thought to be caused due to mechanical obstruction of pulmonary vessels by amniotic fluid embolus consisting of fetal squames (squamous cells), vernix caseosa, lanugo hair, trophoblasts, fetal gut mucin, and bile stained meconium. At present, AFE is thought to result from an immune-mediated mechanism, given its similarity to septic shock or anaphylactic shock. It results from an abnormal immunological response of the mother following exposure to fetal antigens leading to the release of various pro-inflammatory mediators. The exact immunological mechanism is still unknown. Complement activation as the primary mechanism has been proposed. The levels of complement factors C3 and C4 have been found to be reduced in patients with AFE. Furthermore, mast cells can be secondarily activated after complement activation. The reason for activation of the coagulation cascade is incompletely understood. Tissue factor in amniotic fluid and apoptotic amniotic cells may initiate the coagulation cascade, but it is still doubtful if the small quantities of these factors could lead on to the disseminated intravascular coagulation (DIC) picture that is seen in AFE. Recently, an integrated mechanism was proposed. According to this theory, activation of the coagulation cascade can lead to microthrombi in pulmonary vessels and add on to the mechanical obstruction by amniotic fluid components. This, along with the various inflammatory mediators like leukotrienes can cause the complete picture of the syndrome.

Sadera G, Vasudevan B. Amniotic fluid embolism. J Obstet Anaesth Crit Care. 2015;5:3-8.

QK14. Answer TTFT

Absolute contraindications to nasotracheal intubation are as follows: (1) Suspected epiglottitis; (2) Midface instability; (3) Coagulopathy; (4) Suspected basilar skull fractures; (5) Apnea or impending respiratory arrest.

Relative contraindications are as follows: (1) Large nasal polyps; (2) Suspected nasal foreign bodies; (3) Recent nasal surgery; (4) Upper neck hematoma or infection; (5) History of frequent episodes of epistaxis; (6) Prosthetic heart valves (increased risk of bacteremia during the insertion).

Chauhan V, Acharya G. Nasal intubation: A comprehensive review. Indian J Crit Care Med. 2016;20(11):662-7.

QK15. Answer TTFT

Aedes aegypti is a small mosquito responsible for transmitting the Zika virus, dengue virus, yellow fever virus and chikungunya virus as a primary vector in certain parts of the world. Mosquito-borne virus infections are on the raise, expanding its geographical range into new areas. The spread of infections from Africa and Asia to other continents is thought to be due to extensive travelling, trade, population growth in high-risk areas, globalization of vectors, urbanization, climatic change, as well as virus genome evolution.

Muktar Y, Tamerat N, Shewafera A. *Aedes aegypti* as a Vector of Flavivirus. J Trop Dis. 2016;4:223.

QK16. Answer TTFT

All patients should receive a second-line Group 2 injectable agent in the intensive phase of MDR-TB treatment unless resistance is documented or highly suspected. Either kanamycin, amikacin or capreomycin can be used as a first choice if all meet the criteria of "likely to be effective". Ciprofloxacin has weaker efficacy against TB than other fluoroquinolones and is not recommended as an anti-TB drug.

> Companion Handbook to the WHO Guidelines for the Programmatic Management of Drug-Resistant Tuberculosis. Geneva: World Health Organization; 2014. 5, Treatment strategies for MDR-TB and XDR-TB.

QK17. Answer FTTT

No clinical trials have evaluated the management of PRES, but rapid withdrawal of the trigger appears to hasten recovery and to avoid complications: for example, aggressive blood pressure management (which may include increased ultrafiltration), withdrawal of the offending drug, or delivery in eclampsia. Antiepileptic drugs should be used to treat seizures, and anesthesia and ventilation should be instituted in generalized status epilepticus and to protect the airway in obtunded patients. Corticosteroids should theoretically improve vasogenic edema, but there is no evidence for their use in PRES.

> Hobson EV, Craven I, Blank SC. Posterior Reversible Encephalopathy Syndrome: A Truly Treatable Neurologic Illness. Peritoneal Dialysis International : Journal of the International Society for Peritoneal Dialysis. 2012;32(6):590-4.

QK18. Answer TTTT

Refractory SE is defined as SE which is refractory to two intravenous AEDs, one of which is a benzodiazepine. Some authorities have also defined RSE on the basis of the duration of seizure for 1 or 2 hours. Early induction of pharmacological coma has been practiced in generalized-convulsive SE using midazolam, propofol, or barbiturates. Several other treatments such as inhalational anesthetic, oral antiepileptic drugs, immunomodulatory compounds, or nonpharmacological approaches (electroconvulsive treatment, hypothermia, ketogenic diet, transcranial magnetic stimulation) have been used in resistant SE. Ketamine has been used to control prolonged SE since 2000, although there has been no randomized trial conducted till now.

> Dubey D, Kalita J, Misra UK. Status epilepticus: Refractory and super-refractory. Neurol India 2017;65(Suppl S1):12-7.

QK19. Answer TFTT

Data suggests that toxicity as well as relative deficiencies of parenteral nutrition components can lead to TPN associated injury. Aluminum, chromium and manganese have all been implicated. Aluminum present in the TPN solution is known to cause metabolic bone disease as well as neurological impairment. Concerns have also been raised for organ damage secondary to chromium delivery during parenteral nutrition. Chromium plays a role in regulation of the action of insulin. Additionally, peripheral neuropathy, weight loss as well as kidney damage have been reported in patients receiving TPN. Over the past several years there has been an effort to decrease chromium concentration in parenteral nutrition solutions. Anemia, cholestasis as well as neurotoxicity have been noted with manganese provided as part of TPN. Recent guidelines recommend monitoring of manganese levels if TPN has been provided for longer than 30 days.

> Kumar JA, Teckman JH. Controversy in the mechanism of total parenteral nutrition induced pathology. Children. 2015;2:358-70.

QK20. Answer TFTT

Special approaches for preventing CLABSI
1. Use antiseptic- or antimicrobial-impregnated CVCs in adult patients (quality of evidence: I).
2. Use chlorhexidine-containing dressings for CVCs in patients over 2 months of age (quality of evidence: I).
3. Use an antiseptic-containing hub/connector cap/port protector to cover connectors (quality of evidence: I).
4. Use silver zeolite–impregnated umbilical catheters in preterm infants (in countries where it is approved for use in children; quality of evidence: II).
5. Use antimicrobial locks for CVCs (quality of evidence: I).

> Yokoe DS, Anderson DJ, Berenholtz SM et al. A Compendium of Strategies to Prevent Healthcare-Associated Infections in Acute Care Hospitals: 2014 Updates. Infection control and hospital epidemiology : the official journal of the Society of Hospital Epidemiologists of America. 2014;35(8):967-77.

QK21. Answer TTFT

It is a novel topical antibiotic and the first approved member in this new class. It is approved for the treatment of skin and soft tissue infections caused by *S. pyogenes* and *S. aureus* which are resistant to the most commonly used topical antibiotics. It is ineffective against gram-negative organisms. Retapamulin is a semisynthetic pleuromutilin derivative isolated from *Clitopilus scyphoides* (an edible mushroom). It is a protein synthesis inhibitor which acts by binding to 50-S subunit of bacterial ribosomes.

Plasma protein binding of Retapamulin is 94% and it is metabolized mainly in liver by CYP3A4 to numerous metabolites. The most common adverse effect is pruritus at the application site.

Rai J, Randhawa GK, Kaur M. Recent advances in antibacterial drugs. International Journal of Applied and Basic Medical Research. 2013;3(1):3-10.

QK22. Answer TTTT

The following have been shown to control hemorrhage and avoid the need for hysterectomy: (1) Intra-uterine balloon tamponade, (2) Uterine compression sutures, (3) Interventional radiology (IR) -(intra-arterial balloon occlusion and arterial embolization), (4) Pelvic vessel ligation (internal iliac, uterine, hypogastric, or ovarian arteries). IR intra-arterial balloons may be placed prophylactically. The balloons can be inflated after delivery while the bleeding is controlled. In ongoing hemorrhage, IR may be used to embolize arteries. Such techniques may help preserve fertility and halt hemorrhage but are only available in a limited number of institutions.

Plaat F, Shonfeld A. Major obstetric hemorrhage .Continuing Education in Anaesthesia Critical Care & Pain. 2015;15(4):190-3.

QK23. Answer FFFF

Unfortunately, no pharmacologic therapy for ARDS has been shown to reduce either short-term or long-term mortality. Inhaled nitric oxide transiently improves oxygenation and may improve long-term lung function among patients who survive, but it does not reduce mortality and is associated with acute kidney injury. Glucocorticoids may improve oxygenation and airway pressures and, in patients with pneumonia, may hasten radiographic improvement, but these agents are not associated with a consistent survival benefit and are harmful if started 14 days or more after ARDS has been diagnosed. Surfactant replacement, neutrophil elastase inhibition, and anticoagulation have failed in clinical trials, as have nonsteroidal anti-inflammatory agents (ketoconazole and lysofylline), statins, albuterol, and antioxidants (procysteine [L-2-oxothiazolidine-4-carboxylic acid]), though many of these trials had relatively small samples, and in some cases, the doses tested did not modulate the intended biologic targets.

Thompson BT, Chambers RC, Liu KD. Acute Respiratory Distress Syndrome. N Engl J Med. 2017;377:562-72.

QK24. Answer TFTT

Indeed, the use of a low tidal volume, with the aim to reduce the risk of VILI, may cause the development of hypercapnia. However, arterial carbon dioxide levels up to 70 mm Hg with a pH of 7.20 were found to be safe in the absence of pathological condition such as raised intracranial pressure or right heart failure. The rationale of a more liberal CO_2 management (permissive hypercapnia) lies in the well-known positive effects of hypercapnic acidosis on arterial and tissue oxygenation: the potentiation of hypoxic pulmonary vasoconstriction, the inhibition of airway tone, the increase in cardiac output, the anti-inflammatory effect and the rightward shift in the oxygen-hemoglobin dissociation curve .

Umbrello M, Formenti P, Bolgiaghi L, et al. Current Concepts of ARDS: A Narrative Review. International Journal of Molecular Sciences. 2017;18(1):64.

QK25. Answer FTTT

Disadvantages of combination therapy: (1) Increased drug toxicity, particularly when aminoglycosides are used. Although this increased risk may be acceptable in a critically ill population with a high risk of MDR organisms, it is likely less acceptable in more stable patient populations or where the risk of β-lactam resistance is lower. (2) Risk of superinfection with resistant bacteria or fungal infections. (3) Increased cost may not have clinical significance.

Vincent JL, Bassetti M, François B, et al. Advances in antibiotic therapy in the critically ill. Crit Care. 2016;20:133.

QK26. Answer TFTT

However, various technical issues need to be addressed. During mechanical ventilation, large droplets (>5 μm) are more likely to be trapped in the circuit, whereas smaller particles (<0.5 μm) are more likely to be expulsed during expiration, so that the size of the particles generated should optimally be between 1 and 3 μm. Particle size depends on the aerosol generator and ventilator settings. On ultrasonic nebulizers, aerosol particle size is inversely proportional to the piezoelectric crystal vibration frequency, and drug output is directly proportional to the amplitude of crystal vibration. On vibrating mesh nebulizers, droplet size is more homogeneous and easier to calibrate. To increase lung deposition, tidal volume has to be set at 500 mL (or more) in adults, with a long inspiratory time (which can be obtained by increasing the I:E ratio) and reduced inspiratory flow. When using a heat/moisture exchanger, it has to be removed during nebulization (and replaced at the end of the aerosol treatment). When using a heated humidifier, it should be switched off during nebulization or the amount of drug should be increased.

Vincent JL, Bassetti M, François B, et al. Advances in antibiotic therapy in the critically ill. Crit Care. 2016;20:133.

QK27. Answer TTTF

Upon arrival to the ICU it is essential for the ICU physician to understand where the patient is in the continuum of both surgical management and ongoing resuscitation, and to assess overall stability and the extent of unresolved shock. Because shock is a cumulative phenomenon in which the depth and duration determine the total "dose" in an integrative fashion, the timeliness of resuscitation may have a significant impact on subsequent morbidity and mortality. Virtually all critically injured patients require some degree of immediate physiologic support on arrival to the ICU. This includes assurance of adequate respiratory and ventilator support as well as aggressive intervention to minimize secondary central nervous system (CNS) injury, resolve critical acid–base and electrolyte disorders and restore normothermia. Not all patients respond to aggressive resuscitative measures. This can be due to occult injury or poor physiologic response. A recent review of undiagnosed injuries and outcomes, suggested up to 6.5% of all trauma-related deaths were attributable to clinically undiagnosed injury.

Shere-Wolfe RF, Galvagno SM, Grissom TE. Critical care considerations in the management of the trauma patient following initial resuscitation. Scandinavian Journal of Trauma, Resuscitation and Emergency Medicine. 2012;20:68.

QK28. Answer TTTF

ICU clinicians must ensure that patients die with dignity. The definition of "dying with dignity" recognizes the intrinsic, unconditional quality of human worth but also external qualities of physical comfort, autonomy, meaningfulness, preparedness, and interpersonal connection. Respect should be fostered by being mindful of the "ABCDs" of dignity-conserving care (attitudes, behaviors, compassion, and dialogue).

Cook D, Rocker G. Dying with Dignity in the Intensive Care Unit. N Engl J Med. 2014;370:2506-14.

QK29. Answer TTTF

Four families of enveloped RNA viruses, filoviruses, flaviviruses, arenaviruses, and bunyaviruses, cause hemorrhagic fevers. These viruses are maintained in specific natural cycles involving nonhuman primates, bats, rodents, domestic ruminants, humans, mosquitoes, and ticks. Vascular instability varies from mild to fatal shock, and hemorrhage ranges from none to life threatening. The pathogenic mechanisms are extremely diverse and include deficiency of hepatic synthesis of coagulation factors owing to hepatocellular necrosis, cytokine storm, increased permeability by vascular endothelial growth factor, complement activation, and disseminated intravascular coagulation in one or more hemorrhagic fevers.

Paessler S, Walker DH. Pathogenesis of the Viral Hemorrhagic Fevers. Annual Review of Pathology: Mechanisms of Disease. 2013;8(1):411-40.

QK30. Answer FTTT

Causes of fatigue in heart failure:
- Drug causes
  - Overdiuresis
  - Hypokalemia from loop diuretics

- β-blockers
- Blood loss due to aspirin
- Anaemia
  - See aspirin
  - Anemia of chronic disease
  - Comorbidities—for example, pernicious anemia, malignancy
- Sleep problems
  - Orthopnea
  - Paroxysmal nocturnal dyspnea
  - Periodic respiration ± sleep apnea
  - Anxiety/depression
- Psychological
  - Depression
  - Anxiety

Johnson MJ. Management of end stage cardiac failure. Postgraduate Medical Journal. 2007;83(980):395-401.

QK31. Answer TFTT

Signs of aortic dissection on chest X-ray
Mediastinal widening
Disruption of normally distinct contour of aortic knob
Calcium sign—separation of intimal calcification from the vessel wall > 5 mm.
Double density appearance within aorta
Tracheal deviation to the right
Deviation of nasogastric tube to the right

Strayer RJ, Shearer PL, Hermann LK. Screening, Evaluation, and Early Management of Acute Aortic Dissection in the ED. Current Cardiology Reviews. 2012;8(2):152-7.

QK32. Answer FFTF

Our analysis implies that intravenous and nebulized magnesium sulfate could be additional standard treatments for children and adults respectively, especially for the patients with acute asthma that has not responded to initial treatments, while the roles of both intravenous magnesium sulfate in adults and nebulized magnesium sulfate in children require further investigation. Considering the low risk of serious side effects from magnesium sulfate and readily availableness it would seem reasonable to use intravenous and nebulized magnesium sulfate to treat patients with life threatening features. Further studies with larger sample sizes, especially involving nebulized magnesium sulfate in children, should be warranted. Meanwhile, large randomized controlled trials are required to compare nebulized and intravenous magnesium sulfate with each other and with placebo, in patients with acute asthma, to establish the optimal dosage and the most effective route of administration.

Shan Z, Rong Y, Yang W, et al. Intravenous and nebulized magnesium sulfate for treating acute asthma in adults and children: A systematic review and meta-analysis. Respiratory Medicine. 2013;107:321-30.

QK33. Answer FTTT

Pharmacologic therapy for acute termination of SVT is appropriate in patients when vagal maneuvers fail. The preferred initial agents are intravenous (IV) adenosine or a nondihydropyridine calcium channel blocker. Adenosine's effects are mediated by membrane hyperpolarization that typically occurs within 15–30 seconds after administration. Adenosine has a powerful effect on the atrioventricular node and is highly effective in causing temporary, complete atrioventricular nodal block. Because propagation of the action potential through the atrioventricular node is calcium-channel dependent, the nondihydropyridine calcium channel blockers verapamil and diltiazem are highly effective in the termination of AVNRT and AVRT. Beta blockers such as IV metoprolol or esmolol infusion are often used in acute SVT, but data regarding this practice are limited.

Sohinki D, Obel OA. Current Trends in Supraventricular Tachycardia Management. The Ochsner Journal. 2014;14(4):586-95.

QK34. Answer TTFT

Any type of ileus may promote abdominal fluid sequestration with severe systemic hypovolemia, intestinal bacterial overgrowth with the evolution of bacterial translocation and systemic invasive infections and inflammation of the intestinal wall with concomitant release of cytokines and the development of the systemic inflammatory response syndrome. The most serious complications of ileus are mediated by an increase in IAP. Intra-abdominal hypertension has been found in up to 20% of critically ill patients and may lead to a broad pattern of systemic consequences with multiple organ dysfunction, including cardiovascular, hepatic, pulmonary, renal and neurological function. The abdominal compartment syndrome is an emergency condition which is defined as elevation of IAP above 20 to 25 mmHg and the presence of systemic consequences.

Madl C, Druml W. Gastrointestinal disorders of the critically ill: Systemic consequences of ileus. Best Pract Res Clin Gastroenterol. 2003;17(3):445-56.

QK35. Answer FFFT

There is no evidence to support the use of omega 3 fatty acids in ARDS, hence it is not recommended. Standard enteral formulations are recommended in ICU patients with acute and chronic liver disease. There is no evidence of further benefit of branched-chain amino acid formulations (BCAA) on coma grade in the ICU patient with encephalopathy who is already receiving first-line therapy with luminal-acting antibiotics and lactulose. The rationale for the use of high fat pulmonary formulae has been found to be erroneous. The respiratory quotient increases because of overfeeding and not due to carbohydrates. The high content of omega 6 fatty acids may drive up inflammatory processes.

Tayloe BE et al. Guidelines for the Provision and Assessment of Nutrition Support Therapy in the Adult Critically Ill Patient: Society of Critical Care Medicine (SCCM) and American Society for Parenteral and Enteral Nutrition (ASPEN). Critical Care Medicine. 2016;2:438.

QK36. Answer FTTT

Asymptomatic bacteriuria

Duration of catheterization is the most important determinant of bacteriuria. The daily risk of acquisition of bacteriuria when an indwelling catheter *in situ* is 3-7%. The rate of acquisition is higher for women and older persons. Bacteriuria is universal once a catheter remains in place for several weeks. Patients with chronic indwelling catheters are assumed to be continuously having bacteriuria. From 60-80% of hospitalized patients with an indwelling catheter receive antimicrobials, usually for indications other than urinary tract infection. This intense antimicrobial exposure means antimicrobial resistant organisms are frequently isolated from the urine of catheterized individuals. Statewide surveillance of carbapenemase resistant Enterobacteriaceae (CRE) in Michigan reported 61% of isolates were from urine cultures, and a urinary catheter was present in 48% of these patients. Bacteria colonizing the drainage bags of catheterized patients have been reported to be a source for outbreaks of resistant organisms in acute care facilities. In the nursing home setting, the urine of residents with chronic indwelling catheters is the most common site of isolation of resistant gram negative organisms.

Nicolle LE. Catheter associated urinary tract infections. Antimicrobial Resistance and Infection Control. 2014;3:23.

QK37. Answer TFTT

The tracheal tube prevents closure of vocal cords, and represents an access for bacteria to progress in the trachea through the folds of high-volume low-pressure tracheal tubes into the lower respiratory tract. Underinflation of the tracheal cuff under 20 cmH$_2$O results in microaspiration, and was identified as an independent risk factor for VAP. However, this cut-off is based on one single center study including few patients. Therefore, microaspiration could probably occur at highest or lowest levels of cuff pressure. Mechanical ventilation plays an important role in microaspiration, and cuff pressure is tightly correlated with airway pressure. The application of a positive end expiratory pressure was identified as protective from microaspiration and VAP. Tracheal suctioning could be associated with higher risk for microaspiration, because of negative pressure applied during this procedure. It has been demonstrated that leakage rate around the cuff depends on the difference in pressure between the two areas above and below the cuff.

Jaillette E, Martin-Loeches I, Artigas A, et al. Optimal care and design of the tracheal cuff in the critically ill patient. Annals of Intensive Care. 2014;4:7.

QK38. Answer TTTF

Respiratory failure in PE is predominantly a consequence of hemodynamic disturbances. Low cardiac output results in desaturation of the mixed venous blood. In addition, zones of reduced flow in obstructed vessels, combined with zones of overflow in the capillary bed served by nonobstructed vessels, result in ventilation–perfusion mismatch, which contributes to hypoxemia. In about one-third of patients, right-to-left shunting through a patent foramen ovale can be detected by echocardiography: this is caused by an inverted pressure gradient between the right atrium and left atrium and may lead to severe hypoxemia and an increased risk of paradoxical embolization and stroke. Finally, even if they do not affect hemodynamics, small distal emboli may create areas of alveolar hemorrhage resulting in hemoptysis, pleuritis, and pleural effusion, which is usually mild. This clinical presentation is known as 'pulmonary infarction'. Its effect on gas exchange is normally mild, except in patients with pre-existing cardiorespiratory disease.

> 2014 ESC Guidelines on the diagnosis and management of acute pulmonary embolism: The Task Force for the Diagnosis and Management of Acute Pulmonary Embolism of the European Society of Cardiology (ESC).European Heart Journal, 2014;35(43):3033-73.

QK39. Answer TFTT

A normal D-dimer value has the same exclusion value for PE in pregnant women as for other patients with suspected PE but is found more rarely, because plasma D-dimer levels physiologically increase throughout pregnancy. The diagnostic yield of scintigraphy is around 80%, with 70% of tests yielding normal perfusion scans and 5–10% yielding high-probability scan. This is at least as high as that of CT in this particular population, due to a higher proportion of inconclusive CT scans during pregnancy.

Conventional pulmonary angiography carries a significantly higher radiation exposure for the fetus (2.2–3.7 mSv) and should be avoided during pregnancy.

> 2014 ESC Guidelines on the diagnosis and management of acute pulmonary embolism: The Task Force for the Diagnosis and Management of Acute Pulmonary Embolism of the European Society of Cardiology (ESC).European Heart Journal. 2014; 35(43):3033-73.

QK40. Answer FTTT

CID is caused by changes in intestinal absorption and might be accompanied by excessive electrolyte and fluid secretion. Furthermore, this type of diarrhea may be a consequence of biochemical changes caused by chemotherapy. Depending on the chemotherapeutic regimen, rates of severe or life-threatening CID can be up to 30% (grade 3-5 diarrhea), especially with 5-FU bolus or combination therapies of irinotecan and fluoropyrimidines (IFL, XELIRI). Regarding the tremendous effects on patients' safety and quality of life, the possible occurrence of CID has to be carefully considered. Current research focuses on establishing predictive factors for toxicities caused by therapeutic agents like UGT1A1-polymorphisms for irinotecan or DPD-insufficiency for fluoropyrimidines. Despite the amount of clinical trials evaluating therapeutic or prophylactic measures in CID, there are just three drugs recommended in current guidelines: loperamide, deodorized tincture of opium and octreotide. Further evaluation of treatment options is absolutely essential for the management of this debilitating toxicity.

> Stein A, Voigt W, Jordan K. Chemotherapy-induced diarrhea: pathophysiology, frequency and guideline-based management. Therapeutic Advances in Medical Oncology. 2010;2(1):51-63.

QK41. Answer TTTF

The chances of survival are affected by several clinical factors. Acute renal failure, being on mechanical ventilation, refractory shock, performance status, and CPR duration are predictive of resuscitation failure. Patients with cancer who had sudden, unexpected cardiac arrest had a substantially higher chance of survival until discharge than patients in whom cardiac arrest was anticipated.

> Shimabukuro-Vornhagen A, Böll B, Kochanek M, et al. Critical care of patients with cancer. CA: A Cancer Journal for Clinicians. 2016;66:496-517.

QK42. Answer TFTT

However, when ICU patients are also receiving, among other vital support, full enteral and/or parenteral nutrition for several weeks or longer, the alterations within the thyroid axis appear different. In this phase of critical illness, low plasma T3 concentrations now coincide with low plasma T4 concentrations and low-normal TSH concentrations in a single morning sample. Moreover, overnight repeated sampling revealed that the pulsatility of the TSH secretory pattern is virtually lost, which relates to low plasma thyroid hormone levels, a presentation resembling central hypothyroidism. In line with this interpretation, Fliers *et al.* demonstrated in postmortem brain samples of chronic critically ill patients that thyrotropin releasing hormone (*TRH*) gene expression in the hypothalamic paraventricular nuclei was much lower than in patients who died after acute insults. Furthermore, a positive correlation was observed between the *TRH* mRNA expression and the plasma concentrations of TSH and T3. Together, these data indicate that production and/or release of thyroid hormones is reduced in prolonged critical illness due to reduced hypothalamic stimulation of the thyrotropes, in turn leading to reduced stimulation of the thyroid gland.

Van den Berghe G. Non-Thyroidal Illness in the ICU: A Syndrome with Different Faces. Thyroid. 2014;24(10):1456-65.

QK43. Answer FFTT

A critically ill patient with an established coagulopathy may not be able to provide any history, and the diagnosis may only be questioned in the light of an abnormal coagulation profile. It is imperative to appreciate that a significant coagulopathy may exist even in the presence of a 'normal' coagulation profile. The classical clinical manifestations of impaired hemostasis are conditions that affect platelets and disorders of coagulation. Patients with platelet abnormalities or severe thrombocytopenia typically bleed immediately after trauma, whereas patients with coagulation abnormalities exhibit more delayed bleeding. Petechiae are commonly seen with disorders of platelet function and are small discrete areas of capillary hemorrhage that develop due to increased venous pressure. Classically, they are located on dependent areas of the body and in ambulatory patients the feet, ankles and legs are the commonest sites. In supine ITU patients, they tend to be more widespread. Ecchymoses are caused by the escape of blood into tissues and usually develop without a history of local trauma. They are soft tissue hematomas that develop in patients with significantly impaired coagulation.

Retter A, Barrett NA. The management of abnormal hemostasis in the ICU. Anesthesia. 2015;70:121-e41.

QK44. Answer FFFT

Neither the Glasgow Coma Scale (GCS) nor the Coma Remission Scale (*Koma Remissions Skala*, KRS, a scale widely used in Germany) enables a clear, operationalized distinction between PVS and MCS. An internationally established instrument for this purpose is the revised Coma Recovery Scale (CRS-R), which contains an ordinal scale ranging from zero (deepest possible coma) to 23 points (awake and fully capable of contact) and permits a clear differentiation of PVS from MCS and from the successful emergence from MCS to a still higher level of consciousness.

Bender A, Jox RJ, Grill E, et al. Persistent Vegetative State and Minimally Conscious State: A systematic review and meta-analysis of diagnostic procedures. Deutsches Ärzteblatt International. 2015;112(14):235-42.

QK45. Answer FTFF

Increasing dose intensity of CRRT above 20-25 mL/kg/hr does not deliver clinical benefits to critically ill patients with severe AKI. High intensity CRRT is associated with electrolyte disturbances such as hypophosphatemia or hypokalemia, which may do harm to renal, cellular, respiratory or cardiac function. Increasing the intensity of RRT may double or triple the amount of amino acid or protein losses as well as many micronutrient losses such as vitamins, selenium and folic acid. Many antibiotics can be cleared significantly by RRT, and high-intensity RRT would make it more complicated to adjust the dose of antibiotics and could potentially generate periods of inadequate antibiotic levels, which, in turn, may impede the efficacy of antimicrobial therapy. Lastly, the RENAL study found that high-intensity CRRT required more filters per day, indicating more clotting events and frequent interruption occurred during therapy. 90-day mortality of RRT-treated AKI patients was higher in the presence of fluid overload in RENAL and FINNAKI studies. Studies comparing CRRT versus IHD in AKI have not shown any mortality benefit. Meta-analyses have found both IHD and CRRT to have comparable mortality outcomes. No real proven benefit for endotoxin removal on outcome has been reported until now.

Bellomo R et al. Acute kidney injury in the ICU: from injury to recovery—reports from the 5th Paris International Conference. Ann Intensive Care. 2017;7:49.

QK46. Answer TTFF

Clinically important posttraumatic stress disorder symptoms occurred in one fifth of critical illness survivors at 1-year follow-up, with higher prevalence in those who had comorbid psychopathology, received benzodiazepines, and had early memories of frightening ICU experiences. In European studies, ICU diaries reduced posttraumatic stress disorder symptoms.

> Parker AM, Sricharoenchai T, Raparla S, et al. Posttraumatic stress disorder in critical illness survivors: a metaanalysis. Crit Care Med. 2015;43(5):1121-9.

QK47. Answer TFTT

Acute graft versus host disease generally occurs after allogeneic hematopoietic stem cell transplant (HSCT). It is a reaction of donor immune cells against host tissues. The three main tissues that acute GVHD affects are the skin, liver, and gastrointestinal tract.

> Jacobsohn DA, Vogelsang GB. Acute graft versus host disease. Orphanet Journal of Rare Diseases. 2007;2:35.

QK48. Answer FFTF

A patient's baseline condition begins to deteriorate a mean of 6.5 hours before an unexpected critical event or actual cardiac arrest. Seventy percent of such events are preventable. An RRT is intended to prevent deaths outside the intensive care unit (ICU) by providing a resource team that can be called to a patient's bedside 24 hours a day, 7 days a week. RRTs may consist of different structured groups: physician and nurse, intensivist and respiratory therapist, physician assistant alone, critical care nurse and respiratory therapist, or clinical specialist alone. The hospital wide operational and financial benefits of implementation of an RRT greatly outweigh the challenges of starting up an RRT. Benefits include improved safety of patients, shorter hospital stays, fewer code blues, fewer transfers to the ICU, increased awareness and identification by nurses of signs and symptoms leading to deterioration in a patient's condition, decreased mortality and morbidity, increased satisfaction of physicians with nurses, increased satisfaction of patients with their care, and increased job satisfaction among nurses. Developing a structured RRT for patients' safety empowers all staff to operate at a higher competence level.

> Thomas K, Force MV, Rasmussen D, et al. Rapid Response Team: Challenges, Solutions, Benefits. Crit Care Nurse. 2007; 27:20-27.

QK49. Answer FFTT

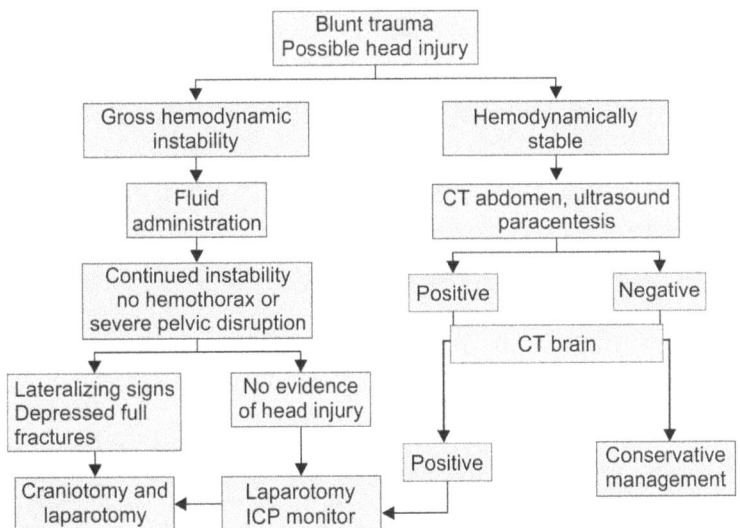

> Prabhu AJ, Matta BF. Anesthesia for extra-cranial surgery in patients with traumatic brain injury. Continuing Education in Anaesthesia Critical Care & Pain. 2004;4(5):156-9.

QK50. Answer TFFT

FIRST LINE THERAPY of symptomatic CCB poisoning (1) High-dose insulin therapy as a monotherapy in the presence of myocardial dysfunction (2) High-dose insulin therapy in the absence of documented myocardial dysfunction if used in combination with IV fluids, calcium, and vasopressors (3) Dobutamine or epinephrine in the presence of cardiogenic shock (4) Atropine in the presence of symptomatic bradycardia or conduction disturbances.

CONTRAINDICATIONS to use (1) Dopamine in the presence of shock (2) Vasopressin as a single vasoactive agent in the presence of documented cardiogenic shock. SECOND LINE TREATMENTS (1) Incremental doses of high-dose insulin therapy (up to 10 U/kg/hr) if evidence of myocardial dysfunction is present (2) Pacemaker in the presence of unstable bradycardia or high-grade AV block, without significant alteration in cardiac inotropism (3) IV lipid-emulsion therapy.

St-Onge M, Anseeuw K, Cantrell FL et al. Experts Consensus Recommendations for the Management of Calcium Channel Blocker Poisoning in Adults. Critical Care Medicine. 2017;45(3):e306-e315.

MODEL QUESTION PAPER II

Nita George, Kamal Lashkari

A Type Questions
(One best answer)

A1. The first line vasopressor for the treatment of acute circulatory failure in adult critically ill patients is:
   a. Dopamine
   b. Vasopressin
   c. Phenylephrine
   d. Adrenaline
   e. Norepinephrine

A2. Regarding cerebral perfusion pressure (CPP) which one is correct?
   a. CPP is defined as MAP (measured at the right atrium) – Intracranial pressure (ICP)
   b. Under normal conditions cerebral blood flow (CBF) varies with CPP
   c. Is defined as MAP (measured at the tragus of the ear)–ICP
   d. In traumatic brain injury (TBI) augmentation of CPP is done by administering more IV fluids
   e. In order to maintain CPP all patients with TBI should have ICP monitoring

A3. In TBI which is most acceptable:
   a. Prophylactic hyperventilation to $PaCO_2$ of 25 to 30 mm Hg
   b. Application of prophylactic moderate hypothermia from 32 to 35°C for 48 hours
   c. Giving systemic steroids
   d. Hypertonic saline is recommended over mannitol to control ICP
   e. Decompressive craniectomy improves outcomes in TBI

A4. Regarding aneurysmal subarachnoid hemorrhage (SAH) select the most appropriate amongst the following:
   a. Early and short course of antifibrinolytic therapy should be considered for patients who are at high risk of rebleeding
   b. The optimal timing for treatment is 7–10 days after the bleed
   c. Prophylactic hypervolemia is recommended to prevent delayed cerebral ischemia (DCI) and vasospasm
   d. Initiation of statin therapy is recommended
   e. IV Nimodipine is recommended for treatment

A5. Regarding ICP monitoring which one is correct?

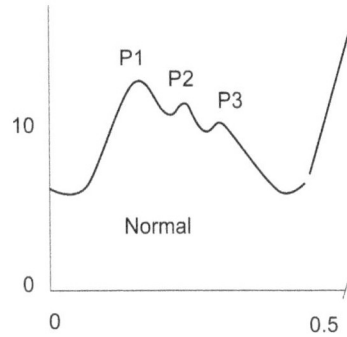

   a. Normal ICP waveform consists of 3 peaks called Lundberg waves
   b. Rising amplitude of P3 indicates decreasing intracranial compliance
   c. P1 reflects CVP
   d. Lundberg A waves are always pathological
   e. Respiratory cycle has no effect on the ICP waveform

A6. Regarding criteria for brainstem death testing:
   a. Cardiorespiratory stability is a prerequisite
   b. Patients on depressant drugs cannot be tested for brain death
   c. Sr. Sodium above 160 mEq/L is an absolute contraindication to BD testing
   d. EEG is a confirmatory test for brain death
   e. Infants less than 2 months of age and preterm babies can be tested for brain death

A7. In a CVP waveform giant V wave is indicative of

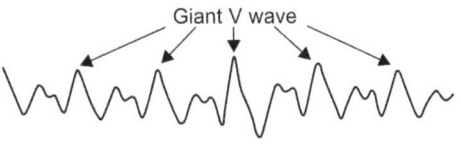

   a. Tricuspid stenosis
   b. Pulmonary hypertension
   c. Complete heart block
   d. Severe tricuspid regurgitation
   e. Right ventricular infarction

A8. Regarding Extravascular Lung Water (EVLW) all the following are true *except*:
   a. EVLW is an estimation of pulmonary edema
   b. It is measured by transpulmonary thermodilution
   c. It is the difference between intrathoracic thermal volume and intrathoracic blood volume
   d. EVLW can predict fluid responsiveness
   e. In ARDS high values of EVLW are significantly associated with mortality

A9. A 40-year-old male patient was admitted to a tertiary care hospital with history of crushing chest pain, diaphoresis and difficulty in breathing. ECG shows acute ST elevation inferior wall myocardial infarction (IWMI). Management includes all the following *except*:
   a. Aspirin 325 mg chewed and clopidogrel 600 mg PO
   b. Fibrinolytic therapy within 30 minutes
   c. IV Nitroglycerin
   d. IV Morphine sulphate 2–4 mg
   e. Primary percutaneous intervention (PCI)

A10. High priority investigations in patients with inhalational injury include all of the following *except*:
   a. Arterial blood gas analysis
   b. RBC cyanide levels
   c. Bronchoscopy
   d. Chest X-ray
   e. Flow volume loops on pulmonary function tests

A11. A 73-year-old male who has history of diabetes and hypertension underwent transthoracic oesophagectomy under combined general and epidural anesthesia. Postoperatively he is in fast atrial fibrillation with hypotension. Treatment includes all the following *except*:
   a. Adequate pain relief
   b. Correction of electrolyte abnormalities
   c. Assess fluid status and maintain normovolemia
   d. Administration of beta blockers
   e. Electrical cardioversion

A12. Prevention measures against *Clostridium difficile* infection include all of the following *except*:
   a. Prohibiting the use of Ceftriaxone, Fluoroquinolones and Clindamycin
   b. Strict hand hygiene with alcohol based hand sanitizers
   c. Isolation of the infected/ colonized patient
   d. Using probiotics
   e. Antibiotic stewardship

A13. Noise pollution in the ICU can be managed by all of the following methods *except*:
   a. Use of noise level monitors
   b. Behavior modification programs for nurses
   c. Headsets for patients
   d. Music therapy
   e. Sound absorbent surface coverings

A14. With regards to the stress dose of steroids in septic shock:
   a. It decrease mortality
   b. Increases the risk of secondary superinfection
   c. The benefit of steroids is limited to patients with vasopressor refractory shock
   d. It reduces the duration of shock
   e. Methylprednisolone is more likely to cause shock reversal than hydrocortisone

A15. Regarding glucose control in the critically ill:
   a. Glycemic variability is independently associated with mortality
   b. Intensive insulin therapy improves mortality
   c. Blood sugar target should be 120–140 mg%
   d. Once blood sugar values are stable with insulin infusion, blood sugar should be checked every 2 hours
   e. Insulin should be administered subcutaneously in diabetic patients

A16. Treatment of multiple organ dysfunction syndrome (MODS) includes all of the following *except*:
   a. Multi organ support
   b. Nutrition
   c. Steroids
   d. Seek and treat the underlying cause
   e. Glucose control

A17. Mosquito borne diseases include all the following *except*:
   a. Dengue
   b. Leptospirosis
   c. Japanese encephalitis

d. Malaria
e. Filariasis

A18. **Treatment of H1N1 pneumonia includes all of the following *except*:**
a. Tab Oseltamivir
b. H1N1 vaccine
c. ECMO
d. Isolation measures
e. Steroids

A19. **A 25-year-old female presents with history of diarrhea. On examination she is tachycardic with a heart rate of 130/min, blood pressure is 90/60 mm Hg and JVP is low. Her ABG shows a pH—7.39, PaO_2—85 mm Hg on room air, $PaCO_2$—39 mm Hg and HCO_3—24. Na/K/Cl—140/3.5/90 and HCT 0.6.**
a. Her ABG is normal
b. She has respiratory alkalosis
c. ABG shows anion gap metabolic acidosis and metabolic alkalosis
d. Non anion gap acidosis and respiratory alkalosis
e. This ABG is not a valid report

A20. **The Berlin definition for ARDS includes all *except*:**
a. Acute onset
b. Bilateral infiltrates on chest X-ray
c. PAWP ≤ 18
d. Divided into mild, moderate and severe category based on PaO_2/FiO_2 (PF ratio)
e. PF ratio < 300 mm Hg with a minimum of 5 cm H_2O PEEP (or CPAP)

A21. **Dehydration that is common in hot environments results in maximal utilization of endogenous:**
a. Corticosteroids
b. Vasopressin
c. Melatonin
d. Thyroxin
e. None of the above

A22. **Regarding ventilator associated event (VAE), all are true *except*:**
a. Can be applied to a patient who is mechanically ventilated for at least 4 days
b. A sustained increase in the daily minimum PEEP of ≥ 3 cm H_2O following a period of stability
c. Positive culture of endotracheal aspirate is a must
d. A sustained increase in the daily minimum FiO_2 of ≥ 0.20 (20%) following a period of stability
e. VAE is used for surveillance purpose

A23. **Regarding ventilator associated pneumonia (VAP) select the best choice:**
a. In all suspected cases of VAP, empiric gram-negative antipseudomonal, MSSA and/or MRSA cover is required
b. For patients with suspected HAP/VAP, antibiotic therapy should be initiated based on Modified Clinical Pulmonary Infection Score (CPIS) plus clinical criteria
c. Patients with ventilator associated tracheobronchitis (VAT) should be started on antibiotic therapy
d. In Acinetobacter VAP sensitive only to polymyxins- inhaled colistin need not be given along with IV polymyxin
e. In Acinetobacter VAP IV tigecycline is recommended

A24. **Contraindications to non-invasive ventilation (NIV) include all the following *except*:**
a. Decreased level of consciousness
b. Marked hemodynamic instability
c. Respiratory arrest
d. Intestinal obstruction
e. Bronchial asthma

A25. **Treatment of cyanide toxicity includes all the following *except*:**
a. Sodium nitrite
b. Thiamine
c. Sodium thiosulphate
d. Amyl nitrite
e. Hydroxycobalamin

A26. **Oxygen therapy:**
a. Is indicated to treat breathlessness
b. Should be given in carbon monoxide (CO) poisoning even though the saturation is 100% and PaO_2 is normal
c. Should be started only after taking an oximetry measurement on room air
d. Should be given in all patients with stroke
e. In metabolic acidosis with tachypnea

A27. **A 20-year-old male with suspected drug overdose was admitted to the emergency department with decreased level of consciousness, pin point pupils and a respiratory rate of 8/min. What is the most likely diagnosis?**

a. Tricyclic antidepressant overdose
b. Benzodiazepine overdose
c. Alcohol intoxication
d. Cocaine toxicity
e. Heroin overdose

A28. Features of heat stroke may include all of the following *except*:
a. Coma
b. Rhabdomyolysis
c. Fulminant hepatic failure
d. Hypotension
e. Hot moist skin

A29. Regarding Noise levels in the ICU:
a. Hospital noise levels should average 85 dBA during the day and 80 dBA at night
b. Noise in ICU have no effect on respiratory function
c. Can trigger ICU delirium
d. Sleep duration increases and quality decreases
e. Reduces total sleep time with excessive rapid eye movement (REM) sleep

A30. All the following are true about normal pregnancy *except*:
a. Oxygen consumption increases by 15–20%
b. Normal maternal pH is 7.40–7.47
c. Maternal bicarbonate value is 18–22 mEq/L
d. Normal maternal serum creatinine is 1.0–1.2 mg/dL
e. Blood pressure is 10–15 % less than the non-pregnant state

A31. Biomarkers of acute kidney injury includes all the following *except*:
a. Kidney injury molecule-1 (KIM-1)
b. Neutrophil gelatinase associated lipocalin (NGAL)
c. Cystatin C
d. Tissue inhibitor of metalloproteinases-2 (TIMP-2)
e. Interleukin 10 (IL10)

A32. A 20-year-old, 18 weeks pregnant lady was admitted to the ICU with severe nausea and vomiting. Her ABG shows a pH of 7.15, $PaCO_2$ = 25, PaO_2 = 100 and HCO_3 = 15. Lactate = 8. Urine ketones +++. Her management includes all the following *except*:
a. IV fluids
b. IV ondansetron
c. Fetal monitoring
d. IV insulin
e. Thiamine

A33. In obese ICU patients:
a. Enteral nutrition can be delayed up to one week
b. Normal caloric requirement should be targeted
c. Caloric requirements are based on ideal body weight in all obese patients
d. Protein requirements are similar to their non obese counterparts
e. Patients with a history of bariatric surgery should be supplemented with thiamine prior to initiating dextrose containing IV fluids or nutrition therapy

A34. In acute severe pancreatitis:
a. Surgical debridement for infected necrosis should be done as soon as possible
b. Abdominal ultrasound should be done to rule out gallstones
c. All pancreatic pseudocysts have to be drained
d. Prophylactic antibiotics are recommended
e. Patients should be kept nil by mouth for 48 hours

A35. In abdominal compartment syndrome (ACS):
a. Decompressive laparotomy is recommended immediately after the onset of ACS
b. Elevating the head of the bed reduces IAP
c. Overzealous fluid resuscitation can cause ACS
d. Inferior vena cava collapsibility and size correlates well with fluid status
e. ACS is defined as intra-abdominal pressure (IAP) > 20 mm Hg

A36. Noninvasive ventilation (NIV) failure is unlikely in critically ill cancer patients with:
a. Acute respiratory distress syndrome
b. Rapidly reversible respiratory failure
c. Renal replacement therapy
d. Infective acute respiratory failure
e. Vasopressor therapy

A37. Thrombotic thrombocytopenic purpura (TTP) is characterized by all of the following *except*:
a. Deranged coagulation profile—prolonged prothrombin time, activated partial thromboplastin time, and thrombin time

b. Microangiopathic hemolytic anemia
c. Renal failure
d. Altered mental status
e. Fever

A38. **Emergency laparotomy is indicated in the following in trauma:**
a. Stab wound penetrating the anterior peritoneum in hemodynamically stable patient without peritoneal signs or evisceration
b. Gunshot wounds penetrating the anterior peritoneum in a hemodynamically stable patient
c. Blunt abdominal trauma with a positive FAST in a hemodynamically stable patient
d. Abdominal pain and tenderness in a hemodynamically stable patient
e. Pelvic fracture with hypotension

A39. **Fluid resuscitation in burns:**
a. Should be initiated as per the Parkland formula
b. In pediatric patients fluids per kg body weight should be less than the adult patients
c. Tachycardia is a useful parameter to guide fluid resuscitation
d. In electrical injuries is the same as in a thermal injury
e. Lactated Ringer's solution (LR) or Hartmann's solution is most preferred fluid

A40. **Goals in the treatment of head injury includes all of the following *except*:**
a. $PaCO_2$ = 35–45 mm Hg
b. CPP ≥ 60 mm Hg
c. Platelets ≥ 75,000/mm^3
d. Sr. Na 145–155 meq/L
e. Temp 36–38°C

A41. **Anticoagulation in continuous renal replacement therapy (CRRT) includes all the following *except*:**
a. Low-molecular-weight heparin (LMWH)
b. Dabigatran
c. Argatroban
d. Heparin
e. Regional citrate anticoagulation

A42. **Regarding the model for end stage liver disease (MELD) score in liver transplantation all the following are true *except*:**
a. MELD determines priority in the waiting list for cadaveric liver transplant
b. Helps predict survival in cirrhotic patients
c. Is more accurate than Child-Pugh scoring in predicting outcome in cirrhotic patients
d. MELD score is superior to Child-Pugh for management and comparisons at a population level
e. Child-Pugh classification has been a reference for more time and MELD was introduced later

A43. **The following is true about immunosuppressants *except*:**
a. Anti-thymocyte globulin (ATG) is a monoclonal antibody
b. Rituximab is used to suppress antibody formation
c. Cyclosporin is a calcineurin inhibitor
d. Sirolimus is an MTOR inhibitor
e. Mycophenolate Mofetil (MMF) is a prodrug

A44. **All of the following are true about diabetic ketoacidosis (DKA) *except*:**
a. DKA is associated with anion gap metabolic acidosis
b. Bicarbonate therapy should be given to treat metabolic acidosis
c. Lactated ringers solution can be given to treat DKA
d. Hyperchloremic acidosis can occur in the recovery phase if only normal saline is used for resuscitation
e. Potassium infusions have to be given for treatment

A45. **A 29-year-old woman presented with bloody diarrhea, abdominal pain, hemolytic anemia, thrombocytopenia, and acute renal failure. *Escherichia coli* O104:H4 was identified in the stool culture. Her management includes all the following *except*:**
a. Fluid resuscitation
b. Plasma exchange
c. Hemodialysis
d. IV Ciprofloxacin
e. Platelet transfusion

A46. **A 56-year-old patient is admitted with disseminated carcinoma colon with obstructive uropathy, renal failure and sepsis. He had already been evaluated and was unfit for any surgical procedure. His management includes:**
a. Full active management including all organ supports

b. Withhold all life support therapies despite families' insistence on continuing care
c. Refuse admission to ICU
d. Discuss the poor prognosis and implications of forgoing aggressive interventions and work towards a shared decision making process
e. Transfer patient against medical advice

A47. **Discontinuing the ventilator from a brain dead patient is:**
a. Witholding therapy
b. Withdrawing therapy
c. Euthanasia
d. Non escalation of therapy
e. Is legally possible only after either consent for organ donation or after obtaining legal clearance

A48. **In snake bites:**
a. Applying a tourniquet proximal to the site of bite helps reduce the amount of venom absorbed
b. Signs of envenoming can recur after initial response to antivenom after 24 hours
c. Transfusion of blood products is indicated in the treatment of coagulopathy in snake bites
d. Dose of antivenom is related to the body weight of the victim
e. Killing the snake and bringing it to the hospital for identification is very important

A49. **A 48-year-old laborer has presented to the ED after having fallen from 15 feet at a construction site.**

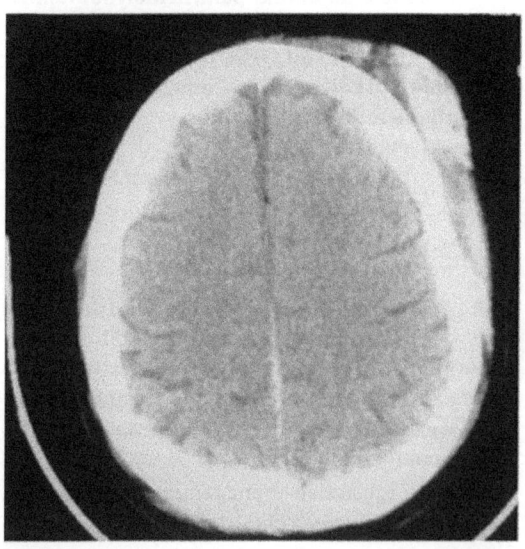

His CT head (plain) is shown. The findings are suggestive of:
a. Scalp hematoma
b. Acute subdural hematoma
c. Chronic subdural hematoma
d. Intracerebral hematoma
e. Normal scan

A50. **Critical incident reporting in ICU's should NOT have the following attribute:**
a. The persons involved in the incident should be named
b. They should emphasize a systems approach to error analysis
c. Rapid feedback to all involved and interested parties
d. Evidence that incident reporting is used to make system improvements
e. Culture of discussion and learning from incidents

K Type Questions
[Mark True (T)/False (F)]

K1. **Regarding fluid resuscitation in sepsis:**
a. Blood pressure is a good indicator of successful fluid resuscitation
b. Increased venous-to-arterial carbon dioxide difference (Pv-aCO$_2$) is a sign of hypoperfusion
c. Passive leg Raising (PLR) test is done by assessing the effect of raising both legs on the blood pressure
d. Inferior vena cava (IVC) size is a static measure of preload

K2. **Acute kidney injury (AKI) may occur with bites from:**
a. Cobra
b. Russell's viper
c. Krait
d. Hump nosed viper

K3. **Regarding mixed venous oxygen tension:**
a. Under normal physiological conditions, ScvO$_2$ is more than SvO$_2$
b. In patients with prolonged cardiac arrest ScvO$_2$ higher than 80% is indicative of good prognosis
c. Low ScvO$_2$ values indicate an oxygen debt
d. ScvO$_2$ should not be used alone in the assessment of the cardiopulmonary system in shock states

K4. **Patients with acute ischemic stroke (AIS):**
   a. Should be treated with aspirin 325 mg along with clopidogrel 150 mg within 1 hour after stroke symptom onset
   b. In AIS, decompressive craniectomy within 48 hours of onset for block of proximal middle cerebral artery (MCA) territory or internal carotid artery (ICA) decreases mortality
   c. IV Streptokinase is recommended within 4.5 hours of symptom onset
   d. Antiepileptic drugs should be administered prophylactically.

K5. **A 76-year-old was admitted with ataxia and dysarthria. CT brain showed cerebellar infarct with hydrocephalus. Management includes:**
   a. IV rt-PA (Alteplase)
   b. Aspirin 325mg within 24–48 hours
   c. Placement of an external ventricular drain
   d. Suboccipital decompressive craniectomy

K6. **Status epilepticus:**
   a. Is defined as continuous clinical and/or electrographic seizures lasting at least 5 minutes or recurrent discrete seizures without interictal recovery of consciousness
   b. The drug of choice for termination of seizures is IV Phenytoin
   c. In status epilepticus with fever a lumbar puncture should be done
   d. IV Ketamine can be used for treatment

K7. **In a patient with acute demyelinating polyneuropathy with impending respiratory compromise:**
   a. Noninvasive ventilation (NIV) is a useful alternative to invasive ventilation
   b. Rapid sequence intubation with succinylcholine is indicated
   c. Severe hypotension at intubation is common
   d. Neurally assisted ventilation (NAVA) is superior to other modes of ventilation

K8. **GBS:**
   a. Plasma exchange is the treatment of choice
   b. Treatment with steroids are useful
   c. Aggressive treatment of hypertension with antihypertensives is indicated
   d. Syndrome of inappropriate antidiuretic hormone secretion (SIADH) is a known complication

K9. **A 60-year-old female was admitted to the ICU 2 days after a left hemicolectomy with complaints of severe breathlessness. Her ABG on 15 liters/min oxygen by mask was pH—7.0, $PaCO_2$—102 mm Hg, paO_2—69 mm Hg and HCO_3—14. Echocardiography revealed an EF of 20% with global hypokinesia and apical ballooning. ECG showed global T wave inversion and chest X ray revealed pulmonary edema. Management includes:**
   a. Ventilatory support
   b. IV Furosemide
   c. Beta blockers
   d. Angiotensin-converting enzyme inhibitors (ACEI)

K10. **A 65-year-old male presented on postoperative day 2 after gastrectomy with hypotension, shortness of breath and cardiovascular collapse. He did not have any bleeding and was hemodynamically stable prior to this. His workup may include:**
   a. Electrocardiogram
   b. Transthoracic echocardiography
   c. CT pulmonary angiogram (CTPA)
   d. Compression ultrasound of the lower limb veins

K11. **Regarding the use of vasopressors and inotropes in ICU:**
   a. Low dose dopamine helps to prevent renal failure in shock
   b. Phenylephrine can be used in septic shock
   c. Milrinone is a calcium sensitizer
   d. Norepinephrine is the vasopressor of choice in all types of shock

K12. **Procalcitonin (PCT):**
   a. Can be used to assist in differentiating infectious and noninfectious causes of systemic inflammatory response syndrome (SIRS)
   b. The use of PCT reduces the risk of antibiotic-related diarrhea from *C. difficile*
   c. PCT levels can be used to support the discontinuation of empiric antibiotics in sepsis
   d. PCT elevation may prognosticate increasing severity of illness and mortality

K13. **Regarding antibiotic therapy:**
   a. Empiric broad spectrum therapy is recommended in sepsis or septic shock

b. At least 2 weeks of systemic antibiotic therapy is recommended for severe pancreatitis
c. The loading dose of antibiotics should be reduced in renal failure
d. Empiric combination therapy is recommended in septic shock but not in bacteremia/sepsis without shock

K14. **In neutropenic fever:**
a. First line therapy may include monotherapy with a fluoroquinolones
b. In high risk patients if neutropenia persists but fever resolves antibiotic therapy can be discontinued
c. Empiric antifungal therapy should be started along with broad spectrum antibiotics as first line therapy
d. Myeloid colony stimulating factor is recommended in a setting of established fever and neutropenia

K15. *Clostridium difficile* **colitis:**
a. Is caused by toxin from gram negative organisms
b. Destruction of normal fecal microbiota by antibiotics is the major risk factor for this disease
c. Infants cannot get *C. difficile* infection
d. Testing for *C. difficile* toxin in stool after treatment is used to confirm eradication of infection

K16. **Pneumocystis pneumonia (PCP):**
a. Is caused by a bacteria *Pneumocystis jiroveci*
b. Is characterized by severe respiratory distress and hypoxia but normal findings on auscultation and percussion.
c. Is characterized by high fever
d. Patients with hypoxia should be treated with corticosteroids

K17. **Strategies that are beneficial in the treatment of ARDS include:**
a. Steroids
b. Inhaled nitric oxide
c. Extracorporeal membrane oxygenation (ECMO)
d. High frequency oscillatory ventilation (HFOV)

K18. **Time constant of a lung unit:**
a. Time constant= Compliance × Resistance
b. Is the time taken for the lung unit to inflate 63% of its volume
c. In ARDS the lungs have a long time constant
d. Ventilatory strategies are not affected by time constants

K19. **Regarding ventilator strategies in COPD:**
a. Volume controlled ventilation is as effective as pressure controlled ventilation
b. Externally applied PEEP is harmful
c. Extubation to NIV can facilitate early extubation
d. Extubation failure is an indication for tracheostomy

K20. **Prevention of the occurrence of acute kidney injury in sepsis includes:**
a. Aminoglycoside to treat sepsis empirically
b. Appropriate antibiotics and source control
c. Early goal directed therapy (EGDT)
d. Hetastarch administration to treat hypovolemia

K21. **Weaning from mechanical ventilation:**
a. Should begin by assessing readiness for spontaneous breathing trials (SBT)
b. The duration of SBT should be at least for 4 hours
c. Protocolized weaning led to shorter duration of mechanical ventilation
d. Automated systems which used closed loop circuits to automatically adjust the level of support required showed shorter duration of weaning and shorter duration of mechanical ventilation

K22. **Tracheostomy:**
a. Should be used for prolonged weaning
b. Early tracheostomy improves short-term mortality
c. Percutaneous tracheostomy results in fewer complications than open surgical technique
d. Early tracheostomy allows patients to be transferred out of the ICU setting earlier

K23. **A 23-year-old female, a known asthmatic on steroids comes to casualty with severe breathlessness and a silent chest. She is unconscious. Her ABG reveals a respiratory acidosis. Her initial management includes:**
a. Restricted oxygen therapy to target a saturation of 90–92%.

b. Continuous nebulization of B agonists.
c. Noninvasive ventilation
d. Fluid resuscitation

K24. Examine the following ECG, and mark TRUE/FALSE in the flowing options:

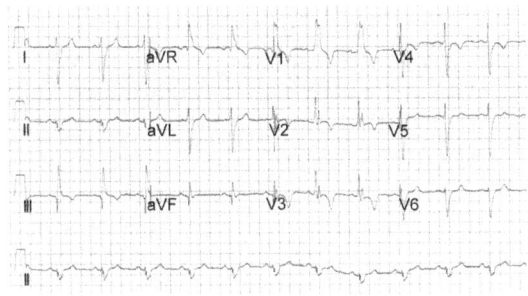

a. Cor pulmonale
b. Hyperkalemia
c. Pulmonary embolism
d. Hypothermia

K25. Criteria for provision of extracorporeal CPR (ECPR) include:
a. Witnessed circulatory arrest
b. Bystander CPR
c. Prolonged CPR
d. Early availability and institution of ECMO after cardiac arrest

K26. A 70-year-old female with bipolar disorder on treatment with lithium since many years was admitted with seizures, renal failure and hypotension. Which of the following is appropriate?
a. She should be treated with activated charcoal
b. Treatment of choice is RRT
c. Is associated with a decreased anion gap
d. Whole bowel irrigation with polyethylene glycol is indicated

K27. Regarding gamma hydroxybutyrate (GHB) also called the date rape drug:
a. It cannot be detected by toxicological analysis
b. Its antidote is naloxone
c. It acts as an inhibitory neurotransmitter to GHB and GABA receptors
d. Recovery is usually rapid

K28. Infection control in ICU should include:
a. Minimum of six total air changes per room per hour are required, with two air changes per hour composed of outside air
b. Waste segregation at source
c. Policies for cleaning and decontamination
d. Temperature regulation has no effect on infection

K29. Regarding antibiotic therapy in the ICU:
a. Minocycline can be given as monotherapy
b. Tigecycline is a bacteriostatic drug
c. Fosfomycin sodium is effective against Acinetobacter baumannii
d. Daptomycin can be used to treat endocarditis of the mitral valve

K30. A full term pregnant lady has been involved in a high-speed road traffic accident. She is unresponsive and hypotensive on arrival in Accident & Emergency (A & E). Her treatment involves:
a. Intubation and ventilation
b. Immediate CT scan of the brain and C-spine
c. Immediate delivery of the baby
d. Elevate the right hip

K31. A 30-week pregnant lady is admitted to your ICU with a diagnosis of probable H1N1 pneumonia and her oxygen saturation is reading 54%. Her management may include:
a. Elective cesarean section in the operation theater
b. Protective lung ventilation
c. ECMO support
d. Prone ventilation

K32. The contraindication(s) to enteral nutrition include:
a. Lack of bowel sounds
b. Gastric tube aspirate of > 250 mL
c. If patients are on vasopressors
d. In prone position

K33. In massive hemorrhage due to polytrauma:
a. Blood tests to prove coagulopathy has to be done before administering blood products
b. Penetrating injury and a positive FAST scan in a hemodynamically unstable patient should trigger a massive transfusion protocol
c. The use of recombinant factor VIIa can improve morbidity and mortality in acutely bleeding trauma patients
d. Hemoglobin concentration is a good guide to assess blood loss

K34. **In a critically ill adult:**
   a. The caloric requirement is approximately 25 kcal/kg/day actual body weight
   b. The daily protein requirement is 1.5 g/kg/day ideal body weight
   c. It is safe to provide 25% of the caloric goal for the first five days.
   d. Diverting tube feeds from gastric to post pyloric in patients with high risk of regurgitation reduces the incidence of VAP

K35. **Factors that predispose a patient to chronic radiation enteritis include:**
   a. Obesity
   b. Concomitant chemotherapy
   c. Radiation dose
   d. Previous perianal surgery

K36. **Parenteral nutrition (PN):**
   a. Is recommended to be started immediately in patients at high nutrition risk who are unable to be initiated on EN
   b. In patients with high nutritional risk supplemental PN should be started immediately if patients are unable to meet their caloric requirements by the enteral route
   c. Hypocaloric PN dosing with adequate protein has been recommended over the first week of ICU admission
   d. Parenteral glutamine should be administered along with PN

K37. **In acute severe pancreatitis:**
   a. Immune enhancing formulae are recommended
   b. All patients should be started on nasojejunal tube feeding
   c. Use of probiotics should be considered
   d. If EN is not tolerated within 48 hours despite measures to improve tolerance PN should be started

K38. **Transfusion related acute lung injury (TRALI):**
   a. Occurs within 48 hours of transfusion
   b. Is more common with transfusion of packed red cells
   c. Steroids are useful in treatment
   d. Is caused by antibodies to recipient Red blood cells

K39. **For patients with deep vein thrombosis (DVT) in the ICU:**
   a. Workup for hypercoagulable states should be done immediately
   b. All patients need to be worked up for an underlying hypercoagulable state
   c. The diagnosis of DVT can be predicted by the Wells Score
   d. A negative value of D-dimer may safely rule out both DVT and PE

K40. **Regarding cervical spine (C-spine) injuries:**
   a. Atlanto-occipital dislocation is a common cause of death in shaken baby syndrome
   b. Hangman's fracture usually involves the odontoid process
   c. Plain X-rays of the cervical spine are sufficient to rule out cervical spine injury
   d. Cervical spine fracture can be ruled out in a fully conscious patient having no neck pain but having fracture ribs and fracture femur

K41. **Indications for involving the thoracic surgeon in chest trauma include:**
   a. Blood loss over the chest Tube Drainage > 1,500 mL initially or >200 mL/hour over 2–4 hours
   b. Flail chest with hypoxemia
   c. Hemoptysis
   d. Hemopneumothorax

K42. **In postoperative renal failure:**
   a. S. creatinine is helpful in differentiating prerenal failure from acute tubular necrosis
   b. Dopamine can be used for treatment
   c. N acetyl cysteine should be used to prevent renal failure in high risk patients
   d. Hetastarch is useful in treating hypovolemia in prerenal failure

K43. **Hepatorenal syndrome (HRS):**
   a. Can occur in patients who are not cirrhotic
   b. Histopathological abnormalities in the kidney are seen on biopsy
   c. Proteinuria is not present
   d. Is reversible with dialysis

K44. **Regarding acute kidney injury (AKI):**
   a. Community acquired AKI has a worse prognosis than hospital acquired AKI

b. Renal biopsy is indicated in prolonged AKI as a routine
c. Doppler ultrasonography is a useful tool to detect patients at risk of developing AKI
d. A positive fluid balance helps in recovery from AKI

K45. **Eye signs seen in a patient with pituitary apoplexy are:**
a. Visual field defects
b. Blindness
c. Ipsilateral mydriasis
d. Ptosis

K46. **The treatment of hepatorenal syndrome includes:**
a. Liver transplant
b. Albumin
c. Terlipressin
d. Diuretics

K47. **A 20-year-old male is admitted with accidental ingestion of large quantities of digoxin. He presents with headache, drowsiness, nausea, vomiting and cardiac arrhythmias. Serum potassium was 7.2 mEq/L. Treatment of hyperkalemia includes:**
a. IV Sodium bicarbonate
b. IV Calcium gluconate
c. Digoxin Fab fragments
d. Insulin-dextrose infusion

K48. **A 80-year-old female patient was admitted in a confused state and her serum sodium was 101 mEq/L. Her HR was 78/ min and blood pressure was 106/70 mm Hg. Her treatment may include:**
a. Tolvaptan
b. Hypertonic saline infusion
c. Thiazide diuretics
d. Fluid restriction

K49. **Benchmarking of markers of ICU care should be done:**
a. To predict mortality
b. To improve quality of care delivered
c. To compare adherence to standards of care in different ICU's
d. To help with predicting costs

K50. **Stress ulcer prophylaxis (SUP):**
a. Reduces the incidence of VAP
b. Proton pump inhibitors may increase the incidence of *Clostridium difficile* infections (CDI)
c. Should be given in all intensive care patients until discharge
d. Can be stopped in patients tolerating EN

ANSWERS

A Type Answers

QA1. Answer e

The Clinical Practice Committee of the Scandinavian Society of Anaesthesia and Intensive Care Medicine (SSAI) guideline (2016) on choice of first-line vasopressor in adult patients with acute circulatory failure recommended norepinephrine for all causes of shock. Norepinephrine rather than any other vasopressors was recommended as first-line treatment for the majority of adult critically ill patients with acute circulatory failure.

> Møller MH. et al. Scandinavian SSAI clinical practice guideline on choice of first-line vasopressor for patients with acute circulatory failure. Acta Anaesthesiologica Scandinavica. 2016;60:1347-66.

QA2. Answer c

MAP measured at the level of the right atrium may be very different from that measured at the level of the tragus when the head end of the bed is elevated. To avoid this variability, the Neuroanesthesia Society of Great Britain and Ireland and the Society of British Neurologic Surgeons issued a joint position statement advocating for measurement of CPP at the level of the tragus in patients with TBI. Under normal conditions, CBF remains constant despite changes in CPP. This is due to cerebral autoregulation. Augmentation of CPP with fluids will increase incidence of ARDS. Vasopressors should be used instead. Not all patients with TBI need ICP monitoring. They can be assessed clinically and with imaging.

> Sandzmark DK. et al. Evidence-Based Practice of Critical Care, 2nd edn. Ch 62. 441-449.

QA3. Answer b

Prolonged prophylactic hyperventilation to Paco2 of 25 to 30 mm Hg should be avoided in TBI patients because of risks of cerebral ischemia. It may be justified as a temporary intervention in emergency and temporary sudden increases in ICP such as with life-threatening herniation syndromes. In severe TBI, there is evidence for selective and cautious application of prophylactic moderate hypothermia from 32 to 35°C for 48 hours. There is an increased risk of death associated with the use of corticosteroids, and thus their use is not recommended by the Brain Trauma Foundation. Hypertonic saline (HTS) cannot be recommended over mannitol for the treatment of elevated ICP but HTS may result in better ICP control in patients who no longer respond to mannitol therapy. Surgical decompressive therapy is an effective measure for the management of persistently elevated ICP. However, there is no evidence that decompression improves clinical outcomes.

> Sandzmark DK, et al. Evidence-Based Practice of Critical Care, 2nd edn. Ch 62. 441-9.

QA4. Answer a

The Neurocritical Care Society Consensus Guidelines advise that an early and short course of antifibrinolytic therapy should be considered for patients who are at high risk of rebleeding. The patients with the highest mortality were those whose surgery was planned for days 7 to 10 after bleed, a time when risk of vasospasm and delayed cerebral injury is greatest. Early surgery or endovascular therapy is recommended. Although induced hypertension, hypervolemia, and hemodilution ("Triple-H therapy") have historically been the mainstay of medical treatment for vasospasm and DIND, hypovolemia is associated with worsening vasospasm and DCI and should be avoided; however, volume loading is associated with harm. Therefore prophylactic hypervolemia is not recommended, and patients should be maintained in a euvolemic state. Statins have pleotropic vascular and neuroprotective effects. However, a well-designed multicenter RCT done with 40 mg simvastatin instituted within 96 hours of SAH for up to 21 days was not associated with improved 6-month functional outcome (modified Rankin scale score). Therefore de novo initiation of statin therapy is not recommended. Oral nimodipine improves outcome in SAH and should be given to all patients unless contraindicated. IV Nimodipine did not improve outcomes.

> Bhalla PK. et al. Evidence-Based Practice of Critical Care, 2nd edn. Ch 63. 450-60.

QA5. Answer d

The ICP waveform has three components: (1) The ICP wave is a modified arterial pressure waveform that is transmitted from the large cerebral blood vessels. (2) The baseline of the waveform varies with the respiratory cycle. (3) Slow waves which are changes in the baseline of the ICP trace. They are also called Lundberg waves and are usually indicative of pathology. There are three types of Lundberg waves—A, B and C waves.

Cross ME, Plunket EVE. Physics, Pharmacology and Physiology for Anaesthetists. Key concepts for the FRCA, 2nd edn. 302-22.

QA6. Answer a

According to the depressant drug used reasonable steps should be taken that the drug has been eliminated out of the body-A period of observation that approximates to four times the elimination half-life of the agent involved, administering antidotes to the drug, checking plasma levels or rule out brain death by other ancillary tests such as cerebral angiography. Potentially reversible cause of coma has to be corrected but derangements that are clearly the result of brain death need not be corrected such as hypernatremia due to diabetes insipidus. EEG is the most popular and best validated ancillary test worldwide but is of little value in drug intoxication. In infants younger than 2 months of age, the diagnosis of brainstem death becomes difficult. Coma in this age group is often multifactorial. Although hypoxic encephalopathy remains the most likely cause of devastating brain injury, it is often difficult to demonstrate structural brain damage and thus the preconditions are rarely met. In preterm infants (gestational age below 37 weeks), there is little evidence concerning normal brainstem reflexes and as such their absence is difficult to demonstrate. Diagnosis of brainstem death is inappropriate in this age group.

Oram J, et al. Diagnosis of death. CEACCP. 2011;11(3):77-81.

QA7. Answer d

Pulmonary hypertension and tricuspid stenosis cause a dominant 'a wave'. Cannon a wave caused by complete heart block. RV infarction causes a prominent x and y descent.

CVP Measurement. Available from: https://lifeinthefastlane.com/ccc/cvp-measurement/ (Accessed 13 February 2018).

QA8. Answer d

EVLW may mostly be used to conduct fluid resuscitation in a safe and controlled manner, especially in septic shock combined with ARDS. High EVLW values may indicate that further fluid administration risks fluid overload and, at the post-acute phase, that fluid removal should be initiated. It is not a measure of fluid responsiveness.

Mc Canny. et al. PACT module. Hemodynamic monitoring and management.

QA9. Answer c

IWMI may have right ventricular involvement in up to 60% cases. Nitroglycerin is contraindicated in the setting of an IWMI with right ventricular involvement because, in this specific situation, the heart is dependent on preload. As discussed above, nitroglycerin decreases preload and will induce further hypotension and possible cardiac arrest in patients suffering from a right ventricular MI, volume depletion, or in those who have recently used erectile dysfunction medications. Fibrinolytic therapy should only be considered if there is lack of available PCI facility, delay in transport to PCI facility or any contraindication to PCI. Primary PCI is preferred over fibrinolytics.

Depta JP. The Washington Manual of Critical Care. 125-38.

QA10. Answer c

Laboratory studies include arterial blood gas analysis with carboxyhemoglobin, methemoglobin, and lactate levels; RBC cyanide levels if persistent acidosis occurs; electrocardiographic (ECG) monitoring; and chest X-ray. For severe inhalation exposure or suspected pulmonary aspiration, chest radiography and arterial blood gas analysis are strictly recommended. The presence of hypoxemia despite a normal arterial partial pressure of oxygen suggests carbon monoxide toxicity. Carboxyhemoglobin levels should be obtained for all fire and explosion victims. Metabolic acidosis may indicate cyanide or hydrogen sulfide intoxication. Pulmonary edema, atelectasis or infiltrates may be detected on chest radiographs. As the final step, baseline pulmonary function should be determined through pulmonary function tests. Flow-volume loops are the most sensitive noninvasive indicators of upper and lower airway obstruction. On the other hand, the efficiency of diagnostic bronchoscopy for inhaled toxin exposure remains controversial.

Gorguner M, Akgun M. Acute Inhalation Injury. EAJM 2010;42:28-35.

QA11. Answer d

Postoperative atrial fibrillation can be triggered by pain, electrolyte imbalances, fluid shifts, hypoxia, hypervolemia and type of surgery. Since the patient is hemodynamically unstable electrical cardioversion may be attempted. Beta blockers should be given in hemodynamically stable patients.

Frogel JK, et al. Evidence-Based Practice of Critical Care, 2nd edn. Ch 53. 361-9.

QA12. Answer b

C. difficile is nearly ubiquitous in health care facilities, and viable spores can be identified on all surfaces. Using alcohol-based hand sanitizers does not reduce the number of viable C. difficile spores, whereas washing with soap and water is required.

Leffler DA, et al. *Clostridium difficile* infection. N Engl J Med. 2015;372:1539-48.

QA13. Answer d

Because noise may be the most adverse effect of the ICU environment, efforts need to be directed to limit the noise in the ICU. Paying attention to the behavior of health care providers is the key to noise control. Behavior modification programs have had positive effects on altering the routines of staff related noise in the ICU setting. Using headsets for patients, making periodic assessment of noise through noise level monitors, and selecting sound absorbent surface coverings in the ICU are recommended interventions.

Fontaine DK. *Essentials of Critical Care Nursing: A Holistic Approach.* Impact of the critical care environment on the patient. 2012 Page 42.

QA14. Answer d

There is no convincing data that stress-dose steroids improve mortality or increase the rate of super infection. There is no clear demarcation of which patients may or may not benefit from steroids. Not all therapeutic corticosteroids are the same. Even at dose equivalency, some corticosteroids have more immunosuppressive properties (e.g., dexamethasone), and some have more mineralocorticoid and vasoreactive properties (e.g., hydrocortisone).

There is strong evidence that boluses of methylprednisolone are less likely to result in shock reversal than hydrocortisone boluses.

Gibbison. et al. Corticosteroids in septic shock: a systematic review and network meta-analysis. Critical Care. 2017;21:78.

QA15. Answer a

Following the publication of the two single-center Leuven studies, the preponderance of evidence has strongly indicated that the use of intensive insulin treatment with the goal of tight glycemic management in critically-ill patients at best provides no benefit over moderate or lax glycemic control, and at worst results in markedly increased rates of severe hypoglycemia and possibly even increased mortality. Blood sugar should be kept below 180 mg% and infusion of insulin should be started when blood sugar exceeds 180 mg%. Blood glucose values are monitored every 1 to 2 hours until glucose values and insulin infusion rates are stable, then every 4 hours thereafter in patients receiving insulin infusions. Insulin infusions should be administered for both diabetics and non-diabetics for control of blood sugar.

Clain J, et al. Glucose control in critical care. World J Diabetes. 2015; 6(9):1082-91.

Rhodes A, et al. Surviving Sepsis Campaign: International Guidelines for Management of Sepsis and Septic Shock: 2016. CCM. 2017;45:3.

QA16. Answer c

MODS is a hypometabolic, immunodepressed state with clinical and biochemical evidence of decreased functioning of the organ systems that develops subsequent to an acute injury or illness. There is no evidence for benefit of steroids in MODS.

Multi-Organ Dysfunction Syndrome (MODS). Available from: https://lifeinthefastlane.com/ccc/multi-organ-dysfunction-syndrome-mods/(Accessed 13 February 2018).

QA17. Answer b

Leptospirosis may also be transmitted through direct contact with urine or tissues of infected animals, or by inhalation of aerosols of contaminated fluids, such as may occur in abattoirs. Ingestion of foods contaminated with urine of infected rats is an occasional route of infection.

Singhi S, et al. Tropical fevers: Management guidelines. Indian Journal of Critical Care Medicine. 2014;18(2).

QA18. Answer b

H1N1 vaccine is used for prevention and not treatment of H1N1 pneumonia.

Rewar S, et al. Treatment and Prevention of Pandemic H1N1 Influenza. Annals of Global Health. 2015;81(5):645-53.

QA19. Answer c

Check validity of ABG by checking whether this relationship is true $[H^+ = 24\times(PaCO_2 / HCO_3)] = 24\times39/24= 39$. This value added to the last 2 digits of pH should roughly be equal to 80 or can be checked against table of pH & H^+. Anion gap is $Na-(Cl+HCO_3)= 140-(90+24)= 26$. Coexisting metabolic disorders can be diagnosed by the corrected HCO_3 or delta gap. Corrected HCO_3= Measured HCO_3 + (corrected anion gap for albumin-12)= 24+(26-12)=38. Therefore there is an anion gap metabolic acidosis along with metabolic alkalosis probably due to hypovolemia and contraction alkalosis.

QA20. Answer c

The Berlin definition for ARDS defines ARDS as occurring within 1 week of a known clinical insult or new or worsening respiratory symptoms. Bilateral opacities—not fully explained by effusions, lobar/lung collapse. Chest radiograph criteria clarified and example radiographs created or nodules. Respiratory failure not fully explained by cardiac failure or fluid overload. No need for measuring PCWP. Need objective assessment (e.g., echocardiography) to exclude hydrostatic edema if no risk factor is present. Oxygenation criteria are based on minimum PEEP as well.

Gordon D, et al. The Berlin definition of acute respiratory distress syndrome. JAMA. 2012;307(23):2526-33.

QA21. Answer b

In some cases, injury may result from the pathophysiologic end points of normal processes used to maintain homeostasis rather than elevated core temperature. For example, the dehydration that is common in hot environments can result in maximal utilization of endogenous vasopressin to reclaim free water. Although the goal is to maintain euvolemia, prolonged reclamation of free water out of proportion to sodium with the additional consumption of free water may result in dilutional hyponatremia.

Lipman GS, Eifling KP et al. Wilderness Medical Society Practice Guidelines for the Prevention and Treatment of Heat-Related Illness: 2014 Update. Wilderness & Environmental Medicine. 2014;(25):S55-S65.

QA22. Answer c

The VAE definition algorithm is for use in surveillance; it is not a clinical definition algorithm and is not intended for use in the clinical management of patients. Chest radiograph is not taken for diagnosis of infection. The subjectivity and variability inherent in chest radiograph technique, interpretation, and reporting make chest imaging ill-suited for inclusion in a definition algorithm to be used for the potential purposes of surveillance reporting. Three categories of VAE were identified: Ventilator-associated condition (VAC), Infection-related ventilator-associated complication (IVAC) and Possible or probable VAP. A period of stability on a ventilator for at least 48 hours (as evidenced by unchanged PEEP or FiO_2) must be present before a VAE can be considered. In addition, increased PEEP or FiO_2 must be present for more than 2 days. Hence VAE has to occur after the patient has been on a mechanical ventilator for more than 4 days. VAEs are identified by using a combination of objective criteria: deterioration in respiratory status after a period of stability or improvement on the ventilator, evidence of infection or inflammation, and laboratory evidence of respiratory infection.

Management of Adults With Hospital-acquired and Ventilator-associated Pneumonia: 2016 Clinical Practice Guidelines by the Infectious Diseases Society of America. Available from: http://www.cdc.gov/nhsn/PDFs/pscManual/10-VAE_FINAL.pdf (Accessed 13 February 2018).

QA23. Answer a

As per 2016 IDSA guidelines, for patients with suspected HAP/VAP, clinical criteria alone, rather than using CPIS plus clinical criteria is recommended. Patients with VAT should not receive antibiotic therapy. Empiric anti MRSA cover is recommended only if patients being treated in units where >10%–20% of *S. aureus* isolates are methicillin resistant, and patients in units where the prevalence of MRSA is not known. Empiric antipseudomonal therapy should be started with one or two antibiotics depending on the resistance to the agent (≤ 10% or ≥ 10%) being considered for monotherapy. The antibiotic should cover MSSA if no risk factors for MRSA. In patients with HAP/VAP caused by *Acinetobacter* species that is sensitive only to polymyxins, intravenous polymyxin (colistin or polymyxin B) and adjunctive inhaled colistin is recommended. IV tigecycline is not recommended even if sensitive.

> Kalil AC, et al. Management of adults with HAP/VAP: 2016 Clinical Practice Guidelines by the Infectious Diseases Society of America and the American Thoracic Society. CID

QA24. Answer e

There is a risk of aspiration if NIV is applied to a patient with intestinal obstruction. Patients on NIV should be able to protect the airway and initiate spontaneous breaths. Patients need to be hemodynamically stable. NIV can be used in severe asthma as long as it does not delay intubation when required.

> Non-Invasive Ventilation. Available from: (NIV)https://lifeinthefastlane.com/ccc/non-invasive-ventilation-niv/ (Accessed 13 February 2018).

QA25. Answer b

Antidotes to cyanide include nitrites, which induces methemoglobinemia red blood cells that combines with cyanide, thus releasing cytochrome oxidase enzyme. Sodium thiosulfate donates a sulfur atom necessary for the transformation of cyanide to thiocyanate by rhodanese, thus increasing the activity of the endogenous detoxification system. Thiocyanate is then renally excreted. Hydroxocobalamin is the drug of choice for treating known or suspected cyanide poisoning. Hydroxocobalamin combines with cyanide to form cyanocobalamin (vitamin B-12), which is renally cleared. Alternatively, cyanocobalamin may dissociate from cyanide at a slow enough rates to allow for cyanide detoxification by the mitochondrial enzyme rhodanese.

> Holstege CP, Kirk MA. Cyanide and hydrogen sulfide. Goldfrank's Toxicologic Emergencies, 10th edn. New York, NY: McGraw-Hill Education; 2015. Chapter 126.

QA26. Answer b

Oxygen is a treatment for hypoxemia, not breathlessness. Oxygen has not been proven to have any consistent effect on the sensation of breathlessness in non-hypoxaemic patients. In carbon monoxide poisoning, a normal or high oximetry reading should be disregarded because saturation monitors cannot differentiate between carboxyhemoglobin and oxyhemoglobin, owing to their similar absorbance. The blood gas PO_2 will also be normal in these cases (despite the presence of tissue hypoxia). Oxygen therapy should not be discontinued based on pulse oximetry readings. Most patients with stroke are not hypoxaemic. Oxygen therapy may be harmful for non-hypoxaemic patients with mild–moderate strokes. Patients with metabolic acidosis do not need oxygen unless hypoxemic.

> O'Driscoll BR et al. BTS guideline for oxygen use in adults in healthcare and emergency settings. THORAX. 2017; 72 (1).

QA27. Answer e

Opiods overdose presents with the triad of decreased consciousness, respiratory depression and miosis. Opioid-based drugs include morphine, heroin, oxycodone, and synthetic opioid narcotics. Tricyclic antidepressants and cocaine cause mydriasis. Alcohol and benzodiazepines do not cause any effect on pupil size.

> Mokhlesi B, et al. Adult toxicology in critical care. Part I: General approach to the intoxicated person. Chest. 2003;123:577-92.

QA28. Answer e

Generally with heat exhaustion, a patient is sweating a lot, whereas with heat stroke, they've stopped sweating and are actually dry.

> Cui J, Sinoway LI. Cardiovascular responses to heat stress in chronic heart failure. Curr Heart Fail Rep. 2014;11:139.

QA29. Answer c

Average sleep duration over a 24-hour period may be reduced during hospitalization. For many acutely ill patients, sleep appears to be spread around the clock, with 40 to 60 percent of sleep occurring during typical waking daytime hours. Hospital noise levels should average 35 dBA during the day and 30 dBA at night. Sleep is highly fragmented, with prolonged sleep latencies, frequent arousals, poor nocturnal sleep efficiency, an increase in stage 2 (N2) sleep, a reduction or absence of deep or slow wave (N3) sleep, and a reduction or absence of rapid eye movement (REM) sleep. Acute sleep deprivation impairs several parameters of respiratory function, including chemosensitivity and control of ventilation, genioglossus muscle activity, inspiratory muscle endurance, and spirometry (in patients with chronic obstructive lung disease).

> Darbyshire JL. Excessive noise in intensive care units. BMJ. 2016;353:i1956.

QA30. Answer d

During pregnancy the glomerular filtration rate (GFR) is increased by 40-50% resulting in a concomitant decrease in serum creatinine and values greater than 0.8 should be considered as abnormal.

> Lazarus DR, et al. Approach to critically ill pregnant female. Textbook of Critical Care. 2016. Ch 67. 65-74

QA31. Answer e

IL-10 is a biomarker for respiratory diseases. IL-10 and IL-6 have been reported to be related to hepatocellular carcinoma (HCC) prognosis.

> Alge JL et al. Biomarkers of AKI: A review of mechanistic relevance and potential therapeutic implications. Clin J Am Soc Nephrol. 2015;10:147-55.

QA32. Answer d

Hyperemesis gravidarum with dehydration and starvation can precipitate ketoacidosis. Pregnancy is a diabetogenic state characterized by relative insulin resistance, enhanced lipolysis, elevated free fatty acids and increased ketogenesis. In this setting, short period of starvation can precipitate ketoacidosis. Short periods of starvation during pregnancy may present as severe anion gap metabolic acidosis (AGMA). Dehydration can produce lactic acidosis resulting in combined anion gap and non-anion gap metabolic acidosis. The treatment for this is intensive care management and IV fluids, dextrose, thiamine and folic acid.

> Sinha N, et al. Starvation ketoacidosis: A cause of severe anion gap metabolic acidosis in pregnancy. Case Reports in Critical Care. 2014; Article ID 906283.

QA33. Answer e

Early EN should be started within 24-48 hours of admission to the ICU for obese patients who cannot sustain volitional intake. High protein hypocaloric feeding is associated with better outcomes than use of high protein eucaloric feeding. It helps the care of obese ICU patients to preserve lean body mass, mobilize adipose stores, and minimize the metabolic complications of overfeeding. In adult obese ICU patients target energy and protein requirements vary according to the BMI. Caloric requirements are 11-14 kcal/kg actual body weight/day for patients with BMI in the range 30-50 and 22-25 kcal/kg ideal body weight/day for patients with BMI > 50. Protein should be provided in a range from 2.0 g/kg ideal body weight/day for patients with BMI 30-40 up to 2.5 g/kg ideal body weight/day for patients with BMI ≥ 40. In addition to thiamine, patients who have undergone bariatric surgery should be evaluated and treated for micronutrient deficiencies such as calcium, vitamin B12, fat soluble vitamins (A, D, E, K) and folate, along with the trace minerals iron, selenium, zinc, and copper.

> Tayloe BE, et al. Guidelines for the Provision and Assessment of Nutrition Support Therapy in the Adult Critically Ill Patient: Society of Critical Care Medicine (SCCM) and American Society for Parenteral and Enteral Nutrition (A.S.P.E.N.). Critical Care Medicine. 2016;44(2):390-438.

QA34. Answer b

Carefully done retrospective studies have demonstrated that reoperation rates, morbidity, and mortality are significantly improved when surgical debridement of infected necrosis can be delayed to more than 28-30 days. Pancreatic pseudocysts that are asymptomatic should be managed nonoperatively. Prophylactic antibiotics are not recommended in patients with mild or severe acute pancreatitis. In patients with severe acute pancreatitis, enteral nutrition should be commenced as soon as possible following admission (within 48 hours).

Greenberg JA et al. Clinical practice guideline: management of acute pancreatitis. J canchir. 2016;59(2).

QA35. Answer c

In ACS, as the mortality rate is close to 50% even after surgery, current suggestions are to medically manage intra-abdominal hypertension as much as possible before proceeding to surgery. Nonoperative techniques should be attempted primarily, but if improvement of the abdominal compartment syndrome is not noted, then surgery within five days of ACS onset is suggested. Elevating the head end of the bed is shown in observational studies to increase the pressure in the abdomen; therefore, it is suggested that in a patient who appears to be developing ACS, lowering the head of the bed to a supine position would be a good initial intervention. The IVC is compressed in ACS with significant decrease of both anteroposterior and lateral diameters. So it cannot be used to assess fluid status. ACS is sustained IAP > 20 mm Hg with new organ failure.

Gentils et al. Abdominal Compartment Syndrome in the Emergency Department. Available from: https://www.ahcmedia.com/articles/139855-abdominal-compartment-syndrome-in-the-emergency-department (Accessed 13 February 2018).

QA36. Answer b

FACTORS ASSOCIATED WITH NIV FAILURE: (1) Infection as the cause of acute respiratory failure; (2) high respiratory rate under NIV; (3) a longer delay between admission and initiation of NIV; (4) a need for vasopressors or renal replacement therapy; (5) acute respiratory distress syndrome. Only patients who have isolated respiratory failure that is judged to be rapidly reversible should receive NIV. If NIV is indicated, it should be started early, and NIV success should be reassessed frequently. Intubation should not be further delayed if NIV does not lead to prompt improvement of respiratory distress. NIV also remains a valid option for patients who have cancer with do not intubate (DNI) situations.

Shimabukuro-Vornhagen A, Böll B, Kochanek M, et al. Critical care of patients with cancer. CA: A Cancer Journal for Clinicians. 2016;66:496-517.

QA37. Answer a

The major differential diagnosis is disseminated intravascular coagulation (DIC). Both TTP and DIC are associated with thrombocytopenia, microangiopathic hemolytic anemia, and schistocytes. In DIC, there is often an associated coagulopathy with prolonged prothrombin time, activated partial thromboplastin time, and thrombin time, which should all be normal in TTP.

George JN, Nester CM. Syndromes of thrombotic microangiopathy. N Engl J Med. 2014;371:654.

QA38. Answer b

The incidence of significant intraperitoneal injury approaches 98% when peritoneal penetration is present and is an indication for laparotomy. All other patients may be evaluated further and then managed conservatively or surgically if a surgical indication is found.

Stefanou C, Zikos N, Pappas-Gogos G, et al. Laparoscopic bullet removal in a penetrating abdominal gunshot. Case Rep Surg. 2016;2016:2712439.

QA39. Answer e

Fluid resuscitation of the patient with moderate or severe burns consists of an IV crystalloid solution. The ideal solution has not been determined, but lactated LR or Hartmann's solution is typically preferred; it contains physiologic concentrations of major electrolytes, and lactate may reduce the incidence of hyperchloremic acidosis that may occur with administration of large volumes of isotonic saline (i.e., 0.9% sodium chloride). There have been concerns over resuscitation in burns using the traditional Parkland formula. Current guidelines recommend 2 mL/kg for every percentage total body surface area (TBSA) for second and third degree burns over 24 hours. Pediatric patients need a higher resuscitation volume due to a larger surface area per unit body mass. Tachycardia is a poor marker for fluid resuscitation and other parameters should be followed. In electrical injuries the fluid requirement is 4 mL/kg ringers lactate × TBSA targeting a urine output of 1 mL/kg/hr until urine clears.

Gueugniaud PY, Carsin H, Bertin-Maghit M, et al. Current advances in th nitial management of major thermal burns. Intensive Care Med. 2000;26(7):848.

QA40. Answer d

S. Na target should be 135-145 mEq/L. In severe traumatic brain injury (TBI) patients with increased intracranial pressure (ICP) or brain edema, a serum sodium level Na$^+$ up to 150–155 mEq/L may be acceptable. However, serum electrolytes disturbances are common complications after TBI. Injury to the hypothalamic-pituitary system is a major contributing factor. The most common causes for hypernatremia (Na+ > 150 mmol/L) in patients with TBI are central or neurogenic diabetes insipidus, osmotic diuresis (mannitol), and the use of hypertonic saline solution (HSS).

ATLS, 10th edn.

QA41. Answer b

Dabigatran is orally administered direct thrombin inhibitor (DTI) which has a long half-life and cannot be titrated like the parenteral anticoagulants. Oral anticoagulants are not used during CRRT. Citrate is used for regional anticoagulation. In patients with heparin induced thrombocytopenia (HIT), all heparin must be stopped and we recommend using DTI (such as argatroban) or Factor Xa inhibitors (such as danaparoid or fondaparinux) rather than other or no anticoagulation during CRRT.

KDIGO Clinical Practice Guideline for Acute Kidney Injury. Kidney International Supplements. 2012;2:89-115.

QA42. Answer c

Child-Pugh classification has been a reference for more than 30 years for assessing the prognosis of cirrhosis. MELD score (2000) comes as the most serious challenger for replacing Child-Pugh score and overcoming its limitations. MELD uses the patient's values for serum bilirubin, serum creatinine, and the international normalized ratio for prothrombin time (INR) to predict survival. The principal advantages of MELD score are that (a) it is based on variables selected by statistical analysis rather than clinical judgement, (b) the variables are objective and unlikely to be influenced by external factors, (c) each variable is weighted according its proper influence on prognosis and (d) the score is continuous which helps scoring individuals more precisely among large populations. The accuracy of the MELD score for predicting outcome in cirrhotic patients, is not always superior (and may even be inferior) to that of Child score.

Durand F, et al. Assessment of the prognosis of cirrhosis: Child-Pugh versus MELD. Journal of Hepatology. 2005;42:S100-S107.

QA43. Answer a

The polyclonal antibody preparations: ATG and antilymphocyte globulin (ALG) became available in the 1970s. With ATG or ALG used for induction or for the treatment of steroid-resistant rejection and azathioprine and prednisolone as the baseline regimen, the success rate of kidney transplantation was 50% at 1 year and the mortality rate was 10% to 20%. ATG is a polyclonal antibody. Rituximab (Rituxan, Mabthera) is a monoclonal anti-CD20 antibody, targeted against the CD20-antigen on B lymphocytes. Cyclosporine is a cyclic polypeptide of fungal origin. Tacrolimus or FK506 is a macrolide antibiotic compound isolated from Streptomyces tsukubaensis. Sirolimus is a macrolide antibiotic compound and everolimus is a similar compound with a short half-life. MMF introduced in 1995, was found to be more effective than azathioprine, reducing the incidence of acute rejection when used with cyclosporine (or tacrolimus) and corticosteroids

Muntean A et al. Immunosuppression in kidney transplantation. Clujul Med. 2013;86(3):177-80.

QA44. Answer b

Bicarbonate therapy during DKA has several potentially deleterious effects including worsening of hypokalemia, worsening of intracellular acidosis, and production of paradoxical central nervous system acidosis. There is no evidence for bicarbonate therapy in DKA and it should not be administered if pH>6.9.

Boord JB, et al. Practical Management of Diabetes in Critically Ill Patients. Am J Respir Crit Care Med. 2001;164:1763-7.

QA45. Answer d

Antibiotics might increase the risk of hemolytic uremic syndrome (HUS) because antibiotic induced injury to the bacterial membrane might favor the release of shiga toxin, antibiotics might give Shiga-toxin-producing *Escherichia coli* (STEC) a selective advantage if these organisms are not as readily eliminated from the bowel as the normal intestinal flora, and some antibiotics (such as fluoroquinolones, particularly ciprofloxacin) are potent inducers of shiga toxin gene expression. Platelet transfusions are sometimes needed to diminish the risk of bleeding in those with severe thrombocytopenia, i.e. platelet counts less than 10,000/dL to control bleeding, or in preparation for an invasive vascular procedure that can cause hemorrhage.

Fakhouri, et al. Hemolytic uremic syndrome. Lancet 2017;390:681-96.

QA46. Answer d

Basic principles of clinical ethics such as autonomy, justice, beneficience and non-maleficience should be followed.

John G, et al. Ethics and ethical analysis. Essentials of Critical Care. Ch 24. 24-1 to 24-18.

QA47. Answer e

A patient who is brain dead is legally dead just like cardiac death but ventilator discontinuation in India can only be done after legal permission or if the family has consented for transplantation.

John G, et al. Ethics and ethical analysis. Essentials of Critical Care.Ch 24. 24-1 to 24-18.

QA48. Answer b

Tourniquets are not recommended in snake bite. Signs of envenoming may recur within 24-48 hours after initial response to antivenom due to continuing absorption of venom from the 'depot' at the site of the bite, perhaps assisted by improved blood supply following correction of shock, hypovolemia and redistribution of venom from the tissues into the vascular space, as the result of antivenom treatment. Reversal of coagulopathy in snake bite occurs with antivenom alone without the need for transfusion. Blood products are indicated only if antivenin is not efficacious, for active bleeding, or for specific coagulation abnormalities. The recommended dose of antivenom is often the amount of antivenom required to neutralize the average venom yield when captive snakes are milked of their venom. Snakes inject the same dose of venom into children and adults. Children must therefore be given exactly the same dose of antivenom as adults. If the snake has already been killed, it should be taken to the dispensary or hospital. Attempting to kill the snake may be dangerous as even a snake with a severed head can bite.

Warrell DA. WHO Guideline for the management of snakebites. 2010.

QA49. Answer a

No skull fracture or intracerebral lesion is seen on the CT scan. A big scalp hematoma is visualized on the left frontal side indicating significant blunt trauma. A lot of blood volume can be lost due to scalp lacerations and hematomas so hemodynamic resuscitation is required to prevent hypovolemia. Also, even in the absence of skull fracture or intracranial pathology, patient should be monitored in supervised settings with appropriate head injury advice for at-least 24 hours.

Shukla D, Devi BI. Mild traumatic brain injuries in adults. J Neurosci Rural Pract. 2010;1(2):82-88.

QA50. Answer a

Critical incident reporting should ensure confidentiality and immunity from blame.

Intensive Care Society Standards for critical incident reporting in critical care. 2006.

K Type Answers

QK1. Answer FTFT

Static parameters of fluid status such as blood pressure, central venous pressure (CVP) and pulmonary capillary wedge pressure (PCWP) have been used as indicators and predictors of successful fluid resuscitation. These measures, however, perform no better than chance in patients who are critically ill. PLR responsiveness should be assessed by a direct measurement of cardiac output and not just monitoring of blood pressure. IVC size is a static measure of preload.

Mukherjee V et al. Annual Update in Intensive Care and Emergency Medicine. 2017; 69-80.

QK2. Answer FTFT

Hemostatic abnormalities are the prima facie evidence of a viper bite. Cobras and kraits do not cause hemostatic disturbances. Saw scaled vipers do not cause renal failure where as Russell's viper and hump-nosed pit viper do. Russell's viper can also manifest with neurotoxic symptoms in a wide area of India which can cause confusion. Further work is necessary to determine the areas in which this species exists.

Singh S, Singh G. Snake Bite: Indian Guidelines Protocol, Toxicology 2013 (www.apiindia.org/medicine - update - 2013/Chap.94)

QK3. Answer FFTT

Under normal physiological conditions SvO_2 is more than $ScvO_2$ as the brain consumes more oxygen compared to the lower body and this relationship is reversed in shock states. In the case of arteriovenous shunting on the microcirculatory level or cell death, SvO_2 and $ScvO_2$ may not decrease or even show elevated values despite severe tissue hypoxia as seen in prolonged cardiac arrest. $ScvO_2$ should not be used alone in the assessment of the cardiocirculatory system but combined with other cardiocirculatory parameters and indicators of organ perfusion such as serum lactate concentration and urine output.

Bloos F, et al. Venous Oximetry: Intensive Care Med. 2005; 31:911-3.

QK4. Answer FTTF

Most patients with AIS should be treated with aspirin 325 mg within 24 to 48 hours after stroke symptom onset. For patients who receive thrombolysis, antithrombotic agents must be avoided for the first 24 hours. Aspirin is usually initiated after a head CT obtained 24 hours after recombinant tissue plasminogen activator (rt-PA) administration demonstrates absence of intracerebral hemorrhage. There is no convincing evidence to support the use of other oral/IV antiplatelet agents such as clopidogrel, dipyridamole, ticagrelor, ticlopidine and glycoprotein IIb/IIIa inhibitor (abcixamab). IV rt-PA is recommended within 4.5 hours of symptom onset for eligible patients. Intravenous rt-PA (alteplase) is the only medication approved by the U.S. Food and Drug Administration for the treatment of AIS. It is recommended to treat seizures aggressively if they occur but not to administer prophylactic anticonvulsants. Data from small randomized controlled trials show that hemicraniectomy for malignant hemispheric infarction reduces mortality. However, the ultimate neurologic outcome is less than optimal (moderate or severe disability) in many cases.

Massaro AM, et al. Evidence-Based Practice of Critical Care. 2nd edn. Ch 64. 461-69.

QK5. Answer FFTT

Although Aspirin and IV Alteplase are recommended in AIS it is contraindicated in a case of cerebellar infarct since the risk of bleeding and cerebellar herniation is high. The patient needs to have surgical intervention immediately to reduce ICP.

Massaro AM et al. Evidence based practice of critical care. 2nd edn. Ch 64. 461-9.

QK6. Answer TFTT

Status epilepticus is defined as: (1) continuous seizure activity for 5 minutes or more without return of consciousness, or (2) recurrent seizures (2 or more) without an intervening period of neurological recovery. The initial drug of choice for terminating Status Epilepticus is a short acting benzodiazepine (Lorazepam or Midazolam). The classical symptoms and signs of acute bacterial meningitis may be absent in convulsive status epilepticus (CSE) with fever. The most appropriate management is suggested to be early parenteral antibiotics and a lumbar puncture when there are no contraindications. Ketamine increases the ICP.

Yi DH, et al. Evidence-Based Practice of Critical Care. 2nd edn. Ch 65. 470-4.

QK7. Answer FFTF

There is likely no benefit in using NIV as a bridge or alternative to intubation. Elective intubation and ventilation has been found to be associated with a reduced incidence of pneumonia and shorter duration of mechanical ventilation. Severe hyperkalemia may be associated with the use of succinylcholine in patients with Guillain-Barre Syndrome (GBS), and alternative neuromuscular blocking agents should be used, if necessary. Autonomic dysfunction is a common complication. Patients are at elevated risk of hemodynamic instability at the time of intubation associated with the vasodilatory effects of anesthetic agents and reduced venous return associated with positive pressure ventilation. There is no data to support the use of one ventilator mode above any other.

Tataroglu C, Ozkul A, Sair A. Chronic inflammatory demyelinating polyneuropathy and respiratory failure due to phrenic nerve involvement. J Clin Neuromuscul Dis. 2010;12(1):42-6.

QK8. Answer FFFT

Intravenous immunoglobulin (IVIG) has replaced plasma exchange as the treatment of choice because of its greater convenience and availability. Neither prednisolone nor methylprednisolone can significantly accelerate recovery or improve long-term outcome in patients with GBS. If vasopressors or antihypertensives are to be administered, short-acting agents (e.g., esmolol, nicardipine) are preferable. Care should be taken with dosage because patients with GBS can be extremely sensitive to even small doses of vasoactive agents because of possible denervation supersensitivity. SIADH is seen in up to 50% of patient with GBS.

Willison HJ, Jacobs BC, Doorn PA. Guillain-Barré syndrome. 2016;388:717.

QK9. Answer TTTT

Perioperative stress cardiomyopathy (Apical ballooning or Takotsubo cardiomyopathy) occurs due to high catecholamine state. It is characterized by transient regional systolic dysfunction of the left ventricle (LV), mimicking myocardial infarction. Medications like β-blockers are often advocated to counteract the hypercatecholamine state, while ACEI or angiotensin-receptor blockers (ARB) may improve survival at 1 year.

Agarwal et al. Seminars in Cardiothoracic and Vascular Anesthesia. 2017;21(4):277-90.

QK10. Answer TTTT

Pulmonary embolism (PE) is a common problem but the symptoms are not very specific and there is no single test for the diagnosis. CTPA is the gold standard test for the diagnosis of PE.

Mehrotra R. Textbook of Critical Care. Ch. 7. Page(s): 63-72

QK11. Answer FTFT

Low dose dopamine does not help prevent renal failure in patients with early renal dysfunction and dopamine is associated with higher mortality. Phenylephrine may be used in septic shock when tachyarrhythmias limit therapy with other vasopressors. Levosimendan is a calcium sensitizer and Milrinone acts by increasing the concentration of cyclic AMP by inhibiting phosphodiesterase III enzyme. The Clinical Practice Committee of the Scandinavian Society of Anaesthesia and Intensive Care Medicine (SSAI) guideline (2016) on choice of first line vasopressor in adult patients with acute circulatory failure recommended norepinephrine for all causes of shock rather than other vasopressors as first line treatment for the majority of adult critically ill patients with acute circulatory failure.

Hollenberg S. Inotrope and vasopressor therapy in septic shock. Crit Care Clin. 2009; 25:781-802.

Møller MH, et al. Scandinavian SSAI clinical practice guideline on choice of first-line vasopressor for patients with acute circulatory failure. Acta Anaesthesiologica Scandinavica. 2016;60:1347-66.

QK12. Answer TFTT

PCT is the 166-amino-acid precursor of calcitonin that is produced by the C-cells of the thyroid gland. In bacterial sepsis, PCT levels increase rapidly secondary to its synthesis from almost all parenchymal tissues which lack the ability to cleave PCT. In contrast, viral/ fungal infections or noninfectious inflammatory reactions do not or only result in a moderate increase in PCT levels in blood. Moreover, recovery from bacterial infection with antibiotic therapy resulted in a simultaneous decline in PCT levels. Hence, PCT has been used as a diagnostic and prognostic biomarker in sepsis.

Rhodes A, et al. Surviving Sepsis Campaign: International Guidelines for Management of Sepsis and Septic Shock: 2016. CCM. 2017;45(3).

Rojas-Moreno C, et al. Procalcitonin in sepsis. American Journal of Hospital Medicine. 2016;(8):1.

QK13. Answer TFFT

SIRS without infection (e.g. severe pancreatitis/burns) does not mandate antimicrobial therapy. The required loading dose of any antimicrobial is not affected by alterations of renal function, although this may affect frequency of administration and/or total daily dose.

> Rhodes A, et al. Surviving Sepsis Campaign: International Guidelines for Management of Sepsis and Septic Shock: 2016. CCM. 2017;45(3):486-552.

QK14. Answer FFFF

First line therapy in neutropenic fever must include an agent with antipseudomonal activity. Quinolones and aminoglycosides are not acceptable as monotherapy. In high risk patients if fever resolves but Absolute Neutrophil count (ANC) is <500/µL then antibiotic therapy is continued for 2 weeks or until resolution of neutropenia. Empiric antifungal agents should be used if fever is not resolving after 4-7 days of antibiotics or if there is a clinical suspicion of fungal infection. The use of myeloid colony-stimulating factors is not recommended in the setting of an established fever and neutropenia. Several randomized studies have shown a decrease in the days of neutropenia, duration of fever, and length of hospital stay with the use of myeloid colony stimulating factors. However, none of those studies has shown a survival benefit.

> Bow EJ. Fluoroquinolones, antimicrobial resistance and neutropenic cancer patients. Curr Opin Infect Dis. 2011;24:545.

QK15. Answer FTTF

Clostridium difficile is an anaerobic gram-positive, spore-forming, toxin-producing bacillus that is transmitted among humans through the fecal-oral route. Majority of infants are colonized with C. difficile but are asymptomatic owing to the lack of toxin-binding receptors in the infant gut as shown in animal models. Antibodies to *C. difficile* toxins are often seen in infants without clinical infection. Post-treatment testing has no role in confirming eradication. Many successfully treated patients will continue to test positive for weeks or months after the resolution of symptoms; additional treatment is neither required nor effective.

> Leffler DA, et al. *Clostridium difficile* Infection. N Engl J Med. 2015;372:1539-48.

QK16. Answer FTFT

PCP is an infection of the lung caused by the fungal organism. *Pneumocystis jirovecii* (formerly known as Pneumocystis carinii). In spite of severe respiratory distress the lungs are frequently clear on auscultation. This discrepancy between the severity of pulmonary symptoms and physical findings is typical. Fever is not usually a factor and the temperature rarely goes beyond 100°F. Lung injury and respiratory impairment during pneumocystis pneumonia are mediated by marked inflammatory responses in the host to the organism. Trimethoprim-sulfamethoxazole with adjunctive corticosteroid therapy to suppress lung inflammation in patients with severe infection remains the preferred treatment.

> Thomas CF. et al. Pneumocystis Pneumonia. N Engl J Med. 2004;350:2487-98.

QK17. Answer FFFF

Early administration of corticosteroids to septic patients does not prevent the development of ARDS. A study by Martin-Loeches et al concluded that the early use of corticosteroids was also ineffective in patients with the pandemic H1N1 influenza A infection, resulting in an increased risk of superinfections. The role of low-dose corticosteroids in established ARDS remains uncertain, with one study of 91 patients demonstrating prolonged low-dose methylprednisolone therapy reducing severity of lung injury by Day 7 of treatment. Inhaled nitric oxide did not decrease mortality but results in only a transient improvement in oxygenation. ECMO has not been proven to be significantly better in any of the clinical trials but ECMO controls gas exchange and perfusion, it stabilizes the patient physiologically, reduces the risk of iatrogenic injury (e.g. VILI) and buys time for the clinician to manage the patient. It is not without risk and is very costly. So should be considered on a case-by-case basis. Results of clinical trials comparing HFOV with conventional ventilation in adults have generally demonstrated early improvement in oxygenation but no improvement in survival.

> Harman E, et al. Acute Respiratory Distress Syndrome Treatment & Management. Available from: http://emedicine.medscape.com/article/165139-treatment (Accessed 13 February 2018).

Kumar R, et al. Extracorporeal Membrane Oxygenation for Adults with ARDS-Current Evidence. Insights in Chest Diseases. 2017;2(2):7.

QK18. Answer TTFF

The impact of disease on the time constant of lung units is important to consider. The decreased compliance in ARDS results in a short time constant, whereas the increased resistance in asthma leads to a longer time constant. Ventilatory strategies change according to the time constants of the alveolar units. For a given pressure lung units with long time constants will have larger volumes and short time constants will have smaller volumes.

Cross M, et al. Physics, Pharmacology and Physiology for Anaesthetists. Respiratory physiology. 210-38.

QK19. Answer FFTT

The disadvantage of volume control is the potential for high airway pressures; pressure limitation provides protection and is available on most modern machines. Alternatively, pressure controlled ventilation may be preferred as high airway pressures are avoided and the inspiratory flow pattern, which better resembles normal breathing, tends to equalize ventilation between lung units rather than preferentially ventilating, and possibly overinflating, the less obstructed (or faster filling and emptying) lung units. When small airway collapse develops during expiration from the structural changes associated with emphysema, the application of PEEPe will reduce gas trapping by stenting open the airways. The value of PEEPe to offset intrinsic PEEP is also important. PEEPe should just exceed PEEPi. Aim for early extubation at the 48–72 hours 'window of opportunity' before secondary infections or other complications occur. NIV can be used as a bridge in those patients at risk for extubation failure. Early tracheostomy is indicated in case of extubation failure.

Davidson AC. The pulmonary physician in critical care: Critical care management of respiratory failure resulting from COPD. Thorax. 2002;57:1079-84.

QK20. Answer FTFF

Earlier and appropriate antimicrobial therapy, along with septic source control, has been associated with lower risk of AKI. Nephrotoxic drugs are to be avoided and renal dose adjustment is indicated if required. EGDT failed to show benefit for reducing AKI, utilization of RRT, or kidney recovery. The ProMISe, ProCESS, and ARISE trials demonstrated no difference in mortality or improved renal outcomes with EGDT. Hydroxyethyl starch and gelatin solutions have been associated with an increased risk of AKI in septic patients and an increased risk of mortality in patients with sepsis induced AKI.

Bellomo R, et al. Acute kidney injury in sepsis. Intensive Care Med. 2017;43:816-28.

QK21. Answer TFTT

The duration of SBT should be at least 30 minutes and not longer than 120 minutes.

Zein H, et al. Ventilator weaning and spontaneous breathing trials: an Educational Review. Emergency. 2016;4(2):65-71.

QK22. Answer TFFT

Tracheostomy, by decreasing airways resistance and reducing dead space, may be beneficial for patients with marginal respiratory mechanics, and may lead to quicker discontinuation of mechanical ventilation. Early tracheostomy can improve mobility and may enhance the patient's psychological well-being, which may help with physical therapy. Patients who require sedation to be able to tolerate their translaryngeal tubes may be more comfortable with a tracheostomy, and subsequent discontinuation of the sedative drugs may facilitate earlier discontinuation from mechanical ventilation. Early tracheotomy is associated with a larger number of Ventilator free days, shorter ICU stays, shorter duration of sedation and lower long-term mortality rates than late tracheotomy.

Hosokawa, et al. Timing of tracheotomy in ICU patients: a systematic review of randomized controlled trials. Critical Care. 2015;19:424.

QK23. Answer FFFT

Clinicians must be aware of the need to optimize oxygenation and avoid dehydration and hypokalemia. Unrestricted high concentrations of oxygen (60–100%) must be administered to abolish hypoxemia, unlike the patient with chronic obstructive lung disease where controlled limited oxygen is indicated. Hypokalemia is common and may be exaggerated by fluid resuscitation and the administration of β agonist bronchodilators. Repeated infusions of potassium chloride may be required with careful monitoring of serum levels and continuous ECG monitoring. In severe asthma with obstructed airways inhaled salbutamol may be ineffective and may need to be given IV. IV high dose steroids and IV aminophylline may be given as 2nd line therapy if IV salbutamol is not available. NIV can only be applied in conscious and spontaneously breathing patients.

    Phipps P, et al. The pulmonary physician in critical care: Acute severe asthma in the intensive care unit. Thorax. 2003; 58:81-88.

QK24. Answer FFTF

ECG of PE is characterized by complete or incomplete RBBB, Right ventricular strain pattern, R axis deviation, dominant R in V1, R atrial enlargement (P pulmonale), S1Q3T3 pattern, non specific ST T changes.

    https://lifeinthefastlane.com/ecg-library/pulmonary-embolism/

QK25. Answer TTFT

Extracorporeal life support (ECLS) with ECMO is by provision of VA ECMO for refractory cardiac arrest and resuscitation. To date there is no prospective randomized study on ECMO for this indication. The available literature on ECPR suggests that ECMO is sufficient to ensure systemic circulation in refractory arrest. Factors that determine success are witnessed cardiac arrest, bystander CPR and time from arrest to ECMO. In addition to excellent basic CPR, the successful use of ECMO depends upon appropriate patient selection and skillful implementation (e.g., rapid response ECLS teams). However, the subset of cardiac arrest patients best suited for ECMO treatment is unknown. A shorter period of arrest prior to ECMO appears to improve outcomes; elevated prearrest lactate levels and noncardiac causes of arrest bode poorly. The expense of ECMO must be considered when determining whether to implement this treatment.

    Chen YS, Lin JW, Yu HY, et al. Cardiopulmonary resuscitation with assisted extracorporeal life-support versus conventional cardiopulmonary resuscitation in adults with in-hospital cardiac arrest: an observational study and propensity analysis. Lancet. 2008;372(9638):554.

QK26. Answer FTTT

Lithium is adsorbed poorly by activated charcoal and is not indicated. Lithium is a prototypical dialyzable toxin because of its low molecular weight, lack of protein binding, water solubility, low volume of distribution and prolonged half-life. Lithium is a monovalent cation and therefore causes a decreased anion gap if serum levels are severely elevated and may be a clue to the diagnosis. Whole bowel irrigation with polyethylene glycol is used to decrease absorption of sustained release lithium.

    Mokhlesi B, et al. Adult toxicology in critical care. Part II: Specific poisonings. Chest. 2003;123:897-922.

QK27. Answer FFTT

GHB is also known as liquid ecstasy or fantasy. It is derived from GABA and acts as an inhibitory neurotransmitter to GHB and GABA receptors in the brain. The clinical manifestations depend on the dose and range from euphoria to deep coma and death. Treatment is mainly supportive which may be required only for a short time since rapid recovery is the norm. Naloxone is not helpful. Although normal toxicological screens do not include GHB, specialized laboratories can detect GHB in both urine and blood by gas chromatography- mass spectroscopy. GHB can also be detected by hair analysis.

    Mokhlesi B, et al. Adult toxicology in critical care. Part II: Specific poisonings. Chest. 2003;123:897-922.

QK28. Answer TTTF

Patients on airborne isolation precautions should be placed in a private room with negative air pressure that has a minimum of 6 to 12 air changes per hour. Doors to the isolation rooms must remain closed, and all individuals who enter must wear a respirator with a filtering capacity of 95% that allows a tight seal over the nose and mouth.

The risk waste is separated from non-risk waste which accounts for 20% of the total medical waste. At source segregation minimizes the chances of infection and injury to the persons who handle the waste. Three isolation categories reflect the major modes of pathogen transmission in nosocomial settings: contact, droplet, and airborne spread. The rooms of patients requiring precautions should be clearly marked with signs containing instructions regarding the type of precautions that must be observed. Ample supplies should be readily available outside the patient room to facilitate adherence, and hospital policies should be enforced.

> Anderson DJ. Infection prevention: Precautions for preventing transmission of infection. Available from: https://www.uptodate.com/contents/infection-prevention-precautions-for-preventing-transmission-of-infection?source=search_result&search=Infection%20control%20in%20ICU&selected Title=2~150 (Accessed 3 December 2017).

QK29. Answer FTFF

In common with other tetracyclines such as tigecycline, minocycline inhibits bacterial protein synthesis through binding with the 30S subunit of the bacterial ribosome, most typically resulting in a bacteriostatic effect. However, synergistic and bactericidal activity against MDR *Acinetobacter* has been noted with minocycline in combination with colistin or carbapenems. *Acinetobacter* is not susceptible to fosfomycin. Daptomycin is indicated only for treating right-sided endocarditis.

> Ritchie DJ, et al. A review of intravenous minocycline for treatment of multidrug-resistant *Acinetobacter* infections. Clinical Infectious Diseases. 2014;59(S6):S374-80.

QK30. Answer TFFT

After mid-pregnancy, the gravid uterus should be moved off the inferior vena cava to increase venous return and cardiac output in the acutely injured pregnant woman. This may be achieved by manual displacement of the uterus or left lateral tilt. Care should be taken to secure the spinal cord when using left lateral tilt. In cases of major trauma, the assessment, stabilization, and care of the pregnant women is the first priority; then, if the fetus is viable (≥ 23 weeks), fetal heart rate auscultation and fetal monitoring can be initiated and an obstetrical consultation obtained as soon as feasible .Maternal health should always take priority over interventions for the fetus. Stabilization of the mother is the first priority. Fetal heart rate is a sensitive indicator of maternal blood volume and fetal well-being. CT scan should be done only after stabilization of the mother. If resuscitative efforts in the mother are not effective a perimortem cesarean section can be done within 4 minutes following cardiac arrest.

> Jain V. et al. Guidelines for the management of a pregnant trauma patient. J Obstet Gynaecol Can. 2015;37(6):553-71.

QK31. Answer FTTT

Pregnant women are at high-risk of complications such as ARDS requiring mechanical ventilation from H1N1 influenza. Early termination of pregnancy may result in improvement in the mother's condition. The timing to terminate is a critical decision necessitating proper cooperation with an obstetrician. This patient is too sick to transport to the operation theatre and warrants caesarean section in the ICU itself. ECMO support and prone ventilation have been used as alternative strategies of ventilation in pregnant patients with severe hypoxemia.

> Bhatia PK, et al. Acute respiratory failure and mechanical ventilation in pregnant patient: A narrative review of literature. J Anaesthesiol Clin Pharmacol. 2016;32(4):431-439.

QK32. Answer FFFF

Lack of bowel sounds may simply indicate a lack of air in the bowel. The use of bowel sounds to drive any clinical decision has never been validated. Gastric residual volumes (GRV) should not be used as part of routine care to monitor ICU patients on EN. For those ICUs where GRV are still utilized, holding EN for GRVs < 500 mL in the absence of other signs of intolerance should be avoided. Traditionally, it was feared that providing nutrition in the context of shock could cause intestinal ischemia. However, enteral nutrition actually appears to improve blood flow to the gut and preserve intestinal integrity. Once a patient has been fluid resuscitated and stabilized on vasopressors, enteral nutrition may be started at low rates. Enteral feeding is possible and preferred with prone positioning. To avoid complications associated with enteral feeding, postpyloric feedings or pro-motility agents are recommended to prevent aspiration.

> SCCM/ASPEN 2016: Guidelines for the provision and assessment of nutrition support therapy in the adult critically ill patient.

QK33. Answer FTFF

In massive hemorrhage, it is unwise to withhold coagulation therapy until Trauma induced coagulopathy (TIC) can be detected since in certain populations, the risk of TIC is excessively high and almost inevitably present. There is no current evidence that the use of recombinant factor VIIa can improve morbidity and mortality in acutely bleeding trauma patients. The first hemoglobin concentration taken in trauma patients is often falsely high because fluid resuscitation has not yet been started. Therefore Hb level cannot be used as a guide to assess blood loss in trauma.

PACT. Severe and Multiple trauma. Clinical problems. 2013.

QK34. Answer FTTT

The caloric requirement is approximately 25 kcal/ kg/ day ideal body weight. In the EDEN trial, a multicenter RCT in patients expected to have a duration of ventilation for > 72 hours for acute lung injury comparing full enteral feeding to lower-volume trophic feeding for six days resulted in a lower incidence of GI intolerance and similar clinical outcomes. When providing hypocaloric nutrition it appears important to provide 100% of the daily requirement of protein. Although small bowel feeding reduces the risk of pneumonia, there is no difference in mortality or length of stay in ICU/hospital.

Tayloe BE, et al. Guidelines for the Provision and Assessment of Nutrition Support Therapy in the Adult Critically Ill Patient: Society of Critical Care Medicine (SCCM) and American Society for Parenteral and Enteral Nutrition (A.S.P.E.N.). Criti Care Med. 2016;2:438.

QK35. Answer FTTF

Chronic radiation enteritis has been reported in up to 20% of patients receiving pelvic radiotherapy, although this may underestimate its true prevalence, as not all patients with gastrointestinal symptoms after radiotherapy will seek medical attention. Predisposing factors to chronic radiation enteritis include a low body mass index, previous abdominal surgery and the presence of co-morbid conditions; the radiation dose, fractionation and technique, as well as the concomitant use of chemotherapy, may also play a role. Clinical features of chronic radiation enteritis are multiple as the disease can affect any part of the gastrointestinal tract.

Theis VS, Sripadam R, Ramani V, et al. Chronic radiation enteritis. Clin Oncol (R Coll Radiol). 2010;22(1):70-83.

QK36. Answer TFTF

The recommendation in patients at either low or high nutrition risk is that use of supplemental PN is to be considered after 7 to 10 days if unable to meet > 60%of energy and protein requirements by the enteral route alone. Initiating supplemental PN prior to this 7–10-day period in critically ill patients on some EN does not improve outcomes and may be detrimental. Parenteral glutamine or enteral glutamine is not recommended in the critical care setting except in burns or surgical patients.

QK37. Answer FFTF

There is no evidence for the use of immune enhancing formulae in acute severe pancreatitis. EN should be initiated within 24-48 hours of admission. EN should be provided to the patient with severe acute pancreatitis by either the gastric or jejunal route, as there is no difference in tolerance or clinical outcomes between these two levels of infusion. In patients who have intolerance to EN measures to improve tolerance such as diverting the level of infusion of EN more distally in the GI tract should be tried. PN should be considered after one week from the onset of the pancreatitis episode.

Tayloe BE, et al. Guidelines for the Provision and Assessment of Nutrition Support Therapy in the Adult Critically Ill Patient: Society of Critical Care Medicine (SCCM) and American Society for Parenteral and Enteral Nutrition (A.S.P.E.N.). Criti Care Med. 2016;2:438.

QK38. Answer FFFF

TRALI has an acute onset of lung injury (within 6 hours of transfusion). It is immune mediated caused by donor antibodies targeting recipient leukocyte antigens on neutrophils sequestered in the lungs. It occurs due to transfusion of plasma containing products such as FFP, platelets or whole blood. Treatment is supportive. There is no evidence for steroids.

Triulzi DJ. Transfusion-related acute lung injury: current concepts for the clinician. Anesth Analg. 2009;108(3):770-6.

QK39. Answer FFTT

Laboratory evaluation in the immediate days to weeks following a thrombosis can yield false results because of the increase in acute phase reactants associated with acute clot formation, which can result in false positive tests for hypercoagulable states. Patients in the ICU have many transient risk factors for the development of thromboembolic disease. Because of this, most instances of thromboembolism do not warrant workup for an underlying hypercoagulable state. However, in the setting of recurrent thrombosis, cerebral vein or visceral vein thrombosis, and non-embolic arterial thrombosis, further evaluation is warranted. For the diagnosis of DVT, Wells and colleagues stratified patients into two risk categories: "DVT unlikely" if the clinical score is ≤1 and "DVT likely" if the clinical score is >1.

Wells score

	Points
Active cancer (treatment ongoing or within previous 6 months or palliative)	1
Paralysis, paresis, or recent plaster immobilization of the lower extremities	1
Recently bedridden for 3 days or major surgery within 12 weeks requiring general or regional anesthesia	1
Localized tenderness along the distribution of the deep veins	1
Entire leg swollen	1
Calf swelling 3 cm > asymptomatic side (measured 10 cm below tibial tuberosity)	1
Pitting edema limited to the symptomatic leg	1
Collateral superficial veins (non varicose)	1
Previous DVT	1
Alternative diagnosis as likely as or more likely than DVT	–2

DVT unlikely: ≤1; DVT likely: ≥2

D-dimer assays are highly sensitive (values up to 95%), but have poor specificity to prove VTE. The negative predictive value for patients with a negative D-dimer blood test is nearly 100%.

Kesieme E. Deep vein thrombosis: a clinical review. Blood Med. 2011;2:59-69.

QK40. Answer TFFT

Atlanto-axial and atlanto-occipital dislocation, dens fractures, and cord transections can occur from excessive stretch in shaken baby syndrome. Hangman's fracture involves the C2 fracture accounts for nearly 19% of all spinal fractures and 55% of cervical fractures. Within C2 fractures, the Hangman's fracture accounts for 23% of occurrences while the odontoid or dens fracture accounts for 55% of them. A fracture of the pars interarticularis on the pedicle of the C2 vertebrae (axis) is most common. The primary screening modality for C-spine is multidetector CT (MDCT) from the occiput to T1 with sagittal and coronal reconstructions. MDCT scans may be used instead of plain images to evaluate the C-spine. C-spine injuries can be ruled out only if the patients are awake, alert and neurologically normal with no neck pain/tenderness or a distracting injury.

Hockerberg RS, Kaji AH. Spinal column injuries. In: Hockberger MJ, Walls R 6th (edn.). Rosen's Emergency Medicine: Concepts and Clinical Practice, Mosby, Philadelphia, 2006.

QK41. Answer TFTF

Flail chest and hemopneumothorax should be managed by members of the trauma team. Injuries which require specialist operative intervention should involve the thoracic surgeon.

Ludwig C, et al. Management of chest trauma. J Thorac Dis. 2017;9(Suppl 3):S172-S177.

QK42. Answer FFFF

Serum creatinine levels are not helpful in the immediate post-operative setting to diagnose the cause of renal failure. N-acetylcysteine does not work in renal failure. Dopamine can be used to increase urine output, but does not prevent or treat ARF. Hetastarch is nephrotoxic and should not be used in treating prerenal failure.

Erdbruegger U, Okusa MD. Etiology and diagnosis of prerenal disease and acute tubular necrosis in acute kidney injury in adults. Available from: https://www.uptodate.com/contents/etiology-and-diagnosis-of-prerenal-disease-and-acute-tubular-necrosis-in-acute-kidney-injury-in-adults?source=search_result&search=Uptodate.%20Edbruegger,U%20and%20Okusa,%20M.%20Etiology%20and%20diagnosis%20of%20Acute%20tubular%20Necrosis%20and%20Pre-renal%20disease.%20Oct%202009.&selectedTitle=1~150 (Accessed 3 December 2017).

QK43. Answer TFTF

HRS is the development of renal failure in advanced chronic liver disease (CLD). Occasionally it can develop in fulminant hepatitis patients who have portal hypertension and ascites. The histological appearance of the kidney is normal. HRS is usually irreversible unless liver transplantation is performed.

Ginès P, Schrier RW. Renal failure in cirrhosis. N Engl J Med. 2009;361(13):1279.

QK44. Answer FFTF

Hospital acquired AKI is associated with a worse prognosis than community acquired AKI as is often iatrogenic in nature. Biopsies of the kidney in patients who have died of septic shock have revealed a uniform pattern of acute tubular injury. As no modification of treatment can be derived from this pattern, renal sampling cannot be advocated in such patients in clinical routine. Renal biopsy is associated with a 12–22% serious adverse event rate. The Doppler-based renal-resistive index, which is a simple, rapid, noninvasive and repeatable marker, could be a promising tool to detect early patients, which are the most at risk of developing AKI in ICU and to distinguish transient from persistent AKI. Positive fluid balance is associated with poor outcomes. Renal congestion, interstitial edema and subsequent changes in renal perfusion worsen AKI.

Bellomo R, et al. Acute kidney injury in the ICU: from injury to recovery- reports from the 5th Paris International Conference. Ann Intensive Care. 2017;7:49.

QK45. Answer TTTT

Altered visual field or visual acuity can be due to involvement of the optic nerves, chiasma, or optic tracts. The III, IV, and VI cranial nerves are vulnerable at the cavernous sinus. There can be associated diplopia. The medial aspect of the cavernous sinus corresponds to the lateral aspect of the pituitary fossa and acute hemorrhage or necrosis within this region can shift the oculomotor nerves. There can be ipsilateral mydriasis and ptosis owing to III cranial nerve involvement. In the study by Milazzo et al., oculomotor palsies were more common (82%) than chiasmatic impairment (54.5%). Blindness can develop in one or both eyes.

Ranabir S, Baruah MP. Pituitary apoplexy. Indian Endocrinol Metab. 2011;15(Suppl3):S188-S196.

QK46. Answer TTTF

If patient meets criteria for HRS, diuretics should be stopped and patient should be normovolemic. Early RRT is recommended.

Wong LP, Blackley MP, Andreoni KA, et al. Survival of liver transplant candidates with acute renal failure receiving renal replacement therapy. Kidney Int. 2005;68(1):362.

QK47. Answer TFTT

Digitalis acts by causing increase in intracellular calcium and this causes more calcium to be released by the sarcoplasmic reticulum. Acute digoxin toxicity causes hyperkalemia, which should not be treated with calcium as it will only aggravate the problem.

Bhagwati AM. Metabolic abnormalities in critically ill patients. Med. Update. 2008;18. Ch 66;500-7.

QK48. Answer FTFF

Correction of chronic hyponatremia with hypertonic saline is generally only necessary if the patient is symptomatic. In asymptomatic patients with euvolemic or hypervolemic hyponatremia in which no specific intervention is available (e.g. SIADH), fluid restriction is generally the treatment of choice. When the orally active V2 receptor antagonists are available, they could be used to treat chronic hyponatremia. Tolvaptan is not indicated for use when urgent treatment of hyponatremia is required to prevent or treat serious neurological symptoms. It has not been established that raising serum sodium with tolvaptan provides symptomatic benefit. Thiazide diuretics are useful in the treatment of nephrogenic diabetes insipidus. Fluid restriction to below the level of urine output is indicated for the treatment of symptomatic or severe hyponatremia in edematous states (such as heart failure and cirrhosis), SIADH, and advanced renal impairment. Restriction to 50 to 60 percent of daily fluid requirements may be required to achieve the goal of inducing negative water balance. In general, fluid intake should be less than 800 mL/day. In patients with a highly concentrated urine (e.g., 500 mOsmol/kg or higher), fluid restriction alone may be insufficient to correct hyponatremia.

Adrogué HJ, Madias NE. Hyponatremia. N Engl J Med. 2000;342(21):1581.

QK49. Answer FTTF

Benchmarking has been divided into the broad categories of process, performance, and strategic benchmarking, and has also been classified as internal (within the same institution) or external benchmarking. In relation to critical care medicine, benchmarking involves the use of quantitative, standardized measurements to allow comparison of performance between intensive care units. Bench marking cannot be used for predicting outcomes.

   Salluh JIF, et al. Understanding intensive care unit benchmarking. Intensive Care Med. 2017;43:1703-1707.

QK50. Answer FTFT

Routine administration of SUP to ICU patients is not justified by current evidence. Accumulating evidence suggests that use of PPIs may increase the risk of nosocomial pneumonia, CDIs and cardiovascular events. EN has a protective effect on the gastric mucosa. Studies have shown no benefit to adding proton pump inhibitor (pantoprazole) to early enteral nutrition in mechanically ventilated critically ill patients.

   Marker S, et al. What's new with stress ulcer prophylaxis in the ICU? Intensive Care Med. 2017;43:1132-34.

   El-Kersh K, et al. Enteral nutrition as stress ulcer prophylaxis in critically ill patients: A randomized controlled exploratory study. Criti Care. 2018;43:108-13.

Index

A

Abdominal cavity 196
Abdominal distension 123
Abdominal nodes 214
Abdominal pain 123, 134, 181, 326
   severe 287
Abdominal tenderness 126
Abdominal trauma 323
Abdominal ultrasonography 334
Absolute neutrophil count 215
Acalculous cholecystitis, acute 125, 143, 322
Accidental kerosene ingestion 246
ACE inhibitor 6, 91
Acetaminophen overdose 248
Acetazolamide 210
Acid-base disorder 118
Acquired infections, prevent hospital 441
Acute kidney injury, staging of 165
Acute thrombotic stroke, suspicion of 79
Acute toxic cholangitis, therapy for 118
Adrenal insufficiency 209
Adriamycin 217, 244
Agitation 96
   severe 248
Air filtration 444
Air fluid levels, multiple 123
Albuminuria 167
Alcohol
   abuse, history of 294
   abuser 293
   intoxication, acute 249
Alcoholism, chronic 202
Alkaline phosphatase 121
Alkalosis 201
   severe 208
Alkylating agents 243
Alleged medical negligence 418
Allergic bronchopulmonary aspergillosis 378
Alprazolam develops 291
Alternaria spp. 452
Aluminum phosphide 246, 256
Alveolar opacities 183
Alveolar-arterial oxygen gradient 53, 353

Amebic abscess 124
American College of Chest Physicians guidelines 196
American Heart Association guidelines 30, 319
American Society of Anesthesiologists 317
American Stroke Association guidelines 319
Amikacin 48
Amino acid 149, 154
Aminoglycoside 167, 179
   nephrotoxicity 169
Amiodarone 6
   side effect of 6
Amitryptilline 244
Amniotic fluid embolism 189
   presentation of 185
   syndrome 186
Amphotericin B 379
   nephrotoxicity 169
Ampicillin 210, 272
Analgesia
   implementation of 437
   monitoring of 437
Analogon iloprost 368
Anemia, type of 167
Anesthetic drug 293
Aneurysmal subarachnoid hemorrhage 80, 87
Angiotensin converting enzyme inhibitors 2
Angiotensin II receptor blockers 191
Anion gap 204, 245
   causes of normal 203
   metabolic acidosis 248
Annual flu vaccine 449
Antecedent biliary-enteric fistula 140
Anthracycline 221
Antibody-mediated rejection 367
   management of 360
Antidepressant medication, multiple 245
Antidiuretic hormone 204
Antifungal agent 273
Anti-lymphocyte antibodies 365
Antimicrobial therapy 310, 436
   usage 424
Antiplatelet therapy 29

Anti-pneumocystis therapy 390
Antiretroviral therapy 270, 298
   long-term 383
Anuria 171
Aortic injury 320
Aortic intramural hematoma 3
Apheresis platelet components 404
Apnea test 88
Arginine vasopressin, secretion of 226
Arterial blood
   gas 41
   partial pressure of oxygen in 53
   pressure measurement, physics of direct 28
Arterial hyperenhancement 44
Arterial line 348
Arterial pressure
   mean 81, 101
   waveform 27, 30
Arteriovenous malformation 80
Arthralgias 380
Ascending colon, massive dilation of 123
Ascorbic acid 161
Aspergillosis 382
Aspergillus precipitin test 378
Aspirin 29, 91, 435
   usage in ACS 423
Asthma
   history of 45
   in pregnancy 184
Atherosclerosis bioprosthetic valve 272
Atrial fibrillation 4-6, 27, 28, 202
   postoperative 30
Atrium, dilated left 4
Autologous blood donation 400
Autonomic dysreflexia 90
Axillary line, anterior 294
Axonal injury, diffuse 86, 337
Azathioprine 122, 380, 388
Azithromycin 203, 290

B

Back pain, severe local 229
Bacterial infections 139
Barbiturates 111

Bariatric surgeries 156
Bartonella
　bacteria 386
　henselae 386
Bartter syndrome 210
Basal ganglia bleed 92
Basilar artery 336
Basilar tip aneurysm 104
Basophilic predominant
　　　inflammatory 42
Beauchamp childress system 347
Bedside echocardiography 293
Beta blocker overdose 246
Beta error 355
Bicarbonate-rich electrolyte
　　　solution 119
Bile duct cancers 117, 128
Biliary complications 134
Binary parenteral nutrition bags 150
Biostatistics and research
　　　methodology 392
Bipolar disorder 248
　history of 291
Bishop Cairo classification 214, 226
Bispectral index, use of 247
Blast injury 247
Blast lung injury, management of 251
Bleeding patient 401
Bleomycin 217, 244
Blindness 245
Blood
　bags, Gram stain of 410
　coagulation studies 410
　group 399
　loss, signs of 335
　pressure 45
　stream infection, central line
　　　associated 218
　tests 45
　urea nitrogen 165, 316
Bloodstream infection,
　　　catheter-associated 447
Blunt abdominal trauma 320
Blunt aortic injuries 330
Blunt head injury 89
Blunt thoracic trauma 320
Blunt trauma patients 335
Body fluids 450
Boerhaave's syndrome 122, 138
Bolam test 418, 425
Bolus dose, single 28
Bone marrow
　aspiration 411
　biopsy 416
　transplant 407, 444
Bony pelvis 189
Bouts of confusion 91
Bowel obstruction, small 123
Bowel rest 139

Bradyarrhythmia 364
Bradykinin 406
Brain
　abscess 102
　　diagnosis of 96
　　risk factor for 96
　　surgical drainage of 96
　dead donors, managements
　　　of 361
　death 341
　　certification of 434
　space occupying lesion 90
　stem tests 79
　tissue oxygen 85
Branched chained amino acids 151
Breast cancer 218
Breath, shortness of 378
Broad-spectrum antibiotic 288, 300
Bromocriptine 204
Bronchial asthma 44
Bronchial breath sounds 45
Bronchiectasis 50
Bronchoalveolar lavage 273, 325, 411
Bronchograms 45
Bronchopleural fistula 51
Bronchoscopy 411
　area 449
　infection control policies for 442
Bupivacaine
　infusion 264
　syringe 249
Burkholderia pseudomallei 307
Burkitt's lymphoma 222
Burn wound infections, invasive 452
Burns unit, infection control
　　　practices for 445
Burst suppression 89
　ratio 89

C

Cachexia 367
Calcineurin inhibitor 191, 363
　tacrolimus 280
Calcium
　acetate 175
　channel blocker 3, 249
Calculous cholecystitis, diagnosis
　　　of acute 125
Caloric assessment 150
Caloric source 149
Caloric test 99
Campylobacter 380
Cancer, chemotherapeutic agents
　　　for 239
Candida albicans 285, 378
Candida auris 275
Candida infective endocarditis,
　　　treatment of 273

Candidemia
　empirical antifungal of 273
　management of 273, 274, 306
Candidiasis 220
Capillary blood, end 53
Capillary perfusion 348
Capnogram 354
　represents 347
Capnography 5, 333
Carbapenems 275
Carbohydrate 149
　antigen, stool for 119
　diet, low 155
Carbon dioxide, normal value of 53
Carbon monoxide 252
　poisoning 202
Carboplatin 243
Carcinoma 214
　breast 225
　buccal mucosa 222
Cardiac allograft vasculopathy
　　　362, 367
Cardiac arrhythmias 171
Cardiac care 420
Cardiac etiology 29
Cardiac filling pressures 368
Cardiac ischemia 409
Cardiac output 5
　Fick formula for 1
Cardiac tamponade 5
Cardiac transplant 360
　rejection 361, 367
Cardiogenic shock 3
Cardiology 1, 25
Cardiomegaly, moderate 45
Cardiopulmonary physiology 51
Cardiopulmonary resuscitation 182
Cardiorespiratory function,
　　　assessment of 360
Cardiovascular disease, risk of 174
Care for patients, quality of 435
Cat and dog bite wounds cause
　　　infections 251
Cat scratch disease 386
CAUTI
　bundle implementation 444
　prevention interventions 446
Cavernous venous sinus
　　　thrombosis 87
Cavitary pulmonary aspergillosis,
　　　chronic 382
Ceftriaxone 290
Cell lung carcinoma, small 231
Cellulitis 442
Center of disease control 440
Central diabetes incipidus
　diagnosis of 229
　management of 3
Central venous catheters 449

Cephalosporin 272
Cerbera odollam 246
Cerebral artery, middle 336
Cerebral blood flow 84
   autoregulation of 88
Cerebral irritation, signs of 379
Cerebral microdialysis 85, 105
Cerebral palsy 328
Cerebral perfusion pressure 86
Cerebral salt wasting 200
   syndrome 85, 105, 337
Cerebral saturation 7
Cerebral vasospasm 99
Cerebrospinal fluid 301
Cerebrovascular disease, severe 367
Cervical spine injury, low risk for 319
Charcoal 249
Charcot's triad 130
Chemical cardioversion 5
Chest pain 409
   pleuritic 43, 44
Childhood asthma 54
Chlorhexidine-impregnated
   dressings 447
Cholangitis
   acute 326
   ascending 318
   recurrent episodes of 125
Cholecystectomy 129
   indications for 118
Cholecystokinin 119
Cholelithiasis 133
Cholescintigraphy 143
Choriocarcinoma 242
Christmas disease 416
Cisplatin 243
Citrate anticoagulation 166
CLABSI
   for prevention of 441
   problem of 449
Clavulanic acid 286
Clostridium difficile infection 300
   diagnosis of severe 275
CMV disease 275, 285, 375, 383, 389
CNS
   infection, postoperative 444
   toxoplasmosis 274
Coagulase negative staphylococci 441
Coagulation factor deficiency 411
Cocaine abuser 248
Cold antibody hemolytic anemia 389
Cold water caloric reflex test 80
Colistin 222, 271
Collapsibility 2
Colloids 409
Colonic cancer, colectomy for 49
Colonoscopic decompression 140

Comatose patient, management of 88
Community acquired pneumonia
   183, 204, 298
   treated for 43
Complete blood count 401
Computerized tomographic
   pulmonary angiography 41
Congestive heart failure 409
Consent 425
Consumer Protection Acts 434
Contrast enhanced transthoracic
   echocardiogram 52
Contrast induced nephropathy
   167, 205
   chances of 29
   incidence of 348
   risk factor for 166
Corneal reflexes 356
Coronary angiogram 380
Coronary artery disease
   accelerated form of 368
   history of 201
Coronary vasospasm 219
Corticomedullary differentiation,
   loss of 165
Corticosteroids 46, 242, 364
Cough 182
   history of increased 41
Crazy-paving 50
Creatine kinase 326
Criminal negligence
   law pertaining to 426
   qualifies for 419
Critical aortic stenosis 27
Critical care 346
   infection control in 440
   transfusions in 399
Critical illness polyneuropathy
   423, 436
Critically ill
   children 155
   patients 52
Crohn's disease 122
Crush syndrome, management of 251
Cryoprecipitate 401, 402, 404,
   408, 411, 414
   indications of 410
   poor plasma 404
   transfusion 401
Cryptococcal infection 275
Cryptococcus neoformans 296, 311
Crystalloids 294
   rapid infusion of 409
Cushing response, triad of 223
Cyanide toxicity, treatment of 245
Cyclophosphamide 226, 243, 244
Cystic lesions, multiple 378
Cytomegalovirus 401

D

Dacarbazine 217, 244
Damp sweeping 452
Dead-space ventilation 309
Death, diagnosis of 422
Deep vein thrombosis 86
   in pregnancy 182
   prophylaxis 43
Delirium 248, 356
Dementia 307
Dengue
   hemorrhagic fever, diagnostic
     criteria 312
   IgM for 381
   infection, severe 297
   shock syndrome 313
   viral infection 313
Depression 271
Dermatomyositis 380
Diabetes
   insipidus 89
   mellitus 29, 79
     history of 202
     steroid induced 364
Diabetic foot infections,
   treatment of 318
Diabetic ketoacidosis 200, 210
   management of 203
Dialysis
   adequate dose of 171
   indication for urgent 169
Diarrhea, history of 379
Diastolic pulmonary vascular
   pressure gradient 365
Dietary allowances 151
Diethylcarbamazine 273
   adverse effects 282
   single dose of 380
Digital subtraction angiography 82
Digoxin
   sign of 254
   therapeutic window of 26
   toxicity 245
Dilated right ventricle, severely 44
Dilutional coagulopathy 402
Dispersion, measure of 393
Disseminated encephalomyelitis,
   acute 82
Disseminated intravascular
   coagulation 196, 415
Diuretics 169
D-lactic acidosis 349
DNA technology 408
Donor leukocytes 407
Donor platelet concentrate,
   single 404
Dopamine 210, 299
Doxycycline 271

Drug eluting stents 26
Drug fever 349
Drug, prescription of 419
Drugs and Cosmetics Act 427
Dyshemoglobinemia 356
Dyskaryotic cell lines 380
Dysphagia 289
Dyspnea 26, 182, 409

E

Echinocandin 274
Echinococcus granulosus 118
Eclampsia
　cases 189
　diagnostic feature of 181
Electrolyte disorders 183
Emergency room 41
Emphysematous cholecystitis 293
Empiric antibiotic therapy 218
Empiric therapy 278
End of life
　care 343
　decision 340
　　making 340
　pathway, presence of 420
End stage renal disease, single
　　predictor of 167
Endocarditis, treatment of 276
Endocrinology 199
Endogenous candidemia 378
Endophthalmitis 378
Endoscopic procedures 411
Endotracheal tube 354
　position 290
Engraftment syndrome 234
Enhanced crossmatches 409
Enteral nutrition 429
　delivery, quality of 424
Enteral tube feeding 160
Enterobacter cloacae 280
Environmental hazard 244
Enzyme secretion 131
Enzyme-linked immunosorbent
　　assay 387
Epidemic diseases 434
Epidural anesthesia 186, 411
Epidural hematoma, acute 324
Epigastric pain 26, 45, 121
Episodic bradycardia 92
Epithelial cells, areas of necrosis
　　in 378
Erythema 216
　migrans 386
Erythropoietin, initial dose of 167
Escherichia coli 48
　enterohemorrhagic 278
Esophageal Doppler 27, 288
ESPEN guidelines 151, 152

Estimated glomerular filtration
　　rate 171
Ethanol 247
Ethylene glycol poisoning 250
Etomidate 308
Euthanasia 344, 431
　implies 340
Exocrine tissue 119
Expiration, end of 53
Extensor posturing 356
Extracorporeal membrane
　　oxygenation 2, 27, 42, 294, 309
　complications of 6
　signs of membrane failure in 4
Extradural hematomas 88
Extrapulmonary complications 389

F

Family satisfaction 341
Fast hugs bid 349
Fast-flush test 7
Fat embolism syndrome 325
　diagnosis of 317
Fat soluble vitamins 151
Fatal cardiomyopathy
　element causes 149
　risk of 154
Fatty acids 164, 192
Fatty liver of pregnancy, acute
　　188, 191
Febrile illness 379
Febrile neutropenia 218, 221, 273
Fetal loss 189
Fetal movements, absence of 188
Fever 274
　history of 90
Fibrinolytic agent 28
Fibronectin 157
Fiduciary obligation 421
Fluconazole 184, 218, 243
　role of 274
Flumazenil 263
Fluoxetine 291
Flush device, continuous 348
Focal segmental glomerulosclerosis
　　184
Foodstuffs 157
Fosfomycin 222, 272
Free intraperitoneal fluid 331
Fresh frozen plasma 404
　indications of 415
　transfusions 47
Fusarium spp. 452
Fusobacterium necrophorum 302

G

Galactomannan 273
　assay 378

Gallbladder gangrene incidence 334
Gamma hydroxybutyrate 249
Gamma irradiation inactivates
　　lymphocytes 411
Gastric
　antrum 120
　bypass surgery 45
　feeding 151
　lavage 253
Gastrinoma patients 131
Gastrointestinal 117
　bleeding, management of
　　upper 147
　endoscopy 381
Genitourinary injuries 323
Gentamicin 272
Gestation 189
Gestational trophoblastic
　　neoplasms 219
Glasgow coma scale 324, 329, 338
Glasgow outcome scale 79, 86
Glasgow-Blatchford
　bleeding score 125
　score, modified 145
Glucose control in ICU 202
Glutamine 151, 158, 164
　plasma levels of 158
Graft versus host disease, acute 216
Gram negative
　bacilli 271
　meningitis 81
Granulocyte transfusion 451
Granulomatous disease, chronic 386
Guillain-Barré syndrome 79, 87

H

H1N1
　influenza 270
　patient 440
　pneumonia 50, 445
Haemophilia
　earlier effective treatment for 408
　history of 401
　severe 401
Hagen-Poiseuille law flow 359
Halo sign 273
Hang hygiene compliance 420
Hartmaan's solution 205
HBV blood test, results of 445
Head injury 86, 321
　neurological examination 324
Head trauma 310
Health care, medicolegal aspects
　　of 434
Health evaluation
　acute chronic 308
　acute physiology 308

Index

Healthcare-associated
    aspergillosis 445
Heart
    and liver, transplantation 360
    disease 182
        left-sided 365
    failure
        acute 3
        acute decompensated 28, 191
        pathophysiology of acute 6
        survival score 360
        transplant 360, 365, 366
            contraindication for 361, 367
Heat and moisture exchanger 54
Heat stroke, management of 251
Heavy metal poisoning 249
HELLP syndrome
    diagnosis of 188
    laboratory criteria for 185
    management of 185
Hematologist plans 404
Hematopoietic growth factors,
    role of 224
Hemithorax, unilateral 318
Hemobilia 118
    causes of 128
Hemodynamic 294
Hemoglobin 399
Hemolysis, rule out 410
Hemophagocytic
    lymphohistiocytosis 387
Hemophilia B, treatment of 416
Hemoptysis 290
Hemorrhagic infarct 322
Hemorrhagic shock 207
Heparin induced thrombocytopenia
    26, 321, 348
Heparin prophylaxis 221
Hepatic blood flow 121
Hepatic enzyme abnormalities 118
Hepatic processes 135
Hepatic venous wedge pressure 124
Hepatitis
    B 99
        immune globulin 453
        surface antigen 124
        vaccine 453
        viral infection 144
        virus 124, 125
    C 98
        chronic 381
        related cirrhosis 44
        virus 124, 136
    E infection 381
Hepatocellular carcinoma 145
Hepatopulmonary syndrome 52
Hepatorenal syndrome 166, 168, 205
    diagnosis of 166

Hepatosplenomegaly 381
Herceptin receptors 219
Herpes simplex encephalitis 81
High flow nasal cannula 54
    therapy 43
Hind brain, spectrum of 103
Hodgkin's lymphoma 223, 231, 244
Homans' sign 182
Hospital, direct liability of 423
Hounsfield units 322, 334
HSV encephalitis 101
Human disease 384
Human immunodeficiency virus 270
    infected pregnant women 385
    infection, acute 315
Human Resources Department 442
Human tissues 450
Hydatid cysts 144
Hydrocortisone
    stress doses of 208
    use of 201
Hyperbaric oxygen 55
Hypercalcaemia, severe 226
Hypercalcemia 210
    management of 203, 214
    mechanism for 224
    symptoms of 223
Hypercapnia 41
Hypercapnic respiratory failure,
    extrapulmonary causes of 44
Hyperglycemia 264, 309
Hyperglycemic hyperosmolar
    state 212
Hyperkalemia 171
    therapy for 170
Hyperlactatemia 201
Hyperlipidemia, pastmedical
    history of 293
Hyperosmolar hyperglycemic
    state 204
Hyperosmolar therapy 86, 106
Hypersensitivity pneumonitis 390
Hypertension, treatment for 182
Hypertensive response, acute 101
Hyperthermia 248, 249
Hyperthyroidism 203
Hypertonic saline 86
Hypertrophy 183
Hyperuricemia 174
Hyperventilation 207
Hyperviscosity syndrome 224, 240
Hypervolemia 351
    complications of 346
Hypocalcemia 100
    in septic shock 205, 213
Hypocapnia 198
Hypoglycemia 202
Hypokalemia 170, 203
Hypokinesia, severe global 27

Hyponatremia 249
Hypophosphatemia 205, 213, 354
    causative factor for 200
    causes of 347
Hypotension 27
    episodes 171
Hypothesis tests, types of error in 395
Hypothyroid 201
Hypothyroidism 150, 292
Hypoxia, acute 293

I

Idiopathic pulmonary syndrome,
    diagnosis of 223
Idiopathic ventricular fibrillation 4
Ifosfamide 243
Imipenem 48
Immune modulating formula 152
Immune senescence 312
Immune thrombocytopenia,
    treatment of 403
Immunomodulating diet 159
    formula 151
Immunosuppressant 360
Immunosuppression 360
Indian Association of Palliative
    Care 344
Infection
    acquired, rates of 420
    and sepsis, severe 287
    prevention 440
    surgical-site 444
Infectious diseases 378
Infectious mononucleosis 386
Infective endocarditis, diagnosis
    of 317
Influenza
    developed 441
    virus 276
Infratentorial extension 93
Inhalational injury cases, acute 51
Insect bite, treatment of 247
Insect related anaphylaxis,
    etiology for 247
Inspiratory oxygen fraction 48
Institute of healthcare improvement,
    component of 440
Insulin
    administration 180
    with glucose 170
Insulinoma 131
Intensive care unit 449
Intermediate syndrome 250
Intermittent fever 96
International subarachnoid
    treatment 89
Interstitial predominance 44
Intestinal ischemia, acute 334

Intra-abdominal hypertension 301
  grades of 319
Intra-aortic balloon
  counter pulsation 349
  pump, hemodynamic effects of 28
Intracranial aneurysms 80
Intracranial brain hemorrhage 80
Intracranial haemorrhage, acute 81
Intracranial hypertension 166
Intracranial pressure 80, 329
Intrapulmonary vascular
  dilatation 52
Intravenous antibiotics 46
Intravenous aztreonam 46
Intravenous fluids 403
Intraventricular hemorrhage 93
Invasive aspergillosis, treatment
  of 378
Invasive candidemia, risk factor
  for 292
Invasive pulmonary aspergillosis 273
Invasive rhinocerebral
  mucormycosis 81
Investigations, record of 419
Ipsilateral hemiplegia, develops 79
Ischemic infarct, acute 167
Ischemic stroke, acute 351
Isolation facilities 444
Isotonic hyponatremia 175

J

Jaundice 326
  presence of 142
Jugular vein
  central vein cannulation,
    internal 7
  distention 325
  suppurative thrombophlebitis 302

K

Kayexalate 201
Ketamine 293
Ketosis 149
Kidney
  disease 171
  injury, acute 165, 251
Klebsiella pneumonia nosocomial
  infections 441

L

Lactatemia 123
Lactic acidosis 150, 155, 210
Laryngeal nerve, external branch
  of superior 327
Law binds physician 419
Law of confidentiality 419, 426

Left bronchial artery 42
Left ventricular
  assist device 28, 366
  dysfunction 369
  failure, acute 166
Lemierre's syndrome 271, 302
Lethal drug, administration of 421
Leukocyte esterase, false negative
  test for 177
Leukoreduced blood products 401
Levine sign 3
Licorice ingestion 210
Liddle syndrome 210
Life
  and personal liberty, right to 421
  decision making, model for end
    of 339
  support
    forgoing of 340
    treatments, forgoing of 343
Life-threatening
  C. difficile colitis, treatment of 270
  reaction 406
Lignocaine 245
Ligustrazine alleviates acute
  pancreatitis 132
Linezolid 210, 271, 278
Lithium 261
Liver
  benign lesions of 117
  disease 118, 415
    chronic 166
  function tests 148
  malignant neoplasms of 117
  segmental anatomy of 117
  transplant 44
Lobe pneumonia, lower 293
Loiasis, treatment of 387
Loop diuretics 169
Lorazepam tablets 249
Lower lobe pneumonia, right 46
Lower segment cesarean section 123
Lumbar puncture 96, 348, 411
  complications of 349
Lumbar spinal cord, trauma to 79
Lundberg A waves 100
Lundberg B waves 100
Lung
  and bilateral mild pleural
    effusion 222
  bilateral 218
  consolidation 47
  contusion 325
  disease 29
  hyper inflated 55
  injury
    acute 321, 325
    ventilator induced 50

thoracic radiation for 55
transplant 50
ultrasound
  addition of 55
  deciphers 5
Lymphoblastic leukemia, acute
  216, 402
Lymphocytic leukemia, acute 219

M

Magic mushrooms 251
Magnesium
  deficiency 201
  retention test 203
  toxicity 187
Magnetic resonance angiography 82
Malaise, complains of 45
Malaria, severe 273
Mallory-Weiss syndrome 144
Mannitol 106
Massive blood
  loss 317
  transfusion, complications of 335
Massive hemoptysis 42
Massive transfusion 405
  protocol 399
Maternal and child enquiries,
  centre for 198
Maxillofacial trauma 323
Mazzotti reaction 387
MDR-TB, management of 272
Mechanical ventilation 45, 53, 435
  complication rate of 52
  for respiratory failure, quality
    of 423
  liberation from 51
Mediastinitis 332
  acute 321
Medical Council Act 427
Medical jurisprudence 425
Medical law
  and ethics 418
  context of 426
Medical negligence
  allegation of 426
  claim of 418, 425
Medical practitioner 419
Medical professional 426
Medical records, maintenance of 427
Medical research 397
Medication errors 257
Melanoma 242
Melioidosis 277, 307
Meningococcal meningitis,
  diagnosis of 443
Mesenteric artery, origin of
  superior 126

Mesenteric ischemia 139
  acute 126
Mesenteric vasospasm 327
Metabolic acidosis 123, 171, 184, 203, 245
  severe 203
Metabolic alkalosis 128, 210, 354
  causes of 204
  treatment of 210
Metabolic cart 156
Metabolism 199
Metallic body implants 450
Metastatic malignancy 240
Metastatic spinal cord compression, evidence of 219
Metformin 91
  causes type B lactic acidosis 254
  intoxication causes 245
Methanol 253
  intoxication 246
  poisoning, treat 247
Methicillin resistant staphylococcus aureus 302, 442
  modes of spread of 449
  treatment of 271
Microcalorimetry 278
Microdialysis chart 90
Microscopic agglutination testing 386
Midazolam 111
Mid-ureteral calculi 173
Miller-Fischer syndrome 98
Milrinone 30
Minocycline 284
Minocycline over tigecycline, advantage of 274
Mite-borne infectious disease 315
Mitochondrial beta-oxidation 192
Mitral stenosis 202
Mitral valve, systolic anterior motion of 307
Moistens 54
Molecular weight, large 165
Monoclonal antithymocyte antibody-muromonab 364
Mononeuclosis 380
Motorcycle 91
Motorcyclist 91
Moxifloxacin 46, 275
Moyamoya 103
MRI brain 96
Mucinous carcinoma of ovary 220
Mucor spp. 452
Mucositis, evidence of 218
Multi-drug resistant 80
Multiorgan failure 28, 312
Murphy sign 334
Muscle contraction, smooth 50
Mushroom poisoning 209
Mycophenolate mofetil 365

Myeloblastic leukemia, acute 273
Myeloid leukemia, acute 273
Myeloma, multiple 400
Myelosuppression 388
Myocardial infarction, acute 3
Myocardial ischemia 126
Myoglobinuria 326

N

N-acetylcysteine 246
Nasal canulla 292
Nasogastric decompression 139
Nasogastric suction 327
Nasogastric tube placement 328
National Health Safety Network 309
National Healthcare Safety Network 52
National Nosocomial Infections Surveillance System 444
Natriuretic peptides 28
Necrotizing fasciitis, risk indicator for 270
Neonatal exchange transfusion 407
Neonatal intensive care unit 441
Nephrogenic fibrosing cholangitis 167
Neuraxial block 186
Neurocritical care 82, 85
  unit 95
Neurogenic bladder 319
Neurointensive care 79, 92, 93
Neuroleptic malignant syndrome 228, 252
Neuromuscular disorders 307
Neuron specific enolase, level of 347
Neutropenic enterocolitis 224, 242
Neutrophil predominance 294
New York Heart Association 364
NIHSS score 90
Nimodipine 89
Nitroglycerin intravenous infusion 124
Non protein calorie sources 155
Non thyroidal illness syndrome 210
Non-convulsive status epilepticus 85
Non-Hodgkin's lymphoma 223, 231, 389
Noninvasive ventilation 2, 41
Nonocclusive mesenteric ischemia 318
Non-protein caloric sources 149
Non-rebreathing mask 222
Nonverbal communication, soler acronym for 421
NSTEMI management 435
Null hypothesis 394, 395
NUTRIC score 160
Nutrition 152

in acute pancreatitis 152
in burn victims 153
in critical care 149
in hepatic failure patients 152
in open abdomen 153
in traumatic brain injury 152
prescription, monitoring of 437
Nutritional assessment 149
Nutritional support, quality of 420

O

Obesity
  hypoventilation syndrome 44
  severe 367
Obstetric patient, resuscitation of 187
Obstetric sepsis 187, 198
Obstetrics and gynecology 181
Obstructive airway disease 53
Obstructive lung disease, chronic 46
Obstructive pulmonary disease, chronic 41
Obstructive sleep apnea 44
Octreotide 125, 126
Oliguria 27, 124
Oncology 214
Oncovin 244
Optic atrophy 245
Optical and colorimetric techniques 53
Oral anticoagulants, direct 322
Oral calcium acetate 167
Organ donation 423
  consent for 422, 434
Organ failure assessment score 304
Organophosphate insecticides 257
Organophosphorus 248
Orientia tsutsugamushi 315
Oropharyngeal decontamination 441
Orthostatic hypotension 126
Oseltamivir 290
Osmolal gap 202, 250
Osteoporosis 364
  severe 367
Over damped waveform, causes of 348
Overtraining syndrome 206
Oxazolidinone antibiotic 278
Oxygen
  consumption, cerebral metabolic rate of 88
  delivery 46, 346
  dissociation curve 55
  mask 287
  saturation 47
    gap 248
  transport parameters 53
Oxygenation
  defect 52
  stable 309

P

Pain
and distress, freedom from 343
presence of 142
Palliation means 339
Palliative care 340, 439
Pancreas 119
adenocarcinoma of 119, 131
Pancreatic abscesses, causes of 132
Pancreatic ascites 123, 140
Pancreatic exocrine secretory 119
Pancreatic juice, bicarbonate concentrations of 119
Pancreatic pseudocysts, management of 133
Pancreaticoduodenectomy 121, 135
Pancreatitis 293
acute 120, 125, 137, 163
chronic 120
mild 117
Pancreato-duodenectomy 215
Pancytopenia 199, 401
Papillary carcinoma thyroid 217
Papillary thyroid cancer 242
Paracetamol 217
poisoning, transplant center in 244
Paralytic ileus 126, 147
postoperative 126
Paraquat poisoning 246, 264
Parasitic infection 128
Parenchymal changes 325
Parenteral anticoagulation 4
Parenteral intravenous fluids 43
Parenteral nutrition, quality markers for 424
Parkinson disease 328
Paroxysmal nocturnal dyspnea 409
Peak oxygen consumption 361
Peak serum creatine kinase levels 326
Peculiarities 51
Pediatric neurosurgical patients 90
Penicillin 272
resistance 301
Peptides, formulas containing 161
Percutaneous coronary intervention, primary 26
Periampullary carcinoma 215
Perilesional edema 271
Perioperative atelectasis 43
Periorbital cellulitis 224
Peripartum cardiomyopathy 182, 187, 196, 197
diagnosis of 187
incidence of 26
Peripheral blood
culture 274
stem cells 407

Peripheral enhancement 220
Peripheral vascular disease, severe 367
Peripheral vein suppurative thrombophlebitis 278
Peritoneal lavage 132
Peritoneovenous shunt 124
Persistent abdominal pain, causes of 246
Personal protective equipment 440
pH 41, 46
Pharmacology, acute 244
Phenytoin toxicity causes 104
Pheochromocytomas 204
Photopheresis 365
Physiologic scale, acute 308
Piperacillin 218
Pituitary
adenomas 90
apoplexy 204
gland 207
macroadenoma, transsphenoidal resection of 92
Plasma magnesium concentration 197
Plasmapheresis, contraindication of 80
Plateau pressure 49, 308
Plateau wave 80, 100
Platelet
concentrate 404
dose of 416
count 403
for prophylactic therapy, standard dose of 412
irradiation 403
products 404
transfusion 198, 402
Pleural effusion
bilateral mild 200
characteristics of 29
unilateral 231
Pleural sliding, presence of 326
Pneumococcal vaccine 215
Pneumocystis jirovecii 378
pneumonia 236, 297
treatment of 381
Pneumocystis pneumonia in malignancy 221
Pneumonia 296
bilateral 54
severity index 316
ventilator associated 49, 52, 436
Pneumothoraces 53
Pneumothorax 323
develops left-sided 45
diagnosis of 318
Poisoning 244

Poisonous snakes 250
Polyclonal antithymocyte globulin 364
Polymerase chain reaction 295
Polymorphisms, genotyping for 325
Polymyxin 278
B, advantage of 271
Polystyrene sulphonate 201
Portal hypertension, causes of 124
Portal venous pressure 124
Portosystemic venous shunt, indications for 118
Posaconazole 191
Positive serum galactomannan 218
Post-cardiac
arrest patients 356
surgery 2
transplant patient 362
Posterior reversible encephalopathy syndrome 88, 194
Postextubation laryngeal edema 55
Post-heart transplant complications 360
Postintensive care syndrome 293
Postpartum hemorrhage 199
Post-renal transplant 379
Postspinal headache 358
Post-transfusion hepatitis, causes of 124
Post-transplant lymphoproliferative disease 388
Post-transplant persistent pulmonary arterial hypertension, management of 368
Post-traumatic
epilepsy 86
seizure, risk factor for 86
Potential teratogenic 196
Preanesthetic check-up 45
Predeposit autologous donation 406
Prednisone 244
therapy, chronic 293
Preeclampsia 167
severe 187, 197
Pregnancy 166, 181
develops gradual progressive dyspnea 183
managing sepsis in 181
mechanical ventilation in 183
physiologic changes of 190
physiological adaptation of 185
trauma in 181, 187, 322
Premature newborns 407
Pressure support ventilation 288
Prilocaine 245
Prilox cream 245
Primary adjuvant therapy, pillars for 55
Procarbazine 244

Index

Progesterone receptors 219
Promyelocytic leukemia, acute 219
Prone ventilation 42, 436
Propofol, use of 111
Prostacyclin 368
Protein content 157
Prothrombin complex concentrate 404
Proton pump inhibitor 126
Protozoal 390
Pseudocyst 120
   recurrence, risk of 120
Pseudomembranous colitis 146
Psychiatric illness 307
Pulmonary arterial hypertension 332
   characteristic of 321
Pulmonary arterial pressure 47
Pulmonary artery 1, 359
   catheter 53, 350
   hypertension 25, 44
      causes of 25
   massive embolism of common 46
   occlusion pressure 30
Pulmonary aspergillosis, chronic 382
Pulmonary capillary wedge pressure 1
Pulmonary circulation 349
Pulmonary clearance medications 43
Pulmonary contusion 320
   opacities 331
Pulmonary edema 413
   bilateral perihilar 182
   causes of 2
Pulmonary embolism 25, 30, 41
   acute 367
   diagnosis of 221
   risk of 221
Pulmonary function, prevent deterioration of 244
Pulmonary hemorrhages 380
Pulmonary hypertension 365
   evidence of 366
   typical characteristics of 29
Pulmonary oxygen toxicity 52
Pulmonary toxicity 217
Pulmonary tuberculosis, history of treated 289
Pulmonary vascular disease, assessment of 361
Pulmonary vasculature 55
Pulse
   oximeter 353
   pressure
      maximum 306
      mean 306
      minimum 306
      variation 306
Pupillary responses, absence of 356
Purulent sputum 46
Pyoderma gangrenosum 270
Pyogenic abscess of liver 124
Pyogenic hepatic abscess, current therapy for 117
Pyogenic liver abscess 121, 135
   treatment of 121
Pyogenic meningitis, management of suspected 272

Q

qSOFA 291, 295, 304, 311, 347, 352
Qualitative variables 393, 398
Quantitative futility 433
Quantitative serum hemoglobin 410
Quantitative variables 398

R

Radiation induced lung injury 55
Radiation pneumonitis 55, 224
Radiation syndrome, acute 245
Radiator coolant 248
Random donor platelet concentrate 404
Rankin scale, modified 87
Ranson's prognostic signs 123, 143
Recurrent variceal haemorrhage, prevention of 118
Red blood cell 399
Red cell eluate 409
Re-expansion pulmonary edema 50
   predictive of 42
Refeeding syndrome 151, 159, 200, 207, 354
Refractory angina 366
Refractory asthma in ICU 43
Refractory hypoxemia 43
Renal cell carcinoma 242
Renal disease 154, 162
   end stage 183
Renal dose, antibiotics need 169
Renal failure 152, 364
   and hypotension 248
Renal impairment 169
Renal replacement therapy 166
   continuous 151, 154, 166
Renal stone, unilateral 166
Renal tubular acidosis 205, 213
Renal tubulopathy 243
Replacement fluid, dose of 165
Residual bronchiectasis 289
Respiratory 41
   alkalosis 207, 346, 354
      causes of 50
   care 435
   compliance, sudden fall in 42
   cycle 1
   distress 312, 327
   distress syndrome, acute 45, 325
      management of 186
   extracorporeal membrane oxygenation 6
   failure 45, 52
      acute 50, 52, 152
      causes of 52
   infections, prevalence of 447
   muscle weakness 51
   rate 46
Resuscitate order 340
Resuscitation, principles of 197
Retinoic acid 222
Retroviral disease 378
   diagnosis of 379
Retroviral infection 380
   acute 315
Retroviral syndrome, acute 298, 315
Rhabdomyolysis 204, 212, 317, 326
   overdoses causing 249
Rhesus 196
Rheumatic heart disease 94
Rheumatoid arthritis 293
   azathioprine for 380
Rhinocerebral mucormycosis 102
Rhizopus spp. 452
Riboflavin 154
Ribonucleic acids 164
Right ventricular infarction 25
Road traffic accident 79, 399
Rocuronium 293
Room air pressure, negative 451
Root canal treatment 289
Rotavirus 442
Routine liver chemistries 121
Roux-en-Y pancreaticojejunostomy 140
Ruptured mycotic aneurysm 94

S

Salbutamol, inhalation of 46
Salicylate intoxication 248
Salicylate overdose 260
Saliva 450
Salmonella bacteremia 379
Salmonella septicemia 385
Scedosporium prolificans 384
Schistosomiasis 386
Schizophrenia, treatment for 244
Sclerosis, multiple 328
Scorpion envenomation 247
Scrub typhus 315
Scrub typhus infection 298
Seizures, risk factor for 107
Selenium deficiency 154
Selenium supplementation 154
Sella turcica 207
Sent biopsies 289

Sentinel loop 122, 137
Sepsis 28, 312
  prognostic factors of 290
  severe 293
  uncontrolled 130
Septic shock 204, 207, 295
Sequential compression devices 86
Serologic testing 121
Serotonin syndrome 204, 212, 305, 350, 359
Serotonin toxicity 254
Serum
  alanine aminotransferase 188
  amylase test 335
  bilirubin 410
  creatinine 171
  digoxin level 26
  ferritin 274
  iron 29
  lactic dehydrogenase 123
  potassium concentration 180
  procalcitonin 272
  sodium 167
  transaminases 121
  voriconazole 273
Shigella 380
Sickle cell
  anemia 403
  disease 386
Sinus tachycardia 183
Six sigma DMAIC
  format 442
  methodology 448
Smoker, chronic 42
Social justice 339, 342
Sodium
  bicarbonate 207, 261
  nitroprusside 368
Soft tissue infection, necrotizing 300
Solid organ transplant 275
  recipients 297
Somatosensory-evoked potentials 356
Sonography in trauma, focused assessment with 323
Sphincterotomy 287
Spina bifida, diagnoses of 328
Spinal cord
  compression, malignant 223
  injury 90, 328
    acute 320
    leads 100
    sign of 81
Splenorenal shunt, distal 129
Spontaneous bleeding 402
Spontaneous breathing trial 51
Spontaneous intracerebral haemorrhage, management of 319

Spurious hypoxemia 236
Sputum production 46, 289
Staphylococcus aureus 452
Staphylococcus epidermidis 284
Statistical test 392
Status epilepticus 89
Stones obstructing ureteropelvic junction 173
Stones within ureter 173
Storing platelet 417
Streptococcus pneumoniae 388
  infection 301
Streptokinase treatment 3
Stress ulcer prophylaxis 85
Stroke
  index, normal value of 2
  right sided 95
  volume 300
    variation 5
Subdural hematoma
  acute 88
  chronic 88
Subtotal thyroidectomy, postoperative case of 215
Sudden ventricular tachycardia, develops 4
Sulfamethoxazole 222, 224
Sulfite ion 149, 159
Supraventricular arrhythmia 364
Surgery and trauma 317
Surrogate 339, 342
Syndrome of inappropriate antidiuretic hormone secretion 85, 200, 324
  diagnostic criteria of 214
Systemic complications, risk factor for 381
Systemic inflammatory response syndrome 304, 311
Systolic blood pressure 171

T

Tachycardia 27, 126, 248
Tachypnea 119, 182, 248
Tacrolimus 369
  administration 184
Takotsubo cardiomyopathy 29
Targeted temperature management 348
Tazobectum 218
TB meningitis 274
T-cell
  opsonization 364
  response, suppression of 365
Teicoplanin 218
Telescopes 147
Temporary hemodialysis catheter 165

Temporary transvenous pacing
  correct indication for 30
  lead 25
Tenofovir nephrotoxicity, clinical presentations of 277
Terson syndrome 90
Thiamine 155
  deficiency lack
    signs associated with 161
    symptoms associated with 161
Thiazide diuretics 3
Thoracic malignancies 55
Thrombocytopenia 188, 198, 289, 325, 332, 402
  typical heparin induced 26
Thromboembolic events 219
Thromboembolic phenomenon 193
Thrombolytic therapy 30, 51
Thrombotic mesenteric ischemia, chronic 123
Thrombotic stroke
  hyper acute 108
  service, hyperacute 87
Thyroid storm 209
Tidal volume 49
Tigecycline 101
Tocolytic induced pulmonary edema, develops 51
Total abdominal hysterectomy 199
Total lymphoid irradiation 365
Toxoplasma gondii 286
Toxoplasmosis 379
Trachea, acute obstruction of 42
Tracheostomy 86
Transcellular shifts 354
Transesophageal echocardiography 4, 322
Transfusion reaction 399
Transient ischemic attach 3
Transpulmonary thermodilution method 30
Transthoracic echocardiography 4
Transurethral resection 184
Trauma
  lethal triad of 324
  management of 436
  multiple 181
Traumatic acute subdural hematoma, management of 319
Traumatic brain injury 86, 323
  essential diagnostic criteria for 324
  management of 81
  steroid in 87
Traumatic cardiac tamponade 320
Traumatic diffuse axonal injury 324
Tricyclic antidepressant 253
Trimethoprim 222, 224
Tubercular meningitis 80, 90

Tuberculosis, treatment for active 379
Tubular necrosis, acute 176
Tumor lysis syndrome 200, 207, 214, 221, 238

U

Ultrasound femoral vessels 190
Uncal herniation, sign of 79
Unstable angina 27
Upper airway 54
Upper esophagus, carcinoma of 223
Upper gastrointestinal bleeding 29, 123
Upper limb catheter, decreased risk of 49
Upper ureteral stones 173
Ureteral injury, cause of 319
Ureteral stones, distal 173
Urethral injury 320
Uric acid 174
 excretion of 206
Urinary
 angiotensinogen, measurement of 177
 catheters 328
 chloride 208
 fat stains 325
 pneumococcal antigen 316
 tract infection 319
Urine
 analysis 168
 hemoglobin 410
 ketones 202
 legionella antigen 203
 output 201
 specimen, contamination of 167
Urology 181
Uterine rupture 196

V

Vaginal discharge 181
Vaginal fluid 450

Valve infective endocarditis 270
Vancomycin 47, 179, 271, 276
 intermediate staphylococcus aureus 445
 resistant enterococci 445
Variceal bleeding, acute 124
Vascular intestinal ischemia 322
Vascular nonocclusive 334
Vascular occlusive 334
Vascular resistance, metric unit for 1
Vasculitis 232
Vasodilatation 207
Vasodilators 7
Vasopressin 124, 312
 acts 141
Vasopressor support 199
Vasospasm, management of 87
Vein of Galen 80
 AVM 100
Vena cava, inferior 215
Venom immunotherapy 250
Veno-occlusive disease 219
Venous air embolism, detection of 90
Venous arterial blood management protection 354
Venous thromboembolic disease 183
Venous thromboembolism 346
 in pregnancy 185
Veno-venous hemodiafiltration, continuous 165
Ventilation, volume control 288
Ventilation–perfusion 185
Ventilator alarms 49
Ventilator-associated
 complication, infection-related 451
 condition 451
 event 309, 443
 tracheobronchitis 445
Ventilatory support 48
Ventricular arrhythmias 249
Ventricular drain, external 82, 87, 295
Ventricular fibrillation 7
Ventricular waveform 1

Vertebral artery 80
Vicarious liability 419
Vinblastine 243, 244
Vinca alkaloids 243
Vincristine 217, 243
Viper bites 247
Viral
 infection 389
 pneumonias 310
Virus mask, aerosolization of 452
Visual disturbances 197
Vital parameters 199
Vital signs 45
Vitamin
 A 154
 B12 29
 C 161
 in ESPEN guidelines 152
 K 154
Voriconazole 382
 prophylaxis 224

W

Wallace "rule of nine" 323
Water soluble occupational chemical 248
Waterhouse-Friderichsen syndrome 199, 206
Weakness, right sided 90
Weight loss 123
Weil disease 386
Wernicke's encephalopathy 89, 110
Western blot 379
Wheezing 378
Whipple's procedure 121, 227
White cell counts 96
World Society of abdominal compartment syndrome 319

Z

Zika virus 274
 disease 285
Zollinger-Ellison syndrome 119

EU GSPR Authorised Reprsentative
Logos Europe, 9 rue Nicolas Poussin
1700, La Rochelle, France
Phone: +33 (0) 6 67 93 73 78
E-mail: contact@logoseurope.eu

www.ingramcontent.com/pod-product-compliance
Ingram Content Group UK Ltd.
Pitfield, Milton Keynes, MK11 3LW, UK
UKHW050042210326
4879IPUK00006B/105